Ignatavicius ■ Workman

MEDICAL-SURGICAL NURSING

Patient-Centered Collaborative Care

Ignatavicius ▪ Workman

MEDICAL-SURGICAL NURSING

Patient-Centered Collaborative Care

8th Edition

CHRIS WINKELMAN, PhD, RN, CNE, CCRN, ACNP, **FCCM, FAANP**
Associate Professor
Frances Payne Bolton School of Nursing
Case Western Reserve University;
Clinical Nurse
Trauma/Critical Care Float Pool
MetroHealth Medical Center
Cleveland, Ohio

ELSEVIER

ELSEVIER

3251 Riverport Lane
St. Louis, Missouri 63043

CLINICAL COMPANION FOR MEDICAL-SURGICAL NURSING: ISBN: 978-0-323-22235-8
PATIENT-CENTERED COLLABORATIVE CARE, EIGHTH EDITION

Notices

International Standard Book Number: 978-0-323-22235-8

Executive Content Strategist, Nursing: Lee Henderson
Content Development Manager: Billie Sharp
Associate Content Development Specialist: Samantha Taylor
Publishing Services Manager: Deborah L. Vogel
Senior Project Manager: Brandilyn Flagg
Design Direction: Margaret Reid

Printed in the United States of America
Last digit is the print number: 9   8   7   6   5   4   3   2   1

Working together
to grow libraries in
developing countries

www.elsevier.com • www.bookaid.org

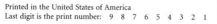

PREFACE

Welcome! This new edition of the *Clinical Companion for Medical-Surgical Nursing: Patient-Centered Collaborative Care* has been updated and streamlined to match content changes in the most current Ignatavicius and Workman textbook. Many changes reflect the increased emphasis in health care on implementing strategies for patient care that have evidence for both safety and effectiveness.

Part One has been revised to emphasize concepts in nursing education and reflects many of the ideas developed in the Ignatavicius and Workman textbook. These concepts are cellular regulation, fluid and electrolyte balance, inflammation and infection, pain, and palliation. Perioperative settings and coordination for discharge/transfer—two transitions in care that are associated with great patient vulnerability and risk for staff error—are also included in this section.

Part Two, the core of the *Clinical Companion,* provides A-to-Z synopses of more than 250 conditions, along with collaborative care. Part Two retains a format that is consistent with that of the Ignatavicius and Workman textbook.

Throughout Parts One and Two, important aspects of care are highlighted, such as Genetic/Genomic Considerations ☧, Considerations for Older Adults, Gender Considerations, and Cultural Considerations ⊕. These considerations help nurses and nursing students offer focused and individualized assessment and intervention. Canadian brand name drugs are represented by a maple leaf icon ♣. Nursing Safety Priority boxes █ highlight important information that nursing students and nurses can use to avoid patient harm. These boxes are further categorized as Drug Alert, Action Alert, or Critical Rescue. New **QSEN** boxes have been created to reflect nursing roles in the health care system such as actions that improve quality and safety. These **QSEN** boxes reflect both competencies described by the Quality and Safety Education for Nurses website (QSEN.org) and quality measures from the Centers for Medicare and Medicaid Services (cms.gov). Effective, safe, efficient, and patient-centered care is delivered individually and across settings.

There are now eight appendixes. Each appendix is designed to provide brief, concentrated capsules related to medical-surgical nursing care. This content provides information about both common and specialized skills that cross settings, diseases, and conditions.

Medical-surgical nursing is a demanding specialty, often considered the foundation of all nursing. Most adults will receive care from a medical-surgical nurse sometime during their life. We hope this book supports our readers' efforts to provide comfort, avoid error, and promote high-quality patient-centered care. Let us know what you think; your feedback is important to the evolution of this succinct reference.

ACKNOWLEDGMENTS

Smart, compassionate clinicians continue to inspire me and nursing students do not allow me to become complacent. Thank you! Linda Workman provides ongoing mentorship with caring, trust, and an eye toward professional development. And my family's humor, patience, and support are essential to my own health and ability to (still) deliver safe, effective patient care.

PART ONE

Concepts of Medical-Surgical Nursing

CANCER PATHOPHYSIOLOGY

Cancer is abnormal cell regulation; the processes of normal cell growth and function are lost and become unpredictable.

OVERVIEW

- *Neoplasia* is any new or continued cell growth not needed for normal development or replacement of dead and damaged tissues. This new growth may be benign or malignant.
- *Benign tumor cells* are normal cells growing in the wrong place or at the wrong time. They are not needed for normal growth and development. Although benign tumors do not invade other tissues, depending on their location, they can damage normal tissue and may need to be removed.
- *Cancer cells,* also called *malignant cells,* are abnormal, serve no useful function, and invade and destroy normal body tissues. Without treatment, cancer leads to death of tissues, organs, and, ultimately, the person with a cancer diagnosis.
- Cancer can develop in any tissue or organ but tends to occur more commonly in tissues that continue to grow by cell division (mitosis) throughout the life span.
- All cancers start from normal cells that undergo changes at the gene level. These changes result in a loss of control over cell growth.
- *Carcinogenesis* and *oncogenesis* are additional names for cancer cell growth and development.
- *Malignant transformation* is the process of changing a normal cell into a cancer cell.
- *Carcinogens* are substances that can damage normal cell DNA and change the activity of genes. Carcinogens may be chemicals, physical agents, or viruses.
- Cellular dysregulation present in cancer cells and malignant tumors is:
  1. Anaplasia or loss of the specific appearance *(morphology)* of the parent cells
  2. A large nuclear-cytoplasmic ratio or a larger-than-normal cell nucleus

1

   3. Loss of specific cell function
   4. Loose adherence resulting in the ability of malignant cells to migrate
   5. Rapid, persistent cell division with loss of contact inhibition
   6. Aneuploidy or abnormal chromosomes
   7. No response to normal cellular signals for programmed cell death (i.e., apoptosis)
- A *primary tumor* is the original tumor, identified by the normal tissue from which it arose.
- When primary tumors are located in vital organs, such as the brain or lungs, they can grow excessively and lethally damage the vital organ or crowd out healthy organ tissue and interfere with that organ's ability to perform its vital function.
- A *metastatic tumor* is one that has spread from the original site, usually through the blood or lymph, into other tissues and organs, where it can establish metastatic or secondary tumors that grow and cause more damage and dysfunction.
   1. When a metastatic tumor is in another organ, it is still a cancer from the original altered tissue.
   2. For example, when breast cancer spreads to the lung and the bone, it is breast cancer in the lung and bone, not lung cancer and not bone cancer.

CARCINOGENESIS/ONCOGENESIS

- The process of carcinogenesis or oncogenesis occurs through the steps of initiation, promotion, progression, and metastasis.
   1. *Initiation* begins the change of a normal cell into a cancer cell. Initiation is the result of the expression of oncogenes (genes that cause normal cells to transform into cancerous cells) or reduced expression of suppressor genes (genes that prevent cancerous transformation of normal cells), altering cell division. If growth conditions are right, widespread metastatic disease can develop from just one cancer cell.
   2. *Promotion* is the enhancement of growth of an initiated cell. Many normal hormones and body proteins, such as insulin and estrogen, act as promoters and make initiated cells divide more often.
   3. *Progression* is the continued change of a cancer, making cells more malignant. One change is the development of a separate blood supply. Over time, changes in cell growth and function provide advantages that allow cancer cells to live and divide, no matter how the conditions around them change.
   4. *Metastasis* is the spread of a tumor or cancer cells from the original site. For example, cancer cells can migrate through the lymph or vascular system to other organs. Common

sites of metastasis are lymph nodes, lungs, bones, and the brain.

- Cancers are classified by the type of tissue from which they arise. For example, glandular cancers are carcinomas and connective tissue cancers are sarcomas.
- Solid tumors develop from specific tissues (e.g., breast cancer and lung cancer). Hematologic cancers (e.g., leukemias and lymphomas) arise from blood cell-forming tissues and lymphatic tissues.
- Systems of cancer grading and staging are used to standardize cancer diagnosis, prognosis, and treatment.
- *Grading* of a tumor classifies cellular aspects of the cancer and ranks cancers for the degree of malignancy based on cancer cell appearance, growth rates, and aggressiveness compared with the normal tissues from which they arose. Low-grade cancers have fewer malignant features and are well differentiated; high-grade cancers have more malignant features, such as anaplasia.
- Tumor *ploidy* classifies tumor chromosomes as normal or abnormal. When cancer cell chromosomes are abnormal they are called *aneuploid.* The degree of aneuploidy usually increases with the degree of malignancy.
- *Staging* describes the extent or severity of a person's cancer. The TNM staging system is based on the size of the primary tumor (T), whether cancer cells have spread to nearby lymph nodes (N), and whether metastasis (M) or spread of cancer to other parts of the body has occurred. Staging is important because for most cancers the smaller the cancer is at diagnosis, the fewer the lymph nodes that are involved; and the less it has spread, the greater the chances are that treatment will result in a cure. Staging also influences selection of therapy.
    1. *Clinical staging* assesses the patient's clinical manifestations and evaluates clinical signs for tumor size and possible spread.
    2. *Surgical staging* assesses the tumor size, number, sites, and spread by inspection at surgery.
    3. *Pathologic staging* is the most definitive type, determining the tumor size, number, sites, and spread by pathologic examination of tissues obtained at surgery.

CANCER ETIOLOGY AND GENETIC RISK

- Carcinogenesis may take years and depends on several tumor and patient factors.
- Three interacting factors influence cancer development: exposure to carcinogens, genetic predisposition, and immune function.
- *Oncogene activation* with overexpression is the main mechanism of carcinogenesis regardless of the specific cause. Oncogenes cause normal cells to transform into cancerous cells.

- The normal cell's suppressor genes (which control cell growth and prevent oncogene overexpression) can be damaged or mutated. As a result, the oncogenes are overexpressed.
- Both external and personal factors can activate oncogenes, damage suppressor genes, or both, leading to cancer development.
- External factors that cause cancer include:
  1. Exposure to chemical carcinogens, including many known chemicals, tobacco, drugs, and other exposures that occur in everyday life, such as air pollution and sun exposure
  2. Exposure to physical carcinogens, such as radiation and chronic irritation
  3. Infection with a carcinogenic virus, such as certain strains of the human papillomavirus (HPV) or hepatitis C (HVC)
  4. Possible dietary factors, such as low fiber intake, high intake of red meat, and high animal fat intake; preservatives, contaminants, preparation methods, and additives (e.g., dyes, flavorings, and sweeteners) also may have cancer-promoting effects
- Personal factors in cancer development include:
  1. Immune function, with decreased immune function increasing cancer risk
  2. Advancing age, the single most important risk factor for cancer
  3. Genetic predisposition, resulting from the inheritance of specific gene mutation(s)

🧬 Genetic/Genomic Considerations

- Genetic risk for cancer occurs only in a small percent of the population; however, people who have a genetic predisposition are at very high risk for cancer development.
- Mutations in suppressor genes or oncogenes can be inherited when they occur in germline cells (sperm and ova) and are then passed on to one's children, in whom all cells contain the inherited mutations. Thus for some people tight cellular regulation is compromised by a mutation in a suppressor gene, which reduces or halts its function and allows oncogene overexpression.
- In other people, the suppressor genes are normal and the oncogene is mutated and does not respond to suppressor gene signals, thus reducing cellular regulation and increasing the risk for cancer development.
- Inherited predisposition for specific cancers, inherited conditions associated with cancer, familial clustering, and chromosomal aberrations demonstrate a pattern of genetic risk for cancer.

🌐 Cultural Considerations

- The incidence of cancer varies among ethnicities. Black Americans have a higher incidence of cancer than white Americans do, and the death rate is higher for African Americans.
- One explanation for this difference is that individuals in an ethnic minority have less access to health care. Black individuals are more often diagnosed with later stage cancer that is more difficult to cure or control. However, this disparity in health care access does not explain all differences.

PATIENT-CENTERED COLLABORATIVE CARE

- Teach patients to use sunscreen and to wear protective clothing during sun exposure.
- Encourage patients to participate in the recommended cancer-screening activities for their age group and cancer risk category.
- Inform all patients who smoke that tobacco use is a causative factor in 30% of all cancers. Assist anyone interested in smoking cessation to find an appropriate smoking cessation program.
- Assess the patient's knowledge about causes of cancer and his or her screening and prevention practices.
- Help patients who fear a cancer diagnosis to understand that finding cancer at an early stage increases the chances for cure.
- Ask all patients about their exposures to environmental agents that are known or suspected to increase the risk for cancer.
- Obtain a detailed family history (at least three generations) and use this information to create a pedigree to assess the patient's risk for familial or inherited cancer.
- Teach anyone, especially older adults, the "seven warning signs of cancer" (indicated by the acronym *CAUTION*):
  1. Changes in bowel or bladder habits
  2. A sore that does not heal
  3. Unusual bleeding or discharge
  4. Thickening or lump in the breast or elsewhere
  5. Indigestion or difficulty swallowing
  6. Obvious change in a wart or mole
  7. Nagging cough or hoarseness

CANCER TREATMENT

- Primary prevention of cancer involves avoiding exposure to known causes of cancer.
- Secondary prevention of cancer involves screening for early detection.
- Tertiary treatment occurs after a cancer diagnosis and the purpose is to prolong survival time or improve quality of life.
- Therapies for cancer include surgery, radiation therapy, cytotoxic agents, biological and immunomodulation drugs, hormonal therapy, and photodynamic therapy.
- Therapies may be used separately or, more commonly, in combination to kill cancer cells.
- The types and amount of therapy used depend on the specific type of cancer, whether the cancer has spread, and the health of the patient.

CANCER SURGERY
OVERVIEW

- Surgery for cancer involves the removal of diseased tissue and may be used for prophylaxis, diagnosis, cure, control, palliation, determination of therapy effectiveness, and reconstruction.
  1. *Prophylactic surgery* is the removal of at-risk tissue to prevent cancer development and is performed when a patient has an existing premalignant condition or a known family history that strongly predisposes the person to the development of a specific cancer.
  2. *Diagnostic surgery (biopsy)* is the removal of all or part of a suspected lesion for examination and testing. It provides proof of the presence of cancer.
  3. *Curative surgery* is focused on removal of all cancer tissue and alone can result in a cure rate of 27% to 30% when all visible and microscopic tumors are removed or destroyed.
  4. Cancer control, or *cytoreductive surgery*, is the removal of part of the tumor and leaving a known amount of gross tumor. It is also known as *debulking surgery*, and it does not alone result in a cure.
  5. *Palliative surgery* is focused on improving the quality of life during the survival time and is not focused on cure.
  6. *Second-look surgery* is used for a rediagnosis after treatment. The results of this surgery are used to determine whether a specific therapy should be continued or discontinued.
  7. *Reconstructive or rehabilitative surgery* increases function, enhances appearance, or both.

PATIENT-CENTERED COLLABORATIVE CARE

- The nursing care needs of the patient having surgery for cancer are similar to those related to surgery for other reasons.
- Surgery usually involves the loss of a specific body part or its function.
- The amount of function lost and how much the loss affects patients depend on the location and extent of the cancer and surgical intervention.
- Some cancer surgery results in major scarring or disfigurement.
- Two additional priority care needs are psychosocial support and assisting the patient to achieve or maintain maximum function.
    1. Assess the patient's and family's ability to cope with the uncertainty of cancer and its treatment and with the changes in body image and role.
    2. Coordinate with the health care team to provide support for the patient and family.
    3. Encourage the patient and family to express their feelings and concerns.
    4. Encourage the patient to look at the surgical site, touch it, and participate in any dressing changes or incisional care required.
    5. Provide information about support groups, such as those sponsored by the American Cancer Society or specialty cancer organizations.
    6. Discuss with the patient the idea of having a person who has coped with the same issues come for a visit.
    7. Teach the patient about the importance of performing and progressing the intensity of any prescribed exercises to regain as much function as possible and prevent complications.
    8. Coordinate with the physical therapist, occupational therapist, and family members to plan strategies individualized to each patient to regain or maintain optimal function.

RADIATION THERAPY

OVERVIEW

- The purpose of radiation therapy for cancer is to destroy cancer cells with minimal exposure of the normal cells to the damaging actions of radiation.
- Because the effects of radiation are seen only in the tissues in the path of the radiation beam, this type of therapy is a local treatment.
- Radiation doses vary according to the size, location, and radiation sensitivity of the tumor and the surrounding normal tissues.
- Radiation therapy is delivered in one of two categories:
    1. *Teletherapy:* The radiation source is external to the patient and remote from the tumor site. It is also called *external beam*

radiation. Because the source is external, the patient is not radioactive and is not a hazard to others. This type of therapy usually is given as a series of divided doses.

2. *Brachytherapy:* The radiation source comes into direct, continuous contact with the tumor tissues for a specific period of time. It is delivered in a solid, sealed form or unsealed within body fluids. *With all types of brachytherapy, the patient emits radiation for a period of time and is a hazard to others.*

- Side effects of radiation therapy are limited to the tissues exposed to the radiation and vary according to the site. Skin changes and hair loss are local but are likely to be permanent. Other common side effects include altered taste sensations and severe fatigue.
- Radiation damage to normal tissues during cancer therapy can start the inflammatory responses that cause tissue fibrosis and scarring. These effects may not be apparent for many years after radiation treatment.

PATIENT-CENTERED COLLABORATIVE CARE
- For teletherapy, teach patients to:
  1. Wash the irradiated area gently each day with water or with a mild soap and water and rinse thoroughly.
  2. Not remove any ink or dye markings that indicate exactly where the beam of radiation is to be focused.
  3. Dry the irradiated area with patting motions rather than rubbing motions; use a clean, soft towel or cloth.
  4. Powders, ointments, lotions, or creams on the skin should not be used at the radiation site unless they are prescribed by the radiologist or the radiation therapy advanced practice nurse.
  5. Wear soft clothing over the skin at the radiation site.
  6. Avoid wearing belts, buckles, straps, or any type of clothing that binds or rubs the skin at the radiation site.
  7. Avoid exposure of the irradiated area to the sun.
     a. Protect this area by wearing clothing over it but *not* by applying sunscreen agents.
     b. Avoid going outdoors between 10:00 AM and 4:00 PM to avoid the more intense sunrays.
  8. Avoid heat exposure.
- For patients receiving brachytherapy:
  1. Assign the patient to a private room with a private bath.
  2. Place a "Caution: Radioactive Material" sign on the door of the patient's room.
  3. If portable lead shields are used, place them between the patient and the door.
  4. Keep the door to the patient's room closed as much as possible.

5. Wear a dosimeter film badge at all times while caring for patients with radioactive implants. Each badge should be used only by one individual.
6. Wear a lead apron while providing care. Always keep the front of the apron facing the source of radiation (do not turn your back toward the patient).
7. Pregnant nurses should not care for these patients; do not allow pregnant women or children younger than 16 years old to visit.
8. Limit each visitor to 30 minutes per day. Be sure visitors are at least 6 feet from the source.
9. Never touch the radioactive source with bare hands. In the rare instance that it is dislodged, use long-handled forceps to retrieve it. Deposit the radioactive source in the lead container kept in the patient's room.
10. Save all dressings and bed linens until after the radioactive source is removed.

CYTOTOXIC SYSTEMIC AGENT THERAPY
OVERVIEW
- *Anti-neoplastic agents* (commonly called *chemotherapy*) are used to cure cancer and to increase survival time. These drugs have some selectivity for killing cancer cells over normal cells.
- The tumors most sensitive to chemotherapy are those that have rapid growth.
- The effects of cytotoxic therapy are systemic, providing the opportunity to kill metastatic cancer cells that may have escaped local treatment.
- The normal cells most affected by chemotherapy are those that divide rapidly, including skin, hair, intestinal tissues, spermatocytes, and blood-forming cells.
- Cytoxic drugs are classified by the specific types of action they exert in the cancer cell and include antimetabolites, antitumor antibiotics, antimitotics, alkylating agents, topoisomerase inhibitors, and miscellaneous agents.
- Successful cancer chemotherapy most often involves giving more than one anticancer drug in a timed manner, known as *combination chemotherapy.*
- Drugs are selected based on known tumor sensitivity to the drugs and the degree of side effects expected.
- Dosages for most chemotherapy drugs are calculated according to the type of cancer and the patient's size, usually based on milligrams per square meter of total body surface area or on weight in kilograms.

- Although most chemotherapy drugs are given IV, they may also be given by the oral, intra-arterial, isolated limb perfusion, intra-cavitary, and intrathecal routes.
- Administration of IV chemotherapy is usually performed by a registered nurse who has completed an approved chemotherapy course.
- *Extravasation,* or *infiltration,* is a serious complication of IV chemotherapy administration that can lead to pain, tissue loss, and in worst-case scenarios, loss of the limb.
  1. The most important nursing intervention for extravasation is prevention by close monitoring of the access site during chemotherapy administration.
  2. Immediate treatment of extravasation depends on the specific drug. Coordinate with the oncologist and pharmacist to determine the type of compress and specific antidote needed for the extravasated drug.
  3. Perform and document the following activities for an extravasation event:
     a. Date and time when extravasation was suspected or identified
     b. Date and time when the infusion was started
     c. Time when the infusion was stopped
     d. The exact contents of the infusion fluid and the volume of fluid infused
     e. The estimated amount of fluid extravasated
     f. A diagram of the exact insertion site, and indication of whether this is a venous access device, implanted port, or a tunneled catheter
     g. The method of administration (e.g., pump, controller, rate of infusion)
     h. The needle type and size
     i. Indication on the diagram of the location and number of venipuncture attempts
     j. The time between the extravasation and the last fully documented blood return
     k. All agents administered in the previous 24 hours through this site (list agent administered, dosage and volume, and order of administration)
     l. Patient's vital signs
     m. Patient's subjective sensations and symptoms
     n. All observations of the site, including size, color, and texture
     o. A photograph of the site
     p. Administration of neutralizing or antidote agents
     q. Application of compresses and their temperature

    r. Other nursing interventions

    s. Patient's responses to nursing interventions

    t. Notification of the prescribing physician (including the time)

    u. Written and oral instructions given to the patient about follow-up care

    v. Any consultation request

- Nurses and other health care workers who prepare or give these drugs or who handle the patient's excreta within 48 hours of the patient receiving IV chemotherapy must use extreme caution and wear personal protective equipment (PPE), including eye protection, masks, double gloves, and gown.
- Side effects of chemotherapy often include bone marrow suppression (e.g., neutropenia, anemia, and thrombocytopenia), nausea and vomiting, mucositis, alopecia, changes in cognitive function, and peripheral neuropathy.

PATIENT-CENTERED COLLABORATIVE CARE

- For patients with neutropenia:
  1. Administer medications that enhance the immune system (e.g., biological response modifiers [BRMs]) as prescribed such as filgrastim (Neupogen, Imu-Max, etc.) to promote the production and release of white blood cells.

Considerations for Older Adults

Older adults are at even greater risk for chemotherapy-induced neutropenia because of age-related changes in bone marrow function. Using growth factors, such as filgrastim (Neupogen) and pegfilgrastim (Neulasta) before neutropenia occurs can reduce the severity of neutropenia and the risk for infectious complications.

  2. Assess the skin and mucous membranes, lung sounds, mouth, and insertion sites for venous access device(s) every 8 hours.
  3. Urge the patient to report any indicator of infection, such as a change in skin and mucous membranes (e.g., pimple, sore, rash, open area), presence of a cough, burning on urination, pain around the venous access site, or new drainage from any location.
  4. Use good handwashing before contact with the patient.
  5. Modify the environment to protect patients who have neutropenia or thrombocytopenia.

6. Ensure that mouth care and washing of the axillary and perianal regions are performed at least every 12 hours to reduce bioburden. Some institutions use daily chlorhexidine cloths.
7. Monitor for manifestations of infection.

! NURSING SAFETY PRIORITY: Critical Rescue

The patient with neutropenia often does not develop a high fever or have purulent drainage, even when a severe infection is present. Consider any temperature elevation in a patient with neutropenia to be an indication of infection. Report it to the provider immediately and anticipate immediate intervention such as implementation of a sepsis protocol.

8. Teach patients and family members precautions to reduce the risk for infection.
- For patients with anemia:
  1. Administer BRMs as prescribed.
  2. Assess for tachycardia and increased respiratory rate.
  3. Encourage the patient to rest.
  4. In collaboration with other members of the health care team, postpone or cancel activities that do not have a direct impact on the health of the patient.
- For patients with thrombocytopenia, provide a safe hospital environment:
  1. Handle the patient gently, such as using a lift sheet when moving and positioning the patient in bed.
  2. Avoid IM injections and venipunctures.
  3. Apply firm pressure to needle stick sites for 10 minutes.
  4. Test all urine and stool for the presence of occult blood.
  5. Observe IV sites every 4 hours for bleeding.
  6. Avoid rectal temperatures, even on unconscious patients.
  7. Administer prescribed suppositories carefully with liberal lubrication.
  8. Instruct the patient and unlicensed assistive personnel to use an electric shaver rather than a razor.
  9. When providing mouth care or supervising others in providing mouth care, instruct about:
     a. Using a soft-bristled toothbrush or tooth sponges
     b. Checking to ensure that dentures fit and do not rub
- For patients with chemotherapy-induced nausea and vomiting (CINV):
  1. Administer prescribed antiemetics on a scheduled, rather than PRN, basis.

2. Ensure that premedication with antiemetics occurs before each session of IV chemotherapy.
3. Assess patients for dehydration and electrolyte imbalances.
4. Teach patients to continue the therapy as prescribed, even when the nausea and vomiting appear controlled.

- For patients with mucositis:
  1. Examine the patient's mouth, including the roof, under the tongue, and between the teeth and cheek, every 4 hours.
  2. Document the location, size, and character of fissures, blisters, sores, or drainage.
  3. Provide or encourage self-managed, frequent oral hygiene:
     a. Use a soft-bristled brush or sponges after meals and before sleeping.
     b. Rinse the mouth with plain water or saline every 2 hours while awake and as often as the patient desires.
     c. Avoid the use of alcohol or glycerin-based mouthwashes.
  4. Administer antimicrobial agents, topical analgesic drugs, and artificial saliva as prescribed.
- For patients with alopecia:
  1. Reassure patients that hair loss is temporary and that hair regrowth usually begins about 1 month after completion of chemotherapy.
  2. Inform the patient that the new hair may differ from the original hair in color, texture, and thickness.
  3. Teach the patient to avoid scalp injury by:
     a. Using head covering to avoid direct sunlight on the scalp
     b. Wearing some head covering underneath helmets, head-phones, headsets, and other items that rub
- For patients with changes in cognitive function ("chemo brain"):
  1. Support the patient who reports this side effect. Listen to the patient's concerns and tell him or her that other patients have also reported such problems.
  2. Warn patients against participating in other behaviors that exacerbate cognitive impairment, such as excessive alcohol intake, recreational drug use, and taking part in activities that increase the risk for head injury.
- For patients with chemotherapy-induced peripheral neuropathy, teach patients to prevent injury by:
  1. Wearing well-fitting shoes with a protective sole
  2. Inspecting feet daily (with a mirror) for open areas or redness
  3. Avoiding extremes of temperature; wearing warm clothing in the winter, especially over hands, feet, and ears
  4. Protecting hands with potholders when cooking and gloves to wash dishes or garden

5. Moving slowly and scanning the ground when changing positions

IMMUNOTHERAPY: BIOLOGICAL RESPONSE MODIFIERS

OVERVIEW

- BRMs modify the patient's biological responses to tumor cells. Some have direct antitumor activity; others interfere with cancer cell differentiation, transformation, or metastasis. BRMs also can improve immune function and enhance the body's ability to repair or replace cells damaged by cancer treatment.
- Two common types of BRMs used as cancer therapy are:
  1. Interleukins (ILs), which help different immune system cells recognize and destroy abnormal body cells; in particular, IL-1, -2, and -6 appear to "charge up" the immune system and enhance attacks on cancer cells by macrophages, natural killer (NK) cells, and tumor-infiltrating lymphocytes. Side effects of ILs include generalized inflammatory reactions that can be severe:
     a. Widespread edema from "capillary leak"
     b. Chills or rigors (severe shaking with chills); rigors is managed with meperidine (Demerol)
     c. Fever with flu-like general malaise, often managed with acetaminophen
  2. Interferons (IFNs), which can slow tumor cell division, stimulate the growth and activation of NK cells, induce cancer cells to resume a more normal appearance and function, and inhibit the expression of oncogenes.

MOLECULARLY TARGETED THERAPY

OVERVIEW

- Technically biological agents, these drugs take advantage of one or more differences in cancer cell growth or metabolism that are not present or are only slightly present in normal cells.
- Agents used as targeted therapies disrupt pathways that lead to excessive cancer cell division/reproduction by:
  1. Targeting and blocking epithelial growth factor receptors (EGFRs) or the vascular endothelial growth factor (VEGF) and receptors (VEGFRs); when a cancer cell's growth depends on having the growth factors bind to their specific receptors, blocking the receptor slows or eliminates the cancer cell's growth.
     NOTE: For therapies that bind to the EGFR and VEGFR receptors, normal cells in the skin, GI tract, and mucous

membranes also express these receptors and may develop open sores, rashes, and acne-type lesions.

2. Blocking signals for cell division and function. These drugs include tyrosine kinase inhibitors (TKIs), multikinase inhibitors (MKIs), and proteasome inhibitors.

3. Blocking many enzymes essential to cancer cell and tumor blood vessel growth; these agents are categorized as multikinase inhibitors.

4. Blocking the growth of blood vessels so that nutrients cannot be delivered to tumors (angiogenesis inhibitors)

5. Inhibiting the formation of proteins in cells, a drug class called proteasome inhibitors

- Targeted therapies work only on cancer cells that overexpress the actual target substance. Each person's cancer cells are evaluated to determine whether the cells have enough of a target to be affected by targeted therapy.

MONOCLONAL ANTIBODY THERAPY

- Monoclonal antibodies bind to specific cell surface membrane proteins, preventing the protein from performing its function, typically promoting cell division. By binding cancer cell proteins, monoclonal antibodies prevent cell division.
- The monoclonal antibodies to the EGFR bind to those specific receptors when the receptors are on normal tissue. Thus side effects occur in those tissues that normally express EGFR, such as the skin, mucous membranes, and lining of the GI tract.

HORMONAL MANIPULATION

- Hormonal manipulation can help control some types of cancer by decreasing the amount of hormones reaching hormone-sensitive tumors.
- Some drugs are hormone antagonists that compete with natural hormones at the tumor's receptor sites, preventing a needed hormone from binding to the receptor.
- Hormone inhibitors suppress the production of specific hormones in the normal hormone-producing organs.
- Androgens and the antiestrogen receptor drugs cause masculinizing effects in women, with increased chest and facial hair, interruption of the menstrual period, and shrinkage of breast tissue.
- Feminine manifestations often appear in men who take estrogens, progestins, or antiandrogen receptor drugs, including thinning facial hair, smoother skin, and gynecomastia. Testicular and penile atrophy also occur to some degree.

PHOTODYNAMIC THERAPY
OVERVIEW
- *Photodynamic therapy (PDT)* is the selective destruction of cancer cells through a chemical reaction triggered by different types of laser light.
- It is most commonly used for non-melanoma skin cancers, ocular tumors, GI tumors, and lung cancers located in the airways.
- An agent that sensitizes cells to light is injected IV along with a dye. These drugs enter all cells but leave normal cells more rapidly than cancer cells. Usually within 48 to 72 hours, most of the drug has collected in high concentrations in cancer cells. At this time, a laser light is focused on the tumor. The light activates a chemical reaction within those cells, retaining the sensitizing drug that induces irreversible cell damage.

PATIENT-CENTERED COLLABORATIVE CARE
- The patient has increased sensitivity to light for up to 12 weeks after the photosensitizing drug is injected, with the most sensitivity in the 48 hours immediately after a treatment.
- The most intense period of light sensitivity is after injection and before the laser treatment. During this time, the patient is at high risk for sunburn and eye pain for 1 to 3 months after therapy. Teach the patient to:
  1. Reduce exposure to light with protective clothing, window shades, and UV-protective sunglasses.
  2. Refrain from taking any newly prescribed or over-the-counter (OTC) drugs without contacting the physician who performed the PDT. Some drugs make the light sensitivity even worse; other drugs interact with the photosensitizing drug.
  3. Start re-exposure to sunlight and other bright lights slowly. Start by exposing only about 1 inch of skin to sunlight at a time. Start with 10 minutes, and increase the time by about 5 minutes each day.
  4. Remember that sunscreen cannot prevent severe sunburn during this time.

ONCOLOGIC EMERGENCIES
- Oncologic emergencies are acute complications associated with cancer and its treatment that often require immediate intervention to avoid life-threatening situations. These complications include sepsis and disseminated intravascular coagulation, syndrome of inappropriate antidiuretic hormone, spinal cord compression, hypercalcemia, tumor lysis syndrome, and superior vena cava syndrome.

- Sepsis and disseminated intravascular coagulation
  1. Microorganisms enter the bloodstream and grow unchecked, because the patient often has low a white blood cell count and impaired immune function. This problem can lead to septic shock and death.
  2. Disseminated intravascular coagulation (DIC) is a clotting problem triggered by sepsis, the release of clotting factors from cancer cells, or blood transfusions. Extensive abnormal clotting occurs throughout the small blood vessels, using up the existing clotting factors and platelets. This process is then followed by extensive bleeding that can range from minimal to fatal hemorrhage.
  3. Management focuses on prevention, early detection, and prompt aggressive treatment.
  4. For prevention:
     a. Identify those patients at greatest risk for sepsis and DIC.
     b. Use aseptic technique during care for open skin areas, nonintact mucosa, or any invasive procedure.
     c. Teach patients and family members the early manifestations of infection and sepsis and when to seek medical assistance.
  5. For treatment:
     a. Administer timely IV antibiotic therapy.
     b. With DIC, anticipate IV administration heparin or clotting factors.
- Syndrome of inappropriate antidiuretic hormone
  1. Certain cancers secrete or stimulate the secretion of antidiuretic hormone (ADH) when it is not needed by the body for fluid and electrolyte balance. The result is retention of pure water and dilution of electrolytes. In addition to lung and other cancers, syndrome of inappropriate antidiuretic hormone (SIADH) can be caused by morphine and cyclophosphamide.
  2. Assess for:
     a. Weight gain daily
     b. Decreased urine output
     c. Weakness and fatigue
     d. Muscle cramps
     e. Low serum sodium levels of 115 to 120 mEq/L (normal range is 135 to 145 mEq/L)
     f. Decreased and altered mentation and seizures when sodium levels are less than 110 mEq/L; this is a medical emergency
  3. Management includes:
     a. Free water restriction
     b. Increased sodium intake

      c. Drug therapy, most often with demeclocycline
      d. Immediate cancer therapy to cause tumor regression
   4. Monitor for fluid overload, including peripheral edema and pulmonary edema (dyspnea, presence of crackles in lungs).
- Spinal cord compression
   1. Spinal cord compression (SCC) and damage occur when a tumor directly enters the spinal cord or when the vertebrae collapse from tumor degradation of the bone. It most commonly occurs with lung, prostate, breast, and colon cancers.
   2. Manifestations include:
      a. Back pain
      b. Numbness or tingling
      c. Paralysis (which may be permanent)

❗ NURSING SAFETY PRIORITY: Action Alert

Early recognition and treatment of spinal cord compression are essential to a good outcome. Assess any cancer patient with new-onset back pain, muscle weakness or a sensation of "heaviness" in the arms or legs, numbness or tingling in the hands or feet, loss of ability to distinguish hot and cold, or an unsteady gait, and report these findings to the oncologist immediately.

   3. Teach patients and families the manifestations of early SCC and instruct them to seek help as soon as problems are apparent.
   4. Management is often palliative and may include:
      a. High-dose corticosteroids to reduce swelling around the spinal cord
      b. High-dose radiation to the site
      c. Intense chemotherapy to reduce tumor size
      d. Surgery to remove the tumor from the area (less common)
      e. External back or neck braces to reduce pressure on the spinal cord or spinal nerves
- Hypercalcemia
   1. Hypercalcemia (high serum calcium level) occurs most often in patients with bone metastasis. Tumors can also secrete parathyroid hormone, causing bone to release calcium.
   2. Management includes:
      a. Oral hydration
      b. Parenteral hydration with normal saline

   c. Drug therapy to reduce calcium levels *temporarily:*
     (1) Oral glucocorticoids
     (2) Bisphosphonates
   d. Dialysis (if renal impairment is present)

- Tumor lysis syndrome
  1. Tumor lysis syndrome (TLS) occurs when large numbers of tumor cells are destroyed rapidly and their intracellular contents, including potassium and purines (DNA components), are released into the bloodstream faster than the body can eliminate them. The purines are converted to uric acid. Untreated TLS can cause renal failure and death by hyperkalemia and cardiac arrest.
  2. TLS is most often seen in patients receiving radiation or chemotherapy for cancers that are very sensitive to these therapies, including leukemia, lymphoma, small cell lung cancer, and multiple myeloma.
  3. Prevention through hydration is the best management for TLS.
     a. Instruct at-risk patients to drink at least 3000 mL (5000 mL is more desirable) of fluid the day before, the day of, and for 3 days after treatment.
     b. Stress the importance of adhering to the antiemetic regimen so that oral hydration can be accomplished.
     c. Instruct patients to contact the cancer clinic immediately if nausea and vomiting prevent adequate fluid intake, so that IV fluids can be started.
     d. Management of actual TLS includes:
        (1) Aggressive fluid resuscitation
        (2) Osmotic diuretics
        (3) Drug therapy to increase the excretion of purines such as allopurinol (Aloprim, Zyloprim); rasburicase (Elitek), or febuxostat (Uloric)
        (4) Drug therapy to reduce serum potassium levels
           i. Sodium polystyrene sulfonate
           ii. IV infusions of glucose and insulin
        (5) Dialysis (for severe hyperkalemia and hyperuricemia)
- Superior vena cava syndrome
  1. Superior vena cava (SVC) syndrome occurs when the SVC is compressed or obstructed by tumor growth or by the formation of clots in the vessel. It is most common in patients with lymphomas, lung cancer, and cancers of the breast, esophagus, colon, and testes.
  2. Manifestations result from blockage of blood flow from the head, neck, and upper trunk. Early manifestations include:
     a. Facial edema, especially around the eyes, on arising
     b. Tightness of the shirt or blouse collar (Stokes' sign)

3. Later manifestations include:
   a. Edema in the arms and hands
   b. Dyspnea
   c. Erythema of the upper body
   d. Epistaxis (nosebleeds)
4. Late manifestations include:
   a. Hemorrhage
   b. Cyanosis
   c. Mental status changes
   d. Decreased cardiac output and hypotension
5. Management includes:
   a. High-dose radiation therapy to the mediastinal area
   b. Stenting of the vena cava
   c. Surgery (rarely)

CELLULAR REGULATION

- Cellular regulation refers to all aspects of cell growth and function. Many different normal cells work together to make the whole person function at an optimal level. For optimal function, each cell must perform in a predictable manner.
- Genes are the coded instructions for the making of all the different proteins the human body produces.
- An allele (pronounced "ah-lee-el") is an alternate form (or variation) of a gene.
- Protein synthesis is the process by which genes are used to make the proteins needed for physiologic function.
- Some genetic variations (also called mutations) can reduce the function of the protein produced, some can eliminate the function of the protein produced, and a few variations enhance the function of the produced protein compared with the function of the normal or typical genetic sequence.
- Gene mutations that increase the risk for a disorder are known as susceptibility genes. Gene mutations that decrease the risk for a disorder are known as protective or resistance genes.
- For optimal function, each cell must perform in a predictable manner:
  1. Specific morphology; each normal cell type has a distinct and recognizable appearance, size, and shape.
  2. A smaller nuclear-to-cytoplasmic ratio; the size of the normal cell nucleus is relatively small compared with the size of the rest of the cell, including the cytoplasm.
  3. Differentiated function; a normal cell has at least one function it performs to contribute to whole-body function. For example, skin cells make keratin and liver cells make bile.

4. Tight adherence; normal cells make proteins that protrude from the membranes, allowing cells to bind closely and tightly together. An example is fibronectin to keep most normal tissues bound tightly to each other. Exceptions are blood cells.
5. Nonmigratory; normal cells do not wander throughout the body (except for blood cells).
6. Orderly and well-regulated growth is a very important feature of normal cells. They divide (undergo mitosis) for only two reasons: (1) to develop normal tissue or (2) to replace lost or damaged normal tissue.

FLUID AND ELECTROLYTE BALANCE

- Body function depends on keeping the fluid and electrolytes within each body fluid compartment (space).
- The compartments are divided into spaces outside the cells (extracellular) and inside the cells (intracellular).
  1. The extracellular compartment is subdivided into blood and other compartments, including lymph, bone, connective tissue, and transcellular spaces such as the cerebrospinal, synovial, peritoneal, and pleural spaces.
  2. The extracellular fluid (ECF) space contains one third (about 15 L) of the total body water. The ECF includes interstitial fluid or fluid between cells, sometimes called the "third space."
  3. ICF has about two thirds (25 L) of the total body water.
- Three processes control fluid and electrolytes so the internal environment remains stable even when the external environment changes:
  1. *Filtration:* The movement of fluid through a biologic membrane as a result of hydrostatic pressure differences on the two sides of the membrane
  2. *Diffusion:* Unimpeded movement of a substance through a permeable membrane between two fluid compartments; occurs down a concentration gradient; does not require the expenditure of chemical energy
  3. *Osmosis:* Diffusion of water (no other substance) through a selectively permeable membrane from an area of lower osmotic pressure to an area of greater osmotic pressure
- Body fluids are composed of water and particles dissolved or suspended in water. The solvent is the water portion of fluids. Solutes are the particles dissolved or suspended in the water.
  1. Solutes vary in type and amount from one fluid space to another.
     a. For example, sodium is the major extracellular cation and potassium is the major intracellular cation.

  b. Common electrolyte derangements are described in Part
      Two:
      (1) Hyper- and hyponatremia
      (2) Hyper- and hypokalemia
      (3) Hyper- and hypocalcemia
2. When solutes express an overall electrical charge, they are
    known as electrolytes.
    a. Cations have a positive charge.
    b. Anions have a negative charge.
    c. An equal number of cations and anions are present within
        the cell, tissue, or fluid except in cells that start or transmit
        impulses like the cardiac pacemaker cells and neurons.
- Fluid and electrolyte balance contribute to perfusion and tissue
  integrity. Imbalances lead to alterations in cell, tissue, and organ
  function that require urgent intervention to avoid harm.

Considerations for Older Adults

Older adults are at risk for electrolyte imbalances as a result of
age-related organ changes, especially reduced kidney function.
They are more likely to be taking drugs that affect fluid or electrolyte balance.

- The cardiac system contributes to fluid and electrolyte balance by
  providing adequate perfusion to the kidneys and gastrointestinal
  system for intake and output of fluid and electrolytes and nutrients to maintain organ health.
- The kidneys are responsible for elimination of excess fluid or
  electrolytes and retention of fluid or electrolytes when intake is
  low such as during illness, NPO (nothing by mouth) status, and
  other conditions.
- The neuroendocrine system contributes to fluid and electrolyte
  balance
  1. Renin-angiotensin aldosterone (RAAS) pathway
      a. The RAAS pathway is activated when specialized cells in
          the kidney sense low blood pressure, low blood volume,
          low blood oxygen, or low blood osmolarity related to
          sodium concentration.
      b. Specialized cells in the kidney secrete renin.
      c. Renin activates angiotensinogen, ultimately resulting in
          converting it into its most active form, angiotensin II.
      d. Angiotensin II acts to:
          (1) Raise blood pressure through vasoconstriction in the
              body's arterioles

       (2) Reduce urine output by constricting renal arterioles, lowering the glomerular filtration

       (3) Stimulate the adrenal glands to secrete aldosterone, a hormone that causes the kidneys to reabsorb water and sodium, increasing blood pressure and blood volume

2. Antidiuretic hormone (ADH), or vasopressin, is released from the posterior pituitary gland in response to changes in blood osmolarity.

   a. The hypothalamus contains the osmoreceptors that are sensitive to changes in blood osmolarity. Increased blood osmolarity (dehydration) triggers ADH release.

   b. The action of ADH only retains water; it does not directly regulate electrolyte retention or excretion.

   c. ADH acts directly on kidney tubules and collecting ducts, making them more permeable to water only. As a result, more water is reabsorbed by these tubules and returned to the blood.

   d. When blood osmolarity decreases with low plasma sodium levels from fluid overload, the osmoreceptors swell slightly and inhibit ADH release. Less water is then reabsorbed, and more is lost from the body in the urine.

       (1) Osmolality is the concentration of particles (solutes) within a solution as measured per kilogram of solution.

       (2) Osmolarity is the concentration of particles (solutes) within a solution as measured per liter of solution.

3. Natriuretic peptides (NPs) are hormones secreted by special cells that line the atria of the heart (atrial natriuretic peptide [ANP]) and the ventricles of the heart (brain natriuretic peptide [BNP]).

   a. Although BNP is secreted by the heart ventricular cells, it is known as brain natriuretic peptide because it was first discovered in the brain.

   b. ANP and BNP are secreted in response to "stretched" heart tissue from excess blood volume and blood pressure.

• ANP and BNP bind to kidney receptors, inhibiting reabsorption of sodium and increasing glomerular filtration, causing increased urine output. Two conditions of **fluid imbalance** are dehydration and fluid overload (overhydration).

1. Dehydration: Fluid volume deficit is a condition caused by too little intake of fluid or too great a loss of fluid. It is manifested by decreased circulating (extracellular) fluid volume.

   a. Dehydration is detailed in Part Two.

   b. Dehydration is associated with low circulating volume and impaired tissue perfusion.

Considerations for Older Adults

Older patients are at high risk for dehydration because they have less total body water than younger adults. In addition, many older adults have decreased thirst sensation and may have difficulty with walking or other motor skills needed for obtaining fluids. They also may take drugs such as diuretics, antihypertensives, and laxatives that increase fluid excretion.

    2. Fluid overload: Fluid volume excess or overhydration is a clinical sign of a problem in which fluid intake or retention is greater than the body's fluid needs. The most common type of fluid overload is hypervolemia from excessive fluid in the ECF space. Both excessive intake and inadequate excretion of fluids cause this condition and it is associated with a variety of diseases.

      a. Fluid overload is detailed in Part Two.

      b. Fluid overload is most commonly associated with hypervolemia or excessive fluid in the ECF space.

INFECTION

OVERVIEW

- An infection is the invasion of a body tissue by microorganisms that allows replication of the microorganism and results in tissue damage.
- A *pathogen* is any microorganism, also called an *agent*, capable of producing disease.
- *Virulence* is the ability of a pathogen to invade the body and cause damage and the frequency with which it causes disease.
- *Normal flora* are microorganisms that live in or on the human host without causing disease. Some beneficial microbes can be pathologic when they move to another body area.
- *Colonization* is the process of having pathogenic organisms living and growing in or on a body area without causing disease or damage.
- *Toxins* are protein molecules released by bacteria to affect host cells at a distant site.
    1. Exotoxins are released by the bacteria into the host's body.
    2. Endotoxins remain within the bacterial cell walls and are released when the bacterium is attacked.
- *Microorganisms* are parasites that live at the host's expense.
- Infectious diseases can be communicable (transmitted from person to person, such as influenza) or not communicable (e.g., peritonitis).

- Transmission of infection requires these factors:
  1. Reservoir (or source) of infectious agents
     a. Animate reservoirs include people, animals, and insects
     b. Inanimate reservoirs include soil, water, other environmental sources, or medical equipment
  2. Susceptible host with a portal of entry
  3. Mode of transmission
  4. Portal of exit (exit of the microbe from the host often occurs through the portal of entry but can exit by other routes)
- Prevention of infection transmission involves disrupting the three factors or breaking the chain of infection at any point.
- Host factors that increase the susceptibility to infection are:
  1. Congenital or acquired immune deficiencies
  2. Alteration of normal flora by antibiotic therapy
  3. Age over 65 years
  4. Hormonal changes (e.g., pregnancy, diabetes, corticosteroid therapy, or adrenal insufficiency)
  5. Defective phagocytosis
  6. Breaks in skin or mucous membranes
  7. Interference with flow of urine, tears, or saliva
  8. Impaired cough reflex or ciliary action
  9. Malnutrition or dehydration
  10. Smoking, alcohol consumption, or inhalation of toxic chemicals
  11. Invasive therapy, chemotherapy, radiation therapy, steroid therapy, or surgery
- Common modes of infection transmission are:
  1. Contact transmission (most common)
     a. Direct (person-to-person) contact, in which the source and host have physical contact and microorganisms are transferred directly (e.g., common cold)
     b. Indirect contact, in which the transfer of microorganisms occurs from a source to a host by passive transfer from a contaminated object (e.g., staphylococcal organisms)
  2. Droplet transmission from contact with infected secretions or droplets (e.g., influenza)
  3. Airborne transmission from small airborne particles containing pathogens that leave the infected source, are suspended in the air, and enter a susceptible host (e.g., *Mycobacterium tuberculosis* or the varicella zoster virus)
  4. Vector transmission, in which insects carry pathogens between two or more hosts, such as the deer tick that causes Lyme disease
- Human physiologic defenses against infection include:
  1. Intact skin and mucous membranes
  2. Normal flora

3. Secretions of the respiratory, GI, and genitourinary tracts
4. Inflammation and phagocytosis (native immunity)
5. AMI and CMI
- A hospital-acquired infection (HAI) is an infection acquired while the patient was in a health care setting. Old terms for this include *nosocomial* and *iatrogenic.*
- HAIs can be prevented or controlled in at least five major ways:
  1. Hand hygiene
     a. Hand hygiene (wetting, soaping, lathering, applying friction under running water for at least 15 seconds, rinsing, and adequate drying)
     b. Alcohol-based hand rubs (ABHRs)
  2. Disinfection/sterilization
  3. Standard precautions
  4. Transmission-based precautions
  5. Staff and patient placement and cohorting

QSEN QUALITY IMPROVEMENT

Infection control within a health care facility is designed to reduce the risk for HAIs and thus reduce morbidity and mortality. Participation in care processes and monitoring methods to design and test changes that reduce HAIs is an essential component of nursing practice.

- Centers for Disease Control and Prevention (CDC) Transmission-Based Guidelines include implementing:
  1. *Standard precautions* assume that all body excretions, secretions, and moist membranes and tissues, excluding perspiration, are potentially infectious; the precautions should be used in the care of all patients.
     a. Respiratory hygiene and cough etiquette (RH/CE) for respiratory illnesses
        (1) Patient, staff, and visitor education
        (2) Posted signs
        (3) Hand hygiene

❗ NURSING SAFETY PRIORITY: Action Alert

Remember that gloves are an essential part of infection control and should always be worn as part of standard precautions. Either handwashing or use of alcohol-based hand rubs is done before donning and after removing gloves. The combination of hand hygiene and wearing gloves is the most effective strategy for preventing infection transmission.

      (4) Covering the nose and mouth with a tissue and prompt tissue disposal or using surgical masks

      (5) Separation from the person with respiratory infection by more than 3 feet (1 m)

      (6) Safe injection practices, using a sterile, single-use disposable needle and syringe for each injection, prevention of contamination of injection equipment and drug, and use of retractable needles

2. Transmission-based precautions

   a. *Airborne precautions* for patients known or suspected to have infections transmitted by the airborne transmission route (e.g., tuberculosis, measles [rubeola], and chickenpox [varicella])

     (1) Negative airflow rooms

     (2) Enclosed booths with high-efficiency particulate air (HEPA) filtration or ultraviolet light

   b. *Droplet precautions* for patients known or suspected to have infections transmitted by the droplet transmission route (e.g., influenza, mumps, pertussis, meningitis)

   c. *Contact precautions* for patients known or suspected to have infections transmitted by direct contact or contact with items in the environment (e.g., significant multidrug-resistant organism [MDRO] infection or colonization, pediculosis, scabies, respiratory syncytial virus [RSV], and *Clostridium difficile*)

A number of microorganisms have become resistant to multiple antibiotics, and once-useful drugs no longer control these infectious agents, including methicillin-resistant *Staphylococcus aureus* (MRSA) and vancomycin-resistant *Enterococcus* (VRE).

! NURSING SAFETY PRIORITY: Action Alert

Patients most at risk for hospital acquired multidrug-resistant organism (MDRO) infections are older adults and those who have suppressed immunity, have a long history of antibiotic therapy, or have invasive tubes or lines. Intensive care unit (ICU) patients are especially at risk. Check with your agency policy regarding specific infection-preventive measures. Examples include bathing patients with chlorhexidine cloths.

• Complications from infection are relapse, cellulitis, pneumonia, abscess formation, sepsis, septic shock, disseminated intravascular coagulation (DIC), multi-system organ failure, and death.

PATIENT-CENTERED COLLABORATIVE CARE
Assessment
* Obtain patient information about:
  1. Age
  2. History of tobacco or alcohol use
  3. Current illness or disease (e.g., diabetes)
  4. Past and current drug use (e.g., prescribed, OTC, recreational, injection)
  5. Nutritional status
  6. Previous vaccinations or immunizations
  7. Exposure to infectious agents
  8. Contact with animals, including pets
  9. Insect bites
  10. Travel history
  11. Sexual history
  12. Transfusion history
  13. Previous infection history
  14. Order of symptom onset
* Assess for and document:
  1. Skin manifestations
     a. Redness
     b. Warmth
     c. Swelling
     d. Drainage or pus
     e. Pain
  2. Generalized manifestations
     a. Fever (usually a temperature above 101°F [38°C] or 99°F [37°C] for older adults)
     b. Chills
     c. Malaise and fatigue
     d. Lymphadenopathy
     e. Joint pain, muscle aches
     f. Photophobia
  3. GI tract manifestations
     a. Nausea and vomiting
     b. Diarrhea
  4. Genitourinary manifestations
     a. Dysuria
     b. Frequency
     c. Urgency
     d. Hematuria
     e. Purulent drainage
     f. Pelvic, flank, or low back pain
  5. Respiratory tract manifestations
     a. Cough
     b. Congestion

      c. Rhinorrhea, sputum
      d. Sore throat
      e. Chest pain
  6. Abnormal laboratory findings
      a. Positive culture
      b. Positive serologic results
      c. High or low WBC count
      d. Elevated erythrocyte sedimentation rate (ESR)
  7. Abnormal imaging findings
      a. Chest x-ray, sinus or joint films, GI studies
      b. Computed tomography (CT)
      c. Magnetic resonance imaging (MRI)
      d. Ultrasonography
  8. Biopsy

Planning and Implementation

- Effective anti-infective therapy requires:
  1. Agent appropriate for the known organism
  2. Sufficient dosage and duration of treatment
  3. Timely administration (avoid delays or skipped doses)
- Nursing interventions include:
  1. Obtaining and reviewing an allergy history before giving antibiotics
  2. Monitoring the patient for side effects of antibiotics, such as nausea, vomiting, or rash
  3. Using best practices to reduce fever; this can vary by age, underlying pathology, or institutional policy
     a. Antipyretics
     b. External cooling measures but avoid shivering
  4. Monitoring for manifestations of dehydration
     a. Thirst
     b. Decreased skin turgor
     c. Dry skin and mucous membranes
  5. Encouraging fluid intake or administering IV fluids
  6. Measuring intake and output
  7. Monitoring vital signs and oxygen saturation
  8. Monitoring skin intactness, color, and temperature

QSEN EVIDENCE-BASED PRACTICE

Fever may increase the potential for pressure ulcer formation. Monitor the patient more often and provide pressure-relieving interventions for vulnerable patients.

  9. Assessing level of consciousness and for seizure activity
  10. Monitoring laboratory values
  11. Providing or assisting with oral and personal hygiene

12. Teaching the patient and family about the mode of transmission of infection and mechanisms that prevent spread to others

Community-Based Care

- Provide vaccination, using guidelines established annually by the CDC.
- Remove indwelling urinary catheters as soon as possible to prevent urinary tract infections.
- Emphasize the importance of a clean home environment, especially for the patient who is immunocompromised or uniquely susceptible to superinfection.
- Demonstrate proper handwashing with patient and family and ask for a return demonstration to assess learning.
- Teach the patient and family about:
  1. What is causing the illness
  2. Modes of transmission if applicable
  3. Specific precautions for transmission prevention, including:
     a. Whether any special household cleaning is necessary and if so, what those special steps include
     b. How to dispose of any used needles and syringes safely and legally
     c. Cleaning clothing soiled with blood or other body fluids by washing them with bleach or disinfectant (e.g., Lysol)
     d. Cleaning measures based on actual equipment and facilities
  4. The importance of adhering to the prescribed antibiotic therapy regimen, including:
     a. Timing of doses
     b. Number of days
     c. Any specific drug administration instructions (e.g., before meals, with meals, without other agents) and the possible side effects
     d. Allergic manifestations and the need to notify a health care provider if an adverse reaction occurs
     e. What to do if a drug dose is missed (e.g., doubling the dosage or waiting until the next dose time)
  5. Managing IV drug therapy
- Refer to home health care agencies as needed.

INFLAMMATION AND IMMUNITY

OVERVIEW

- Inflammation and immunity are provided through the actions and products of white blood cells (WBCs), also called *leukocytes*.
- There are several types of WBCs, and these cell types are the basis of the differential of the WBC count. The differential can be used

to determine the patient's risk for infection, the presence or absence of infection, the presence or absence of an allergic reaction, and whether an infection is bacterial or viral.

- WBCs provide protection through defensive actions such as recognition of self versus non-self. Self-tolerance is the special ability of WBCs to recognize healthy self cells using proteins in cell membranes. WBCs are the only body cells able to recognize non-self cells and to attack them. One example of membrane proteins that provide self-identification is human leukocyte antigens (HLAs) found on the surface of most body cells. HLAs are inherited and determine *tissue type.*
- Other defensive actions by which WBCs provide protection include:
  1. Destruction of foreign invaders, cellular debris, and unhealthy or abnormal self cells
  2. Production of antibodies directed against invaders
  3. Complement activation
  4. Production of cytokines that stimulate WBC production in bone marrow and increase specific leukocyte activity
- Immunocompetence requires that inflammation, antibody-mediated, and cell-mediated responses all have optimal functioning. Inflammation is a general, nonspecific protective response.
  1. Inflammation
     a. Inflammation and infection are not the same thing. Infection almost always is accompanied by inflammation, but inflammation often occurs without infection.
     b. The tissue responses to inflammation are helpful if they are confined to the area of invasion or infection and do not extend beyond the acute phase. Chronic inflammation can damage tissues and reduce function.
     c. Inflammation cannot be transferred from one person to another.
  2. Immunity is an adaptive internal protection that results in long-term resistance to the effects of invading microorganisms. There are two types:
     a. Antibody-mediated immunity (AMI), also known as *humoral immunity*
        (1) Antigen-antibody interactions neutralize, eliminate, or destroy foreign proteins.
        (2) Antibodies are produced by sensitized B-lymphocytes (B-cells).
        (3) AMI can be transferred from one person or animal to another for a short-term effect.
     b. Cell-mediated immunity (CMI) that controls and coordinates the entire inflammatory and immune response

3. Immune function peaks between 20 and 40 years of age; the older adult is at an increased risk for infection and cancer development.

4. Patients who take immunosuppressive drugs for any reason have an increased risk for infection and cancer development.

5. Transplant rejection is a normal response of the immune system that can damage or destroy the transplanted organ. Patients who receive transplanted organs (unless they are from an identical sibling) need to take immunosuppressive drugs daily to prevent transplant rejection.

ORGANIZATION OF THE IMMUNE SYSTEM

- The immune system is not located in any one organ or body area, but most immune system cells come from the bone marrow. Some cells mature in the bone marrow; others leave the bone marrow and mature in different body sites.

- When mature, many immune system cells are released into the blood, where they circulate to most body areas and have specific effects.

- Each WBC has a specific function. The cells of the immune system and their functions are as follows:

  1. *Neutrophils* nonspecifically ingest and phagocytize microorganisms and foreign protein.

  2. *Macrophages* nonspecifically recognize foreign proteins and microorganisms, ingesting and phagocytizing these invaders.

  3. *Monocytes* destroy bacteria and cellular debris; they also mature into macrophages.

  4. *Eosinophils* have weak phagocytic action and release vasoactive amines during allergic reactions.

  5. *Basophils* release histamine and heparin in areas of tissue damage.

  6. *Lymphocytes* have two categories of specialized cells, each with subtypes:

     a. B-lymphocytes are essential to AMI. They sense foreign cells and proteins and exist as either *plasma cells* or *memory cells*, secreting immunoglobulins in response to the presence of a specific antigen.

     b. T-lymphocytes are essential to CMI and are further characterized as *helper or inducer T-cells* (which enhance immune activity through secretion of various factors, cytokines, and lymphokines), *suppressor T-cells* (which regulate immune activity by preventing hypersensitivity), *cytotoxic* or *cytolytic T-cells* (which selectively attack and destroy non-self cells, including virally infected cells, grafts, and transplanted organs), or *natural killer (NK) cells* (which nonselectively attack non-self cells, especially body cells that have undergone mutation and become malignant; they also attack grafts and transplanted organs).

- *Phagocytosis* is the engulfing and destruction of invaders. This action also rids the body of debris after tissue injury. Neutrophils and macrophages are most efficient at phagocytosis. Phagocytosis involves seven steps:
  1. *Exposure and invasion:* For phagocytosis to start, leukocytes must first be exposed to organisms, foreign proteins, or debris from damaged tissues.
  2. *Attraction:* To ensure the WBCs come into direct contact with the target (antigen, invader, or foreign protein), damaged tissues and blood vessels secrete chemotaxins (chemical attractants) that can combine with the surface of invading foreign proteins to improve attraction.
  3. *Adherence:* This process allows the phagocytic cell to bind to the surface of the target.
  4. *Recognition:* This process occurs when the phagocytic cell sticks to the surface of the target cell and recognizes it as non-self. This action ensures that phagocytosis occurs only against non-self or unhealthy self cells.
  5. *Cellular ingestion:* Phagocytosis (engulfment) into the phagocyte is needed because the destruction of the target cell occurs inside the phagocytic cell.
  6. *Phagosome formation:* This occurs when the phagocyte's granules are inside the vacuole and fuse to the invader.
  7. *Degradation:* The phagosome enzymes digest the engulfed target, which is the final step.

INFLAMMATION

- Inflammation, also called *natural* or *innate-native immunity*, provides immediate protection against the effects of tissue injury and invading foreign proteins.
- Inflammation is characterized by blood vessel and tissue reactions to rid the body of harmful microorganisms and other invaders.
- Inflammation differs from immunity in two important ways:
  1. Inflammatory protection is immediate but short term against injury or invading organisms. It does not provide true immunity on repeated exposure to the same organism and cannot be transferred to another person.
  2. Inflammation is a nonspecific body defense to invasion or injury and can be started by almost any event, regardless of where it occurs or what causes it.
- The classic manifestations of inflammation are:
  1. Warmth
  2. Redness
  3. Swelling

    4. Pain

    5. Decreased function

- Symptoms of inflammation can be local or widespread, depending on the intensity, severity, and duration of exposure to the initiating injury or invasion.

- Inflammation occurs in response to tissue injury and to invasion by organisms. Infection is usually accompanied by inflammation; however, inflammation can occur without infection.

  1. Examples of inflammation without infection include sprain injuries to joints, myocardial infarction, sterile surgical incisions, blister formation, and thrombophlebitis.

  2. Examples of inflammation caused by noninfectious invasion by foreign proteins include allergic rhinitis, contact dermatitis, and other allergic reactions.

  3. Examples of inflammation caused by infection include pneumonia, appendicitis, and viral hepatitis.

- Four types of WBCs (leukocytes) are involved in inflammation:

  1. Neutrophils

  2. Macrophages

  3. Eosinophils

  4. Basophils

SEQUENCE OF INFLAMMATORY RESPONSES

- Inflammatory responses occur in a predictable sequence of three stages. The sequence is the same regardless of the triggering event, and the timing may overlap.

  1. *Stage I* is the vascular part of the inflammatory response. Injured tissues and the leukocytes in this area secrete histamine, serotonin, and kinins that constrict the small veins and dilate the arterioles in the area of injury. Increased blood flow and capillary permeability deliver nutrients to injured tissues but also cause redness, swelling, and pain. The duration of Stage 1 depends on the severity of the initiating event, but usually subsides within 24 to 72 hours.

  2. *Stage II* is the cellular exudate part of the response, Neutrophilia (increased number of circulating neutrophils) occurs. Exudate in the form of pus occurs, containing WBCs, the pathogen, necrotic tissue, and fluids.

     a. The neutrophil can increase in count up to five times within 12 hours after the onset of inflammation as a result of cytokine stimulation.

     b. Neutrophils destroy organisms and remove dead tissue through phagocytosis.

     c. The arachidonic acid (AA) cascade contributes to the inflammatory response by converting fatty acids in plasma membranes into AA. Enzymes (including cyclooxygenase) then convert AA into many chemicals that are further processed into the substances that continue the inflammatory response in the tissues. Some of these substances include histamine, leukotrienes, prostaglandins, serotonin, and kinins.

3. *Stage III* features tissue repair and replacement. Although this stage is completed last, it begins at the time of injury and is critical to the healing.

a. Some of the WBCs involved in inflammation start the replacement of lost tissues or repair of damaged tissues by releasing growth factors, inducing the remaining healthy cells to divide.

b. In tissues that are unable to divide, molecules released by WBCs trigger new blood vessel growth (angiogenesis) and scar tissue formation. Because scar tissue does not behave like normal tissue, loss of function occurs wherever damaged tissues are replaced with scar tissue.

CONSEQUENCES OF INFLAMMATION

- When inflammation occurs in response to invasion by infectious microorganisms, its actions can eliminate or destroy the invaders and prevent the person from becoming ill.
- Inflammation is needed to trigger both AMI and CMI.
- When inflammatory responses are prolonged or occur at inappropriate times or in inappropriate places, they can cause tissue damage with extensive fibrosis, scarring, and loss of healthy tissue function.

IMMUNITY

Lymphocytes develop actions and products that provide the protection of true immunity.

ANTIBODY-MEDIATED IMMUNITY

- AMI, also known as *humoral immunity*, involves antigen-antibody interactions to neutralize, eliminate, or destroy foreign proteins. Antibodies are produced by B-lymphocytes (B-cells).
- B-cells become sensitized to a specific foreign protein (antigen) and produce antibodies directed specifically against that protein. The expressed antibody (rather than the B-cell) causes one of several actions to neutralize, eliminate, or destroy that antigen.
- B-cells start as lymphocytes in the bone marrow, the primary lymphoid tissue, and migrate into many secondary lymphoid tissues, where maturation is completed. The secondary lymphoid

tissues for B-cell maturation are the spleen, parts of lymph nodes, tonsils, and the mucosa of the intestinal tract.

- Seven steps are needed to produce a specific, long-lasting antibody directed against a specific antigen whenever the person is exposed to that antigen:

    1. *Exposure or invasion* is needed because antibody actions occur inside the body or on a few body surfaces. Without exposure, an antibody cannot be made.

    2. *Antigen recognition* is the recognition of the invader by an unsensitized B-cell. This process involves macrophages and helper-inducer T-cells.

    3. *Lymphocyte sensitization* occurs when the B-cell recognizes the antigen as non-self and becomes sensitized to this antigen. A single naive B-cell can become sensitized only once.

    4. *Antibody production and release* occurs at a rate as high as 300 molecules of antibody per second by each sensitized B-lymphocyte. These antibody molecules are released and can bind to their specific antigen. *Circulating antibodies can be transferred from one person to another to provide the receiving person with immediate immunity of short duration.*

    5. *Antibody-antigen binding* occurs when the tips of the Y-shaped antibody recognize the specific antigen and bind to it. The binding stimulates reactions to neutralize, eliminate, or destroy the antigen.

    6. *Antibody-binding actions* include agglutination, lysis, complement fixation, precipitation, and inactivation or neutralization, all of which can neutralize, eliminate, or destroy the antigen.

    7. *Sustained immunity (memory)* is critical in providing long-lasting immunity to a specific antigen. It results from memory B-cells made during the lymphocyte sensitization stage. These memory cells remain sensitized to the specific antigen to which they were originally exposed. On re-exposure to the same antigen, the memory cells rapidly respond, and each new cell can rapidly make large amounts of the antibody specific for the sensitizing antigen. This ability of the memory cells to respond on re-exposure to the same antigen that originally sensitized the B-cell allows a rapid and large immune (anamnestic) response to the antigen. Such large quantities of antibody are made that the invading organisms usually are removed completely, and the person does not become ill. Because of this process, most people do not become ill with chickenpox or other infectious diseases more than once, even though they are exposed many times to the causative organism. Without the action of memory, people would

remain susceptible to specific diseases on subsequent exposure to the organisms, and no sustained immunity would be generated.

- All antibodies are immunoglobulins (Ig), also called *gamma globulins*, because they are globular proteins that confer immunity. There are five antibody types:
  1. IgA is the secretory antibody found on body surfaces and secretions to prevent antigen entry.
  2. IgM is the antibody type a sensitized B-cell makes on first exposure to an antigen. It is a large and complex structure with 10 binding sites. IgM is a powerful antibody, even though it is produced in small amounts. This antibody ensures that an initial infectious illness, such as chickenpox, lasts only 5 to 10 days.
  3. IgG is the most common antibody found in the blood. On re-exposure to the same antigen, the already sensitized B-cell makes large amounts of the IgG type of antibody against that antigen. The enormous numbers produced make IgG antibodies efficient at clearing the antigen and protecting the person from again becoming ill with the disease.
  4. IgE is the antibody type that is responsible for many allergic reactions.
  5. IgD activates B-cells and modifies the activity of IgM.

ACQUIRING ANTIBODY-MEDIATED IMMUNITY

- *Adaptive immunity* is the immunity that a person's body learns to make (or can receive) as an adaptive response to invasion by organisms or foreign proteins. AMI is an acquired immunity, is active or passive, and is acquired naturally or artificially.
  1. *Active immunity* occurs when antigens enter the body and the body responds by actively making specific antibodies against the antigen.
     a. Natural active immunity occurs when an antigen enters the body without human assistance and the body responds by actively making antibodies against that antigen (e.g., chickenpox virus). *This type of immunity is the most effective and the longest lasting.*
     b. Artificial active immunity is the protection developed by **vaccination** or immunization. Small amounts of specific antigens are placed as a vaccination into a person and the immune system responds by actively making antibodies against the antigen.
  2. *Passive immunity* occurs when antibodies against an antigen are in a person's body but were transferred to the person's body after being made in the body of another person or

animal. It provides only immediate short-term protection against a specific antigen.

   a. Natural passive immunity occurs when antibodies are passed from the mother to the fetus through the placenta or to the infant through colostrum and breast milk.
   b. Artificial passive immunity involves injecting a person with antibodies that were produced in another person or animal.

- AMI works with inflammation to protect against infection. However, AMI can provide the most effective, long-lasting immunity only when its actions are combined with those of CMI.

CELL-MEDIATED IMMUNITY

- CMI, or cellular immunity, involves many WBC actions and interactions. This type of immunity is provided by lymphocyte stem cells that mature in the secondary lymphoid tissues of the thymus and pericortical areas of lymph nodes. These cells are known as *T-lymphocytes (T-cells)*.
- Certain CMI responses influence and regulate the activities of AMI and inflammation by producing and releasing cytokines. For total immunocompetence, CMI must function optimally.
- Cytokines are small proteins produced by WBCs and other cells. Cytokines have effects on cells of the immune system and on other body cells.
   1. Cytokines act like *messengers* that tell specific cells how and when to respond.
   2. Cytokines include the interleukins, interferons, colony-stimulating factors, and tumor necrosis factor.
- Four T-lymphocyte subsets that are critically important for the development and continuation of CMI are:
   1. *Helper-inducer T-cells* (T4 cells, T_H cells, CD4+ cells) easily recognize self cells versus non-self cells. In response to the recognition of non-self (antigen), helper-inducer T-cells secrete cytokines that can enhance the activity of other WBCs.
   2. *Suppressor T-cells* (T8 cells, CD8+ cells, T_S cells) regulate CMI by preventing hypersensitivity (continuous overreactions) when a person is exposed to non-self cells or proteins. These cells secrete cytokines that inhibit immune-system cell action and work in opposition to helper-inducer T-cells. Immune function is well balanced when T4+ cells outnumber T8+ cells by a 2:1 ratio.
   3. *Cytotoxic or cytolytic T-cells* are a subset of suppressor cells that destroy cells containing a processed antigen's major histocompatibility complex (MHC). This activity is most effective against self cells infected by parasites, such as viruses or protozoa.

4. *NK cells* (CD16 cells) have direct cytotoxic effects on some non-self cells that are independent of the interactions of other WBCs. NK cells conduct "seek and destroy" missions in the body to eliminate non-self cells. NK cells are most effective in destroying unhealthy or abnormal self cells, such as cancer cells and virally infected body cells.

- CMI helps protect the body through the ability to differentiate self from non-self.
- The non-self cells most easily recognized by CMI are cancer cells.
- Self cells infected by organisms that live within host cells and transformed cancer cells are generally recognized as abnormal and are destroyed by CMI.

PAIN

OVERVIEW
Pain is a universal, complex, and unpleasant sensory and emotional experience.
- Self-report is always the most reliable indication of pain.
- Pain is either temporary or not:
  1. *Acute pain* results from sudden accidental trauma or surgery. It is usually temporary, has a sudden onset, and is localized. Features include:
     a. Physiologic responses from activation of the sympathetic nervous system
        (1) Increased heart rate
        (2) Increased blood pressure
        (3) Increased respiratory rate
        (4) Dilated pupils
        (5) Sweating
     b. Common behavioral responses
        (1) Restlessness
        (2) Inability to concentrate
        (3) Apprehension
        (4) Overall distress
  2. *Chronic* or *persistent pain* persists for longer than 3 months, is often poorly localized, and is hard to describe. It may not be associated with tachycardia or hypertension. It is often associated with depression, interference with personal relationships, and inability to maintain activities of daily living. Chronic pain is further divided into two subtypes, cancer and non-cancer pain:
     a. Chronic cancer pain is associated with:
        (1) The cancer itself
        (2) Nerve compression

      (3) Invasion of tissue

      (4) Bone metastasis

      (5) Cancer treatments (e.g., chemotherapy, radiation therapy)

   b. Chronic non-cancer pain is the more common type and is associated with tissue injury that has healed or a chronic non-cancer diagnosis such as arthritis or back pain.

- Pain is also categorized as:

   1. Nociceptive or visceral-somatic, with normal processing of pain signals. This type of pain can be acute or chronic.

   2. Neuropathic, originally the result of nerve injury, the abnormal processing of pain signals. Processing abnormalities may be generated in either the peripheral or central nervous systems. Neuropathic pain is usually chronic.

! NURSING SAFETY PRIORITY: Action Alert

Although many characteristics of chronic pain are similar in different patients, be aware that each situation is unique and requires an individualized plan of care.

The attitudes of health care professionals toward pain influence the way they perceive and interact with patients in pain.

Factors such as age, gender, sociocultural background, and genetics influence the patient's ability to process and react to pain. For example, men have more cluster headaches, back pain, gout, peripheral vascular disease, and postherpetic neuralgia.

Considerations for Older Adults

Pain is not an inevitable consequence of aging; however, there is a higher incidence in older adults. Sensitivity to pain does not diminish with age. Many older adults, even those with mild to moderate dementia, are able to use a self-report assessment tool if nurses and other caregivers take the time to administer it.

Many patients are reluctant to report pain. When they do, they may underreport its severity.

Although pain is familiar to everyone, it is so complex that there is no single universal treatment.

Definitions Important to Pain Management:

   1. *Addiction* is a primary, chronic neurobiologic disease with one or more of the following: impaired control over drug use, compulsive use, continued use despite harm, and craving.

Gender Considerations

Certain chronic painful conditions are more common in women. Women have more migraine headaches, tension headaches, rheumatoid arthritis and osteoarthritis, fibromyalgia, and multiple sclerosis. Consider the implications of chronic pain on the woman's life during assessment when a chronic condition is present even when that condition is not the primary reason for nursing care.

2. *Pseudoaddiction* is a health care–induced syndrome created by the undertreatment of pain. Features include patient behaviors such as anger and escalating demands for more or different medications, and results in suspicion and avoidance by staff.
3. *Tolerance* is a state of adaptation in which exposure to a drug induces changes that result in a decrease in one or more of the drug's effects over time.
4. *Physical dependence* is adaptation manifested by a drug class–specific withdrawal syndrome that can be produced by abrupt cessation, rapid dose reduction, decreasing blood level of the drug, or administration of an antagonist. It occurs in everyone who takes opioids over an extended period.
5. *Withdrawal* or *abstinence syndrome* results when a patient who is physically dependent on opioids abruptly ceases using them.
6. *Placebo* is any medical treatment or nursing care that produces an effect in a patient because of its therapeutic intent and not because of its actual physical or chemical properties.

❗ NURSING SAFETY PRIORITY: Drug Alert

Carefully explain the difference between physical dependence and addiction when a patient starts on opioid therapy. **NOTE:** tolerance, physical dependence, and addiction can coexist.

❗ NURSING SAFETY PRIORITY: Drug Alert

Deceitful administration of a placebo violates informed consent law and jeopardizes the nurse-patient therapeutic relationship. Never administer a placebo to a patient. Promptly contact your nursing supervisor if you are given an order to do so.

PATIENT-CENTERED COLLABORATIVE CARE
Assessment

* Assess and record pain history information:
  1. Pain experience, including the sequence of events (precipitating and relieving factors, localization, character and quality of pain, and duration of pain)

    2. Nature of adjustments, if any, in life or in the family
    3. Beliefs about the cause of the pain and what should be done about it (patient's expectations)
- Assess for physical and clinical manifestations:
    1. Patient's statement of pain
    2. Tachycardia and increased or decreased blood pressure (heart rate and blood pressure are less likely to be altered with chronic pain)
    3. Altered movement, such as splinting or listlessness
    4. Functional status impairment
    5. Location of pain
       a. Localized (pain is confined to the site of origin)
       b. Projected (pain occurs along a specific nerve or nerves)
       c. Radiating (diffuse pain occurs around the site of origin that is not well localized)
       d. Referred (pain is perceived in an area distant from the site of painful stimuli)
    6. Intensity and quality of pain
       a. Pain intensity (e.g., number rating scale of 0 to 10, with 10 being the worst possible pain)
       b. Verbal descriptions to convey the quality of pain or descriptive scales, such as "none" to "moderate" to "severe"
       c. Wong-Baker FACES Pain Rating scale of smile to frown
- To assess pain in cognitively impaired or nonverbal patients:
    1. Use self-report (when possible).
    2. Use a valid and reliable tool to assess nonverbal behaviors such as the Checklist of Nonverbal Pain Indicators or Pain Assessment in Advanced Dementia Scale and document with vital signs and after a pain intervention.
    3. Use surrogate reporting (e.g., from a family member).
    4. Attempt an analgesic trial.

Interventions

Nonsurgical Management

- Drug therapy: selection of drugs is based on level of pain, drug effects and adverse effects, and knowledge of the advantages and disadvantages for each route of administration.
    1. The non-opioid analgesics are the first-line therapy for mild to moderate pain. They are typically available without a prescription and administered orally, rectally, or topically.
    2. Examples of non-opioid analgesics include acetaminophen (Tylenol).
       a. Nonsteroidal anti-inflammatory drugs (NSAIDs) such as:
          (1) Aspirin
          (2) Ketorolac (Toradol)
          (3) Ibuprofen (Motrin, Advil, other names)

    (4) Naproxen (Naprosyn)
    (5) Ketoprofen (Orudis)
    (6) Celecoxib (Celebrex)

> **!** **NURSING SAFETY PRIORITY: Drug Alert**
>
> Teach patients to take no more the 4000 mg daily (2400 mg for older adults) of acetaminophen and for no longer than 4 weeks without informing their health care provider about the amount of acetaminophen they take each day. Remind them to have liver and renal function laboratory tests done on a regular basis as prescribed to monitor for early indicators of adverse drug events.

> **!** **NURSING SAFETY PRIORITY: Drug Alert**
>
> Aspirin and other NSAIDs can cause GI bleeding and interfere with renal function. Many short-acting NSAIDs interfere with the anti-platelet activity of prescribed cardiovascular agents. Therefore observe the patient for gastric discomfort, edema, hypernatremia, stroke or acute coronary syndrome, bleeding, or bruising. Teach the patient and family to report these problems to the health care provider immediately if they occur.

  3. Opioid analgesics are used to manage moderate to severe pain. They can be administered by any route. Examples include:
    a. Hydromorphone (Dilaudid)
    b. Morphine (Roxanol, Avinza, Kadian)
    c. Fentanyl (Sublimaze)
    d. Hydrocodone
    e. Oxycodone
    f. Oxymorphone (Opana, Numorphan)
    g. Methadone (Dolophine)
    h. Codeine

🧬 Genetic/Genomic Considerations

It has long been known that the cytochrome (CY) P450 enzyme system is important to the metabolism of some opioids. Inter-ethnic variations in phenotypes of the CYP450 enzymes are common, causing decreased metabolism of selected analgesics in a small percentage of white and Asian individuals. These variations have clinical implications when the opioid codeine, which is metabolized by the CYP450 enzyme system, is administered. Slow metabolizers may not respond well to codeine, and ultra-rapid metabolizers may have an exaggerated response.

> ### ❗ NURSING SAFETY PRIORITY: Critical Rescue
>
> The key to assessing opioid-induced adverse effects is to monitor for sedation. After the first dose of an opioid, determine how easily the patient is aroused. *Stop the medication if the patient is difficult to arouse.* Be sure to assess the patient's level of consciousness with subsequent doses. Monitor respiratory rate and depth, especially while the patient is sleeping, and reduce the dose or stop the drug if respiratory compromise occurs during initial dosing.

- Nursing care issues related to opioid therapy:
    1. Consider onset and duration of drug before administration.
    2. Monitor and prevent complications from side effects. Side effects, in order of seriousness, can include respiratory depression, sedation, constipation, nausea and vomiting, urinary retention, and pruritus (itching).
        a. Monitor respiratory rate and depth, especially when the patient is sleeping.
        b. Sedation occurs before opioid-induced respiratory depression, so nurse-monitored sedation levels are recommended by use of a sedation scale for opioid-naive (not currently on an opioid) patients or those receiving opioids IV or epidurally. The key to assessing sedation is determining how easily the patient is aroused.
        c. Prevent constipation with concurrent administration of a stool softener or bowel stimulant.
- Nursing care issues with patient-controlled analgesia (PCA):
    1. PCA delivers a set amount of drug through IV access, allowing the patient to control the dosage of opioid received, improving pain relief and increasing patient satisfaction.

> ### ❗ NURSING SAFETY PRIORITY: Critical Rescue
>
> An accurate respiratory assessment during opioid use requires watching the rise and fall of the patient's chest to determine the depth and regularity of respirations in addition to counting the respiratory rate for 60 seconds. Listening to the sound of the patient's respiration is also critical; snoring indicates airway obstruction and must be attended to promptly with repositioning, and depending on severity, a request for respiratory therapy consultation and further evaluation. For accuracy, respiratory assessment is done prior to arousing the sleeping patient.

! NURSING SAFETY PRIORITY: Drug Alert

Respiratory depression is managed with an opioid antagonist, naloxone (Narcan). It is a fast-acting drug given IV to reverse the opioid effect. The respiratory-depressant effect of the opioid usually acts longer than naloxone. Continue to monitor the patient after giving the drug, because respiratory depression can recur, necessitating additional naloxone.

2. Morphine, fentanyl, and hydromorphone are the most commonly used drugs for PCA.
3. Drug security is achieved through a locked syringe pump system or locked drug reservoir system.
4. When the patient presses the button or pendant (on ambulatory pumps), the appropriate bolus or demand dose is delivered. A basal rate may also be continuously administered.
5. Teach patients how to use PCA and to report side effects, such as dizziness, nausea and vomiting, and inability to void.
6. Monitor the patient's vital signs, particularly respirations, and check his or her sedation level at least every 2 hours initially or per agency protocol.
7. Do not allow a proxy or staff to administer a bolus or push the button. If the patient is unable to use the PCA device effectively, discontinue PCA and use another mode of drug delivery.

• Nursing care issues for epidural or intraspinal analgesia are:
   1. Collaborate with the pain specialist or anesthesia provider and patient to set pain relief and safety goals.
   2. Epidural analgesia is the instillation of a pain-blocking agent, usually an opioid analgesic alone or in combination with a local anesthetic, such as bupivacaine, into the epidural space.
   3. Epidural analgesia is most commonly used for the management of acute pain.
   4. Morphine (preservative-free), hydromorphone (Dilaudid), and fentanyl (Sublimaze) are the most commonly used opioids for epidural administration.
   5. Pruritus (itching), nausea, and vomiting are common side effects of epidural opioids.
   6. A temporary, externalized epidural catheter is used for acute pain control. This device is not sutured to the skin and is easily dislodged. Be sure to tape the catheter in two places to anchor it properly.
   7. Complications that occur with epidural analgesia are directly related to catheter placement, catheter maintenance, and the type of analgesic.

8. Infection is rare but can occur as a result of failure to maintain aseptic technique during catheter placement, through direct drug instillation, during infusion of solution and tubing changes, and from a failure to maintain aseptic conditions for indwelling catheters at the site of insertion or at the site of tube junctions.

! NURSING SAFETY PRIORITY: Action Alert

To prevent infections, ensure that all catheter line connections are secure and that an occlusive sterile dressing is maintained over the catheter site.

9. There is a risk for respiratory depression resulting from high plasma or cerebrospinal fluid concentrations of the instilled drug. Monitor the patient's respirations and sedation level at frequent intervals during and after the administration of epidural opioids and immediately report any concerns to the health care provider.
10. Urinary retention is a common problem associated with epidural analgesia and is more likely to occur in men than in woman.
11. Lower motor weakness is common when an epidural local anesthetic is used in combination with an opioid. Assist patients who get out of bed for the first time to determine the degree of leg weakness and risk for a fall.

- Adjuvant analgesics may be used to relieve pain alone or in combination with other analgesics by potentiating or enhancing the effectiveness of the analgesic.
  1. Antiepileptic drugs (AEDs or anticonvulsants)
     a. Gabapentin (Neurontin)
     b. Pregabalin (Lyrica)
     c. Topiramate (Topamax)
  2. Tricyclic antidepressants
     a. Amitriptyline (Elavil)
     b. Nortriptyline (Pamelor)
     c. Imipramine (Tofranil)
  3. Other antidepressants
     a. Trazodone (Desyrel)
     b. Paroxetine (Paxil)
     c. Sertraline (Zoloft)
  4. Antianxiety drugs
     a. Alprazolam (Xanax)
     b. Lorazepam (Ativan)
     c. Oxazepam (Serax, Zapex)
     d. Clonazepam (Klonopin)

5. Local anesthetics may be given orally (systemic effects), topically, and via epidural routes. Examples include:
   a. Epidural bupivacaine
   b. Oral mexiletine
   c. Xylocaine
   d. Lidocaine patch (Lidoderm patch)
   e. Lidocaine and prilocaine (EMLA cream)
   f. Lidocaine (ELA-Max cream)
6. Multimodal (balanced) analgesia for epidural pain management is a combination of opioids, non-opioids, and/or local anesthetics to relieve acute pain, usually postoperative pain.
7. Local short-acting gels and creams for cryotherapy. Examples include:
   a. Biofreeze
   b. Bengay
- Nonpharmacologic interventions
  1. Physical measures
     a. Cutaneous (skin) stimulation strategies
        (1) Application of heat, cold, and pressure
        (2) Therapeutic touch
        (3) Massage
        (4) Vibration
     b. Physical and occupational therapy
        (1) Exercise to strengthen muscles or to provide alternative approaches to avoid painful maneuvers
        (2) Massage or manipulation
        (3) Splinting of joints
     c. Transcutaneous electrical nerve stimulation (TENS)
  2. Cognitive-behavioral measures
     a. Distraction
     b. Imagery
     c. Relaxation (may be combined with music therapy)
     d. Hypnosis
  3. Complementary and alternative therapies
     a. Music therapy
     b. Acupuncture and acupressure
     c. Prayer and meditation
- Invasive techniques for chronic pain
  1. Nerve blocks
  2. Spinal cord stimulation

Community-Based Care

- Pain can be managed in any setting, including the home. Some patients require parenteral pain medications at home, thus health teaching should be provided to ensure continuity of care.

- Patients whose pain is difficult to manage should be referred to pain specialists and/or pain centers.
- Communicate and coordinate the plan of care for pain management as the patient transfers between health care agencies and home.
- Make appropriate referrals for physical therapy, a clinical nurse specialist in pain management, a social worker, and hospice or palliative care.
- Plan a home care nurse referral for patients who will require assistance or supervision with the pain relief regimen at home.
- Home agency practices and professional support at home are required if patients leave the hospital with infusion therapy for pain management.
- Ensure that the patient, especially one who is on opioids, has enough pain medication to last at least until the first follow-up visit.
- Teach the patient and family about analgesic regimens, including any technical skills needed to administer or deliver the analgesic, the purpose and action of various drugs, their side effects or adverse reactions, and the importance of dosage intervals.
- If the patient is on a flexible analgesic schedule, teach the patient and family how to safely increase and decrease the drug within the prescribed dosing guidelines.

QSEN SAFETY

Nurses are essential not only to meet the direct care needs of patients but also to ensure patient safety across settings. A fundamental attribute to safe, high-quality care is measurement; one cannot improve if one does not measure. Delivering safe, effective, efficient care is inherent to all nursing environments. In some environments and during transitions between care settings, the risk for error is great. This section highlights care competencies and concepts in three high-risk situations: perioperative, discharge, and end-of-life care.

PALLIATION AND END-OF-LIFE CARE

OVERVIEW

- Palliation is the relief or management of symptoms, particularly symptoms that are distressing to the patient or caregivers.
    1. Palliative care is not limited to care at the end of life. Palliative care is associated with positive patient outcomes of restored function, high patient satisfaction, cost reductions in health care, and slowing the progression of disease.

2. Palliative care can restore function, engage patients and families in meaningful discussions about preferences and values in care, and slow the progression of disease.

- End-of-life care is often used synonymously with hospice care.
  1. Hospice care implies a prognosis of 6 months or less; end-of life care implies weeks to days of life.
  2. Hospice care uses a coordinated, interdisciplinary approach to focus on quality of life among patients at the end of life and their family. This approach neither hastens nor postpones death; hospice staff provides interventions to meet the needs of a dying patient.
- Although dying is part of the normal life cycle, it is often feared as a time of pain, isolation, and suffering.
- *Death* is the cessation of integrated tissue and organ function, manifested by lack of heartbeat, absence of spontaneous respirations, or irreversible brain dysfunction.
- A *good death* is one that is free from avoidable distress and suffering for patients, families, and caregivers, in agreement with patients' and families' wishes, and consistent with clinical practice standards.
- *Advance directives* are legal documents that detail preferences for health care, including care at the end of life. Advance directives can be instructional (e.g., medical directives, living wills) or establish proxy decision makers (i.e., durable power of attorney for health care). The Patient Self-Determination Act of 1990 requires that all patients admitted to any health care agency be asked if they have advance directives.

PATIENT-CENTERED COLLABORATIVE CARE
Assessment
- Obtain patient information to identify the risks for and symptoms of distress:
  1. Diagnosis
  2. Medical history
  3. Recent state of health
- Assess distressing symptom(s) by intensity, frequency, duration, quality, and exacerbating (worsening) and relieving factors.
- Use a consistent method for rating the intensity of symptoms to facilitate ongoing assessments and evaluate treatment response.
- Assess and document the effects of an intervention on distress and comfort.
- Assess the patient for:
  1. Physical manifestations of approaching death
     a. Cold, mottled, discolored extremities
     b. Increased sleeping

    c. Food and fluid decrease
    d. Incontinence
    e. Congestion and gurgling
    f. Breathing pattern change
    g. Disorientation
    h. Restlessness
2. Emotional manifestations of approaching death
    a. Withdrawal
    b. Vision-like experiences
    c. Letting go
    d. Saying goodbye

! NURSING SAFETY PRIORITY: Action Alert

Do not deny or argue with what the dying person claims about talking to people you cannot see or hear and seeing objects and places not visible to you.

3. Family's perception of patient's symptoms
4. Vital signs: anticipate hypotension, slow, fast, or irregular heartbeat, and fast, shallow, or irregular respiratory rate
5. Psychosocial issues that may have an influence on the dying experience, control of symptoms, and family bereavement
    a. Cultural considerations, values, and religious beliefs of patient and family
    b. Fear, anxiety
    c. Knowledge deficits regarding the process of dying
    d. Coping problems
6. Signs that death has occurred
    a. Breathing stops
    b. Heart stops beating
    c. Pupils become fixed and dilated
    d. Body color becomes pale and waxen
    e. Body temperature drops
    f. Muscles and sphincters relax
    g. Urine and stool may be released
    h. Eyes may remain open and there is no blinking
    i. Jaw may fall open
    j. Trickling of fluids internally may be heard

Planning and Implementation
- Prioritized care focuses on symptom management or palliation. Palliative care is not limited to end-of-life care. End-of-life care uses palliation to reduce distress from pain, weakness, dyspnea, nausea and vomiting, agitation and delirium, seizures, and psychosocial reactions to dying.

🌐 Cultural Considerations

- Death-related beliefs and practices vary by ethnicity, religion, and race.
  1. Christianity
     a. There are many Christian denominations, which have variations in beliefs regarding medical care near the end of life.
     b. Roman Catholic tradition encourages individuals to receive the Sacrament of the Sick, administered by a priest at any point during an illness. This sacrament may be administered more than once. Not receiving this sacrament will *not* prohibit them from entering heaven after death.
     c. People may be baptized as Roman Catholics in an emergency situation (e.g., the person is dying) by a layperson. Otherwise, they are baptized by a priest.
     d. Christians believe in an afterlife of heaven or hell once the soul has left the body after death.
  2. Judaism
     a. The dying person is encouraged to recite the confessional or the affirmation of faith, called the *Shma*.
     b. According to Jewish law, a person who is extremely ill and dying should not be left alone.
     c. The body, which was the vessel and vehicle to the soul, deserves reverence and respect.
     d. The body should not be left unattended until the funeral, which should take place as soon as possible (preferably within 24 hours).
     e. Orthodox Judaism does not allow autopsies except under special circumstances.
     f. The body should not be embalmed, displayed, or cremated.
  3. Islam
     a. Islam is based on belief in one God Allah and his prophet Muhammad. The Qur'an is the scripture of Islam, composed of Muhammad's revelations of the Word of God (Allah).
     b. Death is seen as the beginning of a new and better life.
     c. God has prescribed an appointed time of death for everyone.
     d. The Qur'an encourages humans to seek treatment and not to refuse treatment. The belief is that only Allah cures, but that Allah cures through the work of humans.

- Pain management
  1. Patients who have had their pain controlled with long-acting opioids should continue their scheduled doses of opioids to prevent pain recurrence.
  2. Depending on the brand of long-acting opioid, oral capsules may be given rectally, sublingually, or through the buccal mucosa when swallowing is impaired.
  3. Nonpharmacologic pain management strategies can be incorporated with pharmacologic therapy and include:
     a. Massage
     b. Music therapy
     c. Therapeutic touch
     d. Aromatherapy

Considerations for Older Adults

Pain relief is often the priority need of older adults and is often underreported and undertreated. Do not withhold opioid drugs from older adults. Instead, reduce starting doses, make dose increases slowly, and monitor for changes in mental status or excessive sedation.

- Weakness management: Patients commonly experience weakness and fatigue as death nears, which may impair the ability to swallow.
  1. After the patient is unable to swallow, oral intake should be stopped to prevent aspiration.
  2. Educate families about the risk for aspiration, and reinforce that anorexia is a part of the dying process and that giving fluids can actually *increase* discomfort.
  3. Apply emollient to the lips, and moisten the mouth and lips with ice chips or swabs.
  4. In collaboration with a pharmacist experienced in palliative care, identify alternative routes and/or alternative drugs to maintain control of symptoms, choosing the least invasive route, such as oral, buccal mucosa, transdermal, or rectal.
- Breathlessness and dyspnea management: Dyspnea is a subjective experience in which the patient has an uncomfortable feeling of breathlessness that is described as terrifying.
  1. Treatment is based on physical assessment and the underlying condition. *Pharmacologic interventions should begin early in the course of dyspnea.* Nonpharmacologic interventions can be used in conjunction with, but not in place of, drug therapy.

! NURSING SAFETY PRIORITY: Action Alert

Dysphagia near death presents a problem for oral drug therapy.

- Some tablets may be crushed but sustained-release capsules should not be taken apart. Collaborate with the prescriber about discontinuing drugs that are not needed to control pain, dyspnea, agitation, nausea, vomiting, cardiac workload, or seizures.
- Collaborate with a pharmacist experienced in palliation to identify alternative routes and/or alternative drugs to maintain control of symptoms.
- Choose the least invasive route such as oral, buccal mucosa (inside cheek), transdermal (via the skin), or rectal. Some oral drugs can be given rectally. Depending on the patient needs, the subcutaneous or IV routes may be used if access is available. The IM route is almost never used at the end of life because it is considered painful and drug distribution varies among patients.

2. Morphine is the standard treatment for dyspnea near death. Patients who have not been receiving opioids are given starting doses of 10 to 30 mg orally. Those who have taken morphine or other opioids for pain may need much higher doses of morphine (up to 50% more than their usual dose) for relief of dyspnea.
3. Bronchodilators may be used for bronchospasms, and corticosteroids may be used for inflammatory problems.
4. Diuretics may be given for vascular overload with pulmonary edema.
5. Antibiotics may be indicated for dyspnea from a respiratory infection.
6. To reduce oral and respiratory secretions administer anticholinergic medications, such as atropine (packaged as ophthalmic drops but given sublingually) or hyoscyamine. Scopolamine (1 to 3 transdermal patches every 72 hours) can also be used.
7. Administer oxygen and continue this therapy if dyspnea is relieved.
8. Use nonpharmacologic interventions to relieve dyspnea, including:
   a. Circulating cool air (e.g., with an air conditioner and fan)
   b. Applying wet cloths on the patient's face
   c. Positioning the patient (head of bed elevation) to facilitate chest expansion

- Nausea and vomiting management: The dying process, pain, urinary retention and constipation, and drugs can contribute to nausea and vomiting.
  1. When constipation is the cause of nausea and vomiting, administer a biphosphate enema for immediate fecal release.
  2. Determine whether opioids or anticholinergics (new drugs or new doses) are contributing to nausea and/or vomiting, and consider stopping or decreasing the drug.
  3. Administer prescribed antiemetic drugs.
  4. Remove sources of odors and keep the room temperature at a level that the patient desires.
  5. For some patients, aromatherapy with peppermint, fennel, camphor, lavender, or rose may relieve nausea.
- Agitation and delirium management: Agitation at the end of life is common and may be caused by pain, urinary retention, constipation, or another reversible cause.
  1. Determine whether the patient is in pain and treat accordingly.
  2. Determine whether the patient is experiencing urinary retention and if so, insert a straight or Foley catheter.
  3. Treat constipation with a stimulant or bisphosphonate enema.
  4. For severe restlessness, consider haloperidol (0.5 to 2 mg orally, IV, subcutaneously, or rectally).
  5. Music therapy or aromatherapy may produce relaxation; consider patient preferences.
- Seizure management: Seizures may occur with brain tumors, advanced AIDS, and pre-existing seizure disorders.
  1. If the patient has been taking antiepileptic drugs, give drugs around the clock to maintain a high seizure threshold.
  2. Drug therapy may include benzodiazepines or barbiturates given by the oral or rectal routes.
- Psychosocial management: The personal experience of dying or of losing a loved one through death can be extremely difficult. Help the patient and family identify the desired outcomes for care in the context of terminal illness.
  1. Offer physical and emotional support by "being with" the patient.
  2. Respect cultural preferences.
  3. Be realistic.
  4. Encourage reminiscence.
  5. Promote spirituality.
  6. Foster hope by listening and caring.
  7. Assist with grief, the emotional feeling related to loss.
- Provide for the care of the patient after death.
  1. Provide all care with respect to communicate that the person was important and valued.
  2. Notify mortality services and the local organ procurement agency if this step is hospital or agency policy.

3. Ask the family or significant others if they wish to help wash the patient, comb his or her hair, or otherwise prepare the body.
   a. If no autopsy is planned, remove or cut all tubes and lines according to agency policy.
   b. Determine whether any organs will be donated after death (e.g., bone, corneas, or body for research or education).
   c. Close the patient's eyes.
   d. Insert dentures if the patient wore them.
   e. Straighten the patient and lower the bed to a flat position.
   f. Place waterproof pads under the patient's hips and around the perineum to absorb any excrement.
4. Allow the family or significant others to see the patient in private and to perform any religious or cultural customs they wish (e.g., prayer).
5. Ensure that the nurse or physician has completed and signed the death certificate.
6. Prepare the patient for transfer to either a morgue or funeral home; wrap the patient in a shroud and attach identification tags per agency policy.

PERIOPERATIVE CARE

The Joint Commission, partnered with other groups and agencies, has developed the Surgical Care Improvement Project (SCIP), a plan for the reduction and elimination of preventable surgical complications. Implementation of these core measures for patient safety is now mandatory. The measures focus on surgical complications from infection and venous thromboembolism (VTE). Perioperative care includes pre-, intra-, and postoperative management.

PREOPERATIVE MANAGEMENT

OVERVIEW
- The preoperative period begins when the patient is scheduled for surgery and ends at the time of transfer to the surgical suite.
- The primary roles of the nurse are educator, patient advocate, and promoter of health.
- *Inpatient* refers to a patient who is admitted to a hospital the day before or the day of surgery and requires hospitalization after surgery.
- *Outpatient* and *ambulatory* refer to a patient who goes to the surgical area the day of the surgery and returns home on the same day (same-day surgery [SDS]).
- The primary reasons for surgery are:
  1. Diagnostic
  2. Curative
  3. Restorative

     4. Palliative
     5. Cosmetic
- The urgency of surgery may be:
  1. Elective
  2. Urgent
  3. Emergency
- The risk of surgery may be:
  1. Minor
  2. Major
- The extent of surgery can be:
  1. Simple
  2. Radical
  3. Minimally invasive surgery (MIS)

Considerations for Older Adults

- The older adult may have a variety of health-related issues that can have an impact on the planning of care and outcome of surgery, including:
  1. Multiple comorbidities
  2. Malnutrition
  3. Endocrine dysfunction with reduced stress response
  4. High risk for cardiopulmonary complications after surgery
  5. High risk for delirium (e.g., related to unfamiliar surroundings, change in routine, drugs given, and other factors)
  6. Risk of a fall and resultant injury
  7. Dysfunction or impaired self-care abilities
  8. Inadequate support systems

PATIENT-CENTERED COLLABORATIVE CARE
Assessment

- Obtain a focused assessment.
- Take and record vital signs and report:
  1. Hypotension or hypertension
  2. Heart rate less than 60 or more than 120 beats/min
  3. Irregular heart rate
  4. Chest pain
  5. Shortness of breath or dyspnea
  6. Tachypnea
  7. Pulse oximetry reading of less than 94%
- Assess for and report any signs or symptoms of infection, including:
  1. Fever
  2. Purulent sputum

   3. Dysuria or cloudy, foul-smelling urine
   4. Red, swollen, draining wound or vascular access site
   5. Increased white blood cell count
- Assess for and report factors that could contraindicate surgery, including:
   1. Increased prothrombin time (PT), international normalized ratio (INR), or activated partial thromboplastin time (aPTT)
   2. Abnormal electrolytes, particularly hypokalemia or hyperkalemia
   3. Patient report of possible pregnancy or positive pregnancy test
- Assess for and report clinical conditions that may need to be evaluated by a provider before proceeding with the surgical plans, including:
   1. Change in mental status
   2. Vomiting
   3. Rash
   4. Recent administration of an anticoagulant drug
   5. Family or personal history of malignant hyperthermia with anesthesia
- Use a standardized list to ensure the following items are available before surgery starts:
   1. History and physical
   2. Signed, dated, and witnessed procedure consent form
   3. Nursing assessment
   4. Preanesthesia assessment
   5. Labeled diagnostic and radiology test results. Two common but not required tests are chest x-ray and electrocardiogram (ECG). Tests specific to the condition or surgical procedure (e.g., CT scan, MRI scans, abdominal films, or orthopedic films) should also be noted.
   6. Any required blood products, implants, devices, and/or special equipment for the procedure

Planning and Implementation
- Explore the patient's level of knowledge and understanding of the planned surgery by having the patient explain in his or her own words the purpose and expected results.
- Ensure informed consent is obtained from the patient (or legal designee) by the surgeon before sedation is given and before surgery is performed. *Consent* implies that the patient has sufficient information to understand:
   1. The nature of and reason for surgery
   2. Who will perform the surgery and whether others will be present during the procedure
   3. All available options and the risks associated with each option

4. The risks associated with the surgical procedure and its potential outcomes
5. The risks associated with the use of anesthesia

> **! NURSING SAFETY PRIORITY: Action Alert**
>
> If you believe that the patient has not been adequately informed, contact the surgeon and request that he or she see the patient for further clarification. Document this request in the medical record.

- A competent adult has the right to refuse treatment for any reason, even when refusal might lead to death.
- Routine preoperative care includes:
  1. Determining the existence and nature of the patient's advance directives
  2. Implementing dietary restrictions
     a. Recommendations include NPO status (no eating or drinking), typically for 6 or more hours for easily digested solid food and 2 hours for clear liquids.
     b. Failure to adhere to NPO status can result in cancellation of surgery or increase the risk for aspiration during or after surgery.
  3. Administering regularly scheduled drugs
     a. Many oral drugs are held the morning before surgery or given IV.
     b. Others, especially for cardiac disease, respiratory disease, seizures, and hypertension, are usually allowed before surgery with a sip of water.
  4. Ensuring intestinal preparation
     a. Before abdominal, bowel, or intestinal surgery, a simple enema, "enemas until clear," or mild or potent laxatives (polyethylene glycol electrolyte solution [GoLYTELY] is an example of a potent laxative) may be prescribed to empty the large intestine to reduce the potential for contamination of the surgical field.
     b. Antibiotics may be administered immediately before abdominal surgery to reduce bacterial load in the gastrointestinal tract.
  5. Performing skin preparation
     a. Confirm or assist the patient in the use of an antiseptic solution while showering and removal of oil and skin debris. This intervention reduces the number of organisms on the skin and the potential for a site infection.
     b. Remove hair at the surgical site with clippers.

6. Preparing the patient for tubes, drains, and vascular access
   a. Describe the purpose and placement of each device.
   b. Show the devices to the patient and family.
   c. Reassure the patient that these are temporary and that efforts will be made to reduce discomfort.
   d. Common devices include:
      (1) Foley catheter
      (2) Nasogastric (NG) tube
      (3) Drains (e.g., Penrose, Jackson-Pratt, Hemovac)
      (4) Vascular access
7. Teaching about postoperative interventions to prevent respiratory complications
   a. Deep diaphragmatic and expansion breathing
   b. Incentive spirometry
   c. Coughing and splinting
   d. Turning and positioning
8. Teaching about identification and prevention of cardiovascular complications
   a. Assess for venous thromboembolism (VTE) as swelling in one leg and/or presence of calf pain that worsens with ambulation.
   b. Use antiembolism stockings (TEDs or Jobst stockings), elastic (Ace) wraps, or pneumatic compression devices to prevent superficial venous stasis.
   c. Use leg exercises and early ambulation to promote venous return.
9. Minimizing anxiety
   a. Assess the patient's knowledge about the surgical experience.
   b. Allow ample time for questions.
   c. Respond to questions accurately or facilitate communication with the knowledgeable care provider.
   d. Incorporate family or supportive persons in communications.
   e. Provide prescribed antianxiety drugs.
   f. Promote rest and relaxation.
   g. Provide opportunity for distraction.

Final Preoperative Preparation

- Review the preoperative chart for:
  1. Completion of surgical informed consent form and any other special consent forms
     a. Patient's signature
     b. Date
     c. Witnesses' signatures
  2. Confirmation that the scheduled procedure is what is listed on the consent form

❗ NURSING SAFETY PRIORITY: Critical Rescue

At a minimum, the patient's identity, correct side and site, correct patient position, and agreement on the proposed procedure must be verified by all members of the surgical team.

3. Documentation of allergies
4. Accurate height and weight
5. Documentation of the results of all laboratory, radiographic, and diagnostic tests in the chart
6. Presence of autologous blood donor or directed blood donations slips (if appropriate)
7. Documentation of current vital signs, within 1 to 2 hours of the scheduled surgery time
8. Documentation of any significant physical or psychosocial observations

❗ NURSING SAFETY PRIORITY: Action Alert

Ask about a history of joint replacement, and document the exact location of any prostheses. Communicate this information to operating room personnel to ensure that electrocautery pads, which could cause an electrical burn, are not placed on or near the area of the prosthesis. Other areas to avoid electrocautery pad placement include on or near bony prominences, scar tissue, hair, tattoos, weight-bearing surfaces, pressure points, or metal piercings.

9. Communication of special needs, concerns, and instructions to the surgical team such as:
   a. Advance directives
   b. No use of blood products
   c. Presence of autologous blood products
   d. Communication difficulties (e.g., visually impaired, hearing impaired, does not speak the main language of the institution)
- Review patient preparation:
   1. Appropriate clothing removal
   2. Application of prescribed antiembolism stockings or pneumatic compression devices
   3. Storage of valuables
   4. Visible patient identification (e.g., identification band)
   5. Removal and safekeeping of dentures, dental prostheses (e.g., bridges, retainers), jewelry (including body piercing), eyeglasses, contact lenses, hearing aids, wigs, and other prostheses.

6. Removal of nail polish and artificial nails if agency policy
7. Assurance that the patient has emptied his or her bladder
8. Siderails raised immediately before transport or after giving drugs that affect cognition or judgment
9. The call system within easy reach of the patient
10. The bed in a low position except during transport

- Correctly administer prescribed preoperative drugs:
  1. Positively identify the patient (using the armband and asking the patient to state his or her name).
  2. Ensure the correct drugs in the correct dosages via the correct route at the correct time are given and documented.
- Transfer the patient to the surgical suite.

INTRAOPERATIVE MANAGEMENT

OVERVIEW

- The intraoperative period begins when the patient enters the surgical suite (operating room [OR]) and ends at the time of transfer to the postanesthesia recovery area, SDS unit, or ICU.
- Nursing priorities in the OR are safety and patient advocacy by reducing, controlling, and managing many hazards.
- Surgical team members include:
  1. The *surgeon*, a physician who assumes responsibility for the surgical procedure and any surgical judgments about the patient
  2. One or more *surgical assistants* who might be another physician (or resident or intern), an advanced practice nurse, physician assistant, certified registered nurse first assistant (CRNFA), or surgical technologist
  3. The *anesthesia provider*, who gives anesthetic drugs to induce and maintain anesthesia and delivers other drugs as needed to support the patient during surgery
     a. The *anesthesiologist*, a physician who specializes in giving anesthetic agents
     b. The *certified registered nurse anesthetist (CRNA)*, who is a registered nurse with additional education and credentials and who delivers anesthetic agents under the supervision of an anesthesiologist, surgeon, dentist, or podiatrist
  4. *Perioperative nursing staff*, who may undergo orientation for 6 to 12 months
     a. The *holding area nurse*, who coordinates and manages the care of the patient in the presurgical holding area next to the main OR. This nurse assesses the patient's physical and emotional status, gives emotional support, answers questions, and provides additional education as needed.

> ! **NURSING SAFETY PRIORITY: Action Alert**
>
> Once the patient has been moved into the holding area or the OR, do not leave him or her alone.

    b. The *circulating nurse*, who is responsible for coordinating all activities within that particular OR. He or she sets up the OR and ensures that supplies, including blood products and diagnostic support, are available as needed. This nurse positions the patient, assists the anesthesia provider, inserts a Foley catheter if needed, and scrubs the surgical site before the patient is draped with sterile drapes. In the absence of a holding area nurse, the circulating nurse also provides holding area tasks. Other responsibilities include:

       (1) Monitoring traffic in the room

       (2) Assessing the amount of urine and blood loss

       (3) Reporting findings to the surgeon and anesthesia provider

       (4) Ensuring that sterile technique and a sterile field are maintained

       (5) Communicating information about the patient's status to family members

       (6) Documenting care, events, interventions, and findings

       (7) Completing documentation in the OR and nursing records about the presence of drains or catheters, the length of the surgery, and a count of all sponges, "sharps" (needles, blades), and instruments

    c. The *scrub nurse* sets up the sterile field, drapes the patient, and hands sterile supplies, sterile equipment, and instruments to the surgeon and the assistant. This person also maintains an accurate count of sponges, sharps, instruments, and amounts of irrigation fluid and drugs used. An OR technician may also perform these tasks.

    d. The *specialty nurse* may be in charge of a particular type of surgical specialty (e.g., orthopedic, cardiac, ophthalmologic) and is responsible for nursing care specific to patients needing that type of surgery.

- Types of anesthesia and complications
  1. *General anesthesia* is a reversible loss of consciousness induced by inhibiting neuronal impulses in several areas of the central nervous system (CNS). The patient is unconscious

and unaware and has loss of muscle tone and reflexes. Agents are administered by inhalation and IV injection.

   a. Complications include malignant hyperthermia (MH), an acute, life-threatening complication of certain drugs in which skeletal muscle exposed to specific agents increases calcium levels and metabolism leading to acidosis, cardiac dysrhythmias, and a high body temperature.

      (1) MH is a genetic disorder with an autosomal dominant pattern of inheritance and is most common in young, well-muscled men.

      (2) Drugs most associated with MH are halothane, enflurane, isoflurane, desflurane, sevoflurane, and succinylcholine.

      (3) When MH occurs, the treatment is intravenous dantrolene.

   b. An overdose of anesthesia can occur when the patient's metabolism and elimination are slower than expected, such as an older adult or one with liver or kidney dysfunction.

   c. Unrecognized hypoventilation with failure to exchange gases adequately can lead to cardiac arrest, permanent brain damage, and death.

   d. Intubation complications from improper neck extension or anatomic differences in a patient can lead to broken or injured teeth and caps, swollen lips, or vocal cord trauma.

   e. Hemodynamic instability from medications, fluid loss, or dysrhythmias can contribute to brain or other organ damage.

2. *Local or regional anesthesia* disrupts sensory nerve impulse transmission from a specific body area or region. The patient remains conscious and able to follow instructions.

   a. Local anesthesia is delivered topically (applied to the skin or mucous membranes of the area to be anesthetized) and by local infiltration.

   b. Regional anesthesia is a type of local anesthesia that blocks multiple peripheral nerves in a specific body region. Regional anesthesia includes field block or nerve block and spinal or epidural routes of delivery.

   c. Complications are associated with overdoses, inadvertent systemic drug delivery, or patient allergic reactions to the agent.

3. *Conscious sedation* is the IV delivery of sedative and opioid drugs to reduce the level of consciousness but allow the patient to maintain a patent airway and to respond to verbal commands. It is used most often in the emergency department or in procedure rooms before short but uncomfortable procedures.

PATIENT-CENTERED COLLABORATIVE CARE
Assessment
- Correct identification of the patient is the responsibility of every member of the health care team.
  1. Verify the patient's identity with two types of identifiers (e.g., name, birth date, medical record number, Social Security number) using the patient's identification bracelet.
     a. Ask the patient, "What is your name?" and "What is your birth date?"
  2. Validate that the surgical consent form has been signed and witnessed.
     a. Ask the patient, "What kind of operation are you having today?"
     b. Compare patient responses to the information on the operative permit and the operative schedule.
     c. When the procedure involves a specific site, validate the side on which a procedure is to be performed.
     d. Investigate any discrepancy and notify the surgeon.
- Validate that all aspects of the checklist are complete.
  1. Ask the patient about any allergies.
  2. Determine whether autologous blood was donated.
  3. Check the patient's attire to ensure adherence with facility policy.
  4. Ensure that all prostheses have been removed, including dentures, dental bridges or retainers, jewelry, contact lenses, and wigs.
- Review the medical record for:
  1. Advance directives (be prepared to implement do-not-resuscitate orders)
  2. Allergies or adverse reactions to anesthesia, blood transfusion, iodine, drugs, and latex
  3. Laboratory and diagnostic test results
  4. Medical history and physical examination findings

QSEN SAFETY

Correct identification of the patient is the responsibility of every member of the health care team to avoid mistakes in surgery. Make sure that a least two ways are used to identify the patient.

Planning and Implementation
- Ensure proper positioning and prevent injury or pressure ulcer formation by:
  1. Padding the operating bed with foam or silicone gel pads, or both

2. Properly placing the grounding pads
3. Assisting the patient to a comfortable position
4. Assessing the skin for pre-existing conditions and applying protective measures such as DuoDERM, Tegaderm, or other skin protective product
5. Modifying the patient's position according to the patient's safety and special needs
6. Avoiding excessive joint abduction
7. Securing the arms firmly on an armboard, positioned at shoulder level
8. Supporting the wrist with padding and not overtightening wrist straps
9. Placing safety straps above or below the nerve locations
10. Maintaining minimal external rotation of the hips
11. Supporting the lower extremities
12. Not placing equipment on lower extremities
13. Urging OR personnel to avoid leaning on the patient's lower extremities
14. Maintaining the patient's extremities in good anatomic alignment by slightly flexing joints and supporting the patient with pillows, trochanter rolls, or pads

- Observe for complications of special positioning, such as wrist-drop or footdrop, loss of sensation, changes in extremity temperature or circulation, and inflammation.

QSEN EVIDENCE-BASED PRACTICE

Aseptic technique must be strictly practiced by all OR personnel to ensure that the patient is free from infection.

- Reduce risk for infection by:
  1. Identifying patients with pre-existing health problems such as diabetes mellitus, immunodeficiency, obesity, and renal failure
  2. Performing prescribed skin preparation
  3. Protecting the patient's exposure to cross-contamination
  4. Ensuring the use of sterile surgical technique, protective drapes, skin closures, and dressings
  5. Administering preoperative antibiotics within 30 to 60 minutes of the first incision
- Prevent complications from hypoventilation, hemodynamic instability, and hypothermia by:
  1. Continuously monitoring the patient according to established standards, including:
     a. Breathing
     b. Circulation

    c. Cardiac rhythm
    d. Blood pressure
    e. Heart rate
    f. Oxygen saturation

! NURSING SAFETY PRIORITY: Critical Rescue

Monitor patients for the cluster of elevated end-tidal carbon dioxide level, decreased oxygen saturation, and tachycardia related to malignant hyperthermia. If these changes begin, alert the surgeon and anesthesia provider immediately.

2. Evaluating core body temperature by:
    a. Maintaining core temperature at 95° to 98.6° F (35° to 37° C)
    b. Determining the safe use of warming devices to effectively support normothermia

POSTOPERATIVE MANAGEMENT

OVERVIEW

- Postoperative care begins at the completion of surgery and transfer of the patient to the postanesthesia care unit (PACU) or other area for specialized monitoring and continues until all activity restrictions have been lifted. The purpose of a PACU (recovery room) is the ongoing direct evaluation and stabilization of patients to anticipate, prevent, and manage complications after surgery.
- Postoperative and postanesthesia care is divided into three phases that are based on the level of care needed, not the physical setting. Not every patient will need all three phases:
  1. Phase 1 includes close monitoring of airway, vital signs, and indicators of recovery every 5 to 15 minutes. This phase typically lasts 1 to 2 hours.
     a. Discharge from the postoperative unit is based on the presence of a recovery score rating of at least 9 to 10 on an established recovery scale.
     b. Indicators of readiness for transition to Phase 2 management are a return of preprocedure level of consciousness and cognition, maintenance of baseline oxygen saturation, and stable vital signs.
  2. Phase 2 focuses on preparing the patient for care in another setting such as an acute care unit, ICU, skilled nursing facility, or home.
  3. Phase 3 occurs in the extended care environment (e.g., hospital or residence) with assisted and self-management.
- On arrival to the postoperative care unit, the anesthesia provider and the circulating nurse give the receiving nurse and provider a

verbal hand-off report to communicate the patient's condition and care needs.

QSEN TEAMWORK AND COLLABORATION

A hand-off report requires effective communication between health care professionals, so that the right information is given on time. The language used by the report giver is clear and cannot be interpreted in more than one way. Report critical results from laboratory and diagnostic tests in an urgent time frame (usually within 15 to 30 minutes). Accurately and completely reconcile medications, including short-term medications that will not be continued at discharge from the perioperative area.

- The hand-off report should contain the following information:
  1. Type and extent of the surgical procedure
  2. Type of anesthesia and length of time the patient was under anesthesia
  3. Tolerance of anesthesia and the surgical procedure
  4. Allergies
  5. Pertinent medical history, including condition/diagnosis requiring surgery and substance abuse
  6. Current and trend vital signs including oxygen saturation and core temperature
  7. Intake and output, including current IV fluid administration and estimated blood loss
  8. Any intraoperative complications, such as a traumatic intubation
  9. Drug reconciliation, specifying one-time and ongoing drugs
  10. Primary language, any sensory impairments, any communication difficulties
  11. Functional, cognitive, and anxiety levels before surgery
  12. Communication barriers and special concerns identified preoperatively
  13. Preoperative and intraoperative respiratory function and dysfunction
  14. Location and type of incisions, dressings, catheters, tubes, drains, or packing
  15. Prosthetic devices
  16. Joint or limb positioning or immobility while in the OR, especially in the older patient
  17. Intraoperative occurrences or complications, how managed, patient responses

PATIENT-CENTERED COLLABORATIVE CARE
Assessment

- The initial assessment of the patient immediately after surgery includes the level of consciousness, temperature, pulse, respiration, oxygen saturation, and blood pressure.
- Examine the surgical area for bleeding and drainage.
- Assess vital signs (VS) on admission and then follow agency protocol for frequency. Changes in heart rate, blood pressure, respiratory rate, or peripheral oxygenation (oximetry, Spo_2) that are concerning need to be communicated urgently to the provider or rapid response team. Increase the frequency of VS assessment whenever VS increase or decrease, particularly when there is clinical concern around maintaining a narrow range of values. High or low values in VS can be early indicators of adverse reaction to operative drugs, blood or volume loss, and postoperative complications including myocardial infarction or stroke.
- Routine postoperative monitoring and assessment includes:
  1. Respiratory status
     a. Evaluating airway patency and adequacy of gas exchange by oxygen saturation, end-tidal carbon dioxide levels, respiratory rate, pattern, and effort
     b. Ensuring security and placement (e.g., depth) of an artificial airway (endotracheal tube, nasal trumpet, oral airway)
     c. Maintaining type of oxygen delivery device and the concentration of oxygen delivered

! NURSING SAFETY PRIORITY: Critical Rescue

Respiratory assessment is the most critical assessment to perform after surgery for any patient who has undergone general anesthesia, moderate sedation, or has received sedative or opioid drugs. If the Spo_2 drops below the level of 95% or the patient's baseline, notify the surgeon or anesthesia provider. If it drops by 10 percentage points, call the Rapid Response Team.

     d. Auscultating lung fields for breath sounds
     e. Examining the degree of symmetry of breath sounds and chest movement
     f. Determining the presence of snoring and stridor
     g. Checking skeletal muscle weakness:
        (1) Inability to maintain a head lift
        (2) Weak hand grasps
        (3) Abdominal breathing pattern

2. Cardiovascular status
   a. Evaluating heart rate, quality, and rhythm
   b. Trending blood pressure values

! NURSING SAFETY PRIORITY: Critical Rescue

Report blood pressures below 110/50 mm Hg or changes that are 25% higher or lower than baseline values or values that do not meet the goals described by the surgeon or anesthesia provider immediately to the provider.

---

   c. Monitoring electrocardiography for dysrhythmias
   d. Comparing distal pulses, color, temperature, and capillary refill on extremities
   e. Examining feet and legs for manifestations of deep vein thrombosis (DVT) (e.g., redness, pain, warmth, swelling)
   f. Maintaining prescribed compression devices or antiembolic stockings applied in the preoperative or operative suite
3. Neurologic status
   a. Trending level of consciousness or awareness:
      (1) Presence of lethargy, restlessness, or irritability
      (2) Patient responses to stimuli (calling the patient's name, touching the patient, and giving simple commands such as "Open your eyes" and "Take a deep breath")
      (3) Degree of orientation to person, place, and time by asking the conscious patient "What is your name?" (person), "Where are you?" (place), and "What day is it?" (time)
   b. Comparing the patient's baseline preoperative neurologic status with postoperative findings
4. Motor and sensory function status
   a. Asking the patient to move each extremity
   b. Assessing the strength of each limb and comparing the results on both sides
   c. Gradually elevating the patient's head and monitoring for hypotension
5. Fluid, electrolyte, and acid-base balance
   a. Measuring intake and output (including IV fluid intake, emesis, urine, wound drainage, nasogastric tube drainage)
   b. Checking hydration status (e.g., inspecting the color and moisture of mucous membranes; the turgor, texture, and tenting of the skin; the amount of drainage on dressings; and the presence of axillary sweat)

    c. Comparing total output with total intake to identify a possible fluid imbalance

6. Kidney and urinary status
   a. Measuring intake and output
   b. Assessing for urine retention by inspection, palpation, percussion of the lower abdomen for bladder distension, or use of a bladder scanner
   c. Performing prescribed intermittent catheterization
   d. Assessing urine for color, clarity, and amount

> **❗ NURSING SAFETY PRIORITY: Critical Rescue**
>
> Report a urine output of less than 0.5 mL/kg/hr for 2 or more hours or 0.3mL/kg/hr for 6 or more hours to the surgeon.

7. GI status
   a. Listening for bowel sounds in all four abdominal quadrants and at the umbilicus
   b. Assessing for nausea and vomiting
   c. Administering prescribed antiemetic drugs
   d. Assessing for manifestations of paralytic ileus (few or absent bowel sounds, distended abdomen, abdominal discomfort, vomiting, and no passage of flatus or stool)
   e. Assessing and recording the color, consistency, and amount of the NG tube drainage
   f. Checking NG tube placement

> **❗ NURSING SAFETY PRIORITY: Action Alert**
>
> After gastric surgery, do not move or irrigate the tube without an order from the surgeon.

8. Skin status
   a. Assessing the incision (if visible) for redness, increased warmth, swelling, tenderness or pain, and the type and amount of drainage; be sure to look under the patient for pooling of collection of drainage and blood
   b. Condition of the sutures or staples
   c. Presence of open areas

9. Dressings and drains
   a. Documenting color, amount, consistency, and odor of drainage
   b. Examining for leakage around or under the patient
   c. Determining patency of drains
   d. Performing neurovascular checks to identify restriction of circulation or sensation

10. Pain
    a. Pain usually reaches its peak on the second day after surgery, when the patient is active and the intraoperative anesthetic agents and drugs have been eliminated
    b. Follow best practices for surgical pain management described below
11. Psychosocial issues of anxiety or fear

Planning and Implementation

- Airway management in the PACU or ICU may include:
    1. Monitoring for snoring or stridor, which indicate obstruction
    2. Inserting an oral airway or a nasal airway (nasal trumpet) to keep the airway open
    3. Keeping the manual resuscitation bag and emergency equipment for intubation or tracheostomy nearby
    4. Positioning the patient in a side-lying or elevated back rest position to prevent aspiration
    5. Suctioning the mouth, nose, and throat to keep the airway clear of mucus or vomitus as needed
    6. Applying prescribed oxygen by face tent, nasal cannula, or mask
    7. Assisting the patient to cough (with the incision splinted), breathe deeply, and use the incentive spirometer
    8. Performing mouth care after removing secretions
- Interventions for inpatients after PACU care may include:
    1. Encouraging the patient to continue deep breathing and incentive spirometry exercises
    2. Assisting the patient to reposition himself or herself every 2 hours and to ambulate as soon as possible
    3. Offering prescribed pain medication 30 to 45 minutes before the patient gets out of bed

Nonsurgical Skin Management

- Wound care includes reinforcing the dressing, changing the dressing, assessing the wound for healing and infection, and caring for drains, including emptying, measuring, and documenting drainage features.
    1. The surgeon often changes the initial dressing.
        a. Reinforce the dressing (add more dressing material to the existing dressing) if it becomes wet from drainage.
        b. Document the added material and the color, type, amount, and odor of drainage fluid and time of observation.
    2. Routine wound care and dressing changes include:
        a. Changing gauze dressings at least once during a nursing shift or daily
        b. Cleaning the area with sterile saline or some other solution as prescribed
        c. Assessing the skin in areas where tape has been used for redness, rash, or blisters

    d. Assessing the incision for integrity, condition, and healing stage

    e. Assessing the incision for wound infection:
      (1) Redness, heat, and swelling
      (2) Drainage of purulent or foul-smelling material

    f. Removing sutures or staples according to agency policy and surgeon request

    g. Removing or advancing drains according to agency policy and surgeon request

    h. Administering prescribed antibiotic therapy

Surgical Management

- Management of *dehiscence*, which is opening all or part of a wound down to the visceral peritoneum:
  1. Apply a sterile nonadherent (e.g., Telfa) or saline dressing to the wound and notify the surgeon.
  2. Instruct the patient to bend the knees and to avoid coughing.
  3. The surgeon may reclose the wound or leave it open to heal by second intention.

- Management of *evisceration*, which is a wound opening with protrusion of internal organs. *This condition is a surgical emergency.*
  1. *Call for help.* Instruct the person who responds to notify the surgeon or Rapid Response Team immediately and to bring any needed supplies into the patient's room.
  2. Stay with the patient.
  3. Cover the wound with a nonadherent dressing premoistened with warmed, sterile normal saline.
  4. If premoistened dressings are not available, moisten sterile gauze or sterile towels in a sterile irrigation tray with sterile saline, and then cover the wound.
  5. If saline is not immediately available, cover the wound with gauze and then moisten with sterile saline using a sterile irrigation tray as soon as someone brings saline.
  6. Do not attempt to reinsert the protruding organ or viscera.
  7. While covering the wound, observe the patient's response and assess for manifestations of shock.
  8. Place the patient in a supine position with the hips and knees bent.
  9. Raise the head of the bed 15 to 20 degrees.
  10. Take vital signs and document them.
  11. Provide support and reassurance to the patient.
  12. Continue assessing the patient, including assessment of vital signs, every 5 to 10 minutes until the surgeon arrives.
  13. Keep dressings continuously moist by adding warmed sterile saline to the dressing as often as necessary. *Do not let the dressing become dry.*

14. When the surgeon arrives, report your finding and your interventions. Then follow the surgeon's directions.
15. Document the incident, the activity the patient was engaged in at the time of the incident, your actions, and your assessments.
16. The surgeon performs surgery in the OR with the patient under general, regional, or local anesthesia to close the wound. Stay or retention sutures of wire or nylon are usually used in addition to or instead of standard sutures or staples.

Management of Surgical Pain
- Opioids and non-opioids are typically given in the early postoperative period.
- Drugs are given IV initially and then are administered orally.
- Around-the-clock scheduling is more effective than on-demand scheduling because more constant blood levels are achieved.
- PCA by IV infusion or internal pump (the catheter is sutured into or near the surgical area) may be used.
- Epidural analgesia can be given intermittently by the anesthesia provider or by continuous drip through an epidural catheter left in place after epidural anesthesia.

See the "Pain" section in Part One for pain assessment and management.

Prevent Hypoxemia
- The highest incidence of hypoxemia after surgery occurs on the second postoperative day. Those at highest risk are older adults and patients with lung disease.
- Monitor the patient's oxygen saturation (Spo_2) with pulse oximetry.
- Apply prescribed oxygen as needed.
- Prevent hypothermia.
- Implement a respiratory therapy assessor protocol to determine the need for respiratory treatments. Position the patient with the head of the bed elevated at 30 to 45 degrees unless contraindicated.
- Implement early progressive mobility within 6 to 48 hours of surgery.

Community-Based Care
- Discharge planning, teaching, and referral begin before surgery and continue after surgery.
- Provide written discharge instructions for the patient to follow at home.
- Assess the need for assistance with wound care and activities of daily living (ADLs).
- The teaching plan for the patient and family after surgery includes:
  1. Prevention of infection
  2. Care and assessment of the surgical wound

3. Management of drains or catheters
4. Nutrition therapy
5. Pain management
6. Antibiotic or surgery-specific drug therapy
7. Progressive increase in activity
8. Follow-up with the surgeon

! **NURSING SAFETY PRIORITY: Action Alert**

Always ensure that the patient and family receive written dis-charge instructions to follow at home. Assess the understand-ing of the patient and family by having them explain the instructions in their own words.

- Ensure that appropriate referrals are made to a case manager, social worker, home care agency, or other community resources.

PLANNING FOR DISCHARGE

- Discharge planning is an example of care coordination. It is a patient-centered, interdisciplinary approach that provides conti-nuity of care across setting. Success in care coordination includes assessment of patient needs, preferences, and values and sharing information across people, functions, and sites. Ultimately, care coordination for discharge has goals of promoting health and independence for each patient.
- Information to ask the patient to assist with discharge planning:
  1. Where do you live?
  2. How will you get home?
  3. Can you describe your home?
  4. How many stairs must you climb to get into your house?
  5. Are your bedroom, bathroom, laundry, and kitchen on the same floor, or will you need to use steps?
  6. Do you live alone, or does someone live with you?
      a. Who lives with you? Will they need help with caregiving?
      b. Will the person be able to help you after your discharge?
      c. Is there a neighbor or church member who can help you after you are discharged?
      d. Is anyone available to help you with grocery shopping, laundry, or driving to doctors' appointments?
- Collaborate with physician(s), physical therapist, occupational therapist, speech therapist, dietitian, pharmacist, stoma/skin care specialist, diabetic educator, social worker, case manager, or dis-charge planner to identify the patient's needs related to care after hospitalization, including education, meal preparation, support

to complete activities of daily living and personal hygiene, wound care, acquisition of durable medical goods, supplies, and prescriptive drugs.

- Provide written and verbal information about referrals for housing, finances, insurance, legal services, funeral arrangements, and spiritual counseling if they are part of the discharge plan.

QSEN INFORMATICS

Correct information about patient medications is essential so that correct administration of drugs occurs. Accurately and completely reconcile drugs that the patient will take at home following discharge. Ensure both *new* and *established* drug regimens are clear. Emphasize the importance of prescribed drugs and regimens. Provide an up-to-date list of medications and document communication of this list to the patient or family. Ensure that this list is accessible to the health care provider(s) who will provide follow-up care. Remind the patient or family members to call the primary care provider to report side effects or challenges to drug adherence.

- Provide patient and family education:
  1. Provide spoken and written information about the disease process, how to recognize complications (if appropriate), and how to manage the disease at home.
  2. Provide spoken and written information to reinforce the need to contact the primary care provider for ongoing care, and to schedule and attend follow-up care. Include contact information (e.g., phone number for appointments, clinic name, and specialty provider name).
  3. Teach the patient about drugs:
     a. Names of drugs
     b. Purpose of drugs
     c. Dosage
     d. Side effects
     e. Interactions, if any, with foods or other drugs
     f. Importance of taking drugs as prescribed
     g. Schedule follow-up labs and ensure skills and supplies are in place for checking blood sugar as prescribed at home; instruct the patient to report any abnormal values and trends to the primary care provider
     h. Provide and help the patient evaluate reliable sources of information and to avoid altering or stopping prescribed treatment without informing the primary care provider

QSEN INFORMATICS

Drugs used for anticoagulation are associated with significant harm if patient responses are not regularly monitored and patient compliance is suboptimal. Provide specific education regarding anticoagulant therapy to patients and families. At discharge, give written information about the following:
- The importance of follow-up monitoring
- The dose and frequency of the drug(s)
- Drug-food interactions
- The potential for adverse drug reactions and interactions

4. Teach the patient about the use of supplies or equipment prescribed for use after discharge, such as dressing changes, suctioning, tube feeding, or other special care that may be required at home.
5. Explain signs and symptoms of adverse drug events that should be reported to the health care provider and the urgency with which bleeding and clotting signs and symptoms should be reported.
- Use established guidelines and teaching tools from reliable sources to reinforce teaching.
- Use institutional forms and policies to document discharge instructions and obtain the patient's or a family member's signature to acknowledge receipt of written instructions for the patient record.

PART TWO

Diseases and Disorders

ABSCESS

An abscess is an enclosed collection of pus. Swelling, erythema, and pain are common symptoms. This local infection is surrounded by inflamed tissue and can occur in a variety of sites. Almost all abscesses require an intervention of systemic antibiotics.

- An anorectal abscess results from obstruction of the ducts of glands in the anorectal region by feces, foreign bodies, or trauma.
  1. The diagnosis is made by physical examination and history with rectal pain as a common initial symptom.
  2. Most perianal and ischiorectal abscesses can be excised and drained with local anesthesia; more extensive abscesses require incision using regional or general anesthesia.
  3. Interventions include assisting the patient to maintain comfort and optimal perineal hygiene by providing warm sitz baths and analgesics, and encouraging the patient to avoid constipation through use of bulk-forming agents, osmotic laxatives, or stool softeners.
- A brain abscess occurs as encapsulated pus in the extradural, subdural, or intracerebral area and most commonly in frontal or temporal lobes.
  1. A brain abscess is more likely to occur in patients with immunosuppression.
  2. The causative organisms are most often bacteria, such as *Streptococcus* and *Staphylococcus.*
  3. A brain abscess typically manifests with symptoms of a mass and of mildly increased intracranial pressure, including:
     a. Headache
     b. Fever
     c. Focal neurologic deficits
     d. Lethargy and confusion
     e. Visual field deficits
     f. Nystagmus and disconjugate gaze
     g. Generalized weakness, hemiparesis
     h. Ataxic gait
     i. Seizures

      j. Various degrees of aphasia with a frontal or temporal lobe abscess

      k. Elevated white blood cell (WBC) count

  4. Interventions include:

      a. Antibiotics, typically administered IV or intrathecally

      b. Antiepileptic drugs, as ordered, to prevent or treat seizures

      c. Analgesics, as ordered, to treat the patient's headache

      d. Surgical drainage of an encapsulated abscess, or an exploratory craniotomy may be performed

- Hepatic (liver) abscess formation is a result of invasion of the liver by bacteria or protozoa. While liver abscess is uncommon, it is associated with a high mortality.

  1. Abscesses can result from acute cholangitis, liver trauma, peritonitis, or sepsis; or an abscess can extend to the liver after pneumonia or bacterial endocarditis.

  2. Pyrogenic abscesses are caused by bacteria such as *Escherichia coli, Klebsiella, Enterobacter, Salmonella, Staphylococcus,* and *Enterococcus.*

  3. Amebic hepatic abscesses occur after amebic dysentery as a single abscess in the right upper quadrant of the liver.

  4. Assessment findings include:

      a. Right upper quadrant abdominal pain with a tender, palpable liver

      b. Anorexia

      c. Weight loss

      d. Nausea and vomiting

      e. Fever and chills

      f. Shoulder pain

      g. Dyspnea

      h. Pleural pain if the diaphragm is involved

      i. Jaundice

  5. Hepatic abscesses are usually diagnosed by contrast-enhanced computed tomography (CT) or ultrasound.

  6. Surgical drainage is usually required.

- A lung abscess is a localized area of subacute infection and necrosis that is usually related to pyogenic bacteria.

  1. Common causes are tuberculosis, fungal infections of the lung, pneumonia, aspiration of mouth or stomach contents, and obstruction as a result of a tumor or foreign body.

  2. A lung abscess also can be caused by dysphagia and aspiration, such as occurs with alcoholic blackouts, seizure disorders, other neurologic deficits, and swallowing disorders.

  3. Assessment findings include:

      a. Recent history of pulmonary infection

      b. Fever, fatigue, and unplanned weight loss

      c. Cough and foul-smelling sputum

    d. Decreased breath sounds on affected side, crackles
    e. Pleuritic pain
    f. Abnormal chest x-ray
  4. Nursing diagnoses and interventions are similar to those for pneumonia.
  5. Management includes percutaneous drainage of the abscess and antibiotic therapy.
- Pancreatic abscess consists of infected, necrotic pancreatic tissue and may follow acute necrotizing pancreatitis.
  1. Antibiotic therapy alone does not resolve the infection; drainage via percutaneous or laparoscopic approaches is performed soon after diagnosis to prevent sepsis and multiple drainage procedures may be necessary.
  2. Temperature spikes may be as high as 104°F (40°C).
  3. Insulin-secreting beta cells may be destroyed with infection, leading to hyperglycemia.
  4. Pleural effusions can accompany pancreatic abscess.
- Peritonsillar abscess (PTA), or *quinsy,* is a complication of acute tonsillitis. The infection spreads from the tonsil to the surrounding tissue, forming an abscess.
  1. The most common cause is infection with group A beta-hemolytic streptococci.
  2. Signs of infection are pronounced on examination. Pus forms behind the tonsil and causes one-sided swelling with deviation of the uvula toward the unaffected side. The swelling causes drooling, severe throat pain radiating to the ear, a voice change, and difficulty swallowing.

❗ NURSING SAFETY PRIORITY: Critical Rescue

Check the patient for airway obstruction, which may occur from swelling. If obstruction is present, notify the Rapid Response Team.

  3. Management includes:
    a. Percutaneous needle aspiration to drain and culture the abscess
    b. Antibiotics
    c. Analgesics
    d. Intravenous corticosteroid to reduce swelling if the airway is compromised
    e. Tonsillectomy after the abscess has healed
- Renal abscess is a collection of fluid and cells resulting from an inflammatory response to bacteria in the renal parenchyma, renal fascia, or flank. Symptoms include:
  1. Fever unresponsive to antibiotic therapy with an established kidney infection

2. Flank pain
3. General malaise
4. Local edema
5. Treatment includes:
   a. Broad-spectrum antibiotics
   b. Drainage by surgical incision or needle aspiration

ACIDOSIS, METABOLIC

OVERVIEW

- Acidosis is not a disease; it is a condition caused by a metabolic problem, a respiratory problem, or both.
- Four processes can result in metabolic acidosis: overproduction of hydrogen ions, underelimination of hydrogen ions, underproduction of bicarbonate ions, and overelimination of bicarbonate ions.
- It is reflected by the following arterial blood gas (ABG) values: pH below 7.35 and bicarbonate (HCO_3^-) values below the normal range (below 22 mEq/L [mmol/L]).
- Metabolic acidosis often is accompanied by potassium excess (hyperkalemia).
- Common causes of metabolic acidosis include:
  1. Conditions that overproduce hydrogen ions:
     a. Diabetic ketoacidosis
     b. Fever
     c. Heavy exercise
     d. Hypoxia, anoxia, or ischemia as a result of lactic acid production (anaerobic metabolism)
     e. Starvation, carbohydrate-free diets
     f. Aspirin or other salicylate intoxication
     g. Ethanol, methanol, or ethylene glycol intoxication
  2. Conditions that cause underelimination of hydrogen ions (renal failure)
  3. Conditions that underproduce bicarbonate ions (liver failure, pancreatitis, or dehydration)
  4. Conditions that overeliminate bicarbonate (diarrhea)

PATIENT-CENTERED COLLABORATIVE CARE

Assessment

- Assessment findings include:
  1. Central nervous system (CNS) changes
     a. Decreased mentation (confusion, lethargy, stupor, and coma)
  2. Neuromuscular changes
     a. Hyporeflexia
     b. Skeletal muscle weakness leading to flaccid paralysis

  3. Cardiovascular changes
     a. Delayed electrical conduction (bradycardia and heart block), manifested by prolonged PR interval and widened QRS complex
     b. Tall T waves
     c. Hypotension
     d. Thready peripheral pulses
  4. Respiratory changes
     a. Increased respiratory rate
     b. Kussmaul pattern of respirations (greatly increased rate and depth of ventilation)
  5. Skin changes
     a. Warm, flushed

Interventions
- Management focuses on:
  1. Correcting the underlying cause of metabolic acidosis
  2. Administering IV fluids and maintaining IV access
  3. Monitoring ABG and serum potassium results and reporting critical values within 30 minutes to physician or prescribing health care provider
  4. Evaluating rate, rhythm, intervals and other components of the electrocardiogram (ECG)
  5. Evaluating the balance of fluid intake and output and reporting significant imbalances (a difference greater than 500 to 1000 mL) over an 8-hour shift

ACIDOSIS, RESPIRATORY

OVERVIEW
- Acidosis is not a disease; it is a condition caused by a metabolic problem, a respiratory problem, or both.
- Respiratory acidosis results when respiratory function is impaired, leading to CO_2 retention.
- Respiratory acidosis results from only one mechanism: retention of CO_2, causing increased production of free hydrogen ions. It is always an *acid excess* acidosis.
- It can be an acute condition or a chronic condition.
- Acute respiratory acidosis is reflected by ABG values indicating a pH below 7.35, normal HCO_3^-, and high PCO_2 values above 45 mm Hg.
- Chronic respiratory acidosis is reflected by ABG values indicating a pH below 7.35, high HCO_3^- above 28 mm Hg, and high PCO_2 above 45 mm Hg.
- Common causes of respiratory acidosis include:
  1. Respiratory depression
     a. Anesthetics
     b. Drugs (especially opioids and benzodiazepines)

    c. Brain injury
    d. Electrolyte imbalance
  2. Reduced alveolar-capillary diffusion
    a. Disease (emphysema, pneumonia, tuberculosis, fibrosis, or cancer)
    b. Pulmonary edema
    c. Atelectasis
    d. Pulmonary emboli
    e. Chest trauma
  3. Airway obstruction
    a. Foreign object in airway
    b. Disease (asthma, epiglottitis)
    c. Strangulation
    d. Regional lymph node enlargement
  4. Inadequate chest expansion
    a. Skeletal deformities (kyphosis, scoliosis), trauma (flail chest, broken ribs), spinal cord injury
    b. Hemothorax or pneumothorax
    c. Respiratory muscle weakness
    d. Obesity
    e. Abdominal or thoracic masses
    f. Ascites

Considerations for Older Adults

- The older adult is at higher risk for respiratory acidosis in the presence of comorbidities of cardiac, respiratory, and kidney disease.
- The older adult is more likely to be taking drugs that interfere with acid-base balance, such as diuretics, nonsteroidal anti-inflammatories, laxatives, and antihypertensives.

PATIENT-CENTERED COLLABORATIVE CARE
Assessment
- Assessment findings include:
  1. CNS changes
    a. Decreased mentation (confusion, lethargy, stupor, and coma)
  2. Neuromuscular changes
    a. Hyporeflexia
    b. Skeletal muscle weakness leading to flaccid paralysis
  3. Cardiovascular changes
    a. Delayed electrical conduction (bradycardia or heart block manifested by prolonged PR interval or widened QRS complex)

       b. Tall T waves
       c. Hypotension
       d. Thready peripheral pulses
   4. Respiratory changes
       a. Rapid, shallow respirations
       b. Diminished respiratory effort
       c. Concurrent hypoxemia
   5. Skin changes
       a. Cool, pale to cyanotic

Interventions

- Management focuses on:
   1. Ensuring adequate oxygenation:
       a. Assessing the airway and breathing effectiveness
       b. Administering oxygen as prescribed
       c. Positioning to provide maximal lung excursion, usually with a back rest elevation greater than 60 degrees
   2. Administering inhaled bronchodilator drugs to improve ventilation and gas exchange, such as albuterol (Proventil, Ventolin), ipratropium (Atrovent, Apo-Ipravent ✿), theophylline (e.g., Elixophyllin, Theo-Dur, Uniphyl, Theolair)
   3. Administering corticosteroids (also called glucocorticoids) to reduce inflammation; these drugs may be administered intravenously for fastest action, orally, or when the condition is no longer acute, as an inhaled agent to prevent future exacerbation.
   4. Monitoring respiratory status at least every 2 hours for response to therapy or worsening of breathing effectiveness
       a. Respiratory rate and depth
       b. Oxygen saturation (Spo_2) and ABG values to maintain a normal range of oxygenation (Spo_2 greater than 90% to 92% and partial pressure of arterial oxygen [Pao_2] greater than 90 mm Hg)
       c. Effort of breathing, including use of accessory muscles
       d. Breath sounds
       e. Color of nail beds and mucous membranes
       f. Level of consciousness and mentation
       g. Fraction of inspired oxygen (Fio_2) with oxygen delivery system or ventilator settings

❗ NURSING SAFETY PRIORITY: Critical Rescue

Assess the cardiovascular system first in any patient at risk for acidosis because acidosis can lead to cardiac arrest from the accompanying hyperkalemia.

ACUTE CORONARY SYNDROMES

- The term *acute coronary syndrome* (ACS) is used to describe patients who have either unstable angina or an acute myocardial infarction (MI).
- *Unstable angina* is chest pain or discomfort that occurs at rest or with exertion and causes severe activity limitation.
- MI occurs when myocardial tissue is abruptly and severely deprived of oxygen. When blood flow is quickly reduced by 80% to 90%, ischemia can lead to injury and necrosis of myocardial tissue if blood flow is not restored.
- In ACS, atherosclerotic plaque in the coronary artery ruptures, resulting in platelet aggregation ("clumping"), thrombus (clot) formation, and vasoconstriction.
- For more information about assessment and management, go to "Coronary Artery Disease."

ACUTE RESPIRATORY DISTRESS SYNDROME/ACUTE LUNG INJURY
OVERVIEW

- Acute respiratory distress syndrome (ARDS) is a lung condition with the following features:
  1. Hypoxemia that persists even when 100% oxygen is given
  2. Decreased pulmonary compliance
  3. Dyspnea
  4. Noncardiac-associated bilateral pulmonary edema
  5. Dense pulmonary infiltrates on x-ray (ground-glass appearance)
- ARDS can occur from both pulmonary and nonpulmonary causes such as sepsis, pneumonia, pulmonary embolism, shock, aspiration, acute pancreatitis, or inhalation injury.
- An inflammatory response injures the alveolar-capillary membrane, causing protein-containing fluid to leak into alveoli. Fluid-filled alveoli cannot exchange oxygen and carbon dioxide.
- Fluid also leaks into the spaces between alveoli (interstitial edema), further compressing alveoli and reducing the capacity to exchange gases.
- ARDS also results in damage to the alveoli and respiratory bronchioles. Alveolar surfactant production is reduced, making the alveoli unstable and at risk for collapse, even when they are not filled with fluid.
- Lung volume and compliance are dramatically reduced with alveoli damage resulting in long-term consequences of prolonged illness and recovery.

⬛ Genetic/Genomic Considerations

An increased genetic risk is suspected in the development and progression of ARDS. Variations in the genes responsible for surfactant production appear to increase the predisposition to developing ARDS as does variation in the genes responsible for cytokine production during inflammatory events associated with sepsis. Ask about the patient's previous responses to infection or injury. If the patient has consistently had greater-than-expected inflammatory responses, he or she may be at increased risk for ARDS and should be monitored for manifestations of the disorder.

- The course of ARDS and its management are divided into three phases:
  1. *Exudative phase:* This phase includes early changes of dyspnea and tachypnea resulting from the alveoli becoming fluid-filled and from pulmonary shunting and atelectasis. Early interventions focus on supporting the patient and providing oxygen.
  2. *Fibroproliferative phase:* Increased lung damage leads to pulmonary hypertension and fibrosis. The body attempts to repair the damage and increasing lung involvement reduces gas exchange and oxygenation. Multiple organ dysfunction syndrome can occur. Interventions focus on delivering adequate oxygen, preventing complications, and supporting the lungs.
  3. *Resolution phase:* Usually occurring after 14 days, resolution of the injury can occur; if not the patient either dies or has chronic disease. Fibrosis may or may not occur. Research indicates that patients surviving ARDS have neuropsychological deficits and poor quality-of-life scores.

❗ NURSING SAFETY PRIORITY: Action Alert

Early identification of patients at high risk for ARDS can allow the nurse to plan interventions for prevention of this serious condition. Both aspiration and systemic infection increase ARDS risk. Use aspiration precautions such as elevating the head of bed greater than 30 to 45 degrees for patients receiving enteral feeding. Avoid oral intake in patients with problems that impair swallowing and gag reflexes. To reduce sepsis, follow meticulous infection control guidelines, including handwashing, invasive catheter and wound care, and body substance precautions.

PATIENT-CENTERED COLLABORATIVE CARE
Assessment
* Assessment findings include:
  1. Identifying patients at high risk for developing this condition
  2. Recognizing decreasing Spo_2 or Pao_2 and related symptoms such as anxiety, restlessness, or confusion
  3. Observing trends for increased effort with breathing manifested by tachypnea, grunting respiration, cyanosis, pallor, and intercostal retractions or substernal retractions
  4. Documenting and communicating severely decreased breath sounds or new onset of diffuse crackles, rhonchi, and wheezing
  5. Communicating associated findings, if accompanied by sepsis or other systemic inflammatory disease: hypotension, tachycardia and/or dysrhythmias, and symptoms of infection (fever, increased sputum, elevated WBC count)

Interventions
* Management includes:
  1. Endotracheal intubation and mechanical ventilation
  2. Antibiotics to manage identified infections
  3. Conservative IV fluid volume administration to prevent excess lung tissue fluid while managing hypotension and inadequate perfusion

! NURSING SAFETY PRIORITY: Critical Rescue

For the patient requiring emergency intubation and ventilation, bring the code (or "crash") cart, airway equipment box, and suction equipment (often already on the code cart) to the bedside. Maintain a patent airway through positioning (head tilt, chin lift) and the insertion of an oral or nasopharyngeal airway until the patient is intubated. Delivering manual breaths with a bag-valve-mask may also be required.

  4. Enteral nutrition or parenteral nutrition as soon as possible to prevent malnutrition, loss of respiratory muscle function, and reduced immune response

ADRENAL INSUFFICIENCY (ADRENAL HYPOFUNCTION)
OVERVIEW
* Adrenal insufficiency is the loss of cortisol and aldosterone.
  1. Low cortisol results in glucose dysregulation and hypoglycemia.
  2. Low aldosterone causes fluid and electrolyte imbalances, especially hyperkalemia, hyponatremia, and hypovolemia.

A

- Decreased production of these adrenocortical steroids occurs as a result of:
  1. Inadequate secretion of adrenocorticotropic hormone (ACTH) (hypopituitarism)
  2. Dysfunction of the hypothalamic-pituitary control mechanisms
     a. The most common cause of this type of dysfunction is the sudden cessation of long-term, high-dose corticosteroid (also called glucocorticoid) therapy.
     b. Other causes include cancer and severe, high acuity illness (sepsis, shock).
  3. Direct dysfunction of adrenal gland tissue that typically occurs gradually
     a. Causes include tuberculosis, autoimmune factors, HIV/AIDS, adrenal tumors, low perfusion states, and irradiation of the adrenal glands.
     b. Adrenalectomy with sudden loss of hormones is also an example of direct dysfunction.
- Acute adrenal insufficiency or *Addisonian crisis* is a life-threatening event in which the need for cortisol and aldosterone is greater than the available supply.
  1. It often occurs in response to a stressful event like surgery, trauma, and severe infection when the adrenal hormone output is already reduced.
  2. Death from hypoglycemia, shock, and hyperkalemia-associated cardiac problems can occur unless interventions are implemented rapidly.

PATIENT-CENTERED COLLABORATIVE CARE
Assessment
- Obtain patient information about:
  1. Change in activity level, or lethargy and fatigue
  2. Increased salt craving or intake
  3. GI problems, such as anorexia, nausea, vomiting, diarrhea, and abdominal pain
  4. Unplanned weight loss
  5. History of irradiation to the abdomen or head
  6. Past or current medical problems (e.g., tuberculosis, previous intracranial surgery)
  7. Past and current drugs, especially steroids, anticoagulants, opioids, or cytotoxic drugs
- Assess for and document:
  1. Manifestations of hypoglycemia (low blood glucose level, sweating, headaches, tachycardia, and tremors)
  2. Manifestations of hypovolemia (e.g., postural hypotension, dehydration)

3. Cardiac problems from hyperkalemia (e.g., dysrhythmias, T wave changes on ECG)
4. Muscle weakness
5. Electrolyte abnormalities (elevated serum potassium and low serum sodium levels)
6. Areas of increased pigmentation, decreased pigmentation, or patchy pigmentation
7. Decreased alertness, forgetfulness, confusion

- Diagnosis is based on clinical manifestations and:
  1. Laboratory findings of low serum cortisol, low fasting blood glucose, low sodium, and elevated potassium levels
  2. Altered plasma levels of ACTH and melanocyte-stimulating hormone (MSH)
  3. Low urinary 17-hydroxycorticosteroid and 17-ketosteroid levels
  4. CT and magnetic resonance imaging (MRI) scans of brain, abdomen, and pelvis
  5. ACTH stimulation testing

Interventions

- Cortisol and aldosterone deficiencies are corrected by replacement therapy with hydrocortisone (corrects corticosteroid, [glucocorticoid] deficiency) and fludrocortisone (corrects aldosterone deficiency).
  1. For hydrocortisone therapy divided doses are usually given, with two thirds given in the morning and one third in the late afternoon (or as prescribed).
  2. Dosage adjustment of fludrocortisone may be needed, especially in hot weather when more sodium is lost because of excessive perspiration.
- Nursing interventions to promote fluid balance, monitor for fluid deficit, and prevent hypoglycemia include:
  1. Weighing the patient daily and recording intake and output
  2. Assessing vital signs every 1 to 4 hours
  3. Checking for dysrhythmias or postural hypotension
  4. Monitoring glucose with point-of-service testing (glucometer)
  5. Monitoring laboratory values to identify hemoconcentration (e.g., increased hematocrit, blood urea nitrogen [BUN])
- Administer cortisol and aldosterone replacement therapy.
- Teach patients how to self-manage this replacement therapy, including the importance of daily drug use and potential need to alter dose during stressful physical conditions.

! | NURSING SAFETY PRIORITY: Action Alert

Do not implement salt restriction or diuretic therapy for anyone with severe adrenal hypofunction because it may lead to an adrenal crisis.

ALKALOSIS, METABOLIC

OVERVIEW

- Alkalosis is not a disease; it is a condition caused by a metabolic problem, a respiratory problem, or both.
- Metabolic alkalosis is caused by any condition that creates the acid-base imbalance through either an increase of bases (base excess) or a decrease of acids (acid deficit).
- It is reflected by ABG values with a pH above 7.45 and high HCO_3^- above 28 mm Hg.
- Often, metabolic alkalosis is accompanied by a low serum potassium level (hypokalemia).
- An *actual metabolic alkalosis* occurs when a base (usually bicarbonate) is overproduced or undereliminated. This type of alkalosis is known as a *base excess alkalosis.*
- A *relative alkalosis* occurs when the amount or strength, or both, of the acids decreases, making the blood more basic than acidic as a result of overelimination or underproduction of acids. This type of alkalosis is known as an *acid deficit alkalosis.*
- Common causes of metabolic alkalosis include:
  1. Increase of base (especially bicarbonate)
     a. Excessive use of antacids or bicarbonate
     b. Milk-alkali syndrome
     c. Multiple transfusions of blood products
     d. IV administration of bicarbonate
     e. Total parenteral nutrition
  2. Acid loss
     a. Prolonged vomiting
     b. Continuous nasogastric suctioning
     c. Dehydration from excess diuretic use
     d. Hypercortisolism
     e. Hyperaldosteronism

PATIENT-CENTERED COLLABORATIVE CARE

Assessment

- Assessment findings include:
  1. CNS changes
     a. Light-headedness
     b. Decreased ability to concentrate
     c. Anxiety, irritability
     d. Paresthesia
     e. Positive Chvostek's sign
     f. Positive Trousseau's sign
     g. Tetany, seizures
  2. Neuromuscular changes
     a. Skeletal muscle weakness
     b. Muscle cramping and twitching

      c. Hyperreflexia

      d. Cardiac changes

      e. Weak, rapid pulse

      f. Hypotension (if hypovolemia is also present)

  3. Respiratory changes

      a. Decreased respiratory effort can occur to compensate for metabolic alkalosis. Monitor the patient for coexisting reduced oxygenation (low SpO_2 or PaO_2) when respiratory rate is slow or breathing is shallow.

Interventions

- Management focuses on:
  1. Drug therapy to resolve the causes of alkalosis (e.g., antiemetics for severe vomiting)
  2. Oral or IV replacement to restore normal fluid, electrolyte, and acid-base balance
  3. Monitoring patient responses to therapy
     a. Respiratory effectiveness (rate, depth, oxygen saturation)
     b. Cardiac effectiveness (pulse, blood pressure)
     c. Intake and output
     d. Serum electrolytes and ABG values
     e. Hand grasps and deep tendon reflexes

ALKALOSIS, RESPIRATORY

OVERVIEW

- Respiratory alkalosis is not a disease; it is a condition caused by a respiratory problem that usually involves an excessive rate or depth of ventilation, or both.
- It is reflected by ABG values indicating a pH above 7.45 and low PCO_2.
- Often it is accompanied by a low serum potassium level (hypokalemia).
- Respiratory alkalosis occurs because of an excess loss of acids in the form of carbon dioxide.
- The main cause of respiratory alkalosis is hyperventilation, which leads to excessive exhalation of carbon dioxide. Common conditions leading to hyperventilation include:
  1. Anxiety or fear
  2. Improper settings on mechanical ventilators (too high a ventilation rate, too great a tidal volume, or both)
  3. Direct stimulation of central respiratory centers
     a. Fever
     b. Hyperthyroidism
     c. Drugs (e.g., salicylates, catecholamines, progesterone)
     d. High altitudes or low atmospheric oxygen levels

PATIENT-CENTERED COLLABORATIVE CARE

Assessment

- Assessment findings include:
  1. CNS changes
     a. Light-headedness
     b. Decreased ability to concentrate
     c. Anxiety, irritability
     d. Paresthesia
     e. Positive Chvostek's sign
     f. Positive Trousseau's sign
     g. Tetany, seizures
  2. Respiratory changes of increased respiratory rate and effort (hyperventilation)
  3. Neuromuscular changes
     a. Skeletal muscle weakness
     b. Muscle cramping and twitching
     c. Hyperreflexia
  4. Cardiac changes
     a. Weak, rapid pulse

Interventions

- Management focuses on:
  1. Ensuring ventilator settings are appropriate
  2. Rebreathing exhaled air to increase carbon dioxide levels
  3. Calming the patient to control ventilation
  4. Administering drug therapy to resolve the causes of alkalosis (e.g., antipyretics for fever, anxiolytics for acute anxiety)
  5. Supporting oral or IV replacement to restore normal fluid and electrolyte levels
  6. Restoring a normal respiratory effort (determined by rate, depth, and oxygen saturation)
  7. Preventing cardiovascular instability (through achieving a normal heart rate and rhythm, pulse quality, and blood pressure)
  8. Achieving intake and output goals

ALLERGY, LATEX

- Latex allergy is a type I hypersensitivity reaction; the specific allergen is a protein found in processed natural latex rubber products. Patients may report an allergy or skin irritation to adhesive bandages and balloons.
- Allergic reactions to latex vary from contact dermatitis (mild) to anaphylaxis (severe).
- People at the greatest risk for latex allergy are those with a high-level exposure to natural latex products, such as patients with spina bifida or congenital urinary tract abnormalities and health

care workers who use latex health care products (e.g., gloves, syringes, blood pressure cuffs).
- Individuals with a latex allergy often have a history of other allergies, especially to specific foods (e.g., banana, avocado, and some nuts).

> **! NURSING SAFETY PRIORITY: Critical Rescue**
>
> Use only latex-free products in the care of a patient with a known latex allergy.

- Teach patients who are sensitive to latex to avoid products containing latex.
- When caring for a patient with a known latex allergy, the health care provider should:
  1. Remove any latex-containing product from his or her person (e.g., erasers, tourniquets, blood tubes)
  2. Use paper tape or other low-irritation adhesive products
  3. Check syringes, medication vials, and IV tubing for latex and use alternatives if latex is present
  4. Wash hands with soap and water (not alcohol-based rub) before entering the room or touching the patient to remove latex residue on the skin from health care products

AMPUTATION

OVERVIEW
- Amputation is the removal of a part of the body.
- The psychosocial aspects of the procedure are often more devastating than the physical impairments that result. The loss is complete and permanent and causes a change in body image and often in self-esteem.
- *Traumatic amputation* occurs when a body part is severed unexpectedly, most often resulting from accidents. Depending on the extent of damage, body parts that are severed may be reattached or reimplanted.

> **! NURSING SAFETY PRIORITY: Critical Rescue**
>
> For prehospital care with any traumatic amputation:
> - Call 911.
> - Assess the patient for airway or breathing problems.
> - Apply direct pressure to amputation site with layers of dry gauze or other cloth.

- Elevate the extremity above the patient's heart to decrease the bleeding.
- Wrap the completely severed digit or limb in a dry, sterile gauze or clean cloth.
- Put the digit or limb in a watertight, sealed plastic bag.
- Place the bag in ice water—never directly on ice. Use one part ice and three parts water.
- Be sure that the amputated part goes with the patient to the hospital.

- *Surgical amputations* are planned, elective procedures performed for a variety of disorders and complications.
- Loss of the great toe is significant, because it affects balance, gait, and push-off ability during walking.
- Midfoot amputations (e.g., Lisfranc, Chopart, or Syme amputation) remove most of the foot but retain the intact ankle so that weight bearing can be accomplished without the use of prosthesis and with reduced pain.
- Other lower extremity amputations are below-knee amputation (BKA), above-knee amputation (AKA), hip disarticulation, or removal of the hip joint, and hemipelvectomy (removal of half of the pelvis with the leg).
- The higher the level of amputation, the more energy is required for ambulation.
- Upper extremity (UE) amputations are rare and usually are more incapacitating than those of lower extremities. Early replacement with a prosthetic device is vital for the patient with UE amputation.
- Complications of elective or traumatic amputation include:
  1. Hemorrhage
  2. Infection
  3. Phantom limb pain
  4. Neuroma
  5. Flexion contractures
  6. Psychological maladjustment

⊕ Cultural Considerations

The incidence of lower extremity amputations is greater in the black, Hispanic, and American Indian populations, because the incidence of major diseases leading to amputation, such as diabetes and arteriosclerosis, is greater in this population. Limited access to health care for these minority groups may also play a major role in limb loss.

PATIENT-CENTERED COLLABORATIVE CARE
Assessment
- Assess:
  1. Neurovascular status of extremity to be amputated
     a. Examine skin color, temperature, sensation, capillary refill, and pulses
     b. Compare findings with those of the unaffected extremity
     c. Check and document the presence of discoloration, edema, ulcerations, hair distribution, and any necrosis
  2. Psychosocial responses
     a. Preparation for a planned amputation
     b. Presence of bitterness, hostility, or depression
     c. Expectations of how the loss of a body part may affect employment, social relationships, and recreational activities
     d. Current self-concept and self-image
     e. Willingness and motivation to withstand prolonged rehabilitation after the amputation
  3. Patient's and family's coping abilities
  4. Patient's religious, spiritual, and cultural beliefs
  5. Diagnostic assessment may include:
     a. Segmental limb blood pressures
     b. Blood flow by Doppler ultrasonography or laser Doppler flowmetry or use of transcutaneous oxygen pressure ($TcPO_2$)

QSEN SAFETY

A high degree of teamwork is essential in the OR to prevent mistakes. With the patient assisting, identify the limb or digit to be amputated preoperatively, and mark it with indelible ink. Follow time-out rules in the operating room, so that the correct patient and digit or limb is identified by at least two people.

Interventions
- Monitor for signs indicating that there is sufficient tissue perfusion but no hemorrhage:
  1. Skin flap at the end of the residual limb should be pink in a light-skinned person and not discolored.
  2. The area is warm, not hot.
  3. Assess the closest proximal pulse for strength and compare it with that in the other extremity.
- Assess and manage pain
  1. Pain management for residual limb pain (RLP) is like that for any patient in pain.

2. Phantom limb pain (PLP) is managed with calcitonin, beta blockade, antidepressants, and antiepileptic drugs.
3. Complementary and alternative therapies for pain following amputation are useful for many patients for both acute and chronic pain syndromes.

! NURSING SAFETY PRIORITY: Action Alert

If the patient reports PLP, recognize that the pain is real and should be managed promptly and completely.

- Prevent infection
  1. Drug therapy with broad-spectrum prophylactic antibiotics may be used before, during, and after surgery.
  2. The initial pressure dressing and drains are usually removed by the surgeon 48 to 72 hours after surgery.
  3. Inspect the wound site for signs of inflammation (e.g., redness, swelling) and monitor the healing process.
  4. Record the characteristics of drainage, if present.
  5. Change the soft dressing every day until the sutures or staples are removed.
  6. Dressings usually include an elastic bandage wrapped firmly around the residual limb after application of a sterile gauze dressing over the incision.
- Promote mobility
  1. Coordinate with the physical therapist to begin exercises as soon as possible after surgery.
  2. For patients with AKAs or BKAs, teach range-of-motion (ROM) exercises for prevention of flexion contractures, particularly of the hip and knee.
  3. Ensure that a trapeze and an overhead frame are used to aid in strengthening the upper extremities and allow the patient to move independently in bed.
  4. Instruct the patient to pull the residual limb close to the other leg and contract the gluteal muscles of the buttocks.
  5. For patients with BKAs, teach how to push the residual limb down toward the bed while supporting it on a pillow.
  6. Follow health care provider and agency policy for elevation of a lower leg residual limb on a pillow while the patient is in a supine position.
- Prepare for prosthesis
  1. Coordinate with a certified prosthetist-orthotist (CPO) for appropriate postoperative planning.
  2. Instruct the patient being fitted for a leg prosthesis to bring a sturdy pair of shoes to the fitting.

   3. After surgery, apply the prescribed device, such as the Jobst air splint, or elastic bandages to shape and shrink the residual limb in preparation for the prosthesis. If elastic bandages are used, reapply the bandages in a figure-eight wrap every 4 to 6 hours or more often if they become loose.
      a. Decrease the tightness of the bandages while wrapping in a distal-to-proximal direction.
      b. After wrapping, anchor the bandages to the most proximal joint, such as above the knee for BKAs.
- Promote positive body image and lifestyle adaptation
   1. If possible, arrange for the patient to meet with a rehabilitated amputee who is about the same age as him or her.
   2. Assess the patient's verbal and nonverbal references to the affected area and determine the patient preference for terminology (e.g., *stump*).
   3. Ask the patient to describe his or her feelings about changes in body image and self-esteem.
   4. Check whether the patient looks at the area during a dressing change.
   5. Document behavior that indicates acceptance or nonacceptance of the amputation.
   6. Teach the patient and family about available resources and support from organizations such as the Amputee Coalition of America (ACA) (www.amputee-coalition.org) and the National Amputation Foundation (NAF) (www.nationalamputation.org).
   7. Stress the patient's personal strengths.
   8. Collaborate with a social worker or vocational rehabilitation specialist to evaluate the skills of a patient who may need to change employment.
   9. If appropriate, refer the patient and family for professional assistance from a sex therapist, intimacy coach, or psychologist.
   10. Help the patient and family set realistic desired outcomes and take one day at a time.
   11. Teach the patient and family how to care for the limb and the prosthesis if it is available.
   12. Teach the patient or family to care for the limb after it has healed by cleaning it each day with the rest of the body during bathing with soap and water.
   13. Teach the patient and family to inspect the limb every day for signs of inflammation or skin breakdown.

AMYOTROPHIC LATERAL SCLEROSIS (ALS)

- Amyotrophic lateral sclerosis (ALS), also known as *Lou Gehrig's disease,* is a progressive degenerative disease involving the motor neurons of the brain, brain stem, and spinal cord.

- As motor neurons are lost, atrophy of muscles occurs, resulting in dysphagia, weakness of the extremities, spasticity, and dysarthria.
- As the disease progresses, flaccid quadriplegia develops. Increased risk for pneumonia and respiratory failure result from paralysis of breathing muscles, including the diaphragm.
- Treatment is symptomatic and directed toward the following: preventing complications of immobility, promoting comfort, providing ongoing support and counseling to the patient and family, and informing the patient about the need for advance directives such as a living will and durable power of attorney.
- The drug riluzole (Rilutek) is associated with increased survival time but there is no cure.

ANAL FISSURE

- An anal fissure is a tear in the anal lining.
- Acute anal fissures are superficial and usually heal spontaneously.
- Diagnosis is made with inspection and palpation of the perianal area.
- Pain during and after defecation is the most common symptom; bleeding may also occur.
- Nonsurgical interventions include local symptomatic relief measures such as warm sitz baths, analgesics, and bulk-forming agents or osmotic laxatives.
- Surgical repair under local anesthesia may be necessary for chronic or recurrent fissures that do not respond to nonsurgical management.

ANAL FISTULA

- An anal fistula, or *fistula in ano,* is an abnormal tract leading from the anal canal to the perianal skin.
- Most anal fistulas result from anorectal abscesses, but they can be associated with tuberculosis, Crohn's disease, or cancer.
- Symptoms include pruritus, purulent discharge, and tenderness or pain aggravated by bowel movements.
- Because fistulas do not heal spontaneously, surgery (fistulostomy) is necessary.
- Measures such as sitz baths, analgesics, and bulking products or stool softeners are used to reduce tissue trauma and discomfort.
- Hygiene is important; patients should be instructed to clean the anal area after each bowel movement.
- Patients should avoid constipation and straining with stool.

ANAPHYLAXIS
OVERVIEW

- Anaphylaxis is the most dramatic and life-threatening example of a type I hypersensitivity reaction.

- It occurs rapidly and systemically, affecting many organs within minutes of allergen exposure.
- Drugs and dyes are common allergens in acute care settings and food and insect/bites/stings are common causes in community settings.
- Anaphylaxis episodes vary in severity and can be fatal, particularly when treatment with epinephrine is delayed.

PATIENT-CENTERED COLLABORATIVE CARE
Assessment
- Diagnosis is based on the presence of two of the three criteria listed below:
  1. Physical findings of:
     a. Skin or mucus problems involving swollen lips, tongue, soft palate, widespread hives, pruritus, or flushing
     b. Respiratory distress or ineffectiveness
     c. Hypotension or reduced perfusion
  2. Onset within minutes to hours after exposure to allergen of more than two of the following symptoms:
     a. Skin or mucous membrane problems
     b. Respiratory distress or ineffectiveness
     c. Hypotension
     d. GI distress
  3. Onset within minutes to hours of systolic blood pressure less than 9 mm Hg or 30% lower than patient's baseline
- Other assessment findings include:
  1. History of anaphylactic response and documentation of allergen
  2. Subjective feelings of uneasiness, apprehension, weakness, and impending doom
  3. Generalized itching and urticaria (hives)
  4. Erythema
  5. Angioedema (diffuse swelling) of the eyes, lips, or tongue
  6. Bronchoconstriction, mucosal edema, and excess mucus production
  7. Nasal congestion and rhinorrhea
  8. Dyspnea, increasing respiratory distress, audible wheezing
  9. Crackles, wheezing, and reduced breath sounds on auscultation
  10. Laryngeal edema (hoarseness and stridor)
  11. Respiratory failure with hypoxemia
  12. Rapid, weak, irregular pulse
  13. Dysrhythmias
  14. Diaphoresis
  15. Increasing anxiety and confusion

A

> ## ❗ NURSING SAFETY PRIORITY: Critical Rescue
>
> If a patient is suspected of having an anaphylactic reaction, immediately call the Rapid Response Team, because most anaphylactic deaths are related to treatment delay. If the patient is not treated immediately, he or she may lose consciousness. Dysrhythmias, shock, and cardiac arrest may occur within minutes. Anticipate the need for immediate administration of epinephrine (1:1000), 0.3 to 0.5 mL IM, IV, interosseous, or via an endotracheal tube.

Interventions
*   Emergency respiratory management
    1. Immediately assess the respiratory status, airway, and oxygen saturation of patients who show any symptoms of an anaphylactic reaction.
    2. If the airway is compromised in any way, call the Rapid Response Team (or anesthesia and respiratory therapy if Rapid Response Team is not available) before proceeding in any other intervention.
    3. Apply oxygen using a high-flow, non-rebreather mask at 40% to 60%.
    4. Ensure that intubation and tracheotomy equipment is ready.
*   Drug therapy

> ## ❗ NURSING SAFETY PRIORITY: Critical Rescue
>
> Administer epinephrine (1:1000) 0.3 to 0.5 mL IM or IV as quickly as possible. Most deaths from anaphylaxis are related to delay in epinephrine administration.

> ## ❗ NURSING SAFETY PRIORITY: Action Alert
>
> Do not remove the IV catheter of a patient experiencing anaphylaxis, but do withdraw fluid from the IV catheter, change the IV tubing, and hang normal saline.

1. Immediately discontinue the drugs of a patient having an anaphylactic reaction.
2. If the patient does not have an IV access, start one immediately, and run normal saline.
3. Anticipate the following:
    a. Epinephrine, 1:1000 concentration: 0.3 to 0.5 mL IV push (immediately); repeat as needed every 10 to 15 minutes until the patient responds

     b. Diphenhydramine: 25 to 50 mg IV push (immediately)

     c. Theophylline: 6 mg/kg IV over 20 to 30 minutes for severe, persistent bronchospasm

     d. Once stabilized, inhaled beta-adrenergic agonist such as metaproterenol (Alupent) or albuterol (Proventil) by means of a high-flow nebulizer every 2 to 4 hours

     e. Corticosteroids (IV) are not effective immediately but given as the patient stabilizes to maintain airway, breathing, and circulation

  4. Document all drugs administered and observe patient responses to drugs.

- Supportive care
  1. Position the patient to maintain airway, breathing, and circulation. Elevate the back rest to 45 degrees unless hypotension is present.
  2. Raise the feet and legs to improve blood return to the heart.
  3. Monitor pulse oximetry and/or ABGs to determine oxygenation adequacy.
  4. Use suction to remove excess oral or nasal mucous secretions.
  5. Continually assess the patient's respiratory rate and depth.
  6. Stay with the patient.
  7. Reassure the patient that the appropriate interventions are being instituted.
  8. Observe the patient for fluid overload from the rapid drug and IV fluid infusions.
  9. Before discharge, instruct the patient to obtain and wear a medical alert bracelet or ID about the specific allergy.
  10. Teach the patient who carries an automatic epinephrine injector (EpiPen) how to care for, assemble, and use the device. Obtain a return demonstration.

ANEMIA

OVERVIEW

- Anemia is a reduction in the number of red blood cells (RBCs), the amount of hemoglobin, or the hematocrit (percentage of packed RBCs per deciliter of blood). *NOTE: A patient who is fluid overloaded may have reduced hematocrit and NOT be anemic. With correction of vascular fluid excess, the hematocrit returns to a normal value.*
- It is a clinical sign, not a specific disease, because it occurs with many health problems.
- Anemia can be caused by increased destruction of RBCs, decreased RBC production, or blood loss.
  1. Examples of conditions that increase RBC destruction are sickle cell disease, glucose-6-phosphate-dehydrogenase

(G6PD) deficiency, and autoimmune hemolytic disease such as Fanconi's anemia.

- a. *Sickle cell disease* is an inherited disorder that results in defective hemoglobin synthesis.
- b. *G6PD deficiency* is an X-linked recessive deficiency of an enzyme needed for RBC glucose metabolism.
- c. *Autoimmune hemolytic anemia* occurs when antibodies attack and destroy one's own RBCs.

2. Examples of conditions that are associated with decreased production of RBCs are iron, vitamin B_{12}, and folic acid deficiencies, or by aplastic anemia from bone marrow injury.

- a. *Iron deficiency anemia* is related to iron-deficient diets, chronic alcoholism, malabsorption syndromes, and partial gastrectomy. It can also occur during periods of rapid metabolism such as during adolescence or pregnancy or with severe infections and injury.
- b. *B_{12} deficiency anemia* can occur with dietary insufficiency and with failure to absorb vitamin B_{12} as a result of reduced intrinsic factor produced by the stomach. Anemia caused by failure to absorb vitamin B_{12} is called *pernicious anemia.*
- c. *Folic acid deficiency anemia* can occur as a result of dietary deficiency and in the presence of certain drugs, including oral contraceptives, antiepileptic drugs, and the immuno-modulator drug methotrexate, which is used to modulate the immune system and treat cancers.
- d. *Aplastic anemia* can occur with exposure to agents that damage the bone marrow such as radiation, insecticides, anti-neoplastic drugs, and some antibiotics.

3. Anemia can also be caused by blood loss, as with gastrointestinal bleeding or after surgery or trauma.

Assessment

- Assessment findings include:
  1. Weakness
  2. Pallor
  3. Shortness of breath from reduced oxygen-carrying capacity
  4. Petechiae or ecchymosis
  5. Chest pain related to reduced oxygen-carrying capacity in the presence of cardiac disease
  6. The complete blood count (CBC) shows reduced RBCs, hemoglobin, and hematocrit
  7. Bone marrow biopsy may show abnormalities within this hematologic cell-forming organ

Interventions

- Management includes:
  1. Blood transfusions when the anemia causes disability, including chest pain at rest or mild activity
  2. Immunosuppressive therapy with drugs such as prednisone and anti-neoplastic or immunomodulation drugs if the case is increased destruction of RBCs
  3. Splenectomy (removal of the spleen) when an enlarged spleen is destroying normal RBCs or suppressing their development
  4. Hematopoietic stem cell transplantation (bone marrow transplantation) to replace defective bone marrow with aplastic anemia (although cost, availability, and complications limit this treatment of aplastic anemia)
  5. Implementation of dietary therapy
     a. For vitamin B_{12} deficiency, teach the patient to eat foods high in vitamin B_{12}, such as animal proteins, eggs, and dairy products. Provide vitamin B_{12} supplements.
     b. For severe deficiency (also known as pernicious anemia), administer vitamin B_{12} injections initially and anticipate ongoing and lifelong oral or parenteral supplementation.
     c. For folic acid deficiency, provide scheduled folic acid replacement therapy.
     d. For iron deficiency, provide a scheduled iron supplement and instruct the patient to increase his or her oral intake of iron from food sources, such as red or organ meat, egg yolk, kidney beans, leafy vegetables, and raisins.
  6. Teach the patient that oral iron supplements can change the color of stool to black and can promote constipation that can be treated with diet, stool softeners, osmotic laxatives, or bulk-forming agents.
  7. Provide transfusion therapy when ordered, using packed RBCs to maintain safe levels of oxygen-carrying hemoglobin.

QSEN SAFETY

Problems in blood transfusion contribute to unintended mortality and morbidity. Use a consistent process to prevent problems in blood transfusion by identifying patients correctly *and* ensuring the correct blood product is administered.

- The nurse who will be administering the blood products must be one of the two persons comparing the patient's identification with the information on the blood component bag.
- Before the transfusion, the priority action is to determine that the blood component delivered is

correct and that identification of the patient is
correct. Check the physician's prescription, the
patient's identity, and whether the identification
band identifiers are identical to those on the blood
component tag.

8. Be familiar with common and severe transfusion reactions. Monitor the patient closely during the first 15 minutes of transfusion therapy to detect adverse reactions.

ANEURYSM, AORTIC

OVERVIEW

- An aneurysm is a permanent, localized dilation of an artery accompanied by weakening of the vessel wall.
- An aneurysm forms when the media, or the middle layer of the artery, is weakened, producing a stretching effect in the intima (the inner layer) and adventitia (the outer layer of the artery).
- The effect of elevated blood pressure on the artery wall enlarges the aneurysm.
- The most common cause is atherosclerosis; atheromatous plaque weakens the intimal surface.
- Hypertension, hyperlipidemia, and cigarette smoking are modifiable contributing factors, whereas age, gender, and family history are nonmodifiable contributing factors.
- Other causes are Marfan syndrome (a genetic connective tissue disease), Ehlers-Danlos syndrome (a rare genetic disorder), chronic inflammation (aortitis), and blunt trauma, usually from motor vehicle crashes.
- Aneurysms can be classified as:
  1. *Saccular,* an outpouching from a distinct portion of the artery wall
  2. *Fusiform,* a diffuse dilation involving the total circumference of the artery
- Aneurysms can also be described as "true," meaning the arterial wall is weakened by congenital or acquired problems. False aneurysms occur as a result of vessel injury or trauma to all three layers of the arterial wall.
- Abdominal aneurysms are located between the renal arteries and the iliac bifurcation.
- Thoracic aneurysms develop between the origin of the left subclavian artery and the diaphragm.
- Aneurysms can thrombose, embolize, or rupture. Rupture, also called dissection, is life threatening.

PATIENT-CENTERED COLLABORATIVE CARE
Assessment
- Most patients with aortic aneurysm are asymptomatic.
- Assess for clinical manifestations of abdominal aortic aneurysms:
  1. Abdominal, flank, or back pain that is usually steady, with a gnawing quality, is unaffected by movement, and may last for hours or days
  2. Prominent pulsation in the upper abdomen (do not palpate)
  3. Abdominal or femoral bruit
- Assess for clinical manifestations of thoracic aneurysms:
  1. Back pain
  2. Shortness of breath
  3. Hoarseness
  4. Difficulty swallowing
  5. Visible mass above the suprasternal notch (occasional)
- Assess for abdominal or thoracic aortic rupture:
  1. Pain that is described as tearing, ripping, and stabbing and located in the chest, back, and abdomen
  2. Symptoms of hypovolemic shock: hypotension, tachycardia, diaphoresis, absent or faint peripheral pulses, and decreased mentation
  3. Nausea, vomiting, and apprehension
- Also assess for:
  1. Presence of a distorted aortic profile on thoracic or abdominal x-ray or CT scan
  2. Enlarged aortic profile by ultrasonography

Planning and Implementation
Nonsurgical Management
- Antihypertensive drugs are prescribed to maintain normal blood pressure and to decrease stress on an aortic aneurysm that is smaller than 2 or 3 inches (6 cm) or when surgery is not feasible.
- Teach the patient the importance of keeping scheduled CT scan appointments to monitor the size of the aneurysm.
- Teach the patient to avoid heavy lifting or activities that increase abdominal and thoracic pressure.
- Review with the patient the clinical manifestations of dissecting the aneurysm and the need to use emergency transportation if symptoms occur.

Surgical Management
- Endovascular stent placement via an intra-aortic catheter avoids the need for an abdominal incision and can be done in the interventional radiology suite or operating room.
- Monitor the patient closely in the hospital and at home for the development of complications, such as bleeding, aneurysm

rupture, peripheral embolization, and misdeployment of the stent graft. All of these complications require surgical intervention.

A

- Surgical removal of the aneurysm is reserved for symptomatic lesions or aneurysms larger than 3 inches (6 cm). The excised portion of the aorta is replaced with a graft. Ruptures always require emergency surgery to replace the damaged aorta.
- Provide perioperative care:
  1. Maintain mean arterial pressure within prescribed ranges to promote tissue perfusion and avoid hypertension.
  2. Assess all peripheral pulses to serve as a baseline for comparison after surgery; mark where the pulse is heard and check peripheral pulses and sensation with vital signs.

QSEN TEAMWORK AND COLLABORATION

Communication is an essential component of safe, effective care. Before any procedure, use a time-out process to conduct a final verification of the procedure, patient, and site using active communication techniques and a checklist.

  3. Assess vital signs every hour to detect early signs of hypotension.
  4. Immediately report to the physician any signs of bleeding, leak, or occlusion at the surgical site or from a drain, such as pulse changes, severe pain, cool to cold extremities below the graft, white or blue extremities or flanks, abdominal distention and decreased urinary output, and decreased or absent motor movement or sensation below the aneurysm or graft site.
  5. Abdominal aortic aneurysm repair can compromise the blood flow to the kidneys and spinal cord.
- Additional postoperative care specific to abdominal aortic repair includes:
  1. Managing pain as for postoperative care by administering opioid analgesics for pain
  2. Avoiding nausea, vomiting, or other occasions of increased thoracic and abdominal pressure
  3. Monitoring ECG, ST segment, and patient symptoms for acute MI; coagulopathy after vascular procedures increases the risk for ACS, including MI
  4. Monitoring for less common complications such as respiratory distress and paralytic ileus
- Care of the patient undergoing thoracic aneurysm repair is similar to that for other thoracic surgeries. Additional postoperative care includes:
  1. Monitoring chest tube drainage for excess drainage such as more than 100 mL for 2 hours

2. Monitoring for cardiac dysrhythmias, paraplegia, acute kidney injury, and respiratory distress
3. Instructing the patient with thoracic aneurysm repair to report back pain, shortness of breath, difficulty swallowing, and/or hoarseness

! NURSING SAFETY PRIORITY: Critical Rescue

Report signs of hemorrhage or graft occlusion to the physician immediately.

Community-Based Care
- Emphasize the importance of compliance with the schedule of CT scanning to monitor the size of the aneurysm in patients who have not had surgery.
- Emphasize the importance of controlling blood pressure.
- Educate the patient and family.
  1. Teach the patient to restrict activities, particularly during recovery from surgery to repair the aortic aneurysm:
     a. Avoiding lifting heavy objects for 6 to 12 weeks postoperatively
     b. Using discretion in activities that involve pulling, pushing, or straining, such as vacuuming, changing bed linens, moving furniture, mopping or sweeping, raking leaves, mowing grass, and chopping wood
     c. Avoiding contact sports or activities that may increase aortic pressures such as horseback riding
     d. Deferring driving a car for several weeks postoperatively
  2. Provide written and oral wound care instructions, if needed.
  3. Provide pain management instruction.
- Refer to home health nursing and other community agencies as needed.

APPENDICITIS

OVERVIEW
- Appendicitis is an acute inflammation of the vermiform appendix, the small finger-like pouch attached to the cecum of the colon.
- Inflammation of the appendix can occur when the lumen of the appendix is obstructed.
- Inflammation leads to infection as bacteria invade the wall of the appendix.
- Appendicitis is the most common cause of pain in the right lower abdominal quadrant.

Considerations for Older Adults

Appendicitis is relatively rare at extremes in age. However, perforation is more common in older people, causing a higher mortality rate. The diagnosis of appendicitis is difficult to establish in older adults because symptoms of pain and tenderness may not be as pronounced in this age-group. This difference results in treatment delay and an increased risk for perforation, peritonitis, and death.

PATIENT-CENTERED COLLABORATIVE CARE

Assessment

- Assessment findings include:
  1. Abdominal pain in the right lower quadrant (McBurney's point); although pain can be anywhere in the abdomen or flank
  2. Abdominal pain that increases with cough or movement and is relieved by flexion of the right hip or knees suggests a perforated appendix with peritonitis
  3. Nausea and vomiting
  4. Muscle rigidity or rebound tenderness may indicate perforation and peritonitis
  5. Normal or slightly elevated temperature
  6. Increased WBC count with neutrophilia, increased segmented neutrophils
  7. Ultrasound or CT scan showing an enlarged appendix

Planning and Implementation

- Provide routine preoperative care; withhold oral fluids 2 to 4 hours preoperatively to surgical appendectomy (removal of the appendix).
- Administer opioid analgesics and antibiotics.
- Keep the patient in a semi-Fowler's position so that any abdominal drainage can be contained in the lower abdomen.
- An appendectomy may be performed as a traditional procedure through external skin incision (laparoscopy or open procedure) or via endoscopy through a natural orifice such as the vagina.
- Provide routine postoperative care as described in Part One, with an anticipated length of stay of less than 24 hours for uncomplicated procedures and 3 to 5 days when perforation or peritonitis are present.
- Administer analgesics and antibiotics to patients with a complicated appendicitis presentation and surgery.

ARTERIOSCLEROSIS AND ATHEROSCLEROSIS

OVERVIEW

- Arteriosclerosis is a thickening or hardening of the arterial wall of the vascular system.

- Atherosclerosis, a type of arteriosclerosis, involves the formation of a plaque within the arterial wall and is the leading cardiovascular disease.
- The exact pathophysiologic mechanism of atherosclerosis is unknown but is thought to occur with inflammation of the vessel.
- Atherosclerosis begins as a fatty streak on the intimal surface of an artery and develops into a fibrous plaque that occludes the blood flow of the artery.
- When plaque ruptures, thrombosis and constriction obstruct the vessel lumen, causing inadequate perfusion and oxygenation to distal tissues. Unstable plaque rupture causes more severe injury.
- After the rupture occurs, the exposed underlying tissue causes platelet adhesion and rapid thrombus formation. The thrombus may suddenly block a blood vessel, resulting in ischemia and infarction (e.g., MI, ischemic stroke).
- The rate of progression of plaque formation and rupture is thought to be influenced by genetic factors, diabetes mellitus and other chronic conditions, and lifestyle (e.g., smoking, dietary intake of fat, sedentary habits).

PATIENT-CENTERED COLLABORATIVE CARE
Assessment
- Assess:
  1. Risk for cardiovascular disease, using history and standard tools
  2. Blood pressure in both arms and note any differences
  3. Pulses at all major sites and note any differences
  4. Presence of prolonged capillary refill
  5. Presence of temperature differences in lower extremities
  6. Presence of arterial bruits at carotid, abdominal, and femoral pulses
  7. Serum cholesterol (total, low-density lipoprotein [LDL], protective high-density lipoprotein [HDL]) and triglyceride levels.

Interventions
- Interventions include:
  1. Teaching the patient to adopt dietary habits to reduce risk, including limiting fat and saturated fat intake and emphasizing the intake of vegetables, fruit, and whole grains
  2. Developing and reinforcing the plan for regular activity with at least 40 minutes three to four times weekly that is aerobic
  3. Administering cholesterol-lowering drugs as prescribed for the patient
  4. Using best practices to assist patients to stop smoking and informing nonsmokers to avoid secondhand smoke

   5. Planning for follow-up and ongoing care with primary care provider at least annually

ARTHRITIS, RHEUMATOID

OVERVIEW

- Rheumatoid arthritis (RA) is a chronic, progressive, systemic inflammatory autoimmune disease process that damages and destroys synovial joints.
- Transformed autoantibodies (rheumatoid factors [RFs]) attack healthy tissue, especially synovium, causing inflammation.
- Onset may be acute and severe or slow and insidious, and the pattern of illness progression includes remissions and exacerbations.
- Permanent joint changes may be avoided or mitigated when RA is diagnosed early. Early aggressive treatment to suppress synovitis may lead to a remission.
- *Systemic* means that inflammatory factors related to this disease affect more than the joints. Affected body systems include cardiovascular (e.g., vasculitis, myocarditis, pericarditis), lung (e.g., pleurisy, pneumonitis), eyes, and skin. Inflammatory factors also contribute to anorexia, weight loss, and nutritional derangements.
- Genetic factors combine with environmental conditions and interact to trigger RA.

PATIENT-CENTERED COLLABORATIVE CARE

Assessment

- Assess for early disease manifestations, including:
   1. Joint stiffness, swelling, pain (especially of the upper extremities); usually bilateral (affecting both sides) and symmetric (same joints) symptoms
   2. Fatigue, generalized weakness
   3. Anorexia, weight loss
   4. Persistent, low-grade fever
   5. Joint infection (one hot, swollen joint that has pain out of proportion to the other joints)

> **❗ NURSING SAFETY PRIORITY: Critical Rescue**
>
> Refer the patient to the health care provider (usually the rheumatologist) immediately if manifestations of joint infection are present.

- Assess for late disease manifestations.
   1. Joints become progressively inflamed, puffy, and quite painful.
   2. Morning stiffness lasts longer than 45 minutes.
   3. Affected joints have a soft or a spongy feeling.

4. Muscles atrophy above and below affected joints.
5. Range of motion (ROM) decreases and can cause pain (e.g., carpal tunnel syndrome).
6. Most or all of the synovial joints are eventually affected.
7. Joint deformity may develop.
8. There may be Baker's cysts (enlarged popliteal bursae behind the knee).
9. There may be bone fractures.
10. Tendon rupture (especially the Achilles tendon) may occur.
11. Cervical vertebrae disease may result in subluxation that may be life threatening.

! NURSING SAFETY PRIORITY: Critical Rescue

Cervical disease may result in subluxation, especially the first and second vertebrae. This complication may be life threatening because branches of the phrenic nerve that supply the diaphragm are restricted and respiratory function may be compromised. The patient is also in danger of becoming quadriparetic (weak in all extremities) or quadriplegic (paralyzed in all extremities). If a person with RA reports cervical pain (may radiate down one arm) or loss of ROM in the cervical spine, notify the health care provider immediately.

- Assess for systemic complications:
  1. Exacerbations, often called *flares,* manifested by increased joint swelling and tenderness
  2. Infection in affected joints and skin
  3. Moderate to severe weight loss
  4. Fever
  5. Extreme fatigue
  6. Subcutaneous nodules along muscles or tendons, which may become open and infected or interfere with activities of daily living (ADLs)
  7. Inflammation of blood vessels, resulting in vasculitis, particularly of small to medium-sized vessels
  8. Ischemic skin and nail lesions that appear in small groups as small, brownish spots
  9. Larger skin lesions, which appear on the lower extremities and may lead to ulceration, and which heal slowly as a result of vascular changes leading to poor peripheral circulation
  10. Peripheral neuropathy, causing footdrop and paresthesias
  11. Respiratory complications, including pleurisy, pneumonitis, diffuse interstitial fibrosis, and pulmonary hypertension
  12. Cardiac complications, including pericarditis and myocarditis

    13. Ocular involvement, such as iritis or scleritis
    14. Sjögren's syndrome (eye, mouth, and vaginal dryness)
    15. Felty's syndrome (enlarged liver and spleen, leukopenia)
    16. Caplan's syndrome (presence of rheumatoid nodules in the lungs and pneumoconiosis), which is found mainly in coal miners and asbestos workers
- Assess for psychosocial issues:
    1. Fear of becoming disabled and dependent, uncertainty about the disease process, altered body image, devaluation of self, frustration, and depression are common.
    2. Physical limitations may result in role changes in the family and society.
    3. Extreme fatigue often causes patients to desire an early bedtime and may result in a reluctance to socialize.
    4. Body changes may also cause poor self-esteem and body image.
    5. The patient may grieve, experience degrees of depression, or have feelings of helplessness caused by a loss of control over a disease that can "consume" the body.
    6. Evaluate the patient's support systems and resources.
- Assess laboratory data (none are specific for RA, but all are associated with it):
    1. Positive RF
    2. Positive antinuclear antibody test (ANA)
    3. Positive anti-Sjögren's syndrome antibodies, especially anti-SS-A (Ro)
    4. Decreased serum complement
    5. Elevated erythrocyte sedimentation rate
    6. Elevated high-sensitivity C-reactive protein (hsCRP) level
    7. Altered CBC and platelet count (low hematocrit and hemoglobin levels, high WBC count)
- Other diagnostic assessments
    1. Joint x-rays
    2. Bone scan or joint scan
    3. MRI
    4. Arthrocentesis, a procedure to aspirate a sample of the synovial fluid to relieve pressure and analyze the fluid for inflammatory cells and immune complexes, including RF

Interventions
- Drug therapy used to treat RA includes:
    1. Disease-modifying antirheumatic drugs (DMARDs) are used to slow the progression of mild rheumatoid disease before it progresses; they include:
       a. Methotrexate (Rheumatrex)
       b. Leflunomide (Arava)
       c. Hydroxychloroquine (Plaquenil)

2. Nonsteroidal anti-inflammatory drugs (NSAIDs) are often the drug of choice to relieve pain and inflammation on a short-term basis
3. Biological response modifiers (BRMs) interfere with the action of different inflammatory mediators
   a. Etanercept (Enbrel)
   b. Infliximab (Remicade)
   c. Adalimumab (Humira)
   d. Anakinra (Kineret)
   e. Abatacept (Orencia)
   f. Rituximab (Rituxan)
   g. Tocilizumab (Actemra)
   h. Tofacitinib (Xeljanz)
4. Steroidal anti-inflammatory drugs
   a. Prednisone (Deltasone, Medrol)
5. Other immunosuppressive drugs
   a. Azathioprine (Imuran)
   b. Cyclophosphamide (Cytoxan)
- Nonpharmacologic management:
  1. Other pain-relief measures: rest, positioning, ice, and heat
  2. Plasmapheresis (or plasma exchange) to remove the antibodies causing the disease
  3. Pain relief methods such as hypnosis, acupuncture, magnet therapy, imagery, or music therapy
  4. Stress management
  5. Nutrition to meet caloric and protein goals
  6. Nutritional supplementation including omega-3 fatty acid and antioxidant vitamins A, C, and E
- Promotion of self-care:
  1. Identify assistive devices to allow the patient as much independence as possible.
  2. Help the patients acquire household items with handles.
  3. Teach the patient to use larger muscle groups to perform tasks usually performed by fine muscle groups (e.g., use the flat of the hand to squeeze toothpaste tubes instead of the fingers).
  4. Refer the patient to an occupational or physical therapist or the Arthritis Foundation for special assistive and adaptive devices.
- Management of fatigue:
  1. Identify factors that contribute to fatigue (e.g., anemia, muscle atrophy, inadequate rest).
  2. Collaborate with the health care team to alleviate or manage contributing factors.
     a. Anemia
        (1) Administer iron, folic acid, vitamin supplements, or a combination of these.

      (2) Assess the patient for drug-related GI bleeding, such as that caused by NSAID therapy, by testing the stool for occult blood.

   b. Muscle atrophy

      (1) Collaborate with a physical therapist to develop and help the patient implement a personalized daily exercise program.

   c. Inadequate rest

      (1) Arrange for a quiet environment.

      (2) Encourage the patient to develop a bedtime routine for sleep hygiene, such as drinking a warm beverage before bedtime.

3. Teach principles of energy conservation.

   a. Pacing activities

   b. Setting priorities

   c. Planning rest periods

   d. Obtaining assistance when possible; delegating activities to the family

- Enhancement of body image:
  1. Identify factors to enhance body image.
  2. Determine the patient's perception of changes and the impact of the reactions of family and significant others.
  3. Communicate acceptance of the patient by establishing a trusting relationship.
  4. Encourage the patient to wear street clothes and his or her own nightclothes or bathrobe.
  5. Assist with grooming, such as shaving and makeup.
- Community-based care considerations for discharge include:
  1. Assisting the patient and family to identify structural changes needed in the home before discharge
  2. Reinforcing information about drug therapy
  3. Teaching the patient to consult with the health care provider before trying any over-the-counter (OTC) or home remedies
  4. Teaching joint protection measures
  5. Teaching the patient to ask for help to prevent further joint damage and disease progression
  6. Reviewing energy conservation measures
  7. Reviewing the prescribed exercise program
  8. Referring the patient to the nutritionist, counselor, home health nurse, rehabilitation therapist, financial counselor, and local and state support groups as needed

ASTHMA

OVERVIEW

- Bronchial asthma is an intermittent and reversible airflow obstruction affecting only the airways, not the alveoli.

- Airway obstruction occurs in two ways:
  1. Inflammation, obstructing the lumen (the inside) of airways, occurs in response to the presence of specific allergens; general irritants such as cold air, dry air, or fine airborne particles; microorganisms; and aspirin.
  2. Airway hyperresponsiveness, obstructing airways by constricting bronchial smooth muscle and causing a narrowing of the airway from the outside, can occur with exercise, an upper respiratory illness, and for unknown reasons.
- Severe airway obstruction from acute asthma can be fatal.
- Although asthma may be classified into different types based on the events known to trigger the attacks, the pathophysiology is similar for all types of asthma regardless of the triggering event.
- Asthma can occur at any age. About half of adults with asthma also had the disease in childhood. Asthma is more common in urban settings than in rural settings.

Considerations for Older Adults

Asthma occurs as a new disorder in about 3% of people older than 55 years. Another 3% of people older than 60 years have asthma as a continuing chronic disorder. Lung and airway changes as a part of aging make any breathing problem more serious in the older adult. One problem related to aging is a change in the sensitivity of beta-adrenergic receptors. When stimulated, these receptors relax smooth muscle and cause bronchodilation. As these receptors become less sensitive, they no longer respond as quickly or as strongly to agonists (e.g., epinephrine, dopamine) and beta-adrenergic drugs, which are often used as rescue therapy during an acute asthma attack. Teaching older patients how to avoid asthma attacks and to use preventive drug therapy correctly are nursing priorities.

Gender Health Considerations

The incidence of asthma is about 35% higher among women than men, and the asthma death rates are also higher among women. Obesity and hormonal fluctuations around the menstrual cycle are thought to contribute to the difference in incidence, and undertreatment of the disease is thought to be a factor in the higher death rate. Teaching women how to be a partner in asthma management and the correct use of preventive and rescue drugs remains a nursing priority in improving the outcomes of the disease.

PATIENT-CENTERED COLLABORATIVE CARE
Assessment

A

- Obtain the patient's personal history
  1. Episodes of dyspnea, chest tightness, coughing, wheezing, and increased mucus production
  2. Specific patterns of dyspnea appearance (at night, with exercise, seasonally, or in association with other specific activities or environments)
  3. Other allergic symptoms such as rhinitis, skin rash, or pruritus, and whether other family members have asthma or respiratory problems
- Clinical manifestations during an attack include:
  1. Decreased peak expiratory flow
  2. Audible wheeze (at first, louder on exhalation)
  3. Increased respiratory rate
  4. Coughing
  5. Inability to complete a sentence of more than five words
  6. Decreased oxygen saturation
  7. Pallor or cyanosis of oral mucous membranes and nail beds
  8. Tachycardia
  9. Changes in level of consciousness
  10. Use of accessory muscles (muscle retraction at the sternum, the suprasternal notch, and between the ribs)
- Physical changes from frequent asthma attacks include:
  1. Increased anteroposterior (AP) chest diameter
  2. Increased space between the ribs
- Laboratory assessment data changes during an asthma attack:
  1. Decreased Pao_2
  2. Decreased partial pressure of carbon dioxide ($Paco_2$) (early in attack)
  3. Elevated $Paco_2$ (later in attack)
- Laboratory assessment data changes from allergic asthma:
  1. Elevated serum eosinophil count
  2. Elevated immunoglobulin E (IgE) levels
  3. Sputum-containing eosinophils, mucous plugs, and shed epithelial cells (Curschmann's spirals)
- Diagnostic assessment:
  1. Pulmonary function tests (PFTs) measured using spirometry, especially:
     a. Forced vital capacity (FVC) (volume of air exhaled from full inhalation to full exhalation)
     b. Forced expiratory volume in the first second (FEV_1) (volume of air blown out as hard and fast as possible during the first second of the most forceful exhalation after the greatest full inhalation)

    c. Peak expiratory flow (PEF) (fastest airflow rate reached at any time during exhalation)

  2. Chest x-ray

Interventions

- The goals of asthma therapy are to improve airflow, relieve symptoms, and prevent episodes by making the patient an active partner in the management plan.
- Priority patient education focuses on:
  1. Teaching the patient to assess symptom severity at least twice daily with a peak flowmeter and adjust drugs to manage inflammation and bronchospasms to prevent or relieve symptoms
  2. Assisting the patient to establish a "personal best" peak expiratory flow (PEF) by measuring his or her PEF twice daily for 2 to 3 weeks when asthma is well controlled and using this value to compare against all other readings
  3. Instructing the patient to evaluate when to use a rescue inhaler ("yellow zone" or PEF is between 50% and 80% of personal best) and when to seek emergency assistance ("red zone" or PEF is below 50% of personal best)

! NURSING SAFETY PRIORITY: Critical Rescue

Teach the patient that if a "red zone" reading occurs when using the peak flowmeter to immediately use the reliever drugs and seek emergency help.

  4. Teaching the patient to keep a symptom and intervention diary to learn his or her triggers of asthma symptoms, early cues for impending attacks, and personal response to drugs

  5. Stressing the importance of proper use of the asthma action plan for any severity of asthma

- Drug therapy focuses on prevention of asthma attacks (preventive therapy) and stopping attacks that have already started (rescue therapy).
- Many preventive and rescue drugs are delivered as dry powder inhalers (DPIs) or as aerosol metered dose inhalers (MDIs). Teach patients the proper ways to use and store these inhalers.
- Preventive therapy drugs are those used to change airway responsiveness to prevent asthma attacks from occurring. They are used every day, regardless of symptoms.

! NURSING SAFETY PRIORITY: Critical Rescue

Teach patients using preventive therapy to take the prescribed drugs daily, even when asthma symptoms are not present.

1. Bronchodilators increase bronchiolar smooth muscle relaxation and include beta$_2$ agonists, cholinergic antagonists, and methylxanthines.
   a. Long-acting beta$_2$ agonists (LABAs) are delivered by inhaler directly to the site of action, the bronchioles. They need time to build up an effect, but the effects are longer lasting. The use of LABAs is recommended to be co-administered with inhaled steroids.

❗ NURSING SAFETY PRIORITY: Drug Alert

These drugs are useful in preventing an asthma attack but have no value during an acute attack. Teach patients *not* to use LABAs to rescue them during an attack or when wheezing is getting worse.

---

   b. Cholinergic antagonists (anticholinergic drugs) are similar to atropine and block the parasympathetic nervous system, causing bronchodilation and decreased pulmonary secretions. Most are used by inhaler:
      (1) Ipratropium (Atrovent)
      (2) Tiotropium (Spiriva)
   c. Methylxanthines are used when other types of management are ineffective:
      (1) Theophylline (Theo-Dur)
      (2) Aminophylline (Truphylline)
      (3) Oxtriphylline (Choledyl)
      (4) Dyphylline (Dilor, Lufyllin)

❗ NURSING SAFETY PRIORITY: Critical Rescue

Teach the patient who takes these drugs daily to keep all appointments for monitoring blood levels of the drug and not to self-increase the dose. These drugs have narrow safety ranges and have many dangerous side effects, especially cardiac and central nervous system stimulation.

---

2. Anti-inflammatory drugs alter the immune and inflammatory responses in the airways. Some are given systemically and have more side effects. Others are used as inhalants and have few systemic side effects.
   a. Inhaled corticosteroids (ICSs):
      (1) Fluticasone (Flovent)
      (2) Budesonide (Pulmicort)
      (3) Mometasone (Asmanex)

b. NSAIDs
   (1) Nedocromil (Tilade)
   (2) Cromolyn sodium (Intal)
c. Leukotriene antagonists:
   (1) Montelukast (Singulair)
   (2) Zafirlukast (Accolate)
   (3) Zileuton (Zyflo)
d. Immunomodulators:
   (1) Omalizumab (Xolair)
- Rescue therapy drugs are those used to stop an attack once it has started. Short-acting beta$_2$ agonists (SABAs) provide rapid but short-term relief. These inhaled drugs are most useful when an attack begins (rescue drug) or as premedication when the patient is about to begin an activity that is likely to induce an asthma attack.
  1. Albuterol (Proventil, Ventolin)
  2. Bitolterol (Tornalate)
  3. Levalbuterol (Xopenex)
  4. Pirbuterol (Maxair)
  5. Terbutaline (Brethaire)

> **! NURSING SAFETY PRIORITY: Critical Rescue**
>
> Teach the patient to always carry the rescue drug inhaler with him or her and to ensure that there is enough drug remaining in the inhaler to provide a quick dose when needed.

- Regular exercise, including aerobic exercise, is a recommended part of asthma therapy.
  1. Teach patients to examine the conditions that trigger an attack and adjust the exercise routine as needed.
  2. Some patients may need to premedicate with inhaled SABAs before beginning activity.
- Supplemental oxygen with a high flow rate or high concentration is often used during an acute asthma attack. Oxygen is delivered by mask, nasal cannula, or endotracheal tube.
- Heliox, a mixture of helium and oxygen (often 50% helium and 50% oxygen) can help improve oxygen delivery to the alveoli.
- *Status asthmaticus* is a severe, life-threatening acute episode of airway obstruction that intensifies once it begins and often does not respond to usual therapy.
  1. Assess for manifestations, including:
     a. Extremely labored breathing and wheezing
     b. Use of accessory muscles
     c. Distention of neck veins

  d. PEF below 50% of expected for patient's age, size, and gender
  e. Oxygen saturation less than 80%
2. Apply oxygen.
3. Anticipate administration of immediate therapy, including:
  a. IV fluids
  b. Repeated doses of inhaled bronchodilators
  c. IV steroids
4. Prepare for emergency intubation.

B

BEDBUGS

- A common emerging parasite is the bedbug, *Cimex lectularius*. Increased infestation is attributed to travel and resistance to pesticides.
- A bedbug bite causes an itchy discomfort. Bedbugs feed on human blood but do not cause disease.
- The adult bedbug is the approximate size, shape, and color of an apple seed.
- Eradicating the infestation and preventing re-infestations requires considerable effort, including the use of multiple powerful pesticides and extreme temperature.

BLINDNESS

See *Visual Impairment (Reduced Vision)*.

BONE MARROW TRANSPLANTATION (HEMATOPOIETIC STEM CELL TRANSPLANTATION)
OVERVIEW

- Hematopoietic stem cell transplantation (HSCT) is the process of collecting stem cells from one person (the donor) and transplanting them into another person (the recipient) or into the same person at a later time.
- *Stem cells* are immature and undifferentiated cells that can mature into any blood cell type.
- Sources of stem cells include the bone marrow, circulating peripheral blood, and cord blood from newborns.
- When stem cells are obtained from the bone marrow, the process is called *bone marrow transplantation (BMT)*.
- When stem cells are transplanted into a recipient, the new cells go to the marrow and then begin the process of hematopoiesis, which results in normal, properly functioning WBCs, RBCs, and platelets.

- Disorders that can be cured by HSCT include acute leukemia, lymphoma, multiple myeloma, aplastic anemia, sickle cell disease, and many solid tumors.
- After successful HSCT, the recipient has the blood type and the immune function of the donor.
- The three types of transplantation are:
  1. *Allogeneic transplantation,* in which the stem cells are taken from a sibling or human leukocyte antigen (HLA)-matched, unrelated donor
  2. *Autologous transplantation,* in which the donor receives his or her own stem cells (collected before any cytotoxic treatment)
  3. *Syngeneic transplantation,* in which the stem cells are taken from the patient's own identical sibling

⊕ Cultural Considerations

About 70% of people on the bone marrow donor lists are white. The chance of finding an HLA-matched, unrelated donor is estimated at 30% to 40% for white individuals, but for black individuals the chance is less than 20%, because there are fewer black Americans among registered donors. Although blood types are common in all racial groups, tissue types can be very different among racial and ethnic groups. Nationally, efforts are made to publicize the need for donors from all cultural and ethnic backgrounds. Research in this area has identified several potential barriers to stem cell donation among black individuals. These include fear of or not trusting the system, concern about costs to the donor, and concern that the recipient may be a drug abuser or a person who would not appreciate the sacrifice of a donation. Targeted education efforts may reduce these barriers.

- HSCT has five phases:
  1. *Stem cell obtainment* involves taking stem cells either from the patient directly (autologous stem cells) or from an HLA-matched person (allogeneic stem cells).
     a. *Peripheral stem cell harvesting* requires mobilization using growth factors to artificially increase stem cells in the donor and collection by apheresis, a form of dialysis.
     b. *Cord blood harvesting* involves obtaining stem cells from umbilical cord blood of newborns.
  2. *Conditioning regimen* involves "wiping out" the patient's own bone marrow, thus preparing the patient for optimal graft take. This process includes giving higher than normal doses of chemotherapy or radiotherapy to rid the person of

cancer cells (myeloablation). Usually a period of 5 to 10 days is required.

3. *Transplantation* is the infusion of the stem cells through the patient's central catheter, similar to the processes for a blood transfusion.

4. *Engraftment* is the process of the transplanted cells moving into the recipient's bone marrow and beginning to make new, functioning blood cells.

5. *Post-transplantation recovery* is the time between when engraftment begins and full recovery of immune function, RBC function, and platelet function occur.

PATIENT-CENTERED COLLABORATIVE CARE

* During apheresis, monitor the donor for:
  1. Hypotension
  2. Catheter clotting
  3. Hypocalcemia
     a. Numbness or tingling in the fingers and toes or around the mouth
     b. Abdominal or muscle cramping
     c. Chest pain
* Patient care for the recipient:
  1. Conditioning:
     a. The day the patient receives the stem cells is day T-0. Before transplantation, the conditioning days are counted in reverse order from T-0, just like a rocket countdown. After transplantation, days are counted in order from the day of transplantation.
     b. The conditioning regimen is individually tailored to each patient and usually includes high-dose chemotherapy and sometimes includes total-body irradiation (TBI) over 3 to 5 days.
     c. Immediate side effects from conditioning are intense or severe and include:
        (1) Nausea and vomiting
        (2) Mucositis
        (3) Capillary leak syndrome
        (4) Diarrhea
        (5) Pancytopenia related to bone marrow suppression

❗ NURSING SAFETY PRIORITY: Critical Rescue

During conditioning and before engraftment, the patient is at great risk for life-threatening infection. Infection protection is the priority for management at this time.

      d. Late effects from the conditioning regimen are also common 3 to 10 years after transplantation. These problems include veno-occlusive disease (VOD), skin toxicities, cataracts, lung fibrosis, second cancers, cardiomyopathy, endocrine complications, and neurologic complications.

  2. Transplantation using best practices for infusion therapy

---

❗ NURSING SAFETY PRIORITY: Action Alert

Do not use blood administration tubing, because the cells can get caught in the filter and not enter the patient's body.

---

      a. Side effects of all types of stem cell transfusions are similar and may include:

        (1) Fever

        (2) Hypertension

        (3) Fluid overload

        (4) Red urine (resulting from RBC breakage in the infused stem cells)

  3. Engraftment:

      a. The successful acceptance of the transplanted cells in the patient's bone marrow is essential to the whole transplantation process.

      b. Engraftment takes 8 to 12 days for peripheral blood stem cell transplantation and 12 to 28 days for bone marrow stem cell transplantation.

      c. To aid engraftment, growth factors such as granulocyte colony-stimulating factor (G-CSF) or granulocyte-macrophage colony-stimulating factor (GM-CSF) may be given. When engraftment occurs, the patient's WBC, RBC, and platelet counts begin to rise.

      d. Nursing care focuses on prevention of complications, which include:

        (1) Infection

        (2) Bleeding

        (3) Failure to engraft (*If the transplanted cells fail to engraft, the patient will die unless another transplantation is successful*).

        (4) Development of graft-versus-host disease (GVHD), in which the immunocompetent cells of the donated marrow recognize the patient's (recipient) cells, tissues, and organs as foreign and start an immunologic attack against them. GVHD occurs most often in the skin, intestinal tract, and liver, and more than 15% of the

patients who develop GVHD die of its complications. Manifestations are:

i. Excessive peeling of the skin

ii. Profuse, watery diarrhea

iii. Liver tenderness, with jaundice

(5) Development of veno-occlusive disease (VOD), which is the blockage of liver blood vessels by clotting and inflammation (phlebitis). Manifestations include:

i. Jaundice

ii. Pain in the right upper quadrant

iii. Ascites

iv. Weight gain

v. Liver enlargement

(6) Depression (contributing factors include prolonged hospitalization, limited activity, intense therapy side effects, and uncertain treatment outcome)

BREAST CONDITION, FIBROCYSTIC
OVERVIEW

- The two main features of fibrocystic breast condition (FBC) are fibrosis and cysts. Areas of fibrosis are made up of fibrous connective tissue and are firm or hard. Cysts are spaces filled with fluid lined by breast glandular cells.
- This condition most often occurs in premenopausal women between 20 and 50 years of age.
- FBC is thought to be caused by an imbalance in the normal estrogen-to-progesterone ratio.
- Typical symptoms include breast pain and tender lumps or areas of thickening in the breasts. The lumps are rubbery, ill defined, and commonly found in the upper outer quadrant of the breast.

PATIENT-CENTERED COLLABORATIVE CARE
Interventions

- Management of FBC focuses on the symptoms of the condition:
  1. Supportive measures such as the use of mild analgesics or limiting salt intake before menses can help decrease swelling.
  2. Wearing a supportive bra can reduce pain by decreasing tension on the ligaments, although some women find that not wearing a bra is more comfortable.
  3. Local application of ice or heat may provide temporary relief of pain.
  4. If drug therapy is indicated, oral contraceptives may be prescribed to suppress oversecretion of estrogen, and progestins may be used to correct luteal insufficiency.

! **NURSING SAFETY PRIORITY: Drug Alert**

Explain to women the benefits and risks associated with drug therapy for FBC, such as stroke, liver disease, and increased intracranial pressure. Teach them to seek medical attention immediately if any signs and symptoms of these complications occur.

5. Vitamins C, E, and B complex may reduce cyst formation.
6. Diuretics may be prescribed to decrease premenstrual breast engorgement.
7. Reduction of dietary fat and caffeine has been suggested, although the role of caffeine and fat in FBC is unclear.
8. Teach patients to follow guidelines for breast self-examination, obtain breast examinations by a health care provider regularly, and undergo mammographic or MRI diagnostic testing.

BURNS

OVERVIEW

- A burn is a complex injury with loss of tissue integrity that results from exposure to temperature extremes, mechanical abrasion, chemical abrasion, radiation, and electrical currents.
- Local and systemic problems resulting from burns include fluid and protein losses, sepsis, and changes in physiologic, metabolic, and psychological function.
- The priorities in care are prevention of infection and closure of the burn wound, because a lack of or delay in wound healing is a key factor for all systemic problems and a major cause of disability and death among patients who are burned.
- Burn severity is determined by the extent to which skin and the underlying tissue is damaged (wound depth) and by how much of the body surface area is involved. Wound depth in burns has four classifications and two classes have subcategories:
  1. *Superficial-thickness wounds* have the least damage, with injury to the epidermis alone occurring. The epithelial cells and basement membrane, needed for total regrowth, remain. Common causes of superficial-thickness wounds are prolonged exposure to low-intensity heat (e.g., sunburn) or short (flash) exposure to high-intensity heat. Redness with mild edema, pain, and increased sensitivity to heat occur as a result. The area heals rapidly in 3 to 6 days without a scar or other complication.
  2. *Partial-thickness wounds* involve the entire epidermis and various depths of the dermis. Depending on the amount of dermal tissue damaged, partial-thickness wounds are further

subdivided into superficial partial-thickness and deep partial-thickness injuries.

   a. *Superficial partial-thickness wounds* are caused by heat injury to the upper third of the dermis, leaving a good blood supply. Wounds are red, moist, and blanch (whiten) when pressure is applied. Blisters often form. Nerve endings are exposed, and any stimulation (touch or temperature change) causes intense pain. With care, these burns heal in 10 to 21 days with no permanent scar, but some minor pigment changes may occur.

   b. *Deep partial-thickness wounds* extend deeper into the skin dermis, and fewer healthy cells remain. Blister formation does not usually occur. The wound surface is red and dry, with white areas in deeper parts. Edema is moderate and reduced blood flow can result in a deeper injury. Pain may be less compared to more superficial burns because more nerve endings have been destroyed. Healing occurs over 3 to 6 weeks with scar formation.

3. *Full-thickness wounds* occur with destruction of the entire epidermis and dermis, leaving no true skin cells to repopulate. The wounded tissue does not regrow, and whatever area of the wound not closed by wound contraction will require grafting. The wound has a hard, dry, leathery eschar that must slough off or be removed from the burn wound before healing can occur. The wound may be waxy white, deep red, yellow, brown, or black. Sensation is reduced or absent in these areas because of nerve ending destruction. Edema is severe under the eschar in a full-thickness wound.

   a. When the injury is circumferential (completely surrounds an extremity or the chest), blood flow and chest movement for breathing may be reduced by tight eschar.

   b. *Escharotomies* (incisions through the eschar) or *fasciotomies* (incisions through eschar and fascia) may be needed to relieve pressure and allow normal blood flow and breathing.

4. *Deep full-thickness wounds* extend beyond the skin into underlying fascia and tissues. Muscle, bone, and tendons are damaged and exposed. The wound is blackened and depressed, and sensation is completely absent. Healing takes weeks to months.

- Common causes of burn injury and emergency interventions to limit injury:

   1. *Dry heat injuries* result from open flames. The patient should stop, drop, and roll to smother the flames.

   2. *Moist heat (scald) injuries* are caused by contact with hot liquids or steam. Clothes that are saturated with hot liquids should be removed immediately.

3. *Contact burns* occur when hot metal, tar, or grease contact the skin, often leading to a full-thickness injury. Removal of the hot substance limits the injury.

4. *Chemical burns* occur as a result of accidents in the home or workplace. The severity of the injury depends on the duration of contact, the concentration of the chemical, the amount of tissue exposed, and the action of the chemical. Dry chemicals should be brushed off the skin and clothing. Wet clothing is removed. Depending on the specific agent, the skin may be flushed with water or covered with mineral oil.

5. *Electrical injury burns* occur when an electrical current enters the body. These injuries have been called the "grand masquerader" of burn injuries, because the surface injuries may look small but the associated internal injuries can be huge. The longer the electricity is in contact with the body, the greater the damage. The patient should be removed from the source of the electricity in such a way that the care provider does not place himself or herself in danger (use a wooden pole, rather than a metal one, to separate the person from the electrical source). *The person must not be touched directly while he or she is in contact with the electrical source!*

6. *Radiation injuries* occur when people are exposed to large doses of radioactive material. The most common type of tissue injury from radiation exposure occurs with therapeutic radiation. More serious injury occurs in industrial settings where radioactive energy is produced or radioactive isotopes are used. Removal of the patient from the source of radiation limits the injury.

• Compensatory responses to the stress of the injury and the direct tissue damage occur through the sympathetic nervous system and inflammatory responses. These result in specific and predictable changes in tissue and organ function:

1. Inflammation

2. Vital sign changes (decreased BP, tachycardia, increased respiratory rate and depth)

3. Capillary leak with a *fluid shift* into the interstitial space. This fluid shift, also known as *third spacing* or *capillary leak syndrome,* is a continuous leak of plasma from the vascular space into the interstitial space. The loss of plasma fluids and proteins decreases blood volume and blood pressure and causes extensive edema, even in areas that were not burned. Fluid shift into tissues with dramatic weight gain usually occurs in the first 12 hours after the burn and can continue for 24 to 36 hours. Fluid returns to the vascular space within 48 to 72 hours.

    4. Decreased urine output
    5. Hemoconcentration (elevated hematocrit and hemoglobin values)
    6. Fluid and electrolyte imbalances (most commonly metabolic acidosis), hyperkalemia (high blood potassium levels), and hyponatremia (low blood sodium levels)
    7. Decreased to absent peristalsis, formation of Curling's ulcer
    8. Elevated blood glucose levels
    9. Hypermetabolism and body temperature variation
- Burn recovery occurs over the course of three phases. Each phase has unique manifestations and care requirements.

RESUSCITATION PHASE OF BURN INJURY
- The resuscitation, or *emergent,* phase is the first phase of a burn injury. It begins at the onset of injury and continues to about 48 hours.
- The goals of management during the resuscitation/emergent phase are to:
    1. Secure the airway
    2. Support circulation and organ perfusion with fluid replacement
    3. Keep the patient comfortable with analgesics
    4. Prevent infection through careful wound care
    5. Maintain body temperature
    6. Provide emotional support

PATIENT-CENTERED COLLABORATIVE CARE
Assessment
- During assessment, obtain the following injury-related information:
    1. Time of the injury
    2. Source of heat or injurious agent
    3. Detailed description of how and where the burn occurred
    4. Any interventions or other actions taken
    5. Whether drugs or alcohol may have been a factor
    6. Events occurring from the time of the burn to admission
    7. Any other events that could increase the burn injury or cause another injury or health problem
- Obtain the following personal patient information:
    1. Age
    2. Height and weight
    3. Medical history (especially cardiac or kidney disease, chronic alcoholism, substance abuse, diabetes mellitus)
    4. Use of prescribed, OTC, or street drugs within the past 24 hours
    5. Smoking history

6. Level of pain
7. Allergies
8. Immunization status (especially tetanus)
* Assess for:
  1. Direct airway injury:
     a. Changes in the appearance or function of the mouth, nose, or throat
     b. Facial burns; singed hair on the head, eyebrows, eyelids, or nose
     c. Blisters or soot on the lips, on oral mucosa, or in sputum
     d. "Smoky" smell of the breath
     e. Progressive hoarseness, wheezing, crowing, stridor
     f. Decreased oxygen saturation
     g. Drooling (inability to swallow oral secretions)

! NURSING SAFETY PRIORITY: Critical Rescue

For a burn patient in the resuscitation phase who is hoarse, has a brassy cough, drools, has difficulty swallowing, or produces an audible breath sound on exhalation, immediately apply oxygen and notify the Rapid Response Team.

  2. Carbon monoxide poisoning:
     a. Headache
     b. Decreased cognitive functioning, confusion, coma
     c. Tinnitus
     d. Nausea
     e. Absence of cyanosis or pallor (lips and mucous membranes may appear bright red)
     f. Elevated carboxyhemoglobin levels
  3. Smoke poisoning/inhalation:
     a. Atelectasis, pulmonary edema
     b. Hemorrhagic bronchitis (6 to 72 hours after injury)
  4. Pulmonary fluid overload:
     a. Dyspnea
     b. Hypoxia
     c. Moist breath sounds and crackles
  5. Cardiovascular changes:
     a. Hypovolemic and cardiogenic shock
     b. Circulatory overload with left-sided congestive heart failure
     c. Rapid, thready pulse
     d. Reduced peripheral pulses
     e. Slow or absent capillary refill
     f. Generalized edema

    g. Weight gain
    h. Baseline and continuous electrocardiographic tracings
  6. Renal or urinary changes:
    a. Decreased urine output (less than 0.5 to 1 mL/kg/hr)
    b. High urine specific gravity
    c. Proteinuria
    d. Absence of urine output
  7. Skin changes:
    a. Depth of injury
    b. Size of injury by the total body surface area (TBSA)
    c. Color and appearance
  8. Gastrointestinal changes:
    a. Decreased or absent bowel sounds
    b. Nausea, vomiting
    c. Abdominal distention
    d. Ulcer formation
    e. Gross or occult blood in vomitus or stool
- Laboratory assessment:
  1. Increased WBCs, with the differential reporting increased neutrophils
  2. Electrolytes
  3. Liver enzyme studies
  4. Clotting studies

🌐 Cultural Considerations

For black individuals with an African heritage, a serum laboratory assay called a sickle cell preparation may be appropriate if sickle status is unknown. The trauma of a burn injury can trigger a sickle cell crisis in patients who have the disease and in those who carry the trait.

Planning and Implementation
- The priority problems for the patient with burn injuries in the resuscitation phase who have sustained a burn injury greater than 25% of the TBSA are:
  1. Potential for inadequate oxygenation related to upper airway edema, pulmonary edema, airway obstruction, or pneumonia
  2. Risk for shock related to increase in capillary permeability, active fluid volume loss, electrolyte imbalance, and inadequate fluid
  3. Potential for organ ischemia (e.g., brain, heart, kidney, gastrointestinal) related to hypovolemia and hypotension
  4. Pain (acute and chronic) related to tissue injury, damaged or exposed nerve endings, débridement, dressing changes, invasive procedures, and donor sites

5. Potential for ARDS related to inhalation injury
6. Risk for infection

INADEQUATE OXYGENATION

Nonsurgical Management

- Interventions include airway maintenance, promotion of ventilation, monitoring gas exchange, oxygen therapy, drug therapy, positioning, and deep breathing.
- Assess hourly for fluid overload (e.g., presence of lung crackles, distended neck veins, decreased cognition, decreased oxygen saturation, and low urine output).
- Coordinate respiratory therapy and ventilation support to maintain airway.
- When the patient is receiving mechanical ventilation or noninvasive ventilator support, interventions are aimed at optimizing oxygenation and avoiding additional lung injury.
  1. Give prescribed positive end-expiratory pressure (PEEP) therapy to provide a continuous positive pressure in the airways and alveoli and enhance the diffusion of oxygen across the alveolar-capillary membrane. PEEP can be combined with intermittent mandatory volume.
  2. Assess and document the patient's response:
     a. Monitor oxygen saturation continuously; communicate decrements greater than 5% or values less than 92% immediately to prescribing health care provider and anticipate oxygen supplementation interventions.
     b. Evaluate ABG levels for low oxygenation (Pao_2 less than 90 mm Hg) or hypercarbia ($Paco_2$ greater than 46 mm Hg).

! NURSING SAFETY PRIORITY: Critical Rescue

Immediately report any signs of respiratory distress or change in respiratory patterns to the health care team and the respiratory therapist.

  3. Administer prescribed neuromuscular blocking drugs to patients receiving mechanical ventilation to reduce oxygen consumption.

Surgical Management

- A tracheotomy may be needed when long-term intubation is expected. This procedure increases the risk for infection in burn patients even more than in nonburned patients. Emergency tracheotomies are performed when an airway becomes occluded and oral or nasal intubation cannot be achieved.

HYPOVOLEMIC SHOCK

Interventions are aimed at increasing blood fluid volume, supporting compensatory mechanisms, and preventing complications. Nonsurgical management is often sufficient for achieving these aims. Surgical management is required most often for full-thickness burns.

Nonsurgical Management

*   Fluid volume and tissue blood flow are restored through IV fluid therapy (rapid IV therapy is called *fluid resuscitation* and is guided by a well-established formula based on the size and depth of burn injury) and drug therapy. Priority nursing interventions are carrying out fluid resuscitation and monitoring for indications of effectiveness or complications.

Considerations for Older Adults

In older patients, especially those with cardiac disease, a complicating factor in fluid resuscitation may be heart failure or MI. Drugs that increase cardiac output (e.g., dopamine [Intropin]) or that strengthen the force of myocardial contraction may be used along with fluid therapy.

Surgical Management

*   An escharotomy may be needed when tight eschar impairs tissue perfusion.
*   A fasciotomy (a deeper incision extending through the fascia) may be needed to relieve constriction from fluid buildup when a burn completely surrounds an extremity.

PAIN MANAGEMENT

Pain management is tailored to the patient's tolerance for pain, coping mechanisms, and physical status. The priority nursing actions include continually assessing the patient's pain level, using appropriate pain-reducing strategies, and preventing complications.

Nonsurgical Management

*   Interventions for the patient having pain include drug therapy, complementary therapy measures, and environmental manipulation.
*   Assess the patient's pain level hourly until pain is well controlled, then every 2 to 4 hours.
*   Administer drug therapy with opioid (e.g., morphine, hydromorphone [Dilaudid], fentanyl) and non-opioid analgesics. For the alert patient, consider using patient-controlled analgesia.

! NURSING SAFETY PRIORITY: Critical Rescue

Give opioid drugs for pain only by the intravenous route during the resuscitation phase. Absorption through the gastrointestinal tract or other tissues may be delayed. Later, as edema resolves, doses can be rapidly absorbed resulting in lethal blood levels of analgesics.

- Provide a quiet environment to promote rest and sleep.
- Coordinate with all members of the health care team to ensure that most procedures are performed during the patient's waking hours.
- Use alternative and complementary pain management techniques, including relaxation techniques, meditative breathing, guided imagery, music therapy, massage, and healing or therapeutic touch.
  Surgical Management
- Surgical management for pain involves early surgical excision of the burn wound.

ACUTE PHASE OF BURN INJURY
- The acute phase of burn injury begins about 48 hours after injury and lasts until wound closure is complete.
- A multidisciplinary approach to care will continue to be needed.
- Care focuses on continued assessment and maintenance of the cardiovascular and respiratory systems, as well as toward GI and nutritional status, burn wound care, pain control, and psychosocial interventions.
- Complications of this phase include pneumonia, malnutrition, loss of musculoskeletal function, infection, and sepsis.

PATIENT-CENTERED COLLABORATIVE CARE
Assessment
- Assess for:
  1. Cardiopulmonary dysfunction:
     a. Pneumonia
     b. Respiratory failure
  2. Neuroendocrine dysfunction:
     a. Hypothermia
     b. Weight loss, negative nitrogen balance, malnutrition
  3. Immune system dysfunction:
     a. Wound healing impairment
     b. Systemic infection and sepsis
  4. Musculoskeletal dysfunction:
     a. Muscle atrophy
     b. Contracture formation manifested by decreased ROM
  5. Pain
  6. Maladaptive psychosocial responses
Planning and Implementation
- Priority nursing problems for patients with burn injuries greater than 25% TBSA in the acute phase of recovery are:
  1. Wound care management related to burn injury, skin grafting procedures, and immobilization

2. Risk for infection related to open burn wounds, the presence of multiple invasive catheters, reduced immune function, and poor nutrition (NANDA-I)
3. Excessive weight loss related to increased metabolic rate, reduced calorie intake, and increased urinary nitrogen losses
4. Impaired mobility related to open burn wounds, pain, and scars and contractures (NANDA-I)
5. Reduced self-image related to trauma, changes in physical appearance and lifestyle, and alterations in sensory and motor function

WOUND CARE MANAGEMENT
Nonsurgical Management
- Assess all burn wounds at least daily for:
  1. Adequacy of circulation
  2. Size and depth of injury
  3. Presence of infection
  4. Evidence of healing: granulation, re-epithelialization, scar tissue formation, decreased wound size
- Participate in wound débridement procedures to remove debris and nonliving tissue from the burn wound.
  1. *Mechanical débridement* can be performed one or two times daily with hydrotherapy. The patient can be immersed in a tub, showered on a specially designed shower table, or have only small areas of the wound washed at the bedside. Nurses and skilled technicians use forceps and scissors to remove loose, nonviable tissue during hydrotherapy. Burn areas are washed thoroughly and gently with mild soap or detergent and water.
  2. *Enzymatic débridement* can occur naturally by autolysis or, more commonly, artificially by the application of exogenous agents. A topical agent is applied directly to the burn wound in once-daily dressing changes. The enzymes digest collagen in necrotic tissues.
  3. Dress the burn wound using standard wound dressings, biologic dressings, synthetic dressings, or artificial skin.
     a. *Standard wound dressings* involve cleansing the wound, applying a topical antimicrobial agent, and then applying multiple layers of gauze over the topical agents. The number of gauze layers depends on the depth of the injury, amount of drainage expected, area injured, patient's mobility, and frequency of dressing changes. The gauze layers are held in place with roller-type gauze bandages applied in a distal to proximal direction or with circular net fabrics. Dressings are reapplied every 8 to 24 hours.
     b. *Biologic dressings* are skin or membranes obtained from human tissue donors or animals. When applied over open

wounds, a biologic dressing rapidly adheres and promotes healing or prepares the wound for permanent skin graft coverage. Types of biologic dressings include:

(1) *Homografts (allografts)* are human skin obtained from a cadaver and provided through a skin bank.

(2) *Heterografts (xenografts)* are skin obtained from another species. Pig skin is the most common heterograft and is compatible with human skin.

(3) *Cultured skin* can be grown from a small specimen of epidermal cells from an unburned area of the patient's body. Cells are grown in a laboratory to produce cell sheets that can be grafted on the patient to generate a permanent skin surface.

(4) *Artificial skin* is an alternative approach to closure of the burn wound. This substance has two layers: a Silastic epidermis and a porous dermis made from beef collagen and shark cartilage.

c. *Biosynthetic wound dressings* are a combination of biosynthetic and synthetic materials. Biobrane is the most common type and is made up of a nylon fabric that is partially embedded into a silicone film. Collagen is incorporated into both the silicone and nylon components. The nylon fabric comes into contact with the wound surface and forms an adherent bond until epithelialization has occurred. The porous silicone film allows exudates to pass through.

d. *Synthetic dressings* are made of solid silicone and plastic membranes (e.g., polyvinyl chloride, polyurethane). They are applied directly to the surface of a clean or surgically prepared wound and remain in place until they fall off or are removed. Many are transparent or translucent, allowing the wound to be inspected without removing the dressing.

Surgical Management

- Surgical management of burn wounds focuses on excision and wound covering. Surgical excision is performed early in the postburn period. Grafting may be performed throughout the acute phase as burn wounds are made ready and donor sites are available. Early grafting reduces the time patients are at risk for infection and sepsis. Wound covering by autografting involves taking healthy skin from an area of the patient's intact skin and transplanting it to an excised burn wound.

INFECTION

- Burn wound infection can occur through *autocontamination,* in which the patient's own normal flora overgrows and invades other body areas, and *cross-contamination,* in which organisms from other people or environments are transferred to the patient.

Nonsurgical Management
- Drug therapy for infection prevention:
    1. Tetanus toxoid, an IM vaccine, is routinely given when the patient is admitted to the hospital. Additional administration of tetanus immune globulin (human) (Hyper-Tet) is recommended when the patient's history of tetanus immunization is not known.
    2. Topical antimicrobial drugs are used at every dressing change or wound cleansing to prevent infection in burn wounds. The goal of this therapy is to reduce bacterial growth into the wound and prevent systemic sepsis. The most commonly used agents are silver sulfadiazine (Silvadene, Flamazine ❦) and mafenide (Sulfamylon).
- Drug therapy for treatment of infection:
    1. Systemic broad-spectrum antibiotics are used when burn patients have symptoms of an infection, including septicemia. After results of blood cultures and sensitivity status are available, specific drugs may be changed to those that are effective against the specific organisms causing the infection.
- Providing a safe environment:
    1. Use aseptic technique with all wound interventions.
    2. Ensure appropriate use of asepsis by all health care team members.
        a. Wear gloves during all contact with open wounds.
        b. Do not share equipment among patients.
        c. Use disposable items as much as possible.
        d. Ensure daily cleaning of patient's room and bathroom.
    3. Do not keep plants or flowers in the patient's room; they are a source of microbes.
    4. Restrict visitors to healthy adults.
    5. Consider reverse isolation therapy.
- Monitoring for early recognition of infection by assessing the burn wounds at each dressing change for:
    1. Pervasive odor
    2. Color changes: focal, dark red, brown discoloration in the eschar
    3. Change in texture
    4. Purulent drainage
    5. Exudate
    6. Sloughing grafts
    7. Redness at the wound edges extending to nonburned skin

Surgical Management
- Infected burn wounds with colony counts of or approaching 10^5 colonies per gram of tissue are life threatening and may require surgical excision to control these infections.

EXCESSIVE WEIGHT LOSS
- Coordinate with the dietitian to calculate the patient's current daily caloric needs and meet his or her desired nutrition status outcomes.
- Nutritional requirements for a patient with a large burn area can exceed 5000 kcal/day and include a diet high in protein for wound healing.
- Nasoduodenal tube feedings are often started within 4 hours of beginning fluid resuscitation to prevent nutritional deficits.
- Encourage patients who can eat solid foods to ingest as many calories as possible.
- Take the patient's preferences into consideration for diet planning and food selection.
- Encourage patients to request food whenever they feel they can eat, not just according to the hospital's standard meal schedule.
- Offer frequent high-calorie, high-protein supplemental feedings.
- Keep an accurate calorie count for foods and beverages that are ingested by the patient.

REDUCED MOBILITY
Nonsurgical Management
- Positioning:
  1. Maintain the patient in a neutral body position with minimal flexion.
  2. Use splints and other devices on the joints of the hands, elbows, knees, neck, and axillae to prevent contractures.
- ROM exercises:
  1. Work with the patient to perform these actively at least three times daily.
  2. Perform passive ROM exercises for patients who are unable to actively perform them.
  3. For burned hands, urge the patient to perform active ROM exercises for the hand, thumb, and fingers every hour while awake.
- Ambulation:
  1. Start ambulation as soon as possible after the fluid shifts have resolved.
  2. Assist patients to ambulate at least twice daily.
  3. Increase ambulation length each time.
- Pressure dressings:
  1. Apply pressure dressings after grafts heal to help prevent contractures and tight hypertrophic scars.
  2. Urge the patient to wear pressure dressings at least 23 hours every day until the scar tissue is mature (12 to 24 months).

Surgical Management
- Surgical management to restore mobility focuses on joint and tendon dysfunction. Surgical release of contractures is most commonly performed in the neck, axilla, elbow flexion areas, and hand.

SUPPORTING POSITIVE SELF-IMAGE

Nonsurgical Management
- Assess which stage of grief the patient is experiencing and help interpret his or her behavior.
- Reassure the patient that feelings of grief, loss, anxiety, anger, fear, and guilt are normal.
- Coordinate with other health care team members (e.g., psychologist, psychiatrist, social worker, clergy or religious leader) in addressing these problems.
- Accept the physical and psychological features of the patient.
- Present patients and families with realistic expected outcomes regarding the patient's functional capacity and physical appearance.
- Plan and encourage the patient's active participation in self-care activities.
- Urge families to include the patient in family decision making to the same degree that he or she participated in this process before the injury.
- Provide information sessions and counseling for the family to help identify effective patterns of support.
- Facilitate the patient's use of these systems and the development of new support systems.
- Make referrals to support groups.

Surgical Management
- Reconstructive and cosmetic surgery can restore function and improve the patient's appearance, often increasing his or her feelings of self-worth and promoting a positive body image. Teach the patient and family about expected cosmetic outcomes.

REHABILITATIVE PHASE OF BURN INJURY
- The technical rehabilitative phase begins with wound closure and ends when the patient returns to the highest possible level of functioning.
- The emphasis during this phase is the psychosocial adjustment of the patient, the prevention of scars and contractures, and the resumption of preburn activity, including resuming work, family, and social roles.
- This phase may take years or even last a lifetime as patients adjust to permanent limitations that may not be apparent until long after the initial injury.

PATIENT-CENTERED COLLABORATIVE CARE
Assessment
- Explore the patient's feelings about the burn injury.
- Ask the patient or a family member whether there is a history of psychological problems.
- Assess and document the type of coping mechanisms the patient has used successfully during times of stress to assist with a future plan of care.
- Assess the patient's family unit and the family members' history of interaction.
- Identify cultural and ethnic factors, and take these into consideration when planning psychosocial interventions.

Community-Based Care
- Discharge planning for the patient with a burn injury begins at the time of admission to the hospital or burn center.
- Help the patient adjust to the reaction of others to the sight of healing wounds and disfiguring scars.
- Teach the patient and family:
  1. How to perform dressing changes
  2. Signs and symptoms of infection
  3. Drug regimens
  4. Proper use of prosthetic and positioning devices
  5. Correct application and care of pressure garments
  6. Comfort measures to reduce pruritus
  7. Dates for follow-up appointments
- Additional common discharge needs of the patient with burns include:
  1. Financial assessment
  2. Evaluation of family resources with possible home assessment (on-site visit)
  3. Psychological referral
  4. Determination of disposition: home, home with home care services, rehabilitation, long-term care, or other setting
  5. Medical equipment or prosthetic training
  6. Referral to community resources
  7. Re-entry programs for school or work environment

C

CANCER, BREAST
OVERVIEW
- Breast cancer is second only to lung cancer as a cause of cancer death in women. Men account for less than 1% of breast cancers.

- Early detection through the regular screening methods of clinical breast examination and mammography can improve survival.
- Breast cancer has many different forms with different clinical presentations and responses to therapy.
- Breast cancer is divided into two broad categories, noninvasive and invasive:
  1. *Noninvasive cancers* remain within the breast ducts and make up 20% of breast cancers. Ductal carcinoma in situ (DCIS) is a common, early, noninvasive breast cancer. Another type is lobular carcinoma in situ (LCIS).
  2. *Invasive cancers* penetrate the tissue surrounding the ducts and make up 80% of all breast cancers. The most common type of invasive breast cancer is infiltrating ductal carcinoma. Another type is inflammatory carcinoma.
     a. When the breast tumor invades lymphatic channels, skin drainage is blocked, causing skin edema, redness, warmth, and an orange peel appearance of the skin ("peau d'orange").
     b. Invasion of the lymphatic channels carries cancer cells to the axillary lymph nodes. Pathologic examination of these nodes helps determine the stage of the disease.
     c. Invasive breast cancer can spread through the blood and lymph systems to distant sites, most commonly the bone, lungs, brain, and liver.
- There is no single cause of breast cancer, but many risk factors are associated with its development:
  1. Female gender
  2. Advancing age
  3. Family history, especially first-degree relatives of individual with breast cancer
  4. Previous exposure to high-dose ionizing radiation to the chest
  5. Early menarche (before 12 years of age) and late menopause (after 50 years of age)
  6. History of previous breast cancer
  7. Nulliparity (no pregnancies) or first birth after 30 years of age

🧬 Genetic/Genomic Considerations

Mutations in several genes, such as *BRCA1* and *BRCA2*, are related to hereditary breast cancer. People who have specific mutations in either one of these genes are at a high risk for developing breast cancer and ovarian cancer. However, only 5% to 10% of all breast cancers are hereditary. Only women with a strong family history and a reasonable suspicion that a

Continued

mutation is present have genetic testing for *BRCA* mutations. Encourage women to talk with a genetics counselor to carefully consider the benefits and potential harmful consequences of genetic testing before these tests are done.

🌐 Cultural Considerations

- One of every eight U.S. women will develop invasive breast cancer by age 70.
- Euro-American women older than 40 years are at a greater risk than other racial/ethnic groups.
- Black American women younger than 40 years have breast cancer more often than others in that age-group.
  Black American women have a higher death rate at any age when compared with other women with the disease.
- Cultural disparities with regard to breast cancer stage and mortality are persistent:
  1. Non-Hispanic white women are more likely to present with an earlier stage breast cancer than American Indian/Alaska Native, Asian Indian/Pakistani, black, Filipino, Hawaiian, Mexican, Puerto Rican, and Samoan women.
  2. Black American and Puerto Rican women have the highest risk for triple negative breast cancer. In this type of breast cancer, cells lack receptors for estrogen, progesterone, and the protein *HER2*.
- Cultural disparities should be addressed with targeted interventions that are appropriate for specific cultural and ethnic groups.

PATIENT-CENTERED COLLABORATIVE CARE
Assessment
- Obtain patient information about:
  1. Age, race, ethnicity
  2. Personal and family history of cancer
  3. Age at menarche and menopause
  4. Number of children and age at first child's birth
  5. Health behaviors, including practice of breast self-exam (BSE), clinical breast examination, and mammography
  6. How the mass was discovered and how long ago
  7. Whether other body changes have been noticed recently, especially bone or joint pain

    8. Brief nutritional history, including intake of fat and alcohol
- Assess for:
  1. Specific information about the mass:
     a. Location of the mass, described using the face-of-the-clock method
     b. Shape, size, and consistency
     c. Assess benign lumps as mobile and round or oval; assess possible malignant lumps as fixed and irregularly shaped, often in the upper outer breast quadrant
     d. Skin changes, such as dimpling, orange peel appearance, redness and warmth, nipple retraction, or ulceration
  2. Presence of enlarged axillary or supraclavicular lymph nodes
  3. Pain or soreness in the affected breast
  4. Psychosocial adjustment:
     a. Patient's current knowledge and need for information
     b. Patient's self-image, sexuality, and current intimate relationships
     c. How the patient has successfully handled stress in the past
     d. Patient's feelings about the disease and expectations of treatment
     e. Myths or misconceptions the patient may have (and how to dispel them)
     f. Need for additional resources
  5. Imaging assessment for diagnosis and staging:
     a. Mammography or digital mammography
     b. Ultrasonography
     c. Breast-specific gamma imaging (BSGI)
     d. Chest x-ray
     e. Bone, liver, and brain scans
     f. Computed tomography (CT) scan of the chest and abdomen
     g. Magnetic resonance imaging (MRI)
  6. Pathologic examination of tissue for diagnosis and prognosis:
     a. Biopsy, which is the definitive test that proves presence or absence of cancer
     b. Presence of tumor hormone receptors (cancers that express receptors have a better treatment response) and protein expression profiling of tumor cell
     c. Lymph node involvement or other sites of metastasis

Planning and Implementation
- Teach women ways to minimize surgical area deformity and enhance body image, such as the use of a breast prosthesis or the option of breast reconstruction.
- Address the reactions of family and significant others to the diagnosis of breast cancer; provide support and education.

- After breast cancer surgery, assess vital signs, dressings, drainage tubes, and amount of drainage.
- Notify the health care team that the arm of the surgical mastectomy side should not be used for blood pressures, blood drawing, or injections.
- Assess the return of arm and shoulder mobility after breast surgery and axillary dissection.
- Teach patient measures to prevent lymphedema after axillary node dissection or assist the patient with measures to reduce lymphedema in the affected arm.
  1. Lymphedema is an abnormal accumulation of protein fluid in the subcutaneous tissue of the affected limb after a mastectomy and is a commonly overlooked topic in health teaching.
  2. Risk factors include injury or infection of the extremity, obesity, presence of extensive axillary disease, and radiation treatment.
  3. A referral to a lymphedema specialist may be necessary for the patient to be fitted for a compression sleeve and/or glove, to be taught exercises and manual lymph drainage, and to discuss ways to modify daily activities to avoid worsening the problem. Management is directed toward measures that promote drainage of the affected arm.
- Observe for and report other complications of breast cancer surgery or breast reconstruction, especially infection and inadequate vascular perfusion.

Surgical Management

- To improve survival and to reduce the risk for local recurrence, the mass itself should be removed by one of several types of surgery.
- A large tumor may be treated with chemotherapy (neoadjuvant therapy) to shrink the tumor before it is surgically removed.
- Surgical approaches include:
  1. *Breast-conserving surgery,* in which the bulk of the tumor is removed (not the entire breast), is used mostly for stages I and II breast cancers and is usually followed with radiation therapy. Types of breast-conserving surgery include lumpectomy, wide excision, partial or segmental mastectomy, and quadrantectomy.
  2. *Modified radical mastectomy,* in which the affected breast, skin, and axillary nodes are completely removed but the underlying muscles remain intact, is indicated when tumor is present in different quadrants of the breast, when the patient may be unable to have radiation therapy, when the tumor is large and the breast is small, and when the patient prefers this approach.
- Provide preoperative care, including psychological preparation:
  1. Review the type of procedure planned.
  2. Assess the patient's current level of knowledge.

3. Teach about perioperative information, including:
   a. The need for a drainage tube
   b. The location of the incision
   c. Mobility restriction, including avoiding blood pressure (BP) in affected arm
   d. Body image issues

- Provide postoperative care described in Part One and:
  1. Place a sign over the patient's bed to inform the staff to avoid using the affected arm for taking BP measurements, giving injections, or drawing blood
  2. Perform wound care:
     a. Observe the wound for signs of swelling and infection.
     b. Assess drainage tubes for patency, color of drainage, and the amount.
  3. Position the patient for best drainage and comfort:
     a. Head of the bed up at least 30 degrees
     b. Arm on the same side as the axillary dissection elevated on a pillow while he or she is awake
  4. Work with the physical therapist to plan progressive exercises:
     a. Squeezing the affected hand around a soft, round object (a ball or rolled washcloth)
     b. Flexion and extension of the elbow

- Breast reconstruction is common for women without complications from the cancer surgery and may be performed during the cancer surgery or at a later time. It may involve one or more stages using skin flaps or prostheses.
- For patients with breast cancer at a stage for which surgery is the main treatment, follow-up with adjuvant radiation therapy, chemotherapy, hormone therapy, or targeted therapy may also be prescribed.
- The decision to follow the original surgical procedure with adjuvant therapy for breast cancer is based on:
  1. Stage of the disease
  2. Patient's age and menopausal status
  3. Patient's preferences
  4. Pathologic examination results
  5. Hormone receptor status
  6. Presence of a known genetic predisposition
- Radiation therapy is administered after breast-conserving surgery and may be delivered by any one of several methods. General management issues for the care of patients undergoing radiation therapy are presented in Part One under *Cancer Treatment*.
  1. Traditional whole-breast irradiation is delivered by external beam radiation over 5 to 6 weeks.

2. *Interstitial brachytherapy,* in which several catheters loaded with a radioactive source are inserted at the lumpectomy cavity and surrounding margin, is given over 4 to 5 days.
3. *Balloon brachytherapy,* also known as *MammoSite,* involves the use of a single balloon-tipped catheter that is surgically placed near the tumor bed. The catheter is loaded with a radiation source and inflated to conform to the total cavity. A total of 10 treatments are given, with at least 6 hours between each treatment.
4. *Intraoperative radiation therapy* uses a high single dose of radiation delivered during the lumpectomy surgery.

- Chemotherapy for breast cancer is delivered over 3 to 6 months in cycles of 2 to 3 weeks each month with a combination of agents. General management issues for the care of patients undergoing radiation therapy are presented in Part One under *Cancer Treatment.*
- Targeted therapy for breast cancer involves the use of drugs that target specific features of cancer cells, such as a protein, an enzyme, or the formation of new blood vessels. These agents are useful only for cancers that overexpress a certain protein or enzyme. For example, a targeted biotherapy drug is trastuzumab (Herceptin), a monoclonal antibody effective against breast cancers that overexpress the *HER2/NEU* gene product.
- Hormonal therapy is used to reduce the estrogen available to breast tumors to stop or prevent their growth. Agents include:
  1. Luteinizing hormone-releasing hormone (LH-RH) gene agonists that inhibit estrogen synthesis
     a. Leuprolide (Lupron)
     b. Goserelin (Zoladex)
  2. Selective estrogen receptor modulators (SERMs) that block the effect of estrogen in the breast but not the ovaries of women who have estrogen receptor (ER)-positive breast cancer; one example is tamoxifen.
  3. Aromatase inhibitors (AIs) to prevent the conversion of androgen to estrogen in the adrenal gland
     a. Anastrozole (Arimidex)
     b. Exemestane (Aromasin)

Community-Based Care
- Make the appropriate referrals for care after discharge:
  1. Home health and social services
  2. Reach to Recovery or other organizations that provide social support
- Teach the patient and family about:
  1. Wound care: drains, dressings, avoidance of lotions or ointments in the area, keeping the affected arm elevated if a lymph node dissection was performed

2. Initial activity restrictions, especially stretching or reaching for heavy objects, while continuing with activity to regain full range of motion (ROM)
3. Measures to improve body image
4. Information about interpersonal relationships and roles
5. Essential follow-up, including annual health care provider visits and mammography or other imaging procedures
6. Measures to avoid injury, infection, and swelling of the affected arm

- Prepare the patient and partner about psychosocial issues:
  1. Describe the expected postoperative appearance.
  2. Reassure her that scars will fade and edema will lessen with time.
  3. Encourage the woman to look at her incision before she goes home and offer to be present when she does so.
  4. Involve the partner or family in teaching.
  5. Discuss sexual concerns before discharge. Sexual dysfunction affects up to 90% of women treated for breast cancer, although it is an issue seldom discussed between patients and health care providers.
  6. Advise sexually active patients receiving chemotherapy or radiotherapy to use birth control during therapy.

CANCER, CERVICAL
OVERVIEW
- Cervical cancer usually arises from the squamous cells on the outside of the uterine cervix.
- It generally takes years for the cervical cells to transform from normal to premalignant to invasive cancer.
- *Invasive* cervical cancer has spread to other pelvic structures by direct extension to the vaginal mucosa, lower uterine segment, parametrium, pelvic wall, bladder, and bowel.
- Risk factors include:
  1. Infection with human papillomavirus (HPV)
  2. History of sexually transmitted disease
  3. Multiple sex partners
  4. Younger than 18 years of age at first intercourse
  5. Multiparity (multiple pregnancies)
  6. Smoking
  7. Oral contraceptive use
  8. Obesity, poor diet
- Vaccination with HPV vaccine, ideally before onset of intercourse, appears to protect against the high-risk HPV strains that are responsible for most cervical cancer.

- Cervical cancer can be detected at early stages, when cure is most likely, through a periodic pelvic examination and Papanicolaou (Pap) test.

PATIENT-CENTERED COLLABORATIVE CARE
Assessment
- Ask the patient about vaginal bleeding. Cervical cancer may manifest as spotting between menstrual periods or after sexual intercourse or douching. The classic symptom of invasive cancer is painless vaginal bleeding. As the cancer grows, bleeding increases in frequency, duration, and amount, and it may become continuous.
- Assess for later manifestations:
  1. Watery, blood-tinged vaginal discharge that becomes dark and foul-smelling (occurs as the disease progresses)
  2. Leg pain (along the sciatic nerve) or swelling
  3. Flank pain indicating hydronephrosis from tumor blocking a ureter, backing up urine into the kidney
- Assess for manifestations of recurrence or metastasis:
  1. Unexplained weight loss
  2. Dysuria (painful urination)
  3. Pelvic pain
  4. Hematuria (bloody urine)
  5. Rectal bleeding
  6. Chest pain
  7. Coughing
- Diagnosis is made by cytologic examination of the Pap smear. Colposcopy examination may be performed to view the transformation zone and biopsy many areas of the cervix.

Interventions
Surgical Management: Early Stage
- Surgical management for small, early-stage cervical cancer include electrosurgical excision, laser therapy, and cryosurgery.
- Teach patients who have these procedures to follow restrictions for about 3 weeks:
  1. Refrain from sexual intercourse.
  2. Do not use tampons.
  3. Do not douche.
  4. Take showers rather than tub baths.
  5. Avoid lifting heavy objects.
  6. Report a fever or any heavy vaginal bleeding or foul-smelling drainage.

Surgical Management: Microinvasive Stage
- Surgical management at the microinvasive stage depends on the patient's health, desire for future childbearing, tumor size, stage, cancer cell type, and preferences.

- A *conization,* in which a cone-shaped area of cervix is removed surgically, can remove the affected tissue while preserving fertility.
    1. Potential complications from this procedure include hemorrhage and uterine perforation.
    2. Long-term follow-up care is needed, because new cancers can develop.
- A *total hysterectomy,* in which the cervix and body of the uterus are removed but the fallopian tubes and ovaries are spared, may be performed if fertility is not an issue. Care for patients undergoing hysterectomy is found in the *Uterine Fibroids (Leiomyomas)* content.
- Refer to *Cancer, Colorectal* for preoperative and postoperative care for the patient undergoing colostomy and to *Cancer, Urothelial (Bladder)* for preoperative and postoperative care for the patient undergoing ileal conduit.

Nonsurgical Management

- Radiation therapy is reserved for invasive cervical cancer.
    1. *Intracavitary* and *external radiation therapies* are used in combination, depending on the extent and location of the lesion.
    2. General management issues for the care of patients undergoing intracavitary (brachytherapy) or external (beam) radiation therapy are presented in Part One under *Cancer Treatment.*
- Chemotherapy with radiation therapy may be also be used for invasive cervical cancer.
    1. The most common agent used is cisplatin (Platinol). Paclitaxel (Taxol), carboplatin, and fluorouracil (5-FU) have also been used.
    2. General management issues for the care of patients receiving combination chemotherapy are presented in Part One under *Cancer Treatment.*

CANCER, COLORECTAL

OVERVIEW

- Colorectal cancer (CRC), or cancer of the colon or rectum, is a common malignancy.
- Most CRCs are adenocarcinomas arising from the glandular epithelial tissue of the colon and developing as a multi-step process.
    1. Abnormal proliferation of the colonic mucosa first forms polyps that can transform into malignant tumors.
    2. Tumors can spread by direct invasion and through the lymphatic and circulatory systems. The most common sites of metastasis are the liver, lungs, brain, bones, and adrenal glands.
- Complications include bowel perforation with peritonitis, abscess or fistula formation, frank hemorrhage, and complete intestinal obstruction.

- Risk factors include:
  1. Age older than 50 years
  2. Genetic predisposition
  3. Personal or family history of cancer or diseases that predispose to cancer (e.g., familial adenomatous polyposis [FAP], hereditary nonpolyposis colorectal cancer [HNPCC])
  4. Crohn's disease or ulcerative colitis

☒ Genetic/Genomic Considerations

- People with a first-degree relative (sister, sibling, or child) diagnosed with CRC have three to four times the risk of developing the disease.
- An autosomal dominant inherited genetic disorder known as familial adenomatous polyposis accounts for 1% of CRCs. People with mutation develop thousands of adenomatous polyps over 10 to 15 years that have an almost 100% chance of becoming malignant.
- Surgical prophylaxis with a colectomy can be performed for cancer prevention.
- HNPCC is another autosomal dominant disorder caused by mutations in the *MLH1* and *MLH2* genes. People with these mutations have an 80% chance of developing CRC at an average of 45 years of age.

PATIENT-CENTERED COLLABORATIVE CARE
Assessment
- Obtain patient information about:
  1. Age
  2. History of inflammatory or familial colon disease
  3. Change in bowel habits with or without blood in stool
  4. Weight loss, pain, and abdominal fullness (late signs)
- Assess for:
  1. Rectal bleeding (the most common manifestation and stool characteristic)
  2. Anemia (low hemoglobin level and hematocrit; stool positive for occult blood)
  3. Cachexia (late sign)
  4. Abdominal distension or mass (late sign)
- Diagnostic assessment includes:
  1. Fecal occult blood test (FOBT)
  2. Carcinoembryonic antigen (CEA) blood test
  3. Colonoscopy
  4. CT or MRI of the abdomen with additional views for evaluation of metastasis (pelvis, thorax, and brain)

Planning and Implementation
Surgical management with tumor removal is the primary approach to treatment. Nonsurgical management reduces the potential for cancer recurrence and metastasis and provides symptom management and psychosocial support.

- Radiation therapy:
    1. Radiation is to reduce tumor size and as a palliative measure to reduce pain, hemorrhage, bowel obstruction, or metastasis.
    2. General management issues for the care of patients undergoing radiation therapy are presented in Part One under *Cancer Treatment.*
- *Chemotherapy* is used after surgery to interrupt cancer cell division and improve survival. General management issues for the care of patients undergoing chemotherapy are presented in Part One under *Cancer Treatment.*
    1. Common drugs include:
        a. 5-FU with leucovorin (folinic acid)
        b. Capecitabine (Xeloda)
        c. Combinations of 5-FU and oxaliplatin (Eloxatin) (FLOFOX4)
    2. Common side effects of this therapy are:
        a. Diarrhea
        b. Mucositis, stomatitis
        c. Leukopenia
        d. Peripheral neuropathy
- *Targeted biotherapy* for advanced CRC includes:
    1. Antiangiogenesis drugs: bevacizumab (Avastin), panitumumab (Vectibix)
    2. Epidermal growth factor antagonist: cetuximab (Erbitux)
- Symptom relief for pain and emesis (opioids and antiemetics)
- Assisting with grieving and allowing patient to verbalize feeling about the diagnosis, treatment, and progression of disease or recovery

Surgical Management
- In a colon resection, the bowel segment containing the tumor is resected (removed) along with several inches of bowel beyond the tumor margin and regional lymph nodes, and an end-to-end anastomosis is performed. This procedure may be performed by the traditional open method or as minimally invasive surgery by laparoscopy.
- A colectomy (colon removal) with temporary or permanent colostomy may be needed.
- In an abdominal peritoneal (A-P) resection, the sigmoid colon and rectum are removed, the anus is closed, and a permanent colostomy is formed.

- Provide preoperative care as described in Part One and:
  1. If a colostomy is planned, consult the enterostomal therapist (ET) to assist in identifying optimal placement of the ostomy and to instruct the patient about the rationale and general principles of ostomies.
  2. Administer laxatives, enemas, or an oral, liquid, large-volume laxative if ordered, the morning of surgery or the day before surgery to mechanically clean the bowel ("bowel prep").
- Provide postoperative care described in Part One and:
  1. Managing the colostomy, if present:
     a. If an ostomy pouch is not in place, cover the stoma with petroleum gauze to keep it moist, followed by a dry, sterile dressing.
     b. Place a pouch system on the stoma as soon as possible and in collaboration with the enterostomal therapist.
     c. Observe the stoma for color, discharge, and intactness of surrounding skin.
     d. Assess for colostomy functioning 2 to 4 days after surgery; stool is liquid immediately after surgery but becomes more solid.
     e. Empty the pouch when excess gas has collected or when it is one third to one half full of stool.

❗ NURSING SAFETY PRIORITY: Action Alert

Report any of these problems related to the colostomy to the surgeon:
- Signs of ischemia and necrosis (dark red, purplish, or black color; dry, firm, or flaccid)
- Unusual or excessive bleeding
- Mucocutaneous separation (breakdown of the suture line securing the stoma to the abdominal wall)

---

  2. Assess the condition of the peristomal skin (skin around the stoma), and frequently check the pouch system for proper fit and signs of leakage. The skin should be intact, smooth, and without redness or excoriation.
  3. Assess for signs of infection, abscess, or other complications.
  4. Consult with the skin care or ostomy specialist early and often during surgical recovery. This may be done as a home health referral for new or ongoing consultation.
  5. Instruct the patient what to expect about the appearance and care of the colostomy.

6. When the patient is physically able, encourage the patient to look at the ostomy (if performed), and to participate in colostomy care.

Community-Based Care
- Provide the patient with these oral and written instructions:
  1. Avoid lifting heavy objects or straining on defecation to prevent tension on the anastomosis site
  2. Avoid driving for 4 to 6 weeks
  3. Note the frequency, amount, and character of the stool
  4. For colon resection, watch for and report manifestations of bowel obstruction and perforation (e.g., cramping, abdominal pain, nausea, vomiting)
  5. Look for signs of incisional healing and infection
- Teach the patient and family colostomy care, including:
  1. Normal appearance of a stoma
  2. Signs and symptoms of complications
  3. How to measure the stoma
  4. The choice, use, care, and application of the appropriate appliance to cover the stoma
  5. How to protect the skin adjacent to the stoma
  6. Dietary measures to control gas and odor
- Provide contacts for community and health resources as needed, particularly ostomy-related information, ostomy support groups, and home health care.

CANCER, ENDOMETRIAL (UTERINE)

OVERVIEW
- Endometrial cancer (cancer of the uterus) is the most common gynecologic cancer.
- Adenocarcinoma is the most common type, accounting for 80% of all cases.
  1. It is slow growing with initial growth in the uterine cavity, followed by extension into the myometrium and cervix.
- Risk factors associated with endometrial cancer include:
  1. Prolonged exposure to estrogen without the protective effects of progesterone
  2. Women in reproductive years
  3. Family history of endometrial cancer or hereditary nonpolyposis colorectal cancer (HNPCC)
  4. Diabetes mellitus
  5. Hypertension
  6. Obesity
  7. Uterine polyps
  8. Late menopause

9. Nulliparity (no childbirths)
10. Smoking
11. Tamoxifen (Nolvadex) given for breast cancer

PATIENT-CENTERED COLLABORATIVE CARE
Assessment
- Obtain patient information about:
  1. Age and ethnicity
  2. Risk factors of family history of cancer
  3. History of diabetes, obesity, or hypertension
  4. Childbearing status, pregnancies, births, infertility
  5. Prolonged estrogen use
- Assess for:
  1. Postmenopausal bleeding (the primary symptom)
  2. Watery, serosanguineous vaginal discharge
  3. Low back, abdominal, or pelvic pain
  4. Enlarged uterus
  5. Anemia from uterine bleeding
  6. CA (cancer antigen)-125 and alpha-fetoprotein (AFP), both of which may be elevated when ovarian (metastatic) cancer is present
  7. The presence of endometrial thickening and cancer; *transvaginal ultrasound* and *endometrial biopsy* are the gold standard tests
  8. Presence of metastatic disease; metastasis outside the uterus can spread cancer through lymph or blood or to the peritoneal cavity

Interventions
  Surgical Management
- Surgical removal and cancer staging of the tumor is first-line therapy. Typically a total abdominal hysterectomy is done (see *Uterine Fibroids [Leiomyomas], Surgical Management, Hysterectomy*). Either a laparoscopic or open approach can be used.
  Nonsurgical Management
- Radiation therapy and chemotherapy are used postoperatively and depend on the surgical staging.
- When intracavitary radiation therapy (IRT) (brachytherapy) is performed, an applicator is positioned within the uterus through the vagina. Implement these interventions for radiation safety and to prevent dislodgment of either the applicator or the radiation source:
  1. Maintain radiation precautions.
  2. Provide bedrest, laying the patient on her back, with her head flat or elevated less than 20 degrees. Restrict active movement to prevent dislodgment.

3. Assess for complications including cystitis, diarrhea, and mucosal or skin irritation.
- Instruct the patient undergoing external beam radiation to:
  1. Observe for signs of skin breakdown.
  2. Avoid sunbathing.
  3. Do not remove the markings that outline the treatment site.
  4. Recognize the complications of treatment, including cystitis, diarrhea, and nutritional alterations.
  5. Recognize that reactions to radiation therapy vary among patients and that some may feel unclean or radioactive after treatments.
- General management issues for the care of patients undergoing intracavitary (brachytherapy) or external (teletherapy) radiation therapy are presented in Part One under *Cancer Treatment.*
- Chemotherapy is used as palliative treatment in advanced or recurrent endometrial cancer.
  1. Chemotherapeutic agents frequently used include doxorubicin (Adriamycin), cisplatin (Platinol), and paclitaxel (Taxol).
  2. General management issues for the care of patients receiving combination chemotherapy are presented in Part One under *Cancer Treatment.*

Community-Based Care
- Provide oral and written instructions on:
  1. Effects or complications from surgery, radiation, or chemotherapy that should be reported to the provider, including vaginal bleeding, rectal bleeding, foul-smelling discharge, abdominal pain or distention, and hematuria
  2. Dosages, scheduling, and side effects of prescribed drugs
- Inform the patient that:
  1. High-dose radiation causes sterility
  2. Vaginal shrinkage or dryness can occur with radiation and chemotherapy
  3. Sexual partners cannot "catch" cancer
  4. The patient is not radioactive (after the intracavitary radiation source is removed)

CANCER, HEAD AND NECK
OVERVIEW
- Head and neck cancers occur in structures within the larynx, the trachea, the throat, the oral cavity, or on the tongue, and they usually arise from the skin or mucosa as squamous cell carcinomas.
- Other origins of head and neck cancers include the salivary glands, the thyroid, and other structures.

- Head and neck cancers are usually squamous cell carcinoma.
- The cancer begins as a loss of cellular regulation characterized by excessive growth of abnormal cells in association with chronic irritation of mucosa and occurring in stages:
  1. Abnormal cells manifested as thick, tough areas of mucosa develop (squamous metaplasia) and appear as white, patchy lesions (leukoplakia) or red, velvety patches (erythroplakia).
  2. Next, mucosal thickening (acanthosis, or hyperplasia) and the development of a keratin layer (keratosis) occur.
  3. With time, the lesions become malignant and may spread (metastasize) first into nearby structures, such as lymph nodes, muscle, and bone, and then to more distant sites, usually the lungs or liver.
  4. The degree of malignancy is determined by cellular analysis:
     a. Early-stage cancers are carcinoma in situ and well differentiated.
     b. Cancers that have progressed are moderately differentiated.
     c. Advanced cancers are poorly differentiated.
- The cause of head and neck cancers is unknown, but the two greatest risk factors are tobacco and alcohol use, especially in combination.
- Other risk factors include voice abuse, chronic laryngitis, exposure to industrial chemicals or hardwood dust, poor oral hygiene, long-term or severe gastroesophageal reflux disease (GERD), and oral infection with HPV.

PATIENT-CENTERED COLLABORATIVE CARE
Assessment
- Obtain patient information about:
  1. Tobacco and alcohol use (quantify these)
  2. History of recurrent acute or chronic laryngitis or pharyngitis, oral sores, and lumps in the neck
  3. Exposure to environmental or occupational pollutants
  4. Infection or vaccination associated with HPV (vaccination is preventative)
- Assess for physical manifestations:
  1. Problems related to risk factors
  2. Dietary habits
  3. Weight loss
  4. Hoarseness
  5. Lumps on the head or in the neck
  6. Mouth sores
  7. Laryngeal abnormalities by laryngeal examination using a laryngeal mirror (physician or advanced practice nurse)

- Assess for psychosocial issues:
  1. Patient or family feelings of denial, guilt, blame, or shame
  2. Adequacy of support systems and coping mechanisms
  3. Patient's use of speech for employment
- Diagnostic assessment may include:
  1. Laboratory tests, complete blood count (CBC), bleeding times, urinalysis, blood chemistries, protein levels, albumin levels, and renal and liver function tests
  2. X-rays of the skull, sinuses, neck, and chest
  3. CT scan or MRI of the head and neck, with or without contrast media
  4. Brain, bone, and liver scans
  5. Positron emission tomography (PET) scans
  6. Direct and indirect laryngoscopy
  7. Panendoscopy (laryngoscopy, nasopharyngoscopy, esophagoscopy, and bronchoscopy)
  8. Biopsy

Planning and Implementation

The goal of treatment is to remove or eradicate the cancer while preserving as much normal function as possible. The specific treatment depends on the extent and location of the lesion.

Nonsurgical Management

- Radiation therapy is used alone or in combination with chemotherapy or surgery. Because radiation therapy slows tissue healing, it may not be performed before surgery.
  1. Complications of radiation therapy for head and neck cancer include increased hoarseness, dysphagia, skin problems, and dry mouth (leading to halitosis, taste changes, increased risk for dental caries and dental infection).
  2. Dry mouth (xerostomia) is a long-term complication and may be permanent. Interventions to improve comfort are:
     a. Providing fluid intake and room or oxygen humidification
     b. Administering artificial saliva, moisturizing gels, or saliva stimulants (e.g., Salagen, cevimeline)
  3. General management issues for the care of patients undergoing radiation therapy are presented in Part One under *Cancer Treatment*.
- Chemotherapy can be used alone or in addition to surgery or radiation for head and neck cancer.
  1. Specific treatment regimens and drug combinations vary, but the most commonly used agents for head and neck cancer include cisplatin (Platinol).
  2. General management issues for the care of patients undergoing chemotherapy are presented in Part One under *Cancer Treatment*.

- Targeted therapy for advanced head and neck cancers may include cetuximab (Erbitux).

  Surgical Management
- Tumor size and location (according to tumor-nodes-metastasis [TNM] classification) determines the type of surgery needed for the specific head and neck cancer.
- Very small, early-stage tumors may be removed by laser therapy or photodynamic therapy, but few head and neck tumors are found at this stage, and most require extensive traditional surgery.
- Traditional surgical procedures for head and neck cancers include:
  1. *Laryngectomy* (total and partial): removal of the larynx
  2. *Tracheotomy:* creation of a new artificial airway by opening the wall of the trachea
  3. Oropharyngeal cancer resections
  4. *Cordectomy:* vocal cord removal
  5. Radical neck dissection, which is removal of the primary tumor along with lymph node dissection. It may involve removing skin, muscle, bone, and other structures.
  6. Composite resections are a combination of surgical procedures, including partial or total glossectomies, partial mandibulectomies, and, if needed, nodal neck dissections.
- Provide preoperative care as described in Part One and:
  1. Teach the patient about the probable location of the surgical incision, self-care of the airway, alternate methods of communication, suctioning, pain control methods, the critical care environment (including ventilators and critical care routines), nutritional support, feeding tubes, and goals for discharge.
  2. Help the patient to practice the use of an alternate form of communication (e.g., pen and pencil, tablet, "magic slate," picture or alphabet board, or computerized word generator).
  3. Determine the communication method most preferred by the patient.
  4. Encourage the patient to express fears and concerns.
  5. Reinforce the surgeon's explanation of the surgical procedure.
- Provide postoperative care as described in Part One and:
  1. Maintain airway and gas exchange by:
     a. Ensuring suction equipment is available
     b. Using suction, deep breathing, and coughing to maintain airway
     c. Dispensing oxygen therapy accurately and with humidification
     d. Evaluating swallowing with respiratory assessment
     e. Providing laryngectomy or tracheostomy care (if surgery included tracheotomy or laryngectomy)

    f. Documenting the quantity and quality of oral and respiratory secretions

! NURSING SAFETY PRIORITY: Critical Rescue

Secretions may remain blood-tinged for 1 to 2 days. Report any increase in bleeding to the surgeon.

C

2. Manage wounds to promote healing and avoid infection:
   a. Evaluate all grafts and flaps hourly for the first 72 hours.
   b. Monitor pain, pulse/perfusion, capillary refill, color, and drainage at the surgical site.
   c. Position the patient so that the side of the head and neck with the flaps is not dependent.
   d. Report increases in blood or quantity of drainage to the surgeon immediately, because surgical intervention may be needed.
3. Prevent hemorrhage:
   a. Observe for carotid artery leakage or rupture.
      (1) Rupture results in large amounts of bright red blood spurting quickly.
      (2) Leakage shows as oozing of bright red blood.

! NURSING SAFETY PRIORITY: Critical Rescue

If a carotid artery leak is suspected, call the Rapid Response Team, and do not touch the area, because additional pressure could cause an immediate rupture. If the carotid artery ruptures because of drying or infection, immediately place constant pressure over the site and secure the airway. Maintain direct manual continuous pressure on the carotid artery and immediately transport the patient to the operating room for carotid resection. Do not leave the patient. Carotid artery rupture has a high risk of stroke and death. Nursing response can save the patient's life.

4. Support nutrition:
   a. Collaborate with the dietitian to provide the patient with at least 35 to 40 kcal/kg of body weight daily.
   b. Anticipate enteral feeding for 7 to 10 days following surgery.
   c. If enteral feeding is delayed for more than 5 days, consider parenteral nutrition.
   d. Assess the patient's ability to swallow before removing the feeding tube.

  5. Speech and language rehabilitation:
     a. Collaborate with the speech and language pathologist.
     b. Work with the patient and family toward developing an acceptable communication method:
        (1) Writing
        (2) Picture board
        (3) Computer
        (4) Artificial larynx
        (5) Esophageal speech
     c. Take time to understand the patient's communication.
     d. Celebrate every success.
     e. Arrange for a visit from a laryngectomee (a person who has had a laryngectomy).

DYSPHAGIA AND RISK FOR ASPIRATION

- Aspiration is not a problem for the patient who has had a total laryngectomy and a permanent tracheostomy.
- Use these precautions for the patient with a feeding tube in place:
  1. Elevate the head of the bed 30 to 40 degrees.
  2. Evaluate the patient's tolerance of the tube feeding every 4 to 6 hours.

> **! NURSING SAFETY PRIORITY: Action Alert**
>
> Do not provide continuous enteral feedings any time the patient must be in a flat, supine position; maintain back rest elevation at 30 to 45 degrees.

- Observe the patient who has had a subtotal, vertical, or supraglottic laryngectomy for aspiration.
- Use these precautions to prevent aspiration when feeding the patient or assisting him or her with eating:
  1. Avoid having meals when the patient is fatigued.
  2. Provide smaller and more frequent meals.
  3. Provide adequate time; do not hurry the patient.
  4. Provide close supervision if the patient is self-feeding.
  5. Keep emergency suctioning equipment close at hand and turned on.
  6. Avoid water and other "thin" liquids.
  7. Thicken all liquids, including water.
  8. Avoid foods that generate thin liquids during the chewing process, such as fruit.
  9. Position the patient in the most upright position possible.
  10. When present, completely (or at least partially) deflate the tracheal tube cuff during meals.
  11. Suction before and after initial cuff deflation to clear the airway and allow maximum comfort during the meal.

12. Feed each bite or encourage the patient to take each bite slowly.
13. Encourage the patient to "dry swallow" after each bite to clear residue from the throat.
14. Avoid consecutive swallows of liquids.
15. Provide controlled small volumes of liquids using a spoon.
16. Encourage the patient to "tuck" his or her chin down and forward while swallowing.
17. Allow the patient to indicate when he or she is ready for the next bite.
18. If the patient coughs, stop the feeding until the patient indicates the airway has been cleared.
19. Continuously monitor tolerance to oral food intake by assessing respiratory rate, ease, pulse oximetry, and heart rate (HR).

- Teach the patient the supraglottic method of swallowing:
  1. Inhaling and holding his or her breath (to close the vocal folds)
  2. Placing food or liquid in swallow position
  3. Swallowing while holding breath
  4. Coughing after swallowing and before inhaling (to clear any residue that may have entered the larynx)

ANXIETY
- Explore the reason for anxiety (e.g., fear of the unknown, lack of teaching, fear of pain, fear of airway compromise, fear of hospitalization, loss of control, fear of death).
- Encourage the patient and family to express their feelings about the cancer diagnosis and the uncertainty of treatment outcome.
- Dispel myths and correct misconceptions.
- Accept that different patients choose to deal with a cancer diagnosis in individual ways.
- Adjust your approach to care as the patient's emotional state changes.
- Integrate outside resources into the plan of care.
- Give prescribed antianxiety drugs.

DISTURBED BODY IMAGE
- The patient with head and neck cancer may have a permanent change in body image because of deformity, the presence of a stoma or artificial airway, speech changes, or a change in the method of eating.
- Help the patient set realistic goals, starting with involvement in self-care.
- Teach the patient alternate communication methods.
- Teach the family to ease the patient into a normal social environment.

- Use positive reinforcement and encouragement while demonstrating acceptance and caring behaviors.
- Refer the patient and family for counseling, as needed.
- Teach the patient tips for an enhanced appearance, including:
  1. The use of loose-fitting, high-collar shirts or sweaters, scarves, and jewelry to cover the laryngectomy stoma, tracheostomy tube, and other changes related to surgery
  2. The use of cosmetics to cover scars and skin disfigurement

Community-Based Care

- Ensure that the patient and family are able to perform tracheostomy or stoma care and participate in nutrition, wound care, and communication methods.
- Coordinate the efforts of the health care team in assessing the specific discharge needs and making the appropriate referrals to home care agencies.
- Coordinate the scheduling for chemotherapy or radiation therapy with the patient and family.
- Ensure that the home environment is assessed for general cleanliness, ease of patient access to toileting and living areas, need for increased humidity, and transportation.
- Teach the patient and family about:
  1. Stoma or tracheostomy or laryngectomy care
  2. Incision and airway care
  3. Safety
  4. Wearing a medical alert (MedicAlert) bracelet and carrying a special identification card
  5. Smoking cessation
  6. Community support agencies

CANCER, LUNG

OVERVIEW

- Lung cancer is a leading cause of cancer-related deaths worldwide.
- The overall 5-year survival rate for all patients with lung cancer is only 16%, because most lung cancers are diagnosed at a late stage, when metastasis is present.
- Lung cancers are classified as small cell lung carcinoma (SCLC) and non–small cell lung carcinoma (NSCLC), which includes epidermoid (squamous cell) cancer, adenocarcinoma, and large cell cancer.
- Metastasis (spread) of lung cancer occurs by direct extension, through the blood, and by invading lymph glands and vessels. Common sites of metastasis for lung cancer are the bone, liver, brain, and adrenal glands.
- Lung cancers occur as a result of repeated exposure to inhaled substances that cause chronic tissue irritation or inflammation.

Cigarette smoking is the major risk factor and is responsible for 85% of all lung cancer deaths.

- Nonsmokers exposed to passive, or secondhand, smoke have a greater risk for lung cancer than nonsmokers.
- Additional environmental causes of lung cancer are chronic exposure to asbestos, beryllium, chromium, coal distillates, cobalt, iron oxide, mustard gas, petroleum distillates, radiation, tar, nickel, uranium, benzopyrone, and hydrocarbons.

C

🧬 Genetic/Genomic Considerations

- Lung cancer development varies among people with similar smoking histories, suggesting that genetic factors can influence susceptibility. Genome-wide association studies have found specific variations in a variety of genes that increase the susceptibility to lung cancer development.
- Differences in a gene that regulates cell division, the Tp53 gene, may be the most important genetic susceptibility link for lung cancer development. Mutations in the alleles of this gene are known to increase the susceptibility to a wide variety of cancers both with and without exposure to environmental risks, including lung cancer development among smokers and nonsmokers.

- Lung cancer interferes with oxygenation and tissue perfusion, including bronchial obstruction, airway compression, compression of alveoli, and compression of blood vessels.
- Common manifestations of lung cancer are associated with respiratory problems and include dyspnea, pallor or cyanosis, tachycardia, bloody sputum, and cough.
- Pain is common when lymph nodes are enlarged and press on nerves.

PATIENT-CENTERED COLLABORATIVE CARE
Assessment
- Obtain patient information about:
  1. Pack-year history and current smoking pattern
  2. Risk factors, including secondhand smoke and environmental exposures
  3. Cough presence and triggers
  4. Sputum:
     a. Amount
     b. Color
     c. Character

    5. Chest pain, tightness, or pressure:
       a. Location
       b. Severity
       c. Duration
       d. Quality
       e. Radiation
    6. Dyspnea:
       a. Duration
       b. Triggers and alleviating factors
- Assess for pulmonary manifestations:
  1. Hoarseness
  2. Wheezing
  3. Decreased or absent breath sounds
  4. Breathing pattern abnormalities:
     a. Prolonged exhalation alternating with periods of shallow breathing
     b. Rapid, shallow breathing
  5. Areas of tenderness or masses palpated on the chest wall
  6. Increased fremitus (vibration) in areas of tumor
  7. Decreased or absent fremitus with bronchial obstruction
  8. Tracheal deviation
  9. Pleural friction rub
  10. Asymmetry of diaphragm movement
  11. Use of accessory muscles manifested by retraction between ribs or at sternal notch
- Assess for nonpulmonary manifestations:
  1. Weight loss
  2. Muffled heart sounds
  3. Dysrhythmias
  4. Cyanosis of the lips and fingertips
  5. Clubbing of the fingers
  6. Bone pain
  7. Fever/chills related to pneumonitis, bronchitis, pneumonia
  8. Paraneoplastic endocrine syndromes caused by hormones secreted by tumor cells, such as syndrome of inappropriate antidiuretic hormone (SIADH)
- Assess for late manifestations, including fatigue, weight loss, anorexia, dysphagia, nausea and vomiting, lethargy, confusion, and personality changes.
- Assess for psychosocial issues of fear, anxiety, guilt, or shame:
  1. Convey acceptance; interact with patient in nonjudgmental way.
  2. Encourage the patient and family to express their feelings about the possible diagnosis of lung cancer.

- Diagnosis of lung cancer is made on the basis of:
  1. Chest x-ray
  2. CT scan
  3. Fiberoptic bronchoscopy
  4. Thoracoscopy or thoracentesis to view and biopsy lung tissue
- Other tests used to determine extent of metastasis include MRI, PET, or radionuclide scans of the liver, spleen, brain, and bone.

Nonsurgical Management

- Chemotherapy is often the treatment of choice for lung cancers, and it may be used alone or as adjuvant therapy in combination with surgery.
- The exact combination of drugs used depends on the response of the tumor and the overall health of the patient; however, most include platinum-based agents.
- Common side effects that occur with chemotherapy for lung cancer include:
  1. Chemotherapy-induced nausea and vomiting (CIN)
  2. Alopecia
  3. Mucositis
  4. Bone marrow suppression resulting in immunosuppression, anemia, and thrombocytopenia
  5. Peripheral neuropathy (PN)
- *Targeted therapy* involves the use of drugs that target specific features of cancer cells, such as a protein, an enzyme, or the formation of new blood vessels. These drugs cause fewer and less severe side effects for most patients compared with traditional anti-neoplastic agents. For lung cancer, targeted therapy drugs include:
  1. Erlotinib (Tarceva), an oral drug
  2. Bevacizumab (Avastin), given IV
  3. Crizotinib (Xalkori), an oral drug
- *Radiation therapy* may be used for locally advanced lung cancers confined to the chest. It is typically used in addition to surgery or chemotherapy and delivered by external beam therapy daily over 5 to 6 weeks. General management issues for the care of patients undergoing radiation therapy are presented in Part One under *Cancer Treatment*.
- Common side effects of radiation therapy for lung cancer are:
  1. Chest skin irritation and peeling
  2. Fatigue
  3. Wheezing from inflamed airways
  4. Esophagitis and changes in taste
- *Photodynamic therapy* (PDT) may be used to remove small bronchial tumors when they are accessible by bronchoscopy. The

patient is first injected with an agent that sensitizes cells to light. This drug enters all cells but leaves normal cells more rapidly than cancer cells, allowing it to concentrate in cancer cells. At about 48 hours, the patient goes to the operating room and is placed under anesthesia and intubated. A laser light is focused on the tumor. The light activates a chemical reaction within the cells, retaining the sensitizing drug that induces irreversible cell damage. Some cells die and slough immediately; others continue to slough for several days.

- The photosensitizing drug has many effects that require special patient teaching and care both before and after the laser treatment. General management issues for the care of patients undergoing PDT are presented in Part One under *Cancer Treatment.*
- When PDT is used in the airways, the patient usually requires a stay in the intensive care unit (ICU) for airway management.

Surgical Management

- Surgery is the main treatment for stage I and stage II NSCLC. Total removal of a non–small cell primary lung cancer is undertaken in hope of achieving a cure. If complete resection is not possible, the surgeon removes the bulk of the tumor.
- The specific surgery depends on the stage of the cancer and the patient's overall health and functional status. Surgeries include:
  1. Removal of the tumor only
  2. Removal of a lung segment (segmentectomy)
  3. Removal of a lobe (lobectomy)
  4. Removal of an entire lung (pneumonectomy)
- Procedures can be performed by open thoracotomy or thoracoscopy with minimally invasive surgery in selected patients.
- Provide routine preoperative care as described in Part One and:
  1. Teach the patient about the probable location of the surgical incision or thoracoscopy openings, shoulder exercises, and about the chest tube and drainage system (except after pneumonectomy).
  2. Encourage the patient to express fears and concerns.
  3. Reinforce the surgeon's explanation of the surgical procedure.
- Provide postoperative care as described in Part One with a focus on respiratory and pain management:
  1. Respiratory management
     a. Maintain a patent airway.
     b. Assess respiratory status at least every 2 hours for the first 12 to 24 hours.
        (1) Check the alignment of the trachea.
        (2) Assess oxygen saturation.
        (3) Assess the rate and depth of respiration.

      (4) Listen to breath sounds in all remaining lobes.

      (5) Assess the oral mucous membranes for cyanosis and the nail beds for rate of capillary refill.

  c. Perform oral suctioning as necessary.

  d. Provide oxygen therapy or mechanical ventilation as prescribed.

  e. Assist the patient to a semi-Fowler's position or to sit up in a chair as soon as possible.

  f. For a patient with spontaneous respirations, encourage the patient to use the incentive spirometer every hour while awake.

  g. If coughing is permitted, help the patient cough by splinting any incision and ensuring that the chest tube does not pull with movement.

2. Pain management

3. Apply closed chest drainage (see Appendix 7, *The Patient Requiring Chest Tubes*).

Palliative Interventions

- Treatment may focus on symptom management, rather than cure.
- Dyspnea management is a priority. Dyspnea is reduced with oxygen, drug therapy, radiation, management of pleural effusion, pain relief, and positioning for comfort. For example, the patient with severe dyspnea may be most comfortable sitting in a lounge chair or reclining chair.
- Oxygen therapy with humidification is prescribed to treat hypoxemia or to relieve dyspnea and anxiety.
- Drug therapy to improve oxygenation and relieve dyspnea includes:
  1. Bronchodilators and corticosteroids for the patient with bronchospasm
  2. Mucolytics to ease removal of thick mucus and sputum
  3. Antibiotics when bacterial infection is present
- Radiation therapy helps relieve hemoptysis, obstruction of the bronchi and great veins, dysphagia, and pain resulting from bone metastasis. Usually, radiation for palliation schedules higher doses for shorter periods than curative regimens. Complications are the same as those occurring with radiation therapy for cure.
- Thoracentesis and pleurodesis relieve pulmonary symptoms caused by pleural effusion.
  1. *Thoracentesis* is fluid removal by suction from the placement of a large needle or catheter into the intrapleural space.
  2. *Pleurodesis* is the deliberate development of an inflammation in the pleural space to cause the pleura to stick to the chest wall and prevent formation of effusion fluid. Agents such as liquid sclerosing chemicals or talc are instilled in the chest by thoracentesis after the effusion fluid has been removed.

- Pain management may be needed for chest pain and pain radiating to the arm. The goal is to keep the patient as comfortable as possible.
  1. Morphine and related opioids relieve symptoms of dyspnea while also treating pain. Oral, parenteral, or transdermal preparations are all potentially effective.
  2. Analgesics are given around the clock and PRN (for breakthrough pain).
  3. Additional nonpharmacologic measures may include positioning, hot or cold compresses, distractions, and guided imagery.
  4. Perform ongoing pain assessment as described in Part One.
  5. Evaluate the patient's response to the management strategies and collaborate with the health care team to make adjustments as necessary for improved patient comfort.
- Refer the terminal patient to hospice or other palliative care programs.

CANCER, OVARIAN

OVERVIEW

- Ovarian cancer is the leading cause of death from female reproductive cancers. Survival rates are low, because ovarian cancer is often not detected until its late stages.
- Most ovarian cancers are epithelial tumors that form on the surface of the ovaries.
- These tumors grow rapidly, spread quickly, and are often bilateral.
- Ovarian cancers metastasize by direct extension into nearby organs and through blood and lymph circulation to distant sites. Free-floating cancer cells also spread through the abdomen.
- Women who have a mutation in the *BRCA1* or *BRCA2* genes are at high risk for developing ovarian cancer over their lifetime, although the actual number of women with these genes is relatively small.

PATIENT-CENTERED COLLABORATIVE CARE

Assessment

- Obtain patient information about risk factors for ovarian cancer:
  1. Family history of ovarian or breast cancer (*BRACA* gene) or hereditary nonpolyposis colorectal cancer (HNPCC)
  2. Diabetes mellitus
  3. Nulliparity or infertility
  4. Older than 30 years at first pregnancy
  5. Personal history of breast or colorectal cancer
  6. Early menarche or late menopause
  7. Endometriosis
  8. Obesity or high-fat diet

- Ask the patient about manifestations of ovarian cancer:
  1. Abdominal pain, swelling, or bloating
  2. Vague GI disturbances such as dyspepsia (indigestion) and gas
  3. Urinary frequency or incontinence
  4. Unexpected weight loss
  5. Vaginal bleeding
- Assess for complications of metastatic cancer:
  1. Pleural effusion
  2. Ascites
  3. Lymphedema
  4. Intestinal obstruction
  5. Malnutrition
- Diagnosis and staging are performed by surgical exploration and biopsy analysis.
- Other assessment techniques helpful in staging the cancer and monitoring therapy progress include the CA-125 cancer antigen test, transvaginal ultrasonography, chest x-ray, and CT.

Interventions
- Nursing care of the patient with ovarian cancer is similar to that for endometrial or cervical cancer.
- Treatment options depend on the extent of the cancer and usually include surgery first, followed by chemotherapy. Radiation therapy is used for more widespread cancers.

  Surgical Management
- Total abdominal hysterectomy and bilateral salpingo-oophorectomy (BSO) are the surgical procedures for all stages of ovarian cancer.
- When cancer has spread to other abdominal organs or lymph nodes, the tumors can be removed during the surgery.
- After surgery, nursing care is similar to that of the patient undergoing a hysterectomy for uterine leiomyomas or care for the postoperative abdominal surgery patient.

  Nonsurgical Management
- For all stages of ovarian cancer, chemotherapy drugs may be used. Drugs may include cisplatin (Platinol), carboplatin, and paclitaxel (Taxol). They may be given IV or intraperitoneally.

CANCER, PANCREATIC
OVERVIEW
- Pancreatic tumors are highly malignant and originate in the epithelial cells (adenocarcinoma) of the pancreatic ductal system.
- These cancers grow rapidly and spread to surrounding organs (stomach, duodenum, gallbladder, and intestine) by direct extension and invasion of the lymphatic and vascular system.
- Pancreatic cancer may also result from metastasis from cancer of the lung, breast, thyroid, or kidney or from skin melanoma.

- Most pancreatic cancers are not diagnosed until the disease is advanced, and the overall survival rate is low.

PATIENT-CENTERED COLLABORATIVE CARE
Assessment
- Obtain patient information about:
  1. Jaundice (yellow discoloration of skin and sclera) and pruritus (itching)
  2. Clay-colored stool and dark, frothy urine
  3. Abdominal pain described as a vague, constant dullness in the upper abdomen and nonspecific in nature; pain related to eating or activity; or back pain
  4. Weight loss (unplanned)
  5. Anorexia accompanied by early satiety, nausea, flatulence, and vomiting
- Assess for:
  1. High blood glucose levels
  2. Splenomegaly
  3. GI bleeding
  4. Leg or calf pain (from thrombophlebitis)
  5. Fatigue and weakness
  6. Dull sound on abdominal percussion indicating ascites
- Diagnostic assessment may include:
  1. Elevated levels of serum amylase, serum lipase, alkaline phosphatase, and bilirubin
  2. Elevated level of carcinoembryonic antigen (CEA)
  3. Elevated levels of serum markers: CA-19-9 and CA-242
  4. Abdominal ultrasound or CT
  5. Endoscopic retrograde cholangiopancreatography (ERC)
  6. Aspiration of pancreatic ascitic fluid

Interventions
- Management of the patient with pancreatic cancer is geared toward preventing tumor spread and decreasing pain. These measures are palliative, not curative. Pancreatic cancer is often metastatic and recurs despite treatment.
  #### Nonsurgical Management
- Drug therapy includes:
  1. High doses of opioid analgesia; dependency is not a consideration because of the poor prognosis
  2. Chemotherapy with drug combinations of 5-FU, gemcitabine (Gemzar), capecitabine (Xeloda), and docetaxel (Taxotere) or a target agent erlotinib (Tarceva)
     a. General management issues for the care of patients undergoing chemotherapy are presented in Part One under *Cancer Treatment.*

- *External beam radiation therapy* to shrink pancreatic tumor cells, alleviating obstruction and improving food absorption, may provide pain relief but has not increased survival rates.
- Implantation of radon seeds in combination with systemic or intra-arterial administration of floxuridine (FUDR) has also been used.
- Biliary stents may be inserted to relieve biliary obstruction.

Surgical Management
- Surgery consists of complete or partial pancreatectomy.
- The classic surgery, the Whipple procedure, entails extensive surgical manipulation, including resection of the proximal head of the pancreas, the duodenum, a portion of the jejunum, the stomach (partial or total gastrectomy), and the gallbladder, with anastomosis of the pancreatic duct (pancreatojejunostomy), the common bile duct (choledochojejunostomy), and the stomach (gastrojejunostomy) to the jejunum. The spleen may also be removed (splenectomy). This surgery may be performed by the traditional open abdominal method or by laparoscopic minimally invasive surgery (in select cancers).
- Palliative measures to relieve obstruction, such as cholecystojejunostomy, may be performed.
- Preoperative care and monitoring includes optimizing fluid and electrolyte balance and nutritional status.
- Postoperative care and monitoring occurs as described in Part One and:
  1. Monitoring the drainage tubes and their patency to remove drainage and secretions from the area and to prevent stress on the anastomosis site
  2. Monitoring drainage for color, consistency, and amount
  3. Observing for fistula formation and excoriation (drainage of pancreatic fluids is corrosive and irritating to the skin, internal leakage causes peritonitis)
  4. Placing the patient in a semi-Fowler's position to reduce stress on the incision and anastomosis and to optimize lung expansion
  5. Maintaining fluid and electrolyte balance
  6. Closely monitoring vital signs for decreased BP and increased HR, decreased vascular pressures, decreased hemoglobin and hematocrit levels, and electrolyte imbalances
  7. Assessing blood glucose levels for transient hyperglycemia or hypoglycemia resulting from surgical manipulation of the pancreas
  8. Monitoring the patient for pitting edema of the extremities and dependent edema in the sacrum and back
- Use enteral feeding if the patient cannot meet caloric needs while intestinal function is intact. A jejunostomy tube is inserted for late

stages of pancreatic carcinoma; this method is preferred for less-ening reflux and facilitating absorption.
- Use of hyperalimentation to optimize nutrition may be used as a single measure or in combination with tube feedings; a peripher-ally inserted or tunneled catheter may be required.

Community-Based Care
- Many of the care measures are palliative and aimed at providing symptom relief.

CANCER, PROSTATE
OVERVIEW
- Prostate cancer is the second most common type of cancer in men and most commonly affects men over 65 years with black men having the greatest risk for this cancer.
- Most prostate tumors are adenocarcinomas arising from epithe-lial cells located in the posterior lobe or outer portion of the gland, and most are androgen-sensitive (need testosterone to grow).
- If found early this slow growing cancer has a nearly 100% cure rate.
- In advanced stages of the disease, metastatic sites include lymph nodes, bone, lungs, and liver.

🧬 Genetic/Genomic Considerations

Many gene mutations play a role in various types of prostate cancer. Some men with the most aggressive prostate cancers have *BCRA2* mutations similar to those in women who have *BCRA2*-associated breast and ovarian cancers. The most common genetic factor that increases the risk of prostate cancer is a mutation in the glutathione S-transferase *(GSTP1)* gene. This gene is normally part of the pathway that helps to prevent cancer.

PATIENT-CENTERED COLLABORATIVE CARE
Assessment
- Obtain patient information about:
  1. Age
  2. Race and ethnicity
  3. Family history of cancer
  4. Nutritional habits
  5. Problems with urination
     a. Difficulty in starting urination
     b. Frequent bladder infections
     c. Urinary retention

6. Pain during intercourse, especially when ejaculating
7. Any other pain (particularly bone pain)
- Assess for:
  1. Blood in the urine (hematuria)
  2. Pain in the pelvis, spine, hips, or rib
  3. Swollen lymph nodes, especially in the groin areas
- Assess for psychosocial issues:
  1. Anxiety, fear, and/or depression
  2. Determine what support systems the patient has, such as family, spiritual leaders, or community group support, to help him through diagnosis, treatment, and recovery.
  3. Refer the patient with concerns related to sexuality and erectile dysfunction (ED) to his surgeon (urologist), sex therapist, or intimacy therapist, if available.
- Diagnostic assessment for cancer and metastasis may include:
  1. Digital rectal examination (DRE). A prostate that is found to be stony hard and have palpable irregularities or indurations is suspected to be malignant.
  2. Elevated levels of complexed prostate-specific antigen (cPSA) (greater than 3.4 ng/mL)
  3. Elevated levels of serum acid phosphatase
  4. Transrectal ultrasound (TRUS) of the prostate
  5. Prostate tissue biopsy
  6. Lymph node biopsy
  7. CT scan of the pelvis and abdomen
  8. MRI

Planning and Implementation
- Patients are faced with several treatment options, depending on the stage of the disease and their overall health. A urologist and an oncologist are needed to help them make the best decision.
- Because prostate cancer is slow growing with late metastasis, older men who are asymptomatic may choose observation without immediate active treatment, an option known as *watchful waiting* or *expectant therapy.*
- Active treatment options are classified as local and systemic therapies. Local therapies include surgery and radiation. A variety of drugs are used for systemic therapy. Specific management is based on the extent of the disease and the patient's physical condition.

Surgical Management
- Surgery is the most common intervention for a cure. Minimally invasive surgery (MIS) or an open surgical technique for radical prostatectomy (prostate removal) is most often performed. Other surgeries for palliation may include:
  1. Transurethral resection of the prostate (TURP) to promote urination

   2. Bilateral orchiectomy (removal of both testicles) to slow the spread of cancer by removing the main source of testosterone
- *Laparoscopic radical prostatectomy (LRP)* is an MIS for cure of patients who have a PSA less than 10 ng/mL and who have had no previous hormone therapy or abdominal surgeries.
- *Traditional open radical prostatectomy* can be performed through a retropubic or perineal approach, but the retropubic method is done most often to preserve perineal nerves needed for penile erection.
  1. Provide preoperative care described in Part One and teach the patient about the probable location of the surgical incision, the use of an indwelling urinary catheter, placement of drains, and the possibility of temporary ED.
- Provide postoperative care described in Part One and:
  1. Keep an accurate record of intake and output, including the character and amount of drainage from devices.
  2. Keep the urinary meatus clean using soap and water.
  3. Emphasize the importance of not straining during bowel movements and avoiding suppositories or enemas.

Nonsurgical Management

- Nonsurgical management is usually an adjunct to surgery but may be done as an alternative intervention if the cancer is widespread or the patient's condition or age prevents surgery.
- External or internal radiation therapy may be used in the treatment of prostate cancer or for palliation of late-stage symptoms.
  1. *External beam radiation therapy* (EBRT) comes from a source outside the body. Patients are usually treated 5 days each week for 6 to 9 weeks.
  2. Complications of EBRT may include:
     a. ED
     b. Acute radiation cystitis
     c. Radiation proctitis
  3. *Internal radiation therapy (brachytherapy)* can be delivered by implanting low-dose radiation seeds directly into and around the prostate gland.
  4. General management issues for the care of patients undergoing radiation therapy are presented in Part One under *Cancer Treatment*.
- Hormone therapy is often used for prostate tumors, because many are hormone dependent, and these tumors can be reduced or have their growth slowed through androgen deprivation. Manipulating the patient's hormones may be accomplished in two ways:
  1. The testosterone influence can be removed by a bilateral orchiectomy (surgery).

   2. Luteinizing hormone-releasing hormone (LH-RH) agonists
      or antiandrogens (drugs) can be given.
- Side effects of hormone therapy may include:
   1. Hot flashes
   2. Gynecomastia (breast development)
- *Systemic cytotoxic chemotherapy* is an option for patients whose
  cancer has spread and for whom other therapies have not worked.
   1. Specific treatment regimens and drug combinations vary,
      but the most commonly used agents for prostate cancer
      include docetaxel (Taxotere), cisplatin (Platinol), and etopo-
      side (VP-16, VePesid).
   2. General management issues for the care of patients undergo-
      ing chemotherapy are presented in Part One under *Cancer
      Treatment.*
- *Cryotherapy (cryoablation)* is a minimally invasive procedure
  for patients whose disease is known to be confined to the prostate gland. Transrectal cryoprobes are positioned around the prostate gland. Liquid nitrogen freezes the gland and results in prostate
  cell death.

Community-Based Care
- Include the patient's sexual partner in any teaching and discharge
  planning.
- Assess and address the patient's physical and psychosocial needs
  before hospital discharge and ensure his or her continued management in the community setting.
- Home care management of the patient after a radical prostatectomy includes:
   1. Collaborating with the case manager to coordinate the efforts
      of various health care providers and possibly a home care nurse
   2. Health teaching about:
      a. Indwelling urinary catheter care if recovering from an open
         procedure, including:
         (1) Caring for the catheter and leg bag
         (2) Identifying manifestations of urinary infection and
             other complications
      b. Restriction for activity or weight lifting; these may be as
         brief as 2 to 3 days for minimally invasive procedures and
         as long as 6 weeks for open surgical procedures.
      c. Kegel perineal exercises may reduce the severity of urinary
         incontinence after radical prostatectomy. Teach the patient
         to contract and relax the perineal and gluteal muscles.
      d. Teach the patient to avoid straining at defecation.
      e. Teach the patient how to inspect the incision site daily for
         signs of infection.
      f. Stress the importance of keeping follow-up appointments.

- Refer the patient and partner to agencies or support groups, many of which can be found on the Internet through respected cancer organizations or government sites. Other personal and community support services, such as spiritual leaders or churches and synagogues, are also important to many patients.
- Refer patients with ED or urinary incontinence to a urologist or other specialist.

CANCER, UROTHELIAL (BLADDER)
OVERVIEW

- Urothelial cancers are malignant tumors of the urothelium, which is the lining of transitional cells in the kidney, renal pelvis, ureters, urinary bladder, and urethra.
- Most urothelial cancers occur in the bladder; the term *bladder cancer* is the general term used to describe this condition.
- Most bladder cancers are transitional cell carcinomas of the bladder and are treated with surgical excision and chemotherapy. Chemotherapy is commonly instilled into the bladder and may require additional patient teaching about safe use of toilets for family members.
- New surgical techniques are being used to divert urine flow, including construction of a neobladder to improve function of patients who have their bladder removed as part of cancer treatment.
- If the cancer is untreated, the tumor cells invade surrounding tissues, the cancer spreads to distant sites (liver, lung, and bone), and the condition ultimately leads to death.
- Causes of urothelial cancers include tobacco use; exposure to toxic chemicals used in hair dye, rubber, paint, electric cable, and textile industries; *Schistosoma haematobium* (a parasite) infection; excessive use of drugs containing phenacetin; and long-term use of cyclophosphamide (Cytoxan, Procytox ✦).

PATIENT-CENTERED COLLABORATIVE CARE
Assessment
- Obtain patient information about:
  1. Age and gender
  2. Active and passive exposure to cigarette smoke
  3. Occupation and exposure to toxic chemicals
  4. Description of change in color, frequency, amount of urine
  5. Presence of any abdominal discomfort
  6. Presence of dysuria, frequency, or urgency
- Assess:
  1. Overall appearance of the patient, especially skin color and general nutritional status

   2. Abdomen for asymmetry, tenderness, and bladder distention
   3. Urine for color, clarity, presence of blood (first sign of bladder cancer)
   4. Anxiety or fear
   5. Patient's methods of coping and the degree of support from family members
- Diagnostic assessment includes:
   1. Urinalysis
   2. Cystoscopy with biopsy
   3. CT scan or MRI for deep, invasive tumors

Interventions

Nonsurgical Management
- Prophylactic immunotherapy with intravesical instillation of bacille Calmette-Guérin (BCG) is used to prevent recurrence of superficial bladder cancers.
- Multiagent chemotherapy or radiation therapy may prolong life after metastasis has occurred but rarely results in a cure.

Surgical Management
- The type of surgery for bladder cancer depends on the type and stage of the cancer and the patient's general health.
- Transurethral resection of the bladder tumor (TURBT) or partial cystectomy is performed for small, early, superficial tumors, and only a portion of the bladder is removed.
- Complete bladder removal (cystectomy) with additional removal of surrounding muscle and tissue offers the best chance of a cure for large, invasive bladder cancers. The ureters are diverted into one of several types of collecting reservoirs or a ureterostomy. The common types of urinary drainage following a cystectomy are ileal conduit, continent pouch, bladder reconstruction (also known as *neobladder*), and ureterosigmoidostomy.
   1. *Ureterostomy* (or a *ureteroureterostomy*) results in the ureters placed on the skin surface as one or two stomas that drain urine into an external pouching system. This system is now less common.
   2. *Ileal conduit* results in the ureters surgically placed in the ileum, which is brought to the skin surface as a stoma. Urine is collected in a pouch on the skin around the stoma.
   3. *Ureterosigmoidostomy* results in the ureters surgically placed into a specially constructed segment of the sigmoid colon. No external pouching is needed.
   4. *Continent pouches* (e.g., Kock's pouch) are internal pouches constructed from an ileal segment. Although these pouches open to the outside of the abdomen, a fold prevents urine leakage. Urine is drained with intermittent catheterization, and an external pouch is not needed.

C

5. *Neobladder* is reconstruction of the bladder from bowel tissue and connecting it to the urethra. Many patients learn to control voiding from the neobladder and neither external pouching nor intermittent catheterization is needed.

- Provide preoperative care and postoperative care described in Part One and:
  1. Reinforce the surgeon's explanation of the procedure
  2. Ensure education about the specific urinary diversion and postoperative care requirements for self-care practices, methods of pouching, control of urine drainage, and management of odor
  3. Coordinate with an enterostomal therapist (ET) for wound, skin, stoma, and pouch care
  4. Explore psychosocial concerns, including those about altered body image, sexuality, fear, and uncertainty
  5. Monitor urine output and urine characteristics
  6. Manage the drain and catheter for patients who have had construction of a continent reservoir
  7. Perform initial irrigation and intermittent catheterization of the neobladder
  8. Teach the patient with a neobladder how to use new cues to know when to void, such as voiding at prescribed times or noticing a feeling of neobladder pressure

Community-Based Care
- Provide health teaching to the patient and family about:
  1. Drugs, diet, and fluid therapy; the use of external pouching systems; and the technique for catheterizing a continent reservoir
  2. Avoiding foods that are known to produce gas (if the urinary diversion uses the intestinal tract)
- Assist the patient to prepare for the impact of urinary diversion on self-image, body image, sexual functioning, and self-esteem.
- Refer patients and families to community support and information organizations such as the United Ostomy Association; the American Cancer Society; and the Wound, Ostomy, and Continence Nurses Society.

CARDIAC VALVE DISEASE

See *Stenosis* and *Regurgitation*.

CARDIOMYOPATHY

OVERVIEW

- Cardiomyopathy is a subacute or chronic heart muscle disease.
- Cardiomyopathy is divided into four categories on the basis of abnormalities in structure and function:

1. *Dilated cardiomyopathy* (DCM), the most common type, involves extensive damage to the myofibrils and interference with myocardial metabolism; it is characterized by dilation of both ventricles and impairment of systolic function.
2. *Hypertrophic cardiomyopathy* (HCM) is characterized by asymmetric ventricular hypertrophy and disarray of the myocardial fibers that results in a stiff left ventricle and diastolic filling abnormalities. In about 50% of patients, HCM is transmitted as a single-gene autosomal dominant trait.
3. *Restrictive cardiomyopathy* (RCM), the rarest of the four cardiomyopathies, is caused by ventricles that restrict filling during diastole. It can be a primary endo- or myocardial condition or a result of sarcoidosis or amyloidosis.
4. *Arrhythmogenic right ventricular* (ARV) *cardiomyopathy* is a condition that results from replacement of myocardial tissue with fibrous and fatty tissue, usually as a familial condition.

- Sudden death may be the first and only manifestation of cardiomyopathy.

PATIENT-CENTERED COLLABORATIVE CARE
Assessment
- Assess for clinical manifestations of DCM:
  1. Signs of left ventricular failure at onset of disease progressing to biventricular failure (see *Heart Failure*).
  2. Progressive dyspnea on exertion
  3. Orthopnea
  4. Palpitations
  5. Activity intolerance
  6. Atrial fibrillation
- Assess for clinical manifestations of HCM:
  1. Exertional dyspnea or angina and unexplained syncope
  2. Atypical chest pain that occurs at rest, is prolonged, has no relation to exertion, and is not relieved by nitrates
  3. Ventricular dysrhythmias
- Assess for clinical manifestations of RCM:
  1. Exertional dyspnea
  2. Weakness, activity intolerance
  3. Coexisting connective tissue disease
  4. Symptoms similar to pericardial tamponade or chronic restrictive pericarditis
- Assess for clinical manifestations of ARV cardiomyopathy:
  1. Dizziness, syncope, or palpitations, particularly with aerobic effort
  2. Irregular pulse, abnormal conduction with electrocardiography (ECG)

Interventions

Nonsurgical Management

- Care of the patient with cardiomyopathy is similar to that for patients with heart failure (see *Heart Failure*) and dysrhythmias.
- Treatment includes:
  1. Administering an angiotensin-converting enzyme inhibitor or angiotensin receptor blocker and a beta blocker to block the neurohormonal contributions to cardiomyopathy; diuretics, vasodilators, and cardiac glycosides may be used as the disease progresses
  2. Anticipating procedure to implant automatic cardiac defibrillator to promote synchronous ventricular emptying and control ventricular dysrhythmias
  3. Teaching the patient to abstain from alcohol because of its cardiac depressant effects
  4. Teaching the patient to report any palpitations, dizziness, or fainting that may indicate a dysrhythmia
- Management of HCM includes beta-adrenergic blocking agents (carvedilol); strenuous exercise is prohibited.

Surgical Management

- The type of surgery performed depends on the type of cardiomyopathy.
  1. Ventriculomyotomy is the most common; it is the excision of a portion of the hypertrophied ventricular septum to create a widened outflow tract.
  2. Placement of an implantable defibrillator with or without ablation to manage dysrhythmia
  3. Heart transplantation is the treatment of choice for patients with severe DCM; a donor heart from a person of comparable body weight and ABO compatibility is transplanted into a recipient within 6 hours of procurement.

! NURSING SAFETY PRIORITY: Critical Rescue

After cardiac transplant surgery, perform frequent comprehensive cardiovascular and respiratory assessments according to agency or heart transplant surgical protocol. *Report any of these manifestations to the surgeon immediately.* To detect rejection, the surgeon performs right endomyocardial biopsies at regularly scheduled intervals and whenever symptoms occur.

Community-Based Care

- Support an interdisciplinary approach to promote self-management for the patient with cardiomyopathy:
  1. Teach patient to recognize symptoms of worsening heart failure including fatigue, dyspnea, peripheral edema, and weight gain

2. Identify strategies to increase acceptance of drug regimens to improve cardiac output and slow the progression of heart failure
3. Promote exercise and healthy lifestyle choices

- For the patient who receives a heart transplant:
  1. Provide postoperative care similar to that provided for patients having open heart surgery (see *Surgical Management* under *Coronary Artery Disease*).
  2. Provide discharge teaching:
     a. Teach the patient to report signs and symptoms of rejection, such as hypotension, dysrhythmias, weakness, fatigue, dizziness, respiratory distress, weight gain, or edema.
     b. Inform the patient that the surgeon will perform endomyocardial biopsy at regularly scheduled intervals to detect rejection.
     c. Teach the patient the importance of taking immunosuppressants for life to prevent transplant rejection.
     d. Encourage the patient to follow a lifestyle similar to that of patients with coronary artery disease.
     e. Encourage the patient to participate in an exercise program, allowing at least 10 minutes of warm-up and cool-down for the denervated heart to adjust to changes in activity level.
     f. Provide information about discharge drugs and diet.

CARDITIS, RHEUMATIC (RHEUMATIC ENDOCARDITIS)

- *Rheumatic carditis (rheumatic endocarditis)* develops after an infection with group A beta-hemolytic streptococci in some individuals.
- Inflammation is evident in all layers of the heart and results in impaired contractile function of the myocardium, thickening of the pericardium, and inflamed endocardium, leading to valvular damage.
- Common manifestations include:
  1. Symptoms of streptococcal infection, leading to endocarditis
  2. Evidence of an existing streptococcal infection: fever, sore throat, tachycardia, and elevated serum findings of antideoxyribonuclease B titer, antistreptolysin O titer, complement assay, and C-reactive protein
  3. New-onset murmur, pericardial friction rub, precordial pain, and/or extreme fatigue
- Management includes antibiotic therapy to manage streptococcal infection and follow-up care to manage heart valve or heart damage (see *Regurgitation, Mitral*; and *Cardiomyopathy*).

CARPAL TUNNEL SYNDROME

OVERVIEW

- Carpal tunnel syndrome (CTS) is a condition in which the median nerve in the wrist becomes compressed, causing pain and numbness.
- Risk factors include common repetitive strain injury (RSI), synovitis, excessive hand exercise, edema or hemorrhage into the carpal tunnel, or thrombosis of the median artery, Colles' fracture of the wrist, and hand burns. CTS is also a common complication of certain metabolic and connective tissue diseases.

PATIENT-CENTERED COLLABORATIVE CARE

Assessment

- Assess for:
  1. Nature, location, and intensity of patient-reported pain, paresthesia, and numbness
  2. Positive results for the Phalen maneuver, producing paresthesia in the palmar side of the thumb, index, and middle finger and radial half of the ring finger within 60 seconds; the patient is asked to relax the wrist into flexion or place the back of the hands together and flex both wrists simultaneously.
  3. Positive results for the Tinel sign, which is the same response as for the Phalen maneuver, elicited by tapping lightly over the area of the median nerve in the wrist
  4. Weak pinch, clumsiness, and difficulty with fine movements that progresses to muscle weakness progressing to muscle wasting in the affected hand
  5. Wrist swelling and autonomic changes such as skin discoloration, nail brittleness, and increased or decreased palmar sweating
- Diagnostic assessment may include any of these: standard x-rays, electromyography (EMG), MRI, and ultrasonography.

Interventions

Nonsurgical Management

- Drug therapy with NSAIDs
- Wrist immobilization with a splint or brace to place the wrist in a neutral position or slight extension during the day, during the night, or both

Surgical Management

- Surgery is performed to relieve the pressure on the median nerve by cutting or laser.
- When CTS is a complication of rheumatoid arthritis, a synovectomy (removal of excess synovium) through a small inner wrist incision may be performed.

- Provide preoperative care described in Part One and reinforce teaching about the surgery
- Provide postoperative care described in Part One and:
  1. Check the dressing for drainage and tightness and the hand and fingers for neurovascular status.
  2. Explain to the patient that hand movements may be restricted for 6 to 8 weeks and discomfort can last that long or longer.
- Multiple surgeries may be needed to fully decompress the median nerve.

CATARACTS

OVERVIEW

- A cataract is a lens opacity that distorts the image projected onto the retina.
- Cataracts can occur at any age, be caused by trauma or exposure to toxic agents, or result from comorbidities like diabetes and from eye disorders.
- Surgery is the only cure for cataracts. However, patients often live with reduced vision for years before the cataract is removed. Driving privileges may be restricted or withheld during this period of reduced vision.
  1. The most common surgical procedure is removal of the lens by phacoemulsification and replacement with a clear plastic lens for specific vision correction.
  2. Stress that care after surgery requires the instillation of different types of eye drops several times each day for 2 to 4 weeks.
  3. Instruct the patient on the importance of following the prescribed regimen for eye drops after surgery.
  4. Instruct the patient to notify the ophthalmologist if there is significant swelling or bruising around the eye; pain occurring with nausea or vomiting; increasing redness of the eye, a change in visual acuity, tears, and photophobia; and yellow or green drainage.

❗ NURSING SAFETY PRIORITY: Critical Rescue

Teach the patient to report any reduction in vision immediately to the ophthalmologist.

  5. Teach the patient to avoid activities that can increase intraocular pressure, including:
     a. Bending from the waist
     b. Lifting objects weighing more than 10 pounds (22 kg)
     c. Sneezing, coughing, blowing the nose
     d. Straining to have a bowel movement

- Interventions for enhanced communication, safety, and independence are described later in *Visual Impairment (Reduced Vision)*. The patient with cataracts is at high risk for falls.

CELIAC DISEASE

- Celiac disease is a multi-system autoimmune disease that has cycles of remission and exacerbation.
- Like other autoimmune inflammatory conditions it is thought to be caused by a combination of genetic, immunologic, and environmental factors.
- Symptoms include anorexia; diarrhea and/or constipation; steatorrhea (fatty stools); abdominal pain, distension, and bloating; and weight loss.
- Malabsorption occurs early in the condition and persists.
- Malnutrition symptoms occur over time when nutrients cannot be absorbed due to digestive enzyme deficiencies. Patients may have malnutrition-related muscle weakness, anemia, osteoporosis, peripheral neuropathy, infertility, weight loss, fluid retention, and easy bruising.
- Dietary management with a gluten-free diet promotes disease remission.

CEREBROVASCULAR ACCIDENT (CVA)

See *Stroke (Brain Attack)*.

CHLAMYDIAL INFECTION

OVERVIEW

- *Chlamydial trachomatis* is an intracellular bacterium that causes genital chlamydial infection, which is the most common sexually transmitted disease (STD) in the United States.
- The incubation period ranges from 1 to 3 weeks, but the pathogen may be present in the genital tract for months without producing symptoms.
- The main manifestation in men is urethritis with dysuria, frequent urination, and a watery, mucoid discharge. Complications include epididymitis, prostatitis, infertility, and reactive arthritis (also known as Reiter's syndrome).
- Many women may have no symptoms or a mucopurulent cervicitis that occurs with a change in vaginal discharge, easily induced cervical bleeding, urinary frequency, and abdominal discomfort or pain. Complications include salpingitis, pelvic inflammatory disease (PID), ectopic pregnancy, and infertility.
- Chlamydia infections are reportable to the local health department.

PATIENT-CENTERED COLLABORATIVE CARE
Assessment
- Obtain patient information about:
  1. The presence of symptoms, including vaginal or urethral discharge, dysuria (painful urination), pelvic pain, and irregular bleeding
  2. Any history of STDs
  3. Whether sexual partners have had symptoms or a history of STDs
  4. Whether patient or partner has had any unprotected intercourse

C

> ### ! NURSING SAFETY PRIORITY: Action Alert
>
> For men, ask about dysuria, frequent urination, and a mucoid discharge that is more watery and less copious than a gonorrheal discharge. These manifestations indicate urethritis, the main symptom of chlamydia in men.

- Diagnostic assessment requires sampling cells from the endocervix and/or urethra and laboratory testing:
  1. Gram staining (to rule out gonorrhea)
  2. Tissue culture for *Chlamydia*
  3. Gene amplification tests or DNA amplification tests (ligand chain reaction [LCR] and polymerase chain reaction [PCR])
  4. Enzyme-linked immunoassay (ELISA)
  5. Direct fluorescent antibody (DFA)

Interventions
- Antibiotic therapy provides a cure. The most common, effective antibiotics are azithromycin (Zithromax) or doxycycline but other agents can be used.
- Test and treat sexual partners.
- Educate patients about:
  1. The mode of disease transmission
  2. The incubation period
  3. Manifestation, including the possibility of asymptomatic infections
  4. Essential elements of treatment with antibiotic
  5. The need for abstinence from sexual intercourse until the patient and partner have completed treatment
  6. No test of cure is required, but all women should be re-screened 3 to 4 months after treatment because of the high risk for PID if re-infection occurs
  7. The need for the patient and partner to return for evaluation if symptoms recur or new symptoms develop

8. Possible complications of an untreated or inadequately treated infection, such as PID, ectopic pregnancy, or infertility
9. Recommendation that all sexually active women 25 years or older should be screened annually for chlamydia

CHOLECYSTITIS

OVERVIEW

- Cholecystitis is an inflammation of the gallbladder that can occur as an acute or chronic process.
- Acute calculous cholecystitis usually develops in association with cholelithiasis (gallstones). About one half of the adult population in the United States has asymptomatic gallstones.
- Acalculous cholecystitis occurs in the absence of gallstones and is associated with biliary stasis caused by any condition that affects the regular filling or emptying of the gallbladder, such as decreased blood flow to the gallbladder, or anatomic problems, such as kinking of the gallbladder neck or cystic duct that can result in pancreatic enzyme reflux into the gallbladder.
- Chronic cholecystitis results when repeated episodes of cystic duct obstruction result in chronic inflammation, and the gallbladder becomes fibrotic and contracted, resulting in decreased motility and deficient absorption.
- Complications of cholecystitis include pancreatitis and cholangitis (inflammation and infection of the common bile ducts).
- Cholangitis is usually associated with choledocholithiasis (common bile duct stones).
- Jaundice (yellow discoloration of body tissues) and icterus (yellow discoloration of the sclera) can occur in acute disease but are most commonly seen in the chronic phase of cholecystitis. Jaundice results from increased bilirubin in the body that collects in the skin and sclera. Itching and a burning sensation result.

PATIENT-CENTERED COLLABORATIVE CARE

Assessment

- Record patient information:
  1. Height and weight, body mass index, and waist circumference
  2. Gender, age, race, and ethnic group
  3. Fatty food intolerances and related GI symptoms, including flatulence, dyspepsia (indigestion), eructation (belching), anorexia, nausea, vomiting, and abdominal pain in relation to fatty food intake
  4. Family history of gallbladder disease
  5. In women, history of estrogen replacement therapy

- Assess for:
  1. Abdominal pain of varying intensity in the right upper abdominal quadrant, including radiation to the right upper shoulder; ask the patient to describe the intensity, duration, precipitating factors, and relief measures

! NURSING SAFETY PRIORITY: Critical Rescue

Biliary colic is pain caused by obstruction of the cystic duct by one or more stones. It may be so severe that it occurs with tachycardia, pallor, diaphoresis, and prostration (extreme exhaustion). Assess the patient for possible shock caused by biliary colic. Notify the health care provider or Rapid Response Team if these manifestations occur. Stay with the patient, and lower the head of the bed.

  2. Other GI symptoms, including nausea, vomiting, dyspepsia, flatulence, eructation, and feelings of abdominal heaviness
  3. With right subcostal palpation, increasing pain with deep inspiration (Murphy's sign)
  4. Guarding, rigidity, rebound tenderness (Blumberg's sign)
  5. Sausage-shaped mass in the right upper quadrant
  6. Late symptoms seen in chronic cholecystitis, such as jaundice, clay-colored stools, and dark urine
  7. Steatorrhea (fatty stools)
  8. Elevated temperature with tachycardia and dehydration from fever and vomiting
  9. Results of serum liver enzyme and bilirubin tests (may be elevated); amylase (may be elevated if pancreas is involved)
  10. Increased white blood cell (WBC) count

Considerations for Older Adults

- Older adults and patients with diabetes mellitus have atypical manifestations, including the absence of pain and fever. Localized tenderness may be the only presenting sign.
- The older adult may become acutely confused.

Planning and Implementation
Nonsurgical Management
- Patients with chronic cholecystitis are encouraged to consume small-volume, low-fat meals.
- If gallstones are causing an obstruction of bile flow, fat-soluble vitamins and bile salts may be prescribed to facilitate digestion and vitamin absorption.

- Food and fluids are withheld during nausea and vomiting episodes; nasogastric (NG) decompression is initiated for severe vomiting.
- Drug therapy includes:
  1. Opioid analgesics to relieve pain and reduce spasm
  2. Antiemetics to provide relief from nausea and vomiting

Surgical Management
- A percutaneous transhepatic biliary catheter may be inserted to decompress obstructed extrahepatic ducts so bile can flow.
- An endoscopic retrograde cholangiopancreatography (ERCP) may be performed.
- Cholecystectomy (removal of the gallbladder) using a laparoscopic approach
  1. Traditional open surgical approach for complicated or infected sites
     a. A T-tube drain is surgically inserted when the common bile duct is explored to ensure patency of the duct.
  2. Newer techniques, such as natural orifice transluminal endoscopic surgery (NOTES), are becoming more commonly used in large tertiary care centers.
- Provide routine preoperative care.
- Provide postoperative care for laparoscopic patients:
  1. Teach the patient the importance of early ambulation to absorb the carbon dioxide that is retained in the abdomen after a laparoscopic procedure.
  2. Inform the patient that shoulder pain is both expected and common; the pain decreases as the gases expanding the abdomen are dissipated.
  3. Inform the patient that he or she can return to usual activities 1 to 3 weeks after the procedure.
- Provide postoperative care for traditional surgery patients:
  1. Administer IV (by patient-controlled analgesia [PCA]) for pain relief, as ordered.
  2. Administer antiemetics for relief of postoperative nausea and vomiting, as ordered.
  3. Advance the diet from clear liquids to solid foods, as tolerated by the patient.
  4. Maintain the patient's T-tube:
     a. Keep the drainage system below the level of the gallbladder.
     b. Assess the amount, color, consistency, and odor of drainage (bile output is approximately 400 mL/day).
     c. Administer synthetic bile salts such as dehydrocholic acid (Decholin), as ordered.
     d. Report to the physician sudden increases or output of more than 1000 mL in 24 hours in bile output.

  e. Assess for foul odor and purulent drainage and report changes in drainage to the physician.
  f. Inspect the skin around the T-tube insertion site for signs of inflammation.
  g. Never irrigate, aspirate, or clamp the T-tube without a physician's order.
  h. Assess the drainage system for pulling, kinking, or tangling of the tubing.
  i. Place the patient in a semi-Fowler's position when in bed.
  j. Assist the patient with early ambulation.
  k. Teach patient to observe stools for brown color 7 to 10 days postoperatively.

QSEN TEAMWORK AND COLLABORATION

Before the start of any invasive procedure, conduct a final verification process using active communication to confirm the correct patient, procedure, and site.

CHRONIC OBSTRUCTIVE PULMONARY DISEASE (COPD)

OVERVIEW

- Chronic obstructive pulmonary disease (COPD) is an irreversible chronic lung disease.
- Two common conditions that lead to COPD are emphysema and chronic bronchitis.
- The major features of *emphysema* that lead to dyspnea are:
  1. Loss of lung elasticity
  2. Hyperinflation of the lung (air trapping)
- Emphysema is classified as panlobular, centrilobular, or paraseptal, depending on the pattern of destruction and dilation of the gas-exchanging units (acini). Each type can occur alone or in combination in the same lung. Most are associated with smoking or chronic exposure to other inhalation irritants.

🧬 Genetic/Genomic Considerations

The gene for alpha$_1$-antitrypsin (AAT) has many known variations, and some increase the risk for emphysema. Different variations result in different levels of AAT deficiency and this is a reason why the disease is more severe for some people than for others. The most serious variation for emphysema risk is the Z mutation, although others also increase the risk but to a lesser degree.

- *Bronchitis* is an inflammation of the bronchi and bronchioles caused by chronic exposure to irritants, especially tobacco smoke. It affects only the airways.
- The major features of chronic bronchitis are:
  1. Increased number and size of mucous glands, which produce large amounts of thick mucus
  2. Thickening of bronchial walls that impairs airflow
  3. Poor gas exchange with decreased Pao_2 (hypoxemia) and increased $Paco_2$ (respiratory acidosis)
- Risk factors for COPD include cigarette smoking, asthma, AAT deficiency, and air pollution.
- Complications of COPD include right heart failure, dysrhythmias, and pneumothorax.
- Respiratory infection can cause an acute exacerbation (worsening) in COPD symptoms.

PATIENT-CENTERED COLLABORATIVE CARE
Assessment
- Obtain and record patient information:
  1. Age, gender, occupational history, and family history
  2. Smoking history, including the length of time the patient has smoked and the number of packs smoked daily
  3. Current breathing problems:
     a. Does the patient have difficulty breathing while talking? Can he or she speak in complete sentences, or is it necessary to take a breath between every one or two words?
     b. Ask about the presence, duration, or worsening of wheezing, coughing, and shortness of breath, and what activities trigger these problems.
     c. If the cough is productive, what is the sputum color and amount, and has the amount increased or decreased?
     d. What is the relationship between activity tolerance and dyspnea? How is the patient's activity level and shortness of breath now compared with a month earlier and a year earlier? Is he or she having any difficulty with eating, sleeping, or performing activities of daily living (ADLs)?
  4. How are the patient's weight and general appearance? The patient with increasingly severe COPD is thin with loss of muscle mass in the extremities, has enlarged neck muscles and a barrel-shaped chest, and is slow moving and slightly stooped.
- Assess for:
  1. Respiratory changes:
     a. Rapid, shallow respirations, paradoxical respirations, or use of accessory muscles

   b. Limited diaphragmatic movement (excursion)
   c. Abnormal lung sounds
   d. Increased anterior-posterior chest diameter
   e. Cough with mucus production when chronic bronchitis is the primary disorder
2. Cardiovascular changes:
   a. HR and rhythm
   b. Swelling of feet and ankles
   c. Cyanosis, or blue-tinged, dusky appearance
   d. Delayed capillary refill
   e. Clubbing of the fingers
3. Psychosocial issues:
   a. Social isolation due to decreased mobility and energy
   b. Exposure to smoke or crowded living conditions
   c. Work, family, social, and sexual roles that may change and affect self-esteem
   d. Anxiety and fear related to dyspnea that may reduce the patient's ability to participate in a full life
   e. Patient's and family's expression of their feelings about the limitations on lifestyle and disease progression
   f. Patient's and family's awareness and use of support groups and services
4. Diagnostic and laboratory tests:
   a. Serial arterial blood gas (ABG) values for hypoxemia and hypercarbia
   b. Oxygen saturation by pulse oximetry
   c. Sputum cultures
   d. Hematocrit and hemoglobin for polycythemia
   e. Serum electrolyte levels for hypophosphatemia, hyperkalemia, hypocalcemia, and hypomagnesemia, which reduce muscle strength
   f. Serum AAT levels in patients with a family history of COPD
   g. Chest x-ray
   h. Pulmonary function test (PFT)
   i. Peak expiratory flow rates
   j. Carbon monoxide diffusion test

Planning and Implementation
- Improving oxygenation and reducing carbon dioxide retention
- Hypoxemia with hypercapnia related to alveolar-capillary membrane changes, reduced airway size, ventilatory muscle fatigue, excessive mucus production, airway obstruction, diaphragm flattening, fatigue, and decreased energy

   Nonsurgical Management
- Assess breath sounds and oxygen saturation routinely as part of physical assessment and before and after interventions.

- Maintain a patent airway by assisting the patient to clear the airway of secretions.
- Position to provide lung expansion with elevated back rest, pillows, and chair-sitting.
- Monitor for changes in respiratory status in the hospitalized patient with COPD at least every 2 hours.
- Identify factors that may contribute to the increased work of breathing, such as respiratory infection.
- Teach breathing techniques:
  1. Diaphragmatic or abdominal breathing
  2. Pursed-lip breathing
- Enhance coughing effectiveness:
  1. Assist the patient to a sitting position with head slightly flexed, shoulders relaxed, and knees flexed.
  2. Teach the patient to take a deep breath, hold it for 2 seconds, and cough two or three times in succession.
  3. Teach the patient to follow coughing with several maximal inhalation breaths.
- Provide oxygen therapy to maintain a peripheral oxygenation (Spo_2) of 88% to 92%.
- Ensure that there are no open flames or other combustion hazards in rooms where oxygen is in use.
- Drug therapy includes:
  1. Inhaled bronchodilator drugs, such as albuterol (Proventil, Ventolin), ipratropium (Atrovent, Apo-Ipravent ✿), tiotropium (Spiriva), theophylline (Elixophyllin, Theo-Dur, Uniphyl, Theolair, and many others)
  2. Inhaled or systemic anti-inflammatory drugs, such as fluticasone (Flovent) and prednisone (Deltasone, Medrol)
  3. Mucolytic drugs, such as acetylcysteine (Mucosil, Mucomyst ✿) or dornase alfa (Pulmozyme)
- Teach patients and family members the correct techniques for using inhalers and how to care for them properly.
- Teach patients about value of exercise training or pulmonary rehabilitation to prevent general and pulmonary muscle deconditioning.
  1. Collaborate with the physical therapist and patient to plan an individualized exercise program.
  2. Remind the patient to perform planned exercises at least two or three times each week.

Surgical Management

- Lung transplantation may be performed for select patients with end-stage COPD.
- Lung reduction surgery can improve gas exchange through removal of the hyperinflated lung tissue areas that are useless for gas exchange.

- Preoperative care includes routine preoperative care described in Part One and:
  1. Pulmonary rehabilitation to maximize lung and muscle function
  2. Testing with pulmonary plethysmography, gas dilution, or perfusion scans to determine the location of greatest lung hyperinflation and poorest lung blood flow
- Postoperative care includes routine postoperative care described in Part One and:
  1. Close monitoring for respiratory problems
  2. Chest tube management
  3. Maintenance of bronchodilator and mucolytic therapy
  4. Collaboration with the respiratory therapist to administer inhaled drugs and adjust oxygen therapy prior to activity
- Promote optimal nutrition.
- Weight loss occurs in patients with COPD as a result of dyspnea, anorexia, and fatigue.
- The patient with COPD often has food intolerance, nausea, early satiety, loss of appetite, and meal-related dyspnea.
- The increased work of breathing raises calorie and protein needs.
- Malnourished patients experience loss of total body mass, ventilatory muscle mass and strength, lung elasticity, and alveolar-capillary surface area.
- Collaborate with the dietician to provide sufficient protein and calories to support the work of breathing.
- Monitor patient weight and other indicators of nutrition, such as skin condition and serum prealbumin levels.
- Manage eating to avoid dyspnea and shortness of breath:
  1. Urge the patient to rest before meals.
  2. Teach the patient to plan the biggest meal of the day for the time when he or she is most hungry and well rested. Four to six small meals each day may be preferred to three larger ones.
  3. Suggest the use of a bronchodilator 30 minutes before the meal.
- Encourage the patient to select food that is appealing, easy to chew, and not gas forming.
  1. Suggest dietary supplements, such as Pulmocare, that provide nutrition with reduced carbon dioxide production.
  2. If early satiety is a problem, advise the patient to minimize drinking fluids before and during meals.

MINIMIZE ANXIETY
- Anxiety can be related to dyspnea, a change in health status, and situational crisis.
- Patients with COPD often have increased anxiety during acute dyspneic episodes, especially if they feel as though they are

choking on excessive secretions. Anxiety has been shown to cause dyspnea.

- Help the patient develop a written plan that states exactly what to do if symptoms flare.
- Stress the use of pursed-lip and diaphragmatic breathing techniques during periods of anxiety or panic.
- Recommend professional counseling, if needed, as a positive suggestion. Stress that talking with a counselor can help identify techniques to maintain control over the dyspnea and feelings of panic.
- Explore other approaches to control dyspneic episodes and panic attacks, such as progressive relaxation, hypnosis therapy, and biofeedback.

IMPROVE ACTIVITY TOLERANCE

Activity intolerance is related to fatigue, dyspnea, and an imbalance between oxygen supply and demand

- Teach energy conservation techniques to plan and pace activities for maximal tolerance and minimal discomfort.
  1. Work with the patient to develop a personal daily schedule for activities and rest periods.
  2. Encourage the patient to avoid working with the arms raised or reaching above the head.
  3. Teach the patient to adjust work heights to reduce back strain and fatigue.
  4. Remind him or her to keep arm motions smooth and flowing to prevent jerky motions that waste energy.
  5. Teach about the use of adaptive tools for housework, such as long-handled dustpans, sponges, and dusters, to reduce bending and reaching.
  6. Suggest how to organize work spaces so that items used most often are within easy reach.
  7. Teach the patient not to talk when engaged in other activities that require energy, such as walking.
  8. Teach him or her to avoid breath-holding while performing any activity.
- Assist with ADLs of eating, bathing, and grooming based on assessment of the patient's needs and fatigue level.
- Assess the patient's response to activity by noting skin color changes, pulse rate and regularity, BP, and work of breathing.
- Suggest the use of supplemental oxygen during periods of high energy use, such as bathing or walking.

PREVENT RESPIRATORY INFECTION

- Patients with COPD who have excessive secretions or who have artificial airways are at increased risk for respiratory tract infections.
- Teach patients to avoid large crowds and anyone who is ill.

- Stress the importance of receiving a pneumonia vaccination and a yearly influenza vaccination.

Community-Based Care

- Coordinate with all members of the health care team to individualize plans for the patient to be discharged to home.
- Determine what equipment and assistance will be needed in the home setting.
- Teach the patient and family about:
  1. The disease and its course
  2. Drug therapy
  3. Manifestations of infection
  4. Avoidance of respiratory irritants, including smoking cessation
  5. Nutrition therapy regimen
  6. Stress and anxiety management
  7. Breathing and coughing techniques
  8. Energy conservation measures while maintaining self-care activities
- Collaborate with the care manager and social worker to obtain needed home services:
  1. Oxygen and nebulizer
  2. Hospital-type bed
  3. Home health nurse or aide
  4. Financial assistance
- Provide appropriate referrals, as needed:
  1. Home care visits
  2. Housekeeping assistance and meal preparation
  3. Support groups
  4. Smoking cessation programs

CIRRHOSIS

OVERVIEW

- Cirrhosis is extensive, irreversible scarring of the liver, usually caused by a chronic reaction to hepatic inflammation and necrosis. Diffuse fibrotic bands of connective tissue distort the normal architectural anatomy of the liver, resulting in disturbed metabolic processes and circulatory pathology.
- Cirrhosis of the liver can be divided into several common types, depending on the cause of the disease:
  1. *Postnecrotic cirrhosis* is caused by viral hepatitis, especially hepatitis C, and certain drugs or other toxins. Worldwide, hepatitis B and hepatitis D are the leading causes of this condition.
  2. *Laennec's cirrhosis*, or *alcoholic cirrhosis*, is caused by chronic alcoholism. The long-term use of illicit drugs, such as cocaine, has similar effects on the liver.

3. *Biliary cirrhosis*, also called *cholestatic cirrhosis*, is caused by chronic biliary obstruction or autoimmune disease.
- Complications of cirrhosis include:
1. *Portal hypertension:* A persistent increase in pressure within the portal vein develops as a result of increased resistance or obstruction to flow. Blood flow backs into the spleen, causing splenomegaly. Veins in the esophagus, stomach, intestines, abdomen, and rectum become dilated. Dilated vessels develop weakened walls, leading to plasma leak and hemorrhage.
2. *Ascites:* Free fluid accumulates within the peritoneal cavity. Increased hydrostatic pressure from portal hypertension results in venous congestion of the hepatic capillaries, causing plasma to leak directly from the liver surface and portal vein. Other contributing factors include reduced circulating plasma protein and increased hepatic lymphatic formation. Massive ascites can cause abdominal compartment syndrome.
3. *Esophageal varices:* Thin-walled, distended esophageal veins result from increased portal hypertension. Varices occur most often in the lower esophagus, stomach, and rectum. Fragile varices can rupture, resulting in gastrointestinal bleeding.
4. *Coagulation defects:* Decreased synthesis of bile fats in the liver prevents the absorption of fat-soluble vitamins. Without vitamin K, synthesis of clotting factors II, VII, IX, and X is impaired and the patient is susceptible to bruising and bleeding. Splenomegaly (enlarged spleen) results from the pressure of portal hypertension. The enlarged spleen destroys platelets (thrombocytopenia), adding to the increased risk for bleeding.
5. *Jaundice,* which is caused by one of two mechanisms:
   a. In *hepatocellular jaundice,* the liver is unable to effectively excrete bilirubin.
   b. In *intrahepatic obstruction,* edema, fibrosis, or scarring of the hepatic bile duct channels and bile ducts interferes with normal bile and bilirubin excretion. Patients with jaundice often report pruritus (itching).
6. *Hepatic encephalopathy* (also called *portal-systemic encephalopathy* [PSE]): This is a complex, neurologic syndrome. It is associated with elevated serum ammonia levels. Early symptoms include sleep disturbance, mood disturbance, mental status changes, and speech problems. Later, altered level of consciousness, impaired thinking processes, and neuromuscular disturbances (e.g., "liver flap") are common symptoms.
7. *Hepatorenal syndrome:* Progressive, oliguric kidney failure is associated with hepatic failure, resulting in functional impairment of kidneys with normal anatomic and morphologic

features. It is manifested by a sudden decrease in urinary output and elevated serum urea nitrogen and creatinine levels, with abnormally decreased urine sodium excretion and increased urine osmolarity.

PATIENT-CENTERED COLLABORATIVE CARE
Assessment
* Record patient information:
  1. Age, gender, and race
  2. Employment history, including working conditions exposing the patient to toxins
  3. History of individual and family liver disease
  4. Medical conditions, including viral hepatitis (especially B, C, and D), systemic viral infections, biliary tract disorders, auto-immune disorders, and heart failure, respiratory disorders, or liver injury. Blood transfusions and bloodborne infections from tattoos may be associated with hepatitis.
  5. Sexual history
  6. History of or present alcohol or substance use
* Assess for:
  1. Generalized weakness, fatigue
  2. Weight changes (loss or gain)
  3. GI symptoms, including loss of appetite, early morning nausea and vomiting, dyspepsia, flatulence, and changes in bowel habits
  4. Abdominal distension, pain, or tenderness
  5. Jaundice of the skin and sclera
  6. Dry skin, rashes, or pruritus
  7. Petechiae and bruising or excessive bleeding from minor injury
  8. Palmar erythema
  9. Spider angiomas on the nose, cheeks, upper thorax, and shoulders
  10. Hepatomegaly palpated in the right upper quadrant, confirmed by palpation, ultrasound, or radiographic imaging
  11. Ascites revealed by bulging flanks and dullness on percussion of the abdomen
  12. Protruding umbilicus
  13. Dilated abdominal veins (caput medusae)
  14. Hematemesis or melena
  15. Fetor hepaticus (the fruity, musty breath odor of chronic liver disease)
  16. Amenorrhea in women
  17. Testicular atrophy, gynecomastia, and impotence in men
  18. Changes in mentation and personality

19. Asterixis (liver flap), a coarse tremor characterized by rapid, nonrhythmic extension and flexions in the wrist and fingers
20. Elevated serum liver enzymes (aspartate aminotransferase [AST], alanine aminotransferase [ALT], and lactate dehydrogenase [LDH]), biliary biomarkers (alkaline phosphatase, gamma-glutamyl transpeptidase [GGT]), and serum bilirubin levels
21. Decreased hemoglobin, total serum protein, and albumin levels
22. Positive hepatitis A, B, C, or D panel
23. Altered coagulation factors, prolonged bleeding times
24. Elevated serum ammonia level
25. Ultrasound, followed by CT or MRI to determine the hepatomegaly or the cause of cirrhosis
26. Esophagogastroduodenoscopy to visualize the upper GI tract and detect complications of cirrhosis

Planning and Implementation
EXCESS FLUID VOLUME

- Monitor respiratory status to avoid complications from pulmonary edema.
    1. Monitor SpO_2 with vital signs.
    2. Elevate the head of the bed to minimize shortness of breath and position for comfort.
- Provide diet therapy:
    1. Provide a low-sodium diet initially, restricting sodium to 500 mg to 2 g/day.
    2. Suggest alternatives to salt, such as lemon, vinegar, parsley, oregano, and pepper.
    3. Collaborate with the dietitian to explain the purpose of diet and meal planning; suggest elimination of table salt, salty foods, canned and frozen vegetables, and salted butter and margarine.
    4. Restrict fluid intake to 1000 to 1500 mL/day if the serum sodium level falls.
    5. Supplement vitamin intake with thiamine, folate, and multivitamin preparations.
    6. Record the patient's daily weight.
- Provide drug therapy:
    1. Give diuretics to reduce intravascular fluid and to prevent cardiac and respiratory impairment.
    2. Monitor intake and output carefully with daily weight.
    3. Monitor serum electrolytes.
- Paracentesis may be indicated if dietary restrictions and drug administration fail to control ascites:
    1. Explain the procedure and verify informed consent obtained.
    2. Obtain vital signs and weight, and check allergies.

3. Assist the patient to an upright position at the side of the bed.
4. Monitor vital signs every 15 minutes during the procedure; rapid, drastic removal of ascitic fluid leads to decreased abdominal pressure, which may contribute to vasodilation and shock.
5. Measure and record drainage; send samples to laboratory if ordered.
6. Position the patient in a semi-Fowler's position in bed, and maintain bedrest until vital signs are stable.
7. Assess the patient's lung sounds.

- Reduce or manage esophageal bleeding:
    1. Prevent hypertension by determining systemic and mean arterial BP goals. Decreasing systemic BP reduces hepatic pressures and portal vessel leak.
    2. Institute frequent monitoring and communicate observations about bleeding immediately to the provider. Coagulopathy and high BP can place the patient at significant risk for hemorrhage.
    3. Provide protection from gastritis with a proton pump inhibitor or H_2 histamine blocker.
    4. Combine vasoconstrictive drug therapy with endoscopic therapy to reduce hemorrhage.
        a. Octreotide (Sandostatin) causes variceal vasoconstriction
        b. Endoscope variceal banding and sclerotherapy to decrease bleeding
    5. Initiate rescue therapy with esophagogastric balloon tamponade to compress bleeding vessels.
        a. The tube is inserted through the nose and into the stomach. The large esophageal balloon compresses the esophagus; a smaller gastric balloon helps anchor the tube and exerts pressure against bleeding varices at the distal esophagus and the stomach. A third lumen terminates in the stomach and is connected to suction, allowing the aspiration of gastric contents and blood.
        b. Check balloons for integrity and leaks; label each lumen to prevent errors in adding or removing pressure and volume.
        c. Keep tube taped and secure and place scissors at the bedside for emergent situations from a migrating tamponade tube blocking the airway.
        d. Monitor the patient for respiratory distress caused by obstruction from the esophageal balloon or aspiration; if distress occurs, cut both balloon ports to allow for rapid balloon deflation and tube removal.
    6. Provide procedural-related care:
        a. An *endoscopic retrograde cholangiopancreatography* (ERCP) uses the endoscope to inject contrast material via the

sphincter of Oddi to view the biliary tract and allow for stone removals, sphincterotomies, biopsies, and stent placements if required.

b. *Esophagogastroduodenoscopy* (EGD) is used to directly visualize the upper GI tract and to detect the presence of bleeding or oozing esophageal varices, stomach irritation and ulceration, or duodenal ulceration and bleeding. EGD is performed by introducing a flexible fiberoptic endoscope into the mouth, esophagus, and stomach while the patient is under moderate sedation. A camera attached to the scope permits direct visualization of the mucosal lining of the upper GI tract.

c. *Transjugular intrahepatic portal-systemic shunting* is a non-surgical procedure whereby the physician implants a shunt, passed through a catheter, between the portal vein and the hepatic vein to reduce portal venous pressure and therefore control the bleeding.

7. Administer blood products (RBCs and fresh-frozen plasma) and IV fluids to sustain circulation and perfusion during episodes of bleeding.

8. Give vasopressin to promote coagulation.

! NURSING SAFETY PRIORITY: Action Alert

Avoid placing or manipulating the nasogastric or orogastric tube in a patient who is at high risk for or diagnosed with esophageal varices, because tube movement can injure a fragile, dilated vessel, causing it to rupture and bleed.

POTENTIAL FOR HEPATIC ENCEPHALOPATHY
- Provide a safe environment.
  1. Altered mentation places the patient at risk for falls, aspiration, and pressure ulcer formation from prolonged immobility. Institutional interventions should be put in place to avoid these adverse events.
  2. Administer lactulose to promote fecal excretion of ammonia.
- Provide diet therapy:
  1. Patient has increased nutritional requirements: high-carbohydrate, moderate-fat, and high-protein foods.
  2. Patients with PSE usually have protein intake limited in the diet to reduce excess protein breakdown by intestinal bacteria leading to ammonia formation.
  3. Be aware of decreased metabolism of many drugs, especially opioids, sedatives, and other central nervous system (CNS) agents.

Community-Based Care
- Health teaching is individualized for the patient, depending on the cause of the disease.
- Identify if the patient needs a family member or friend to help with drugs, or needs a home health care nurse or aide.
- Teach the patient and family to:
  1. Follow the prescribed diet.
  2. Restrict sodium intake if ascites occur.
  3. Obtain and record daily weights and report increase of 5 pounds or more over any 3-day period.
  4. Restrict protein intake if the patient is susceptible to encephalopathy.
  5. Take diuretics as prescribed, report symptoms of hypokalemia, and consume foods high in potassium.
  6. Take H_2 receptor antagonist agent or proton pump inhibitor.
  7. Avoid all nonprescription drugs.
  8. Avoid alcohol (refer to Alcoholics Anonymous if patient is addicted to alcohol).
  9. Recognize signs and symptoms of PSE.
  10. Notify the patient's health care provider immediately in case of GI bleeding or PSE.
  11. Keep follow-up visits with the physicians.

COLITIS, ULCERATIVE

OVERVIEW
- Ulcerative colitis (UC) creates widespread inflammation of the rectum and rectosigmoid colon but can extend to the entire colon.
- UC is characterized by hyperemic intestinal mucosa (increased blood flow) with resultant edema. In more severe inflammation, the lining can bleed and small ulcers occur.
- Abscesses can form in ulcerative areas and result in tissue necrosis, perforation, and peritonitis.
- Edema and mucosal thickening can lead to a narrowed colon and bowel obstruction.
- Complications of the disease include fistula formation, toxic megacolon, hemorrhage, increased risk for colon cancer, and malabsorption.
- Extraintestinal clinical manifestations include polyarthritis, oral and skin lesions, iritis, and hepatic and biliary disease.
- The patient's stool typically contains blood and mucus. Patients report tenesmus (an unpleasant and urgent sensation to defecate) and lower abdominal colicky pain relieved with defecation. Malaise, anorexia, anemia, dehydration, fever, and weight loss are common.

PATIENT-CENTERED COLLABORATIVE CARE
Assessment
- Record patient information:
  1. Family history of inflammatory bowel disease
  2. Previous and current therapy for illnesses, including surgeries
  3. Diet history, including usual patterns and intolerances of food
  4. History of weight changes
  5. Presence of abdominal pain, cramping, urgency, and diarrhea
  6. Bowel elimination patterns; color, consistency, and character of stools and the presence or absence of blood
  7. Relationship between the occurrence of diarrhea and the timing of meals, pain, emotional distress, and activity
  8. Extraintestinal symptoms such as arthritis, mouth sores, vision problems, and skin disorders
- Assess for:
  1. Abdominal cramping, pain, and distention
  2. Bloody diarrhea, tenesmus
  3. Fever, tachycardia
  4. Patient's understanding of the disease process
  5. Psychosocial impact of the disease; the inability to control symptoms, especially diarrhea, can be disruptive and stress producing
  6. Abnormal laboratory values: hematocrit, hemoglobin, WBC count, erythrocyte sedimentation rate, C-reactive protein, and electrolytes
  7. Results from most recent colonoscopy or magnetic resonance enterography

Planning and Implementation
DIARRHEA AND POTENTIAL FOR INCONTINENCE
Nonsurgical Management
- Management of ulcerative colitis is aimed at relieving the symptoms and reducing intestinal motility, decreasing inflammation, and promoting intestinal healing.
- Diarrhea management:
  1. Record patient responses to interventions, noting changes in the color, volume, frequency, and consistency of stools.
  2. Monitor the skin in the perianal area for irritation and ulceration resulting from loose, frequent stools.
  3. Monitor immune function and results of stool or other cultures.
- Drug therapy:
  1. Aminosalicylates are used to reduce inflammation.
  2. Glucocorticoids are used during exacerbations of the illness.

3. Antidiarrheal drugs are given to provide symptomatic management of diarrhea; they are given cautiously, because they can precipitate colonic dilation and toxic megacolon.
4. Biologic response modifiers alter (modulate) the immune response and are most effective when given with glucocorticoids. Examples include infliximab (Remicade) and adalimumab (Humira).

- Diet therapy may include:
  1. NPO status with total parenteral nutrition (TPN) for the patient with severe symptoms
  2. Elemental formulas, which are absorbed in the small intestine, minimizing bowel stimulation
  3. Avoiding caffeine, alcohol, or foods that cause symptoms
- Ensure that the patient has easy access to the bedside commode or bathroom.
- Explore psychosocial concerns such as body image, fear, and anxiety.
- Complementary and alternative therapies may include flaxseed, selenium, vitamin C, biofeedback, yoga, acupuncture, and Ayurveda (combination of diet, herbs, and breathing exercises).

Surgical Management

- The need for surgery is based on the patient's response to medical interventions.
- Surgical procedures include:
  1. *Total proctocolectomy or colectomy with permanent ileostomy,* in which the colon, rectum, and anus are removed and the anus closed; a loop of the ileum is placed through an opening in the abdominal wall (stoma) for draining of fecal material into a pouching system worn on the abdomen. The stoma is located in the right lower quadrant.
     a. Initial output from the ileostomy is a loose, dark green liquid; over time, the volume decreases, becomes thicker, and turns yellow-green or yellow-brown.
     b. A foul or unpleasant odor may be a symptom of some underlying problem (blockage or infection).
  2. Creation of an ileoanal reservoir, a procedure known as *Restorative Proctocolectomy with Ileal Pouch Anal Anastomosis* (RPC-IPAA); it is usually a two-stage procedure that first includes the creation of an ileostomy and removal of the colon and most of the rectum with preservation of the anus and anal sphincter. The surgeon surgically creates an internal pouch (reservoir) using the last 1.5 feet of the small intestine. The pouch, sometimes called a J-pouch, S-pouch, or pelvic pouch, is then connected to the anus. In the second surgical stage, the ileostomy is closed. The time interval between the first and

second stage varies, but the second surgery can occur as soon as 6 weeks after the first surgery.

3. Specific nursing care interventions, including ostomy or perineal wound care, are determined by the procedure performed.

   a. Provide an opportunity for the patient to interact with the certified wound, ostomy, and continence nurse (CWOCN) or enterostomal therapist (ET) preoperatively and postoperatively and at follow-up appointments or at home.

   b. A visit from a patient with an ostomy may be helpful.

! NURSING SAFETY PRIORITY: Critical Rescue

The ileostomy stoma is usually placed in the right lower quadrant of the abdomen below the belt line. It should not be prolapsed or retract into the abdominal wall. Assess the stoma frequently. It should be pinkish to cherry red to ensure an adequate blood supply. *If the stoma looks pale, bluish, or dark, report these findings to the health care provider immediately.*

PAIN MANAGEMENT
- Assess the patient for changes in pain intensity that may indicate disease or surgical complications, such as increased inflammation, obstruction, hemorrhage, or peritonitis.
- Assess for pain, including its character, pattern of occurrence (e.g., before or after meals, during the night, before or after bowel movements), and duration.
- Assist the patient to reduce or eliminate factors that increase the pain.
- Take measures to relieve irritated skin caused by contact with diarrheal stool or ileostomy drainage.
- Assist the patient to use other pain relief measures such as biofeedback and music therapy.

POTENTIAL FOR LOWER GASTROINTESTINAL (GI) BLEEDING
- Monitor the patient for bright red or black and tarry stools and symptoms of GI bleeding.
- Notify the health care provider immediately of GI bleeding, because blood transfusion or surgical interventions may be necessary.

! NURSING SAFETY PRIORITY: Critical Rescue

Monitor stools for blood loss. The blood may be bright red (frank bleeding) or black and tarry (melena). Monitor hematocrit, hemoglobin, and electrolyte values, and assess vital signs. Prolonged slow bleeding can lead to anemia. Observe for fever, tachycardia, and signs of fluid volume depletion. Changes in mental status may occur, especially among older adults, and may be the first indication of dehydration or anemia.

Community-Based Care
- Health teaching includes the following:
  1. Provide information on the nature of the disease, including acute episodes, remissions, and symptom management.
  2. Self-management strategies to reduce or control pain, promote adequate nutrition, manage clinical manifestations, and monitor for complications
  3. Provide additional information for the patient with an ostomy regarding:
     a. Ostomy or pouch care
     b. Skin care, including anal and peristomal skin
     c. Special issues related to drugs (e.g., to avoid taking enteric-coated drugs and capsule drugs); the patient should inform health care providers and the pharmacist that he or she has an ostomy
     d. Symptoms indicating a need to contact the provider such as increased or no drainage, stomal swelling, or discoloration of the stoma
     e. Activity limitations, including avoidance of heavy lifting
     f. The importance of adequate fluid intake, especially during periods of high ostomy output
- Refer the patient to home health care ostomy or outpatient clinics.
- Refer the patient to support groups such as the United Ostomy Association and the Crohn's and Colitis Foundation of America.

COMPARTMENT SYNDROME

OVERVIEW
- Compartments are areas in the body where muscles, blood vessels, and nerves are contained within fascia, especially in extremities.
- Fascia is an inelastic tissue that surrounds groups of muscles, blood vessels, and nerves in the body.
- *Acute compartment syndrome* (ACS) is a serious condition in which increased pressure from tissue swelling as a result of blood or fluid collection within one or more compartments causes massive compromise of circulation to the area.

- It is usually a complication of musculoskeletal trauma in the lower leg and forearm, but it can be seen with severe burns, extensive insect bites, or massive infiltration of IV fluids and with abdominal swelling.
- Pressure to the compartment can also occur from an external source, such as tight, bulky dressings and casts.
- If the condition is not treated, cyanosis, tingling, numbness, pain, paresis, and permanent tissue damage can occur.
- Complications of ACS can include infection, persistent motor weakness in the affected extremity, contracture, and myoglobinuric renal failure.
- In extreme cases, amputation becomes necessary.

PATIENT-CENTERED COLLABORATIVE CARE

- Nursing care includes:
  1. Identifying patients who may be at risk
  2. Monitoring for early signs of ACS by assessing for the "six Ps," which include:
     a. Pain
     b. Pressure
     c. Paralysis
     d. Paresthesia
     e. Pallor
     f. Pulselessness
  3. Invasive monitoring of compartment pressure in patients at especially high risk for ACS using a handheld device with a digital display or a pressure monitor such as that used for abdominal compartment syndrome evaluation
  4. When external conditions are causing the syndrome, implementing interventions to relieve the pressure:
     a. Loosening dressings or tape
     b. Following agency protocol about cutting a tight cast

! NURSING SAFETY PRIORITY: Critical Rescue

When manifestations indicate compartment syndrome, notify the surgeon immediately, because irreversible damage can occur within a few hours.

- Surgical intervention is a fasciotomy (opening in the fascia) made by incising through the skin and subcutaneous tissues into the fascia of the affected compartment to relieve the pressure and restore circulation to the affected area.
- After fasciotomy, the open wound is packed and dressed on a regular basis until secondary closure occurs.
- Débridement and skin grafting may be required.

CORNEAL ABRASION, INFECTION, AND ULCERATION
OVERVIEW
- A *corneal abrasion* is a painful scrape or scratch of the cornea that disrupts the integrity of this structure, most commonly caused by the presence of a small foreign body, trauma, and contact lens use.
- The abrasion provides a portal of entry for organisms, leading to *corneal infection*.
- *Corneal ulceration* is a deeper disruption of the corneal epithelium, often occurring with bacterial, fungal, or viral infection. *This problem is an emergency and can lead to permanently impaired vision.*

C

PATIENT-CENTERED COLLABORATIVE CARE
Assessment
- Assess for these problems in the affected eye:
  1. Pain
  2. Reduced vision
  3. Photophobia
  4. Eye secretions with cloudy or purulent fluid on eyelids or eyelashes
  5. Hazy, cloudy cornea with a patchy area of ulceration
  6. Damaged areas appear green with fluorescein stain

Interventions
- Drug therapy delivered as eye drops:
  1. Antibiotics, antifungals, and antivirals are prescribed to reduce or eliminate the organisms. Usually, a broad-spectrum antibiotic is prescribed first, and it may be changed when culture results are known.
  2. Usually the anti-infective therapy involves instilling eye drops every hour for the first 24 hours.
  3. Steroids may be used with antibiotics to reduce the inflammatory response in the eye.
  4. Anesthetic drops can be used to decrease pain.
- Educate the patient for self-management:
  1. Teach the patient how to apply the eye drops correctly.
  2. Teach the patient to wash hands after touching the affected eye, including instilling eye drops in the other eye when both eyes are affected.
  3. Teach the patient to not wear contact lenses during the entire time that these drugs are being used.

! NURSING SAFETY PRIORITY: Critical Rescue

Stress the importance of applying the drug as often as prescribed, even at night. Treating the infection can save the patient's vision in the infected eye.

CORNEAL OPACITIES, KERATOCONUS, AND CORNEAL TRANSPLANTATION
OVERVIEW
- The cornea can permanently lose its shape, become scarred or cloudy, or become thinner, reducing useful visual sensory perception.
- *Keratoconus* is the degeneration of the corneal tissue resulting in an abnormal corneal shape that can occur with trauma or may occur as part of an inherited disorder.

PATIENT-CENTERED COLLABORATIVE CARE
- *Keratoplasty* is the surgical removal of diseased corneal tissue and replacement with tissue from a human donor cornea (corneal transplant). For a misshaped cornea that is still clear, surgical management involves a corneal implant that adjusts the shape of the cornea.
- Provide preoperative care as outlined in Part One and:
  1. Assess the patient's knowledge of the surgery and of expected care before and after surgery.
  2. Inform the patient that local anesthesia commonly is used.
- Provide postoperative care described in Part One and:
  1. Maintain the eye protective shield and dressing care as prescribed by the surgeon.
  2. Educate the patient or caregiver about eye drop instillation.
  3. Teach the patient and caregiver to examine the eye daily for the presence of infection, graft rejection, and reduced visual acuity.
     a. Report immediately to the surgeon the presence of purulent discharge, a continuous leak of clear fluid from around the graft site (not tears), or excessive bleeding.
  4. Instruct the patient to avoid activities that promote rapid or jerky head motions or increase intraocular pressure for several weeks after surgery.

CORONARY ARTERY DISEASE
OVERVIEW
- Coronary artery disease (CAD) is a broad term that includes *chronic angina* and *acute coronary syndromes* (ACS) (see also *Acute Coronary Syndromes*).
- CAD affects the arteries that provide blood, oxygen, and nutrients to the myocardium.
- CAD causes ischemia when insufficient oxygen is supplied to meet the requirements of the myocardium. *Infarction* (necrosis or

cell death) occurs when severe ischemia is prolonged, resulting in irreversible damage to tissue.
- The most common cause of CAD is atherosclerosis, which is characterized by a lesion that narrows the vessel lumen or obstructs blood flow (see *Arteriosclerosis and Atherosclerosis*).
- The most common symptom of CAD is angina. *Angina* is chest pain, a sign of myocardial ischemia.
  1. Chronic stable angina is chest discomfort that occurs with exertion in a pattern that is familiar to the patient; the frequency, duration, or intensity of symptoms remains the same for several months. It is usually associated with a fixed or stable atherosclerotic plaque.
  2. Unstable angina is chest pain or discomfort that occurs at rest or with exertion and causes severe activity limitation.

Gender Health Considerations

- Many women experience atypical angina, described as a choking sensation that occurs with exertion, indigestion, pain between the shoulders, or an aching jaw.
- Many women with symptomatic ischemic heart disease or abnormal stress testing do not have normal coronary angiography.
- Studies implicate microvascular disease or endothelial dysfunction or both as the causes for risk for CAD in women. Endothelial dysfunction is the inability of the arteries and arterioles to dilate due to lack of nitric oxide production by the endothelium. Nitric oxide is a relaxant of vascular smooth muscle.
- Women typically have smaller coronary arteries and frequently have plaque that breaks off and travels into the small vessels to form an embolus (clot).
- Women have higher morbidity and mortality rates after myocardial infarction (MI) than men do.

  3. MI occurs when coronary blood flow is stopped and the myocardial muscle is abruptly and severely deprived of oxygen.
     a. Ischemia and necrosis (infarction) of the myocardial tissue result if blood flow is not restored.
     b. Generally, an MI is caused by an unstable plaque that initiates the inflammatory cascade and leads to thrombus formation. The clot is the cause of coronary artery blood flow cessation.

4. The patient's response to an MI depends on which coronary arteries were obstructed and which part of the left ventricular wall was damaged: anterior, lateral, septal, inferior, or posterior.
   a. Patients with obstruction of the left anterior descending artery have anterior or septal MIs, or both; patients with anterior MIs are most likely to experience left ventricular heart failure and ventricular dysrhythmias.
   b. Patients with obstruction of the circumflex artery may experience a posterior wall or a lateral wall MI and sinus dysrhythmias.
   c. Patients with obstruction of the right coronary artery often have inferior MIs; these patients are likely to experience bradydysrhythmias or atrioventricular conduction defects, especially transient second-degree heart block.
5. Nonmodifiable risk factors that contribute to the onset and progression of CAD include age, gender, family history, and ethnic background.
6. Modifiable risk factors include elevated serum cholesterol levels, cigarette smoking, hypertension, impaired glucose tolerance, obesity, physical inactivity, and stress.

PATIENT-CENTERED COLLABORATIVE CARE
Assessment
- Collection of historical data is delayed until interventions for pain, vital sign instability, and dysrhythmias are initiated and the discomfort resolves.
- Record the patient's family history and risk factors.
- Note vital signs: HR, BP, respiratory rate and effort, and SpO_2.
- Assess for clinical manifestations of angina and MI:
  1. Quality, onset, duration, and alleviating and aggravating factors related to chest pain or presence and quality of atypical pain, including jaw pain, back pain, or extreme fatigue
  2. Sudden and severe dyspnea
  3. Diaphoresis dizziness, weakness
  4. Irregular heart rhythm or palpitations
  5. Diminished or absent pulses
  6. S_3 gallop or S_4 heart sound
  7. Fear and anxiety or denial
  8. Elevated serum cardiac enzyme levels:
     a. Myoglobin
     b. Troponin
     c. Creatine kinase (CK-MB isoenzyme)
  9. ECG changes:
     a. In angina, ST depression or elevation or T-wave inversion

b. In MI, ST elevation or abnormal Q wave in two or more contiguous leads (this is also known as an ST elevation MI or *STEMI*)

c. About half of MIs occur without ECG changes (this is known as a non-ST elevation MI or *NSTEMI*)

10. Results of exercise test (stress test), thallium scan, contrast-enhanced magnetic resonance (CMR), multigated acquisition (MUGA) scan, CT coronary angiography, and cardiac catheterization, if performed

Considerations for Older Adults

The presence of associated symptoms without chest discomfort is significant. In up to 40% of all patients with MI, primarily older women and patients with diabetes, chest pain or discomfort may be mild or absent. Instead, they have symptoms of dyspnea or fatigue. Some older patients may think they are having indigestion and therefore not recognize that they are having an MI. Others report nausea, palpitations, or new and sudden weakness. The major manifestation of MI in people older than 80 years may be disorientation or acute confusion because of decreased cardiac output.

⊕ Cultural Considerations

Black Americans and women tend to delay seeking treatment for MI and therefore have higher mortality rates than Euro-Americans and men. One contributing factor to this delay is that dyspnea may be the acute symptom among these groups rather than classic angina or chest pain.

! NURSING SAFETY PRIORITY: Action Alert

Do not delay in reporting the patient's symptoms of unstable angina, especially chest pain. Prompt diagnostic testing and treatment can lead to reperfusion of the myocardium and optimal outcomes.

Planning and Implementation

- For the patient with CAD, planning and intervention focus on restoring perfusion through the coronary arteries.

  1. Supplemental oxygen provides additional oxygen to the ischemic myocardium: a nasal cannula at 2 to 4 L is usually sufficient.

2. Nitroglycerin (sublingual) reduces peripheral vasoconstriction and oxygen demand. If three repeated doses given 5 minutes apart do not relieve discomfort, the patient may be experiencing an MI and needs immediate evaluation in a heart center.

3. Nitroglycerin (IV) should be administered in a specialized unit to carefully monitor the patient's BP; hypotension is a serious side effect of this drug.

4. Morphine sulfate (IV) reduces arterial and peripheral vasoconstriction, further reducing oxygen demand. Morphine also provides pain relief.

5. Aspirin (325 mg, chewed) reduces platelet aggregation and prevents clot extension in coronary arteries.

6. Glycoprotein (GP) IIb/IIIa inhibitors target the platelet component of the thrombus; abciximab (ReoPro), eptifibatide (Integrilin), or tirofiban (Aggrastat) may be administered IV to prevent fibrinogen from attaching to activated platelets at the site of a thrombus.

7. A beta blocker, usually metoprolol or carvedilol, reduces HR and oxygen demand, decreases sympathetic stimulation of the compromised myocardium, and prevents life-threatening dysrhythmias.

- Definitive treatment is percutaneous coronary intervention (PCI), which typically involves placement of a stent to open the clotted coronary artery. Care after PCI includes:

1. Monitoring for potential problems after the procedure, including acute closure of the vessel, reaction to the dye used in angiography, hypotension, hyperkalemia, and dysrhythmias

2. Instructing the patient to report the development of chest pain immediately

3. Frequently monitoring the insertion site for bleeding or vessel occlusion by palpating pulses, observing skin color and warmth of the limb, and marking the circumference of any hematoma where the catheter was inserted

   a. Apply manual pressure if there is bleeding from the insertion site.

   b. Report bleeding or changes in perfusion immediately to the physician.

4. Maintaining immobilization of the affected limb for at least 6 hours

5. Maintaining pressure dressing

6. Elevating the head of the bed slowly, per hospital protocol

7. Instructing the patient to:

   a. Return to usual activities in 1 to 2 weeks or when instructed by the physician

   b. Avoid heavy lifting for several weeks
   c. Apply manual pressure if there is bleeding from the insertion site and notify the physician if the bleeding is extensive or if oozing persists for more than 15 minutes
   d. Take nitrates, aspirin, beta blockers, angiotensin-converting enzyme (ACE) inhibitors, and statin, as prescribed

- If an interventional radiologist is not available to place a stent, then a thrombolytic agent is given to dissolve thrombi in the coronary arteries and to restore myocardial blood flow. Examples include tissue plasminogen activator (TPA), alteplase (Activase), reteplase (Retavase), and tenecteplase (TNKase).
- Like PCI, thrombolytic agents are most effective when used within 6 hours of a coronary event.
- Interventions after administration of thrombolytic agents include monitoring the patient for signs of obvious and occult bleeding and reporting indications of bleeding immediately to the physician (most common in women who receive thrombolytic therapy).
  1. Monitor the patient for indications of cerebrovascular bleeding.
  2. Observe all IV sites for bleeding and patency.
  3. Monitor clotting studies.
  4. Observe for signs of internal bleeding, including decreases in hematocrit and hemoglobin.
  5. Test stool, urine, and emesis for occult blood.
  6. Glycoprotein (GP) IIb/IIIa inhibitors prevent fibrin from attaching to activated platelets at the site of a thrombus after PCI or thrombolysis to ensure patency of the newly opened artery.
- Monitor for indications of coronary artery reperfusion, including abrupt cessation of chest pain or discomfort, sudden onset of ventricular dysrhythmias, resolution of ST segment depression, and reduction of markers of myocardial damage over 12 hours.
- IV heparin and aspirin may be given after thrombolytic therapy to reduce additional clot formation; monitor activated partial thromboplastin time (aPTT).
- Promote rest and provide assistance in ADLs to minimize oxygen demands during episodes of chest pain.
- Progress patient mobility with supervision, starting with sitting at the edge of the bed and progressing to ambulation.
- Assess the patient's vital signs and level of fatigue with each higher level of activity.
- Notify the health care provider if there are indications of activity intolerance such as orthostatic hypotension, hypertension with activity, or complaints of dyspnea, chest pain, or dizziness.

- Consider referral to cardiac rehabilitation if the patient has not participated previously. Cardiac rehabilitation is divided into three phases:
  1. Phase 1 begins with acute illness and ends with discharge from the hospital.
  2. Phase 2 begins after discharge and continues through convalescence at home.
  3. Phase 3 involves long-term conditioning.
- Direct interventions toward assisting the patient to take personal actions to manage lifestyle stressors related to CAD:
  1. Assess the patient's understanding of the disease process.
  2. Assess the patient's coping mechanisms (commonly denial, anger, and depression) and level of anxiety.
  3. Provide simple, repeated explanations of therapies, expectations, and surroundings.
  4. Help the patient identify the information that is most important to obtain.
  5. Denial that results in a patient's "acting out" and refusing to follow treatment regimen can be harmful.
     a. Remain calm and avoid confronting the patient.
     b. Clearly indicate when a behavior is not acceptable and is potentially harmful.
  6. Anger may be the result of a patient's attempt to regain control of his or her life.
     a. Encourage the patient to verbalize frustrations.
     b. Provide opportunities for decision making and control.
  7. Depression may be a patient's response to grief.
     a. Listen to the patient, and do not offer false or general reassurances.
     b. Acknowledge depression, but expect the patient to perform ADLs and other activities within restrictions.
- For the patient who experiences an MI, planning and interventions focus on identifying and treating complications from the damage to the heart. After an MI or PCI, the following drugs are often prescribed:
  1. Aspirin taken daily to reduce platelet activation and new thrombus formation
  2. GP IIb/IIIa inhibitor to prevent platelet activation and aggregation
  3. Beta-adrenergic agents to slow pathologic cardiac remodeling and prevent dysrhythmias
  4. An ACE inhibitor or an angiotensin receptor blocker (ARB) to prevent ventricular remodeling and the development of heart failure

5. A statin (antilipemic) to reduce serum cholesterol, which contributes to plaque formation, and to provide anti-inflammation:
   a. Monitor liver enzymes and serum cholesterol.
6. Calcium channel blockers for patients with variant angina or for those who are hypertensive and continue to have angina despite therapy with beta blockers

- If a dysrhythmia occurs, the following actions are taken:
  1. Identify the dysrhythmia.
  2. Assess the patient's hemodynamic status, including BP and peripheral perfusion along with level of consciousness.
  3. Evaluate the patient for chest discomfort.
- Dysrhythmias are treated when they are causing hemodynamic compromise, are increasing myocardial oxygen requirements, or are predisposing to lethal ventricular dysrhythmias (see *Dysrhythmias, Cardiac*).
- Heart failure is a relatively common complication after MI; cardiogenic shock, the most severe form of heart failure, accounts for most in-hospital deaths after MI. See *Heart Failure* for detailed assessment and management.
  1. Monitor HR and BP to attain treatment goals and avoid symptoms of low cardiac output from CAD treatment, including decreased urinary output, hypotension, fatigue, dyspnea, and pulmonary or peripheral edema.
  2. Ensure fluid and electrolyte balance, particularly potassium levels.
- Medical management of left heart failure includes:
  1. Oxygen therapy (intubation and mechanical ventilation may be necessary)
  2. Diuretics, nitroglycerin, or nitroprusside to reduce preload
  3. IV morphine to decrease pulmonary congestion and relieve pain
  4. Invasive hemodynamic monitoring to titrate drug therapy
- Conditions other than left ventricular failure may result in decreased cardiac output after an ACS. In about a third of patients with inferior MIs, right ventricular infarction and failure develop. In this instance, the right ventricle fails independently of the left.
  1. Enhance right ventricular function by administering fluids to maintain central venous pressure around 20 mm Hg.
  2. Avoid overhydration leading to left or biventricular failure.
- Patients who do not respond to drug therapy may require an intra-aortic balloon pump (IABP) or left ventricular assistive device, which is used to improve myocardial perfusion, reduce afterload, and facilitate ventricular emptying.

C

- Recurrent chest pain despite medical therapy is a major indicator for surgery.

Surgical Management

- PCI, an invasive but technically nonsurgical technique, is performed to provide symptom reduction for patients with chest discomfort within 90 minutes of a diagnosis of acute MI unless there are specific contraindications. PCI is performed by introducing a balloon-tipped catheter into the area of the coronary artery occlusion.
  1. When the balloon is inflated, it presses the atherosclerotic plaque against the vessel wall to reduce or eliminate the occlusion.
  2. Techniques used to ensure patency of the vessel are stent placement, laser angioplasty, and atherectomy.
- Coronary artery bypass graft (CABG) surgery is indicated when other treatments have been unsuccessful in managing CAD and ACS. This procedure is performed while the patient is under general anesthesia and undergoing cardiopulmonary bypass surgery. A graft from the saphenous vein, radial artery, or the internal mammary artery bypasses the occluded coronary vessel to restore blood supply to the myocardium.
- Preoperative care includes:
  1. Familiarizing the patient and family with the cardiac surgical critical care environment if surgery is performed as an elective procedure
  2. Teaching the patient how to splint the chest incision, cough and deep breathe, perform arm and leg exercises, and what to expect during the postoperative period including how pain will be managed
- Cardiopulmonary bypass (CPB) is used to provide oxygenation, circulation, and hypothermia intraoperatively during induced cardiac arrest. Blood is diverted from the heart to the bypass machine, where it is heparinized, oxygenated, and returned to the circulation through a cannula placed in the ascending aortic arch or femoral artery.
- Off-pump coronary artery bypass is open heart surgery performed without the use of CPB. It requires special surgeon training and is not yet common.
- Robotic heart surgery uses small endoscopic incisions rather than a sternotomy to access the heart. It is a longer procedure than traditional approaches and requires specialized surgical teams.
- Provide immediate postoperative care in a specialized unit.
  1. Maintain mechanical ventilation for 3 to 6 hours.
  2. Monitor chest tube output.
  3. Monitor pulmonary artery and arterial pressures.
  4. Frequently assess vital signs and cardiac rate and rhythm.

> 5. Ensure that pain is appropriately managed.
> 6. Treat symptomatic dysrhythmias according to unit protocols or physician's order.
> 7. Monitor for complications of open heart surgery, including:
>   a. Fluid and electrolyte imbalances
>   b. Hypotension and hypertension
>   c. Hypothermia
>   d. Bleeding
>   e. Cardiac tamponade
>   f. Neurologic defects that may include slowness to arouse, confusion, and stroke

- Provide continued postoperative care:
  1. Encourage deep breathing and coughing every 2 hours while awake and splinting the incision.
  2. Assist the patient in resuming activity and ambulation.
  3. Monitor for dysrhythmias, especially atrial fibrillation.
  4. Assess for wound or sternal infection (mediastinitis), such as prolonged fever (more than 4 days), reddened sternum, purulent incisional drainage, and an elevated WBC count.
  5. Observe for indications of postpericardiotomy syndrome: pericardial and pleural pain, pericarditis, friction rub, elevated temperature and WBC count, and dysrhythmias; the problem may be self-limiting or may require treatment for pericarditis.
- Minimally invasive direct coronary arterial bypass (MIDCAB) is indicated for patients with a lesion of the left anterior descending artery. Cardiopulmonary bypass is not required.
  1. Assess the patient for postoperative chest pain and ECG changes, because occlusion of the internal mammary artery graft occurs acutely in 10% of patients.
  2. Encourage the patient to cough and deep breathe (chest tube and thoracotomy incision).
- Transmyocardial laser revascularization, for patients with unstable angina and inoperable CAD with area of reversible myocardial ischemia, involves the creation of 20 to 24 long narrow channels through the left ventricular muscle to the left ventricle, which eventually allows oxygenated blood to flow.

! NURSING SAFETY PRIORITY: Critical Rescue

Monitoring the ECG and using the bedside alarms to notify about changes in ST from baseline can provide an early warning of coronary artery occlusion after any of the radiologic or surgical interventions for CAD. Immediately notify the physician about new-onset dysrhythmias, ST elevation, and other changes in the ECG indicating ischemia, injury, or infarct.

Community-Based Care

- Most patients are still recovering from their illness or surgery when discharged from the hospital; home health services may be required.
- Teach the patient and family about:
  1. The pathophysiology of angina and MI
  2. Risk factor modification
     a. Smoking cessation
     b. Dietary changes (e.g., decreasing fat and sodium intake)
     c. BP control
     d. Blood glucose control
  3. Gradual increase in physical and sexual activity, according to cardiac rehabilitation protocol
  4. Cardiac drugs
  5. Occupational considerations, if any
  6. Complementary and alternative therapies such as progressive relaxation, guided imagery, music therapy, and pet therapy
- Teach patients to seek medical assistance if they experience:
  1. A pulse rate that remains 50 or less while awake
  2. Wheezing or difficulty breathing
  3. Weight gain of 3 pounds (6.6 kg) in 1 week, or 1 to 2 pounds (2.2 to 4.4 kg) overnight
  4. Slow, persistent increase in nitroglycerin use
  5. Dizziness, faintness, or shortness of breath with activity
- Patients should call for emergency transportation to the hospital if they experience the following:
  1. Chest discomfort that does not improve after 20 minutes or after taking three nitroglycerin tablets
  2. Extremely severe chest or epigastric discomfort with weakness, nausea, or fainting
  3. Other angina symptoms that are particular to the patient, such as fatigue or nausea
- Other important discharge plans include:
  1. Teaching for drug adherence and provider follow-up
  2. Referring the patient and caregiver for continued cardiac rehabilitation
  3. Referring the patient who has had CABG surgery to Mended Hearts, a nationwide program that provides education and support to patients and their families

CROHN'S DISEASE

OVERVIEW

- Crohn's disease is a chronic inflammatory disease of the small intestine (most often), colon, or both segments of the GI tract.

- "Skip lesions" with thickened intestinal walls, alternating with healthy tissue, can result in deep fissures and ulcerations predisposing the patient to development of bowel fistulas.
- Narrowing of the bowel lumen (strictures) contributes to GI symptoms and complications.
- Complications of Crohn's disease include malabsorption, fistulas, hemorrhage, abscess formation, and intestinal obstruction. Severe malnutrition and debilitation over time can occur with reduced intestinal absorption of nutrients.

PATIENT-CENTERED COLLABORATIVE CARE
Assessment
- Assess for:
  1. Abdominal pain, distension, or masses
  2. Frequency and consistency of stools; presence of blood or fat (steatorrhea) in the stool
  3. Weight loss (indicates serious nutritional deficiencies)
  4. Diet history or nutritional intake
  5. Family history of the disease
  6. Distention, masses, or visible peristalsis
  7. Ulcerations or fissures of the perianal area
  8. Bowel sounds may be diminished or absent in the presence of severe inflammation; high-pitched over narrowed bowel loops
  9. Psychosocial issues related to coping skills and support systems
  10. Results of diagnostic imaging tests that show narrowing, ulcerations, strictures, and fistulas consistent with Crohn's disease
  11. Results of laboratory studies, especially CBC and electrolytes
      a. Low hemoglobin and hematocrit (anemia) may indicate GI bleeding, malnutrition, or both.
      b. Elevated WBC levels may indicate exacerbation or complications (fistula formation, perforation, or peritonitis).

❗ NURSING SAFETY PRIORITY: Action Alert

For the patient with Crohn's disease, be especially alert for manifestations of peritonitis, intestinal obstruction, and nutritional and fluid imbalances. Early detection of a change in the patient's status helps reduce these life-threatening complications.

Interventions
- The care of the patient with Crohn's disease is similar to care for the patient with ulcerative colitis (see *Colitis, Ulcerative*).

- Drug therapy includes:
  1. Aminosalicylates used for anti-inflammation
  2. Glucocorticoids during disease exacerbation
  3. Immunomodulatory therapy to modulate the WBCs or their inflammatory molecules with subsequent immune suppression and risk for serious infection:
     a. Azathioprine (Imuran), mercaptopurine (Purinethol), or methotrexate may be given to decrease lymphocyte activity.
     b. Infliximab (Remicade), adalimumab (Humira), natalizumab (Tysabri), and certolizumab pegol (Cimzia) are biologic response modifiers that interfere with cytokine-mediated inflammation.
     c. Metronidazole (Flagyl, Novonidazol) can be helpful for patients with fistulas.

> ### ❗ NURSING SAFETY PRIORITY: Action Alert
>
> Adequate nutrition and fluid and electrolyte balance are priorities in the care of the patient with a fistula. GI secretions are high in volume and rich in electrolytes and enzymes. The patient is at high risk for malnutrition, dehydration, and electrolyte imbalance, particularly hypokalemia. Assess for these conditions and collaborate with the health care team to manage them. Decreases in urinary output and daily weights indicate possible dehydration and thus should be monitored.

- Malnutrition can result in poor fistula and wound healing, loss of lean muscle mass, decreased immune system response, and increased morbidity and mortality.
  1. Consult with the dietitian to individualize diet and monitor tolerance to nutritional intake.
  2. Assist the patient to select high-calorie, high-protein, high-vitamin, low-fiber meals.
  3. Offer oral supplements such as Ensure and Vivonex.
  4. Record food intake and accurate calorie count.
  5. TPN may be needed for severe exacerbations while the patient is NPO.
- Electrolyte therapy includes:
  1. Fluid and electrolyte replacement by oral liquids and nutrients, as well as IV fluids
  2. Cautious use of antidiarrheal agents to decrease fluid loss
  3. Monitoring of intake, output, and daily weights
- Impaired skin integrity results from fistula formation. The degree of associated problems is related to the location of the fistula, the

patient's general health status, and the character and amount of fistula drainage.

1. In collaboration with the wound enterostomal therapist, apply a pouch or drain to the fistula to prevent skin irritation and to measure the drainage. Negative pressure wound therapy may promote healing when the fistula is large.
2. Provide skin barriers to prevent skin irritation and excoriation.
3. Protect the adjacent skin and keep it clean and dry.
4. Observe for subtle signs of infection or sepsis such as fever, abdominal pain, or change in mental status.

- Some patients with Crohn's disease require surgery such as a bowel resection and anastomosis with or without a colon resection to improve the quality of life (see *Surgical Management* under *Cancer, Colorectal*).
- Stricturoplasty may be performed for bowel strictures.

CYSTIC FIBROSIS

OVERVIEW

- Cystic fibrosis (CF) is a genetic disease present from birth that affects many organs and lethally impairs pulmonary function.
- The underlying problem of CF is blocked chloride transport in cell membranes, causing the formation of thick and sticky mucus.
- This mucus plugs up glands in the lungs, pancreas, liver, salivary glands, and testes, causing atrophy and organ dysfunction.
- Nonpulmonary problems include pancreatic insufficiency with malnutrition and intestinal obstruction, poor growth, male sterility, and cirrhosis of the liver.
- Life expectancy is over 35 years for a patient with typical manifestations of CF. The primary cause of death in the patient with CF is respiratory failure.
- The disorder is most common among white individuals, and about 4% are carriers. It is very rare among African Americans or Asians. Males and females are affected equally.

✴ Genetic/Genomic Considerations

- CF is an autosomal recessive disorder in which both gene alleles must be mutated for the disease to be expressed. The CF gene is located on chromosome 7 and produces a protein that controls chloride movement across cell membranes.
- People with one mutated allele are carriers and have few or no symptoms of CF but can pass the abnormal allele on to their children.

Continued

- More than 1700 different mutations have been identified. The inheritance of different mutations is responsible for the wide variation in disease severity.

PATIENT-CENTERED COLLABORATIVE CARE
Assessment
- The major diagnostic test is sweat chloride analysis, and additional genetic testing can be performed to determine which specific mutation a person may have.
- Assess for these nonpulmonary manifestations: abdominal distention, gastroesophageal reflux, rectal prolapse, foul-smelling stools, steatorrhea (excessive fat in stools), small stature, and underweight for height.
- Assess for these common pulmonary manifestations: frequent or chronic respiratory infections, chest congestion, limited exercise tolerance, cough, sputum production, use of accessory muscles, and decreased pulmonary function (especially forced vital capacity [FVC] and forced exhalation volume over 1 second [FEV_1]).
Interventions
Nonsurgical Management
- Nutritional management focuses on weight maintenance, vitamin supplementation, diabetes management, and pancreatic enzyme replacement (enzymes must be taken with food).
  1. Pulmonary management is focused on preventive maintenance and management of pulmonary exacerbation.
  2. Preventive or maintenance therapy involves the use of a regimen of chest physiotherapy, positive expiratory pressure, active cycle breathing technique, and an individualized regular exercise program. Drug therapy includes bronchodilators, anti-inflammatory agents, mucolytics, and antibiotics.
  3. Exacerbation therapy is needed when the patient with CF has a change in manifestations from baseline. Management focuses on mucus clearance, oxygenation, and antibiotic therapy:
     a. Supplemental oxygen
     b. Heliox delivery of 50% oxygen and 50% helium
     c. Airway clearance techniques (ACTs) four times each day
     d. Intensified bronchodilator and mucolytic therapies, glucocorticoids, and IV antibiotics
  4. Teach patients about protecting themselves by avoiding direct contact of bodily fluids such as saliva and sputum. Teach them not to routinely shake hands or kiss people in social settings. Handwashing is critical because the organism also can be

! NURSING SAFETY PRIORITY: Action Alert

Procedures approved by the Cystic Fibrosis Foundation should be used when cleaning clinic rooms, pulmonary function laboratories, and respiratory therapy equipment to reduce the risk of contamination between CF patients who are often colonized with pathogens that can contribute to disease exacerbation and mortality.

C

acquired indirectly from contaminated surfaces such as sinks and tissues.

Surgical Management

- The surgical management of the patient with CF involves lung and/or pancreatic transplantation.
- Lung transplantation procedures include two lobes or a single lung transplantation, as well as double-lung transplantation. Most often the patient with CF has a bilateral lobe transplant from a cadaver donor or living related donor.
- Provide preoperative care:
  1. Teach the patient the expected regimen of pulmonary hygiene to be used in the period immediately after surgery.
  2. Assist the patient in a pulmonary muscle strengthening and conditioning regimen.
- Provide postoperative care:
  1. The patient is intubated for at least 48 hours and has chest tubes and arterial lines in place. Much of the care needed is the same as that for any thoracic surgery.
  2. Assess for bleeding, infection, and transplant rejection.
  3. Anti-rejection drug regimens must be started immediately after surgery, which increases the risk for infection. The drugs generally used for routine long-term rejection suppression after organ transplantation are combinations of:
     a. Very specific immunosuppressants (cyclosporine [Sandimmune])
     b. Less specific immunosuppressants (azathioprine [Imuran] or mycophenolate mofetil [CellCept])
     c. One of the corticosteroids: prednisone (Apo-Prednisone ♣, Deltasone ♣) or prednisolone (Delta-per)

CYSTITIS (URINARY TRACT INFECTION)

OVERVIEW

- *Cystitis* is an inflammation or infection of the urinary bladder. Infectious causes are bacteria, viruses, fungi, and parasites. Non-infectious inflammation causes include chemical exposure,

radiation therapy, and immunologic responses in chronic inflammatory disease.
- *Interstitial cystitis* is a chronic inflammation of the entire lower urinary tract (bladder, urethra, and adjacent pelvic muscles) that is not the result of infection and can lead to pyelonephritis and sepsis.
- *Urosepsis* is the spread of infection from the urinary tract to the bloodstream.
- *Escherichia coli* normally found in the GI tract account for most cases of bacterial cystitis.
- Other factors that contribute to the development or recurrence of cystitis, or urinary tract infections (UTIs), include:
    1. Structural or functional abnormalities of the urinary tract
    2. Use of indwelling urinary catheters

❗ NURSING SAFETY PRIORITY: Action Alert

Avoid use of indwelling urinary catheters for longer than 3 days to reduce catheter-related UTIs.

    3. Sexual intercourse, diaphragm use, and pregnancy in women
    4. Prostate disease

Considerations for Older Adults

- UTIs occur more often in older adults than in younger adults, with women more commonly affected than men.
- Older patients are at greater risk than others of having an overwhelming and generalized infection, known as *urosepsis.*
- Change in mental status is a common symptom of cystitis in the older adult.

QSEN TEAMWORK AND COLLABORATION; INFORMATICS

Timely reporting of abnormal CBC results (especially an elevated WBC count), abnormal urinalysis results (especially positive nitrogen and leukocyte esterase), and positive urine culture reports are essential to initiating and evaluating effective antibiotic treatment.

❗ NURSING SAFETY PRIORITY: Critical Rescue

A decrease in mental status or increase in HR combined with a decrease in BP can indicate clinical instability or urosepsis, requiring immediate intervention.

PATIENT-CENTERED COLLABORATIVE CARE
Assessment
- Record patient information:
  1. History of UTIs
  2. History of renal or urologic problems, such as kidney stones, structural disease, or functional problems with voiding
  3. History of impaired immune response, such as diabetes mellitus or inflammatory and autoimmune disease
- Assess for:
  1. Increased frequency or urgency in voiding
  2. Pain or discomfort on urination
  3. Change in urine color, clarity, or odor; presence of pus (WBCs) or blood (RBCs)
  4. Presence of nitrogen or leukocyte esterase with urinalysis
  5. Positive urine culture
  6. Elevated plasma WBCs
  7. Abdominal or back pain
  8. Bladder distention
  9. Feelings of incomplete bladder emptying
  10. Voiding in small amounts
  11. Difficulty in initiating urination
  12. Complete inability to urinate
  13. Urinary meatus inflammation
  14. Prostate gland changes or tenderness

Considerations for Older Adults

- The symptoms of UTI may be as vague as increasing mental confusion or unexplained falls.
- Sudden onset of or worsening of incontinence may be an early symptom.
- Fever, tachycardia, tachypnea, and hypotension even without any urinary symptoms may be signs of urosepsis.
- Loss of appetite, nocturia, and dysuria are common symptoms.

Planning and Implementation
- Drug therapy includes:
  1. Antibiotics: In uncomplicated, acute bacterial cystitis in healthy, ambulatory patients, a 3-day course of oral antibiotic treatment may be adequate. A 7- to 14-day course of oral or parenteral antibiotics may be needed for complex, chronic, or recurring infections and for urosepsis.
  2. Analgesics or antipyretics may be used to promote comfort.

3. Antispasmodics may be used to decrease bladder spasm and promote complete bladder emptying in certain chronic conditions or with recurrent UTI.
4. Antifungal agents such as amphotericin B in daily bladder instillations and ketoconazole (Nizoral) in oral form may also be used.

- Diet therapy includes:
  1. Ensure sufficient fluid intake to maintain clear or light yellow urine (2.2 to 3 L/day), unless contraindicated in a chronic condition.
  2. Cranberry juice or tablets taken daily may reduce the frequency of recurrent UTIs but should be avoided with interstitial cystitis.
- Other therapy includes providing warm sitz baths to relieve perineal discomfort.

Surgical Management

- Surgical interventions for management of cystitis include urologic procedures for structural abnormalities or endourologic procedures to manipulate or pulverize kidney stones if these conditions are associated with cystitis.

QSEN QUALITY IMPROVEMENT

Anticipate fall prevention interventions for older patients to reduce the risk of patient harm when confusion accompanies cystitis.

Community-Based Care

- Teach the patient to:
  1. Self-administer drugs and complete all of the prescribed drug.
  2. Expect changes in color of urine with some treatments.
  3. Use appropriate techniques to prevent discomfort with sexual activities and how to prevent postcoital infections.
  4. Consume liberal fluid intake to maintain urine color as clear or light yellow.
  5. Clean the perineum after urination.
  6. Empty the bladder as soon as the urge is felt.
  7. Avoid known irritants such as caffeine, carbonated beverages, tomato products, chemicals in bath water (e.g., bubble baths), vaginal washes, and scented toilet tissue.
  8. Seek prompt medical care if symptoms recur.
- Pregnant women with cystitis require prompt and aggressive antibiotic treatment, because this infection can lead to preterm labor and premature birth.
- Refer patients with interstitial cystitis to the Interstitial Cystitis Foundation.

CYSTOCELE

- A cystocele is a protrusion of the bladder through the vaginal wall resulting from weakened pelvic structures.
- Causes include obesity, advanced age, childbearing, or genetic predisposition.
- Assess for:
  1. Difficulty in emptying the bladder
  2. Urinary frequency and urgency or other symptoms of UTI
  3. Stress urinary incontinence
  4. Bulging of the anterior vaginal wall, especially when the woman is asked to bear down during a pelvic examination
- Diagnostic tests may include cystography, measurement of residual urine, IV urography (IVU), voiding cystourethrography (VCUG), cystometrography, and uroflowmetry.
- Management of patients with mild symptoms is conservative and may include:
  1. Use of a pessary for bladder support
  2. Application of intravaginal estrogen to prevent atrophy and weakening of vaginal walls
  3. Kegel exercises to strengthen perineal muscles
- Surgical intervention for severe symptoms is usually a vaginal sling or an anterior colporrhaphy (anterior repair) to tighten the pelvic muscles for better bladder support (see *Prolapse, Pelvic Organ*).

D

DEHYDRATION

OVERVIEW

- Dehydration is a condition in which fluid intake or fluid retention is less than what is needed to meet the body's fluid needs, resulting in a fluid volume deficit.
- It may be an actual decrease in total body water caused by either too little intake of fluid or too great a loss of fluid; or it can occur as a relative dehydration, without an actual loss of total body water, such as when water shifts from the plasma into the interstitial space.
- *Isotonic dehydration* is the most common type of fluid volume deficit, in which fluid is lost only from the extracellular fluid (ECF) space, including both the plasma and the interstitial spaces.
- Circulating blood volume is decreased (hypovolemia) and leads to inadequate tissue perfusion.
- Causes include:
  1. Hemorrhage
  2. Vomiting

Considerations for Older Adults

Older patients are at high risk for dehydration, because they have less total body water than younger adults. Many older adults have decreased thirst sensation and may have difficulty with walking or other motor skills needed for ingesting fluids. Other older adults may voluntarily cut back fluid intake because of concerns about incontinence. Older adults also may take drugs such as diuretics, antihypertensives, and laxatives that increase the amount of fluid excreted.

3. Diarrhea
4. Profuse salivation
5. Fistulas
6. Ileostomy
7. Profuse diaphoresis
8. Burns
9. Severe wounds
10. Long-term NPO status
11. Diuretic therapy
12. GI suction
13. Hyperventilation
14. Diabetes insipidus
15. Difficulty swallowing
16. Impaired thirst
17. Unconsciousness
18. Fever
19. Impaired motor function

PATIENT-CENTERED COLLABORATIVE CARE
Assessment
- Obtain and record patient information:
  1. Nutritional history
  2. Fluid history
     a. Intake and output volumes
     b. Weight (a weight change of 1 pound corresponds to fluid volume change of about 500 mL)
  3. Presence of excessive sweating, diarrhea
  4. Drug therapy (especially diuretics and laxatives)
  5. Medical history
     a. Diabetes
     b. Kidney disease
  6. Level of consciousness and functional status
  7. Amount of strenuous physical activity

8. Exposure to high environmental temperatures
9. Dizziness or light-headedness when standing
- Assess for:
    1. Vital signs, including orthostatic HR and BP if patient is able to sit or stand
    2. Cardiovascular changes:
        a. Tachycardia at rest
        b. Weak peripheral pulses
        c. Low systolic or mean arterial BP
        d. Decreased pulse pressure
        e. Flat neck and hand veins in dependent position
    3. Respiratory changes:
        a. Increased respiratory rate
        b. Increased respiratory depth
    4. Skin changes:
        a. Dry mucous membranes
        b. Tongue has a pastelike coating or fissures
        c. Dry, flaky skin
        d. Poor skin turgor (skin "tents" when pinched)

Considerations for Older Adults

Assess skin turgor in an older adult by pinching the skin over the sternum or on the forehead, rather than the back of the hand, because these areas more reliably indicate hydration. As a person ages, the skin loses elasticity and tents on hands and arms even when the person is well hydrated.

5. Neurologic changes:
    a. Alterations of mental status (especially confusion)
    b. Low-grade fever
6. Kidney function:
    a. Urine output less than 0.5 to 1 mL/kg/hour for 2 or more hours
    b. Increased urine concentration (specific gravity greater than 1.030, dark amber, strong odor)

! NURSING SAFETY PRIORITY: Critical Rescue

Urine output below 500 mL/day for any patient without kidney disease is cause for concern and should be reported to the health care provider.

- Diagnostic assessment: No single laboratory test result confirms or rules out dehydration. Instead, it is determined by laboratory findings along with clinical manifestations. Common laboratory findings for dehydration include:

1. Elevated levels of hemoglobin and hematocrit
2. Increased serum osmolarity, glucose, protein, blood urea nitrogen, and various electrolytes

! NURSING SAFETY PRIORITY: Action Alert

Hemoconcentration is not present when dehydration is from hemorrhage. Therefore do not rely only on laboratory values to identify dehydration.

Interventions

- Management of dehydration aims to prevent injury, prevent further fluid losses, and increase fluid compartment volumes to normal ranges.
  1. Monitor vital signs, especially HR and BP.
  2. Replace fluids.
     a. Oral fluid replacement is used for correction of mild to moderate dehydration if the patient is alert enough to swallow and can tolerate oral fluids. Commercial solutions for adults include Equalyte, Oralyte, and Rehydralyte.
     b. IV fluid replacement is used when dehydration is severe and when the patient cannot safely swallow or cannot tolerate oral fluids.
  3. Measure intake and output.
  4. Assess muscle strength, gait stability, and level of alertness.
     a. Implement fall precautions for safety
     b. Implement interventions to prevent skin injury
  5. Drug therapy may correct some causes of the dehydration:
     a. Antidiarrheal drugs
     b. Antiemetics
     c. Antipyretics

DEMENTIA

OVERVIEW

- Dementia is a chronic, progressive, degenerative disease that is characterized by memory loss and cognitive impairment.
- *Alzheimer's disease* (AD) and *dementia, Alzheimer's type* (DAT) account for 60% of the dementias occurring in persons older than 65 years.
- Dementia is also seen in people in their 40s and 50s, which is referred to as *early dementia,* or *presenile DAT.*
- AD is characterized by neurofibrillary tangles and neuritic plaques of beta-amyloid proteins in the brain.

- The exact cause of AD is unknown; genetic predisposition, chemical changes, environmental agents, and immunologic alterations have been implicated in the pathology.
- Other causes of dementia are stroke or cerebrovascular impairment, head injury, Parkinson's disease, Lewy body formation, and human immune deficiency virus (HIV) infection.

PATIENT-CENTERED COLLABORATIVE CARE
Assessment
- Record patient information:
  1. Age
  2. Current employment status and work history
  3. Self-management skills for daily living
  4. Ability to complete independent activities such as grocery shopping, laundry, meal planning, and financial transactions
  5. Driving ability
  6. Oral and written communication skills
  7. Behavior
  8. Family history of AD
  9. Medical history, with particular attention to head trauma, viral illness, or exposure to metal or toxic waste
  10. Available support systems (spouse, partner, adult children)
- Assess for:
  1. Indicators of the stages of the disease:
     a. *Early (stage I) AD* is characterized by forgetfulness, misplacing household items, mild memory loss, short attention span, decreased performance, loss of judgment, subtle changes in personality and behavior, and the inability to travel alone to new destinations. There are no associated social or employment problems.
     b. *Middle (stage II) AD* is characterized by severe impairments in all cognitive functions; gross intellectual impairments; complete disorientation to time, place, and event; physical impairment; loss of ability to care for self; visual-spatial deficits; speech-language problems; and incontinence.
     c. *Late (stage III) AD* is characterized by lost motor and verbal skills and by severe physical and cognitive deterioration and total dependence for ADLs.
  2. Cognitive changes, such as changes in attention, concentration, judgment, perception, learning, and short-term memory
  3. Alterations in communication and language skills
  4. Changes in behaviors and personality, such as aggressiveness, paranoia, inappropriate social interactions, rapid mood swings, and increased confusion at night or when fatigued

5. Changes in self-management requiring assistance in hygiene, dressing, following directions, or completing familiar activities
- Genetic testing specifically for apolipoprotein E (apo-E) may be helpful as an ancillary test (not a predictive test) for the differential diagnosis of AD.
- A variety of laboratory or radiographic tests are performed to rule out other treatable causes of dementia or delirium, including serum levels of beta-amyloid.

Planning and Implementation

CHRONIC CONFUSION

- Confusion is related to neuronal degeneration in the brain.
- Collaborate with the health care team to prevent overstimulation and provide a structured and orderly environment.
  1. Provide a safe environment with adequate lighting, and remove items that can obstruct walking.
  2. Implement falls precautions in the acute care setting.
  3. Place the patient within easy view of the staff, preferably in a private room.
  4. Arrange the patient's schedule to provide as much uninterrupted sleep at night as possible. Fatigue increases confusion and behavioral problems such as agitation and aggression.
  5. Establish a daily routine, explaining changes in routine before they occur and again immediately before they take place.
  6. Place familiar objects, clocks, and single-date calendars in easy view of the patient. Encourage the family to provide pictures of family members and close friends that are labeled with the person's name on the picture.
  7. Regularly re-orient the patient to the environment (during early stages).
  8. Use validation therapy for later stages of the disease to prevent agitation.
  9. Collaborate with the physical and occupational therapist to assist the patient to maintain independence in ADLs as long as possible through the use of assistive devices (grab bars in the bathroom) and exercise programs.
  10. Develop an individualized bowel and bladder program for the patient.
  11. Attract the patient's attention before conversing, then use short, clear sentences.
  12. Allow sufficient time for the patient to respond.
  13. In the home environment, place complete outfits on a single hanger for the patient to choose from; encourage the family to include the patient in meal planning, grocery shopping, and other household routines as he or she is able.

14. Provide drug therapy:
  a. Cholinesterase inhibitors are approved for symptomatic treatment of AD.
  b. Selective serotonin reuptake inhibitors are used to treat depression; tricyclic antidepressants should not be used because of their anticholinergic effect.
  c. Psychotropic drugs, also called *antipsychotic* and *neuroleptic drugs,* should be reserved for a patient with emotional and behavioral health problems that may accompany dementia, such as hallucinations and delusions.
15. Use activities and recreation such as art, dance, and music in the long-term care setting to minimize agitation.

D

RISK FOR INJURY

- The risk for injury is related to wandering or elder abuse.
- The following nursing planning and implementation steps are used to decrease the risk for injury:
  1. Ensure that the patient always wears an identification bracelet or badge that cannot be removed by the patient. Devices that use global positioning system (GPS) can be embedded in the bracelet or badge to provide tracking abilities.
  2. Ensure that alarms or other barriers to outside doors are working properly at all times.
  3. Check on the patient often.
  4. Take the patient for walks several times each day, and encourage the patient to participate in activities to decrease his or her restlessness.
  5. Talk calmly and softly, redirecting the patient as needed and using diversion.
  6. Keep the patient busy with structured activities such as music, recreation, and art therapy.
  7. Remove and secure all sharp objects and medications.
  8. Implement seizure precautions if there is a history of seizures.
  9. Keep an updated photograph of the patient that can be used if the patient wanders away.
  10. Inform the patient's family about the Safe Return program, a national government-funded program of the Alzheimer's Association that assists in the identification and safe, timely return of individuals with AD and related dementias who wander off and become lost.

CAREGIVER ROLE STRAIN

- The following nursing planning and implementation steps are used to increase family coping and decrease caregiver role strain:
  1. Advise the family to seek legal counsel regarding the patient's competency and the need to obtain guardianship or durable power of attorney.

2. Refer the family to a local support group affiliated with the Alzheimer's Association.
3. Assess the family and other caregivers for signs of stress, such as anger, social withdrawal, anxiety, depression and lack of concentration, sleepiness, irritability, and health problems; refer them to their health care provider.
4. Encourage the family to maintain its own social network and to obtain respite care periodically.
5. Assist the family to identify and develop strategies to cope with the long-term consequences of the disease.

QSEN TEAMWORK AND COLLABORATION

Evaluate and report critical laboratory values in a timely manner so that reversible causes of delirium receive effective interventions, such as hemoglobin or electrolyte replacement therapy.

Community-Based Care

• When possible, the patient should be assigned to a case manager who can assess the patient's need for health care resources and facilitate appropriate placement throughout the continuum of care.
• The patient is usually cared for in the home until late in the disease process. Therefore teach the patient and family:
    1. How to assist the patient with ADLs
    2. How to use adaptive equipment
    3. With dietary consultation, how to select and prepare food that the patient is able to chew and swallow
    4. How to prevent the patient from wandering
    5. What to do if the patient has a seizure
    6. How to protect the patient from injury
    7. Drug information (if drugs are prescribed) and how to secure drugs so the patient does not take them inappropriately
    8. How to implement the diversion, including activity or exercise
    9. How to obtain respite services
    10. Strategies that caregivers can use to reduce their stress, including:
        a. Maintaining realistic expectations for the person with AD
        b. Taking one day at a time
        c. Trying to find positive aspects of each incident or situation
        d. Using humor with the person who has AD
        e. Setting aside time each day for rest or recreation, away from caregiving duties if possible

    f. Seeking respite care periodically

    g. Exploring alternative care settings early in the disease process for possible use later

    h. Establishing advance directives early in the disease process with the person who has AD

    i. Taking care of themselves by watching their diet, exercising, and getting plenty of rest

    j. Being realistic about what they can do, and getting and accepting help from family, friends, and community resources

- Refer the patient's family and significant others to the local chapter of the Alzheimer's Association.

DIABETES INSIPIDUS

OVERVIEW

- Diabetes insipidus (DI) is a water loss problem caused by either a decrease in antidiuretic hormone (ADH) synthesis or an inability of the kidneys to respond to ADH.
- The result of DI is the excretion of large volumes of dilute urine.
- DI is classified into four types, depending on whether the problem is caused by too little ADH or an inability of the kidneys to respond to ADH.

    1. *Nephrogenic DI* is an inherited (genetic) disorder in which the renal tubules do not respond to the actions of ADH, which results in inadequate water absorption by the kidney.

    2. *Primary DI* results from a problem in the hypothalamus or pituitary gland resulting in lack of ADH production or release.

    3. *Secondary DI* results from tumors in or near the hypothalamus or pituitary gland, head trauma, infectious processes, surgical procedures, or metastatic tumors (usually from the lung or breast).

    4. *Drug-related DI* is most often caused by lithium (Eskalith, Lithobid, Carbolith ♣) and demeclocycline (Declomycin), which can interfere with the kidney response to ADH.

PATIENT-CENTERED COLLABORATIVE CARE

Assessment

- Assess patient information:

    1. History of recent brain surgery, head trauma, and current drugs

    2. Excretion of more than 4 L of dilute urine in 24 hours in excess of fluid intake

    3. Dehydration manifestations (e.g., poor skin turgor, dry mucous membranes, or weight loss in excess of 1 pound/day)

    4. Increased or excessive thirst

5. Low urine specific gravity (below 1.005) and urine osmolality (50 to 200 mOsm/kg)
6. Indications of circulatory collapse, shock (e.g., decreased mental status; tachycardia; low BP; rapid, thready pulse; and decreased pulse pressure)
7. Neurologic changes such as irritability, lethargy, or decreased cognition

Interventions

- Drug therapy may include:
    1. Desmopressin (DDAVP), a synthetic form of vasopressin given intranasally in a metered spray or as an oral tablet; frequency of dosing depends on the patient's response
    2. Aqueous vasopressin for short-term therapy or when the dosage must be changed often; given parenterally
- Nursing interventions include:
    1. Replacing fluids by encouraging the patient to drink fluids equal to the amount of urinary output (if the patient is unable to do so, provide IV, as prescribed)

> **! NURSING SAFETY PRIORITY: Critical Rescue**
>
> Patients with this condition are at risk for severe dehydration and circulatory collapse because they cannot reduce urine output. Provide ongoing access to oral or IV fluids and monitor patient response to intake and output every 4 hours around the clock.

2. Monitoring intake and output with daily weights and communicating imbalances in a timely manner; a loss of 1 kg is equivalent to losing 1 liter of fluid
3. Monitoring for vital sign changes indicating poor tissue perfusion (e.g., low BP; rapid, thready pulse; decreased consciousness)
4. Monitoring for indications of dehydration, including dry skin, poor skin turgor, and dry or cracked mucous membranes
5. Monitoring serum and urine lab results for effectiveness of therapy
- Patient education includes:
    1. Teaching the patient that polyuria and thirst are signals for the need for another drug dose
    2. Teaching the patient to use daily weights to estimate dehydration (and the need for additional ADH/vasopressin) or overhydration (reduce drug dose)
    3. Teaching about the side effects of nasal sprays, including ulceration of the mucous membranes, allergy, sensation of chest

tightness, and inhalation of the spray into the lungs, which precipitates pulmonary problems

4. Teaching about side effects and to contact provider if an upper respiratory infection develops during intranasal drug use
5. Teaching the patient going home on vasopressin how to self-inject the drug
6. Encouraging the patient with chronic DI to wear a medical alert bracelet or necklace at all times

DIABETES MELLITUS

OVERVIEW

- Diabetes mellitus (DM) is a metabolic disease that results from problems with insulin secretion, insulin action, or both.
- The main metabolic effects of insulin are to stimulate glucose uptake in skeletal muscle and heart muscle, and to suppress liver production of glucose and very-low-density lipoprotein (VLDL). Overall, insulin keeps blood glucose levels from becoming too high and helps keep blood lipid levels in the normal range. Insulin is needed for metabolism of carbohydrates, proteins, and fats.
- Movement of glucose into some cells requires the presence of specific carriers, glucose transporters (GLUTs), and insulin. As glucose from the blood enters the cells, the blood glucose level goes back to normal (euglycemia). The glucose in the cell can be used immediately to make adenosine triphosphate (ATP) if the cell needs more chemical energy. If the cell already has enough ATP, the glucose is stored for later use.
- The lack of insulin in DM from a lack of production or a problem with insulin use at its cell receptor prevents some cells from using glucose for energy. Without insulin, the body enters a serious state of cellular starvation, breaking down body fat and protein.
- DM is diagnosed with either a blood glucose measurement or a test of glycosylated hemoglobin (A_{1c}) levels.
- Acute manifestations of DM are hyperglycemia (elevated blood glucose levels), polyuria (excessive urination), polydipsia (excessive thirst and drinking), and polyphagia (hunger).
- DM is classified according to the cause of the disease and the severity of insulin lack. The three most common types of DM are type 1, type 2, and gestational diabetes.
  1. *Type 1 diabetes* is an autoimmune disorder in which beta cells of the pancreas are destroyed in a genetically susceptible person and no insulin is produced. Type I diabetes:
     a. Is abrupt in onset
     b. Requires insulin injections to prevent hyperglycemia and ketosis and to sustain health
     c. Represents fewer than 10% of all people who have diabetes

      d. Occurs primarily in childhood and adolescence but can occur at any age

      e. Causes patients to be thin and underweight

      f. May follow viral infection; viral infection can trigger auto-immune destructive actions

2. *Type 2 diabetes* is a problem resulting from a reduction in the ability of most cells to respond to insulin (insulin resistance), poor control of liver glucose output, and decreased beta cell function. Type 2 diabetes:

      a. Is generally slow in onset and may be present for years before it is diagnosed

      b. May require oral antidiabetic drug therapy or insulin to correct hyperglycemia

      c. Is usually found in middle-aged and older adults but may occur in younger people

      d. May be part of metabolic syndrome or obesity

      e. Is usually not associated with ketoacidosis

      f. Represents about 90% of all people who have diabetes

3. *Gestational diabetes mellitus* (GDM):

      a. Is noted with carbohydrate intolerance during pregnancy and confirmed by an oral glucose tolerance test

      b. Is suspected when a first baby weighs more than 9 pounds

      c. Leaves women at high risk for type 2 diabetes after pregnancy

- Acute complications of DM include:

1. Diabetic ketoacidosis (DKA):

      a. DKA occurs in people with type 1 DM and is most often precipitated by illness, especially infection.

      b. Patients have acidosis and severe dehydration.

      c. Laboratory diagnosis is based on serum glucose level equal to or greater than 300 mg/dL (16.7 mmol/L), arterial pH less than 7.35, arterial bicarbonate level less than 15 mEq/L, blood urea nitrogen level greater than 20 mg/dL, creatinine level greater than 1.5 mg/dL, and ketonuria.

      d. Clinical manifestations of dehydration and acidosis include decreased skin turgor, dry mucous membranes, hypotension, tachycardia, tachypnea, Kussmaul respirations, abdominal pain, nausea, and vomiting. Central nervous system depression results in changes in consciousness varying from lethargy to coma.

      e. Death occurs in 1% to 10% of these cases even with appropriate treatment. Mortality is highest for older patients who also have infection, stroke, MI, vascular thrombosis, intestinal obstruction, or pneumonia.

2. Hyperglycemic-hyperosmolar state (HHS):
   a. HHS differs from DKA by the relative absence of ketosis and much higher blood glucose levels (may exceed 600 mg/dL) and osmolarity levels (greater than 320 mOsm/L).
   b. Dehydration is the most common cause of HHS and becomes worse with the disorder.
   c. HHS occurs almost exclusively in patients with type 2 DM.
   d. It occurs most often in older adults and those who are unaware of their diabetic condition.
   e. Conditions such as silent MI, sepsis, pancreatitis, and stroke, and drugs such as glucocorticoids, diuretics, phenytoin sodium, propranolol, and calcium channel blockers may precipitate HHS.

Considerations for Older Adults

Older adults with DM are at the greatest risk for dehydration and subsequent HHS. The onset of HHS is slow and may not be recognized. The older patient often seeks medical attention later and is sicker than younger patients. The mortality rate for HHS in older adults is as high as 40% to 70%.

! NURSING SAFETY PRIORITY: Action Alert

HHS does not occur in people who are adequately hydrated. Take steps to avoid dehydration in susceptible patients.

3. Hypoglycemia:
   a. Hypoglycemia is a blood glucose level lower than 70 mg/dL.
   b. It can be caused by excessive insulin, some oral antidiabetic drugs, insufficient food intake, and increased physical activity.
   c. *Neurogenic symptoms* of hypoglycemia, which result from autonomic nervous system stimulation triggered by hypoglycemia, include hunger, diaphoresis, weakness, and nervousness. These symptoms occur when there is an abrupt decrease in the blood glucose level.
   d. *Neuroglycopenic symptoms,* which result directly from brain glucose deprivation and include headache, confusion, slurred speech, behavioral changes, and coma, occur with a more gradual decline in blood glucose level.
   e. If not managed properly, hypoglycemia can lead to brain damage and death.

   f. The classic signs and symptoms of hypoglycemia may not
      appear in older patients with DM; changes in levels of con-
      sciousness may be slow and progress through confusion and
      bizarre behavior. Coma may come without warning.
- Chronic complications of DM result from changes in large blood
  vessels (macrovascular) and small blood vessels (microvascular)
  in tissues and organs, leading to poor perfusion and cell death.
  1. Macrovascular complications include hyperlipidemia, hyper-
     tension, coronary heart disease, cerebrovascular disease, and
     peripheral vascular disease.
     a. Coronary artery disease includes angina, MI, and heart failure.
     b. Cerebrovascular disease includes stroke and worse outcomes
        following stroke (e.g., greater disability and mortality).
     c. Peripheral vascular diseases include venous leg ulcers and
        arterial insufficiency leading to amputation.
  2. Microvascular complications lead to nephropathy (kidney
     dysfunction), neuropathy (nerve dysfunction), retinopathy
     (vision problems), male ED, and dementia.

⊕ Cultural Considerations

- **DM is a significant problem for blacks, American Indians,
  and Mexican Americans.**
- **In all populations, prevalence of type 2 DM rises with age
  and obesity.**
- **Minority group members have a higher risk for
  complications when compared with white individuals,
  including hypertension, retinopathy, neuropathy, and
  nephropathy, even after adjusting for differences in blood
  glucose control.**

  3. Although nothing prevents the complications, they can be
     slowed significantly by maintaining serum glucose between 60
     and 150 mg/dL ("tight control").

PATIENT-CENTERED COLLABORATIVE CARE
Assessment
- Ask about and record patient information:
  1. Age
  2. Birth weight of children
  3. Weight change
  4. Occurrence of a recent illness or extreme stress
  5. Omission of insulin or oral antidiabetic drugs if the patient
     is known to have DM
  6. Change in eating habits

7. Change in exercise schedule or activity level
8. Presence and duration of polyuria, polydipsia, polyphagia, and loss of energy
9. History of small skin injuries becoming infected more easily or taking a longer time to heal
10. In women, frequency and duration of vaginal infections
11. Presence of cardiovascular disease such as hyperlipidemia, hypertension, heart failure, or stroke
12. Presence of diabetes in a parent or sibling
13. History of high fasting blood glucose levels
- Assess for:
    1. Elevated blood glucose
        a. Fasting blood glucose level higher than 126 mg/dL on two occasions
        b. Oral glucose tolerance test (2 hour post-load test) with glucose greater than 200 mg/dL
        c. Glycosylated hemoglobin assay (HbA$_{1c}$) results greater than 5.5% to 6.0%
    2. Positive results for urinary ketones; presence of albumin and glucose in the urine
    3. Abdominal pain, nausea, and vomiting (in DKA)
    4. Dehydration (e.g., poor skin turgor, dry mucous membranes, hemoconcentration with elevated hematocrit and hemoglobin levels, decreased urine output, dark and strong-smelling urine)

Planning and Implementation
RISK FOR INJURY RELATED TO HYPERGLYCEMIA
   Nonsurgical Management
- Drug or insulin therapy is indicated when a patient with type 2 DM cannot achieve blood glucose control with dietary modification, regular exercise, and stress management.
    1. *Biguanides:* Metformin (Glucophage) is the only drug in this class and acts to increase insulin secretion by pancreatic beta cells. This drug does not cause hypoglycemia.

! NURSING SAFETY PRIORITY: Drug Alert

Metformin can cause lactic acidosis in patients with renal insufficiency and should not be used by anyone with kidney disease. To prevent kidney damage, the drug should be withheld for 48 hours before and after using contrast material or any surgical procedure requiring anesthesia.

2. *Sulfonylureas:* These drugs include glipizide (Glucotrol) and glimepiride (Amaryl). They trigger release of insulin from pancreatic beta cells (secretagogues). Hypoglycemia is the most serious complication.

3. *Meglitinide analogues:* Repaglinide (Prandin) and nateglinide (Starlix) are oral drugs that also trigger insulin release and are associated with hypoglycemia.

4. *Alpha-glucosidase inhibitors:* These oral drugs include acarbose (Precose) and miglitol (Glyset). They reduce hyperglycemia after meals by slowing digestion and absorption of carbohydrate within the intestine. Drugs in this class do not cause hypoglycemia.

5. *Thiazolidinediones (TZDs) or glitazones:* These oral drugs include rosiglitazone (Avandia) and pioglitazone (Actos). They work by increasing the sensitivity of insulin receptors, thereby promoting glucose utilization in peripheral tissues. They are associated with cardiac complications.

6. *Incretin mimetics (GLP-1 agonists):* These act like natural "gut" hormones that work with insulin to lower plasma glucose levels. They lower glucagon secretion from the pancreas, leading to reduced liver glucose production, and reduce blood glucose levels by delaying gastric emptying, slowing the rate of nutrient absorption into the blood, and reducing food intake. These drugs include exenatide (Byetta), exenatide extended release (Bydureon), and liraglutide (Victoza); all are injectables.

7. *DPP-4 inhibitors* are oral agents that include sitagliptin (Januvia), saxagliptin (Onglyza), linagliptin (Tradjenta), and alogliptin (Nesina). DPP-4 is an enzyme that breaks down the natural gut hormones (GLP-1 and GIP). DPP-4 inhibitors increase the amount of substances produced in the small intestine that work with insulin to lower glucagon secretion from the pancreas and reduce glucose production in the liver. They also reduce blood glucose levels by delaying gastric emptying, slowing the rate of nutrient absorption into the blood, and reducing food intake.

8. *Amylin analog* is pramlintide (Symlin) given subcutaneously. Similar to amylin, a naturally occurring hormone produced by beta cells in the pancreas that is co-secreted with insulin and lowers blood glucose levels by delaying gastric emptying and triggering satiety.

9. *Fixed combination agents:* These are combinations from two different classes of drugs, such as Glucovance, which combines glyburide with metformin. Remember that the side effects of combination agents include those of all drugs contained in the combination.

- Insulin therapy is necessary for type 1 DM and for moderate to severe type 2 DM.
  1. Insulin is available in rapid-, short-, intermediate-, and long-acting forms, which may be injected separately, and some can be mixed in the same syringe.

2. Insulin regimens try to duplicate the normal release pattern of insulin from the pancreas, including single daily injections, two-dose protocol, three-dose protocol, four-dose protocol, combination therapy, and intensified insulin regimens.
3. Teach the patient that insulin type, injection techniques, site of injection, and individual response can all affect absorption, onset, degree, and duration of insulin activity and reinforce that changing insulin may affect blood glucose control.
4. Complications of insulin therapy include:
   a. Hypoglycemia
   b. *Dawn phenomenon,* a fasting hyperglycemia thought to result from the nocturnal release of growth hormone secretion that may cause blood glucose elevations around 5:00 to 6:00 AM and is managed or prevented by providing more insulin for the overnight period
   c. *Somogyi's phenomenon,* a morning hyperglycemia resulting from an effective counterregulatory response to nighttime hypoglycemia, which is managed or prevented by ensuring adequate dietary intake at bedtime and evaluating the insulin dose and exercise program
   d. *Hypertrophic lipodystrophy,* a spongy swelling at or around injection sites
   e. *Lipoatrophy,* a loss of subcutaneous fat in areas of repeated injection that is treated by injection of human insulin at the edges of the atrophied area
   f. *Lipohypertrophy,* an increased swelling of fat that occurs at the site of repeated injections and is prevented by rotating injection sites
5. Insulin may be administered by:
   a. Intermittent subcutaneous injection, typically with a syringe; some patients may use a prefilled cartridge or syringe
   b. Continuous subcutaneous infusion of insulin using an externally worn pump containing a syringe and reservoir with rapid- or short-acting insulin connected to the patient by an infusion set
   c. Insulin pumps implanted into the peritoneal cavity where insulin can be absorbed in a more physiologic manner
6. Teach the patient about storage, dose preparation, injection procedures, and complications associated with drug therapy.
7. Instruct the patient to always buy the same type of syringes and use the same gauge and needle length; short needles are not used for an obese patient.
- The patient needs to know how to perform all aspects of self-monitoring of blood glucose (SMBG) and understand several issues:
   1. Accuracy of the results depends on the accuracy of the specific blood glucose meter, operator proficiency, and test strip

quality. Help the patient select a meter based on the cost of the meter and strips, ease of use, and the availability of repair and servicing.

2. Results are influenced by the amount of blood on the strip, the calibration of the meter to the strip currently in use; environmental conditions of altitude, temperature, and moisture; and patient-specific conditions of hematocrit, triglyceride level, and presence of hypotension.

3. Teach the patient how to clean the equipment to prevent infection.

- Nutrition therapy:
  1. Collaborate with the patient, physician, and dietician to formulate an individualized meal plan for the patient.
  2. Day-to-day consistency in the timing and amount of food eaten helps control blood glucose. Patients taking insulin need to eat at consistent times that are coordinated with the timed action of insulin.
  3. Base the meal plan on blood glucose monitoring results, total blood lipid levels, and weight management goals.
  4. Dietary guidelines are based on the individual needs of the patient.
     a. Carbohydrate intake should be 45% of daily calories, with a minimum of 130 g/day.
     b. A protein intake of 15% to 20% of total daily calories is appropriate for patients with normal kidney function. In patients with microalbuminuria or chronic kidney disease, reduction of protein may slow progression of kidney failure.
     c. Limit total fat intake to 20% to 30% of daily calorie intake with less than 200 mg of dietary cholesterol daily. Choose mono- and poly-unsaturated fats over unsaturated and *trans* fats.
     d. Fiber intake improves carbohydrate metabolism and lowers cholesterol levels. Advise a goal of 25 g of fiber daily for women and 38 g for men. Suggest that adding high-fiber foods to the diet gradually can help to prevent cramping, loose stools, and flatulence.
     e. Nonnutritive sweetness that enhances taste without causing hyperglycemia is acceptable. Avoid sugar-sweetened beverages.
     f. Warn the patient that fat "substitutes" or replacements may increase carbohydrate content in foods.
  5. Teach the patient that alcohol may be taken in moderation only if DM is well controlled.
  6. Explain and reinforce how to read food labels.

7. Reinforce dietary teaching such as how to follow the exchange system for meal planning and how to perform carbohydrate counting.
8. Support and reinforce information provided by the dietician regarding how to make adjustments in nutritional intake during illness, planned exercises, and social occasions.

Considerations for Older Adults

- A realistic approach to diet therapy is essential for older patients with DM. Attempts to change long-time eating habits may be difficult.
- Patients who live alone, do their own food preparation, and have physical limitations may have difficulty following the diet recommended by the American Diabetes Association.
- Socioeconomic factors may also affect a patient's ability to prepare the proper foods.

D

- Regular physical exercise is a recommended component of a comprehensive DM treatment plan:
  1. Collaborate with the patient and rehabilitation specialist to develop an exercise program.
  2. Instruct the patient to have a complete physical examination before starting an exercise program at home.
  3. Instruct the patient to wear proper footwear with good traction and cushioning and to examine the feet after exercise.
  4. Discourage exercise in extreme heat or cold or during periods of poor glucose control.
  5. Advise the patient to stay hydrated.
  6. Patients with type 1 DM should perform vigorous exercise only if blood glucose levels are between 80 and 250 mg/dL and no ketones are present in the urine.
  7. Teach the patient about the risks and complications related to exercise, such as prolonged alterations in blood glucose levels, vitreous hemorrhage, retinal detachment in patients with proliferative retinopathy, and increased proteinuria and foot and joint injury in patients with peripheral neuropathy.

Surgical Management
- Surgical interventions for diabetes include pancreas transplantation. When successful, this procedure eliminates the need for insulin injections, blood glucose monitoring, and many dietary restrictions.
  1. Immunosuppressive therapy is needed for life to prevent rejection of the transplanted pancreas.

    2. Complications include venous thrombosis, rejection, and infection.
- Provide preoperative care as described in Part One and:
  1. Monitor hydration and IV fluids and urine output.
  2. Monitor blood glucose results and administer insulin to maintain serum glucose at less than 18 mg/dL.
- Provide postoperative care as described including:
  1. Send scheduled glucose evaluation; physical stress from surgery, anesthesia, or hypothermia may cause hyperglycemia.
  2. Monitor fluid and electrolyte balance; hyperglycemia and kidney conditions may contribute to problems with fluid and electrolyte balance.
  3. Maintain tight glycemic control throughout the postoperative phase.
  4. Monitor for postoperative complications, including:
     a. MI
     b. Hypoglycemia and hyperglycemia; monitor at least four times daily
     c. Hyperkalemia or hypokalemia
     d. Impaired wound healing or wound infection; an unanticipated episode of hyperglycemia may indicate a new infection
     e. Acute kidney injury or progression of chronic kidney disease

RISK FOR INJURY RELATED TO NEUROPATHY
- Nonhealing foot wounds cause more inpatient hospital days than any other complication of diabetes.
- Loss of pain, pressure, and temperature sensation in the foot increases the risk for injury and ulceration.
- Foot deformities common in diabetic neuropathy may lead to callus formation, ulceration, and increased areas of pressure.
- Foot care education includes:
  1. Teaching preventive foot care to the patient; sensory neuropathy, ischemia, and infection are the leading causes of foot disease
  2. Recommending that the patient have shoes fitted by an experienced shoe fitter such as a certified podiatrist, and instructing the patient to change shoes at midday and in the evening and to wear socks or stockings with shoes
  3. Instructing the patient on how to care for wounds
- Refer the patient to a specialist for orthotic devices to eliminate pressure on infected or open wounds of the foot.
- Topical application of growth factors may be used to accelerate tissue healing for long-standing foot ulcers.

- Wound care for diabetic ulcers includes a moist wound environment, débridement of necrotic tissue, and offloading or elimination of pressure.

MANAGING PAIN FROM NEUROPATHY
- Drug therapy may include:
  1. Anticonvulsants such as gabapentin (Neurontin)
  2. Tricyclic antidepressants, particularly amitriptyline (Elavil, Levate ♣), nortriptyline (Pamelor), or selective serotonin and norepinephrine reuptake inhibitors, such as duloxetine (Cymbalta), as prescribed, to alleviate peripheral neuropathic pain
  3. Capsaicin cream, 0.075% (e.g., Axsain ♣, Zostrix-HP) topically to relieve neuropathic pain
- Use non-drug pain management techniques as appropriate, such as bed cradles, warm baths, and back rubs.

PREVENT INJURY FROM REDUCED VISION
- Encourage all patients to have a baseline ophthalmic examination and yearly follow-up examinations.
- Advise the patient to seek a retinal specialist if problems are present.
- Collaborate with the rehabilitation specialist to recommend strategies to improve the patient's visual abilities; strategies include improving lighting, placing dark equipment against a white background, coding objects such as insulin vials with bright colors or felt-tip markers, and using large-type books and newspapers.
- Various stages of diabetic retinopathy can be treated with laser therapy or surgery.
- Teach the patient with limited vision the following strategies for using adaptive devices to self-administer insulin:
  1. Ensuring proper placement of the device on the syringe
  2. Holding the insulin bottle upright when measuring insulin
  3. Avoiding air bubbles in the syringe by pulling a small amount of insulin into the syringe, moving the plunger in and out three times, and measuring insulin on the fourth draw

SLOW ONSET AND PROGRESSION OF CHRONIC KIDNEY DISEASE
- Stress the importance of maintaining a normal blood glucose level, maintaining a BP level below 130/85 mm Hg, and being screened annually for microalbuminuria.
- Teach the patient to limit protein to 0.8 g/kg of body weight per day if he or she has overt nephropathy.
- Teach the patient about the signs and symptoms of UTI.
- Advise the patient not to take any over-the-counter (OTC) drugs, especially NSAIDs, without checking with the health care provider.
- Approach studies that use some contrast dyes with caution due to nephrotoxicity of the dye.

POTENTIAL FOR HYPOGLYCEMIA

Monitor glucose levels before administering hypoglycemic agents, before meals, at bedtime, and when the patient is symptomatic.

* Treat the patient with mild hypoglycemia (hungry, irritable, shaky, weak, headache, fully conscious, blood glucose less than 60 mg/dL [3.4 mmol/L]) and who is able to swallow with 15 to 20 g of glucose, such as *one* of these:
  1. 2 or 3 glucose tablets
  2. 4 oz of fruit drink
  3. 8 oz of skim milk
  4. 6 saltines
  5. 3 graham crackers
  6. 6 to 10 hard candies
  7. 4 cubes or 2 teaspoons of sugar
* The blood glucose level should be tested after 15 minutes.
* Treat the patient with moderate hypoglycemia (cold and clammy skin, pale, rapid pulse, rapid shallow respirations, marked changes in mood, drowsiness, blood glucose less than 40 mg/dL [2.2 mmol/L]) with 15 to 30 g of rapidly absorbed carbohydrates and additional food such as low-fat milk or cheese after 10 to 15 minutes.

> ## ! NURSING SAFETY PRIORITY: Critical Rescue
>
> For the patient with severe hypoglycemia (unable to swallow, unconscious or convulsing, blood glucose usually less than 20 mg/dL [1.0 mmol/L]), treat by this approach:
> * Administer 50% dextrose (25 to 50 mL) IV or glucagon, 1 mg subcutaneously or IM.
> * Repeat the dose in 10 minutes if the patient remains unconscious.
> * Notify the primary health care provider immediately, and follow instructions.

* Teach the patient to prevent the four common causes of hypoglycemia: excess exercise, excess insulin, alcohol use, and deficient food intake.
* Encourage the patient to wear an identification (medical alert) bracelet.

POTENTIAL FOR DIABETIC KETOACIDOSIS

* Monitor the patient for signs and symptoms of diabetic ketoacidosis (DKA).
* Give insulin bolus as indicated, followed by a continuous drip.
* Check the patient's BP, pulse, and respirations every 15 minutes until stable.

- Monitor the patient for hypokalemia (symptoms are muscle weakness, abdominal distention or paralytic ileus, hypotension, and weak pulse); before administering potassium, ensure that the patient's urine output is at least 30 mL/hr.
- Replace both fluid volume and ongoing losses, monitoring for heart failure symptoms and pulmonary edema if large volume of IV fluid is administered.
- Record urine output, temperature, and mental status every hour.
- Assess the patient's level of consciousness, hydration status, fluid and electrolyte balance, and blood glucose levels every hour until stable; once stable, assess every 4 hours.
- Instruct the patient about how to prevent future episodes of DKA by contacting the primary health care provider when the blood glucose is greater than 250 mg/dL, when ketonuria is present for more than 24 hours, when he or she is unable to take food or fluids, and when illness persists for more than 1 to 2 days.

POTENTIAL FOR HYPERGLYCEMIC-HYPEROSMOLAR STATE (HHS)

- Administer IV fluids and insulin as indicated, and monitor and assess the patient's response to therapy.
- Assess for signs of cerebral edema and immediately report to the physician a change in the level of consciousness; change in pupil size, shape, or reaction to light; or seizure activity.

Community-Based Care

- Discharge planning includes:
  1. Ensuring that the patient understands the significance, symptoms, causes, and treatment of hypoglycemia and hyperglycemia
  2. Assisting the patient to identify the items needed for the administration of insulin and for glucose monitoring
  3. Teaching the patient how to monitor blood sugar level
  4. Teaching the patient how to administer drugs and prevent hypoglycemia
  5. In collaboration with the dietician, teaching the patient the skills associated with food choices and meal planning
  6. Referring the patient to a diabetes educator for the necessary instruction
  7. Helping the patient adapt to DM, including teaching stress management techniques and identifying coping mechanisms
  8. Referring the patient to the American Diabetes Association and its resources
  9. Providing information about community resources, such as diabetic education programs

DIVERTICULA, ESOPHAGEAL

OVERVIEW

- Diverticula are pouchlike herniations of the mucosa through the muscular wall.
- Patients with esophageal diverticula are at risk for esophageal perforation.
- The most common form of diverticulum is Zenker's diverticulum, which is usually located near the hypopharynx and occurs most often in older adults.

PATIENT-CENTERED COLLABORATIVE CARE

Assessment

- Assessment findings include:
  1. Dysphagia
  2. Regurgitation
  3. Feelings of fullness or pressure
  4. Halitosis
  5. Nocturnal cough

Interventions

- Diet therapy and positioning are the primary interventions for controlling symptoms related to diverticula.
- Nursing interventions include:
  1. Collaborating with the dietitian to determine the size and frequency of meals and the texture and consistency that can best be tolerated by the patient
  2. Elevating the head of the bed for sleep to avoid reflux of gastric contents onto diverticula
  3. Teaching the patient to avoid the recumbent position and vigorous exercise for at least 2 hours after eating to prevent reflux
  4. Teaching the patient to avoid restrictive clothing at the abdomen and thorax and to minimize stooping or bending to reduce reflux
- Surgical management is aimed at excision of the diverticula.
- Postoperative care:
  1. Monitor for bleeding and perforation.
  2. Do not irrigate the NG tube used for decompression unless specifically ordered by the physician.
  3. Maintain hydration and nutrition through IV fluids and enteral feedings until oral intake is permitted; NPO status may be several days' duration to allow esophageal healing.
  4. Manage the patient's postoperative pain.
  5. Teach the patient to observe for complications such as infection or poor wound healing.

6. Teach the patient measures to take to reduce reflux (e.g., elevating the head of bed and avoiding a recumbent position).

DIVERTICULAR DISEASE
OVERVIEW
- Diverticular disease includes diverticulosis and diverticulitis.
  1. *Diverticula* are pouchlike herniations of the mucosa through the muscular wall of any portion of the gut.
  2. *Diverticulosis* can occur in any segment of the gut but it most commonly refers to diverticula of the colon. High intraluminal pressure forces the formation of a pouch in the weakened area of the mucosa, commonly near blood vessels.
  3. *Diverticulitis,* or inflammation of one or more diverticula, results when the diverticulum retains undigested food that compromises the blood supply to that area and facilitates bacterial invasion of the diverticular sac.
  4. Complications of diverticula and diverticulitis are abscess formation and perforation followed by peritonitis.

PATIENT-CENTERED COLLABORATIVE CARE
Assessment
- Patients with diverticulosis are usually asymptomatic; a minor history of left quadrant pain or constipation may be reported.
- Diverticula are identified by colonoscopy; a screening abdominal ultrasound may reveal thickened bowel wall.
- Assess for clinical manifestations of diverticulitis:
  1. Abdominal pain that may begin as intermittent and may progress to continuous; pain may be localized to the left lower quadrant and increase with coughing, straining, or lifting
  2. Fever
  3. Nausea and vomiting
  4. Abdominal distention
  5. Blood in the stool (microscopic to larger amounts)
  6. Elevated WBC; reduced hematocrit and hemoglobin if bleeding occurs
  7. Hypotension and dehydration occur if bleeding occurs (see *Shock*)
  8. Signs of septic shock occur if peritonitis has occurred
  9. Serum electrolytes
  10. Intake and output, including NG tube (amount, color and quality) if used for gastric decompression or to manage vomiting

Interventions
- Drug therapy is used to treat infection and inflammation from diverticulitis.
    1. Administer broad-spectrum antibiotics such as metronidazole (Flagyl) plus trimethoprim/sulfamethoxazole (Bactrim, Septra), or ciprofloxacin (Cipro).
    2. Implement management for mild or moderate pain; if pain is severe, use opioids.
    3. Laxatives and enemas are not given, because they increase intestinal motility.
- An NG tube is inserted if nausea, vomiting, or abdominal distention is severe. Report the appearance of output.
- Diet therapy:
    1. Provide IV fluids for hydration during the acute phase of the disease or when the patient is NPO.
    2. Consult with a dietitian to promote healthy food choices.

  Surgical Management
- Patients with diverticulitis need emergent surgery if one of the following occurs:
    1. Rupture of the diverticulum with subsequent peritonitis
    2. Abdominal or pelvic abscess
    3. Bowel obstruction
    4. Fistula
    5. Uncontrolled bleeding
- Surgical management includes a colon resection with an end-to-end anastomosis or temporary or permanent colostomy.
- Preoperative care is provided as described in Part One and includes:
    1. Reinforcing physician teaching about the possible need for a temporary or permanent colostomy
    2. Administering IV fluids, antibiotics, and pain medications, as prescribed
- Postoperative care is routine as described in Part One and includes:
    1. Maintaining a drainage system at the abdominal incision site
    2. If a colostomy was created, monitoring colostomy stoma for color and integrity, anticipating that a gray or black color or separation between the mucous membranes and skin is indicative of poor healing and requires immediate communication with the surgeon
    3. Providing the patient with an opportunity to express feelings about the colostomy
    4. Consulting with the wound or ostomy specialist

  5. Providing written postoperative instructions on:
     a. Wound care
     b. Avoidance of activities that increase intra-abdominal pressure, including straining at stool, bending, lifting heavy objects, and wearing restrictive clothing
     c. Pain management, including prescriptions
- Teach the patient and family to:
  1. Follow dietary considerations for diverticulosis, which include consultation with the dietitian. Keep a food diary to note food associations with symptoms and to implement the following:
     a. Eat a diet high in cellulose and hemicellulose, which are found in wheat bran, whole-grain breads, cereals, fresh fruit, and vegetables.
     b. Use a bulk-forming laxative such as psyllium (Metamucil) to increase fecal size and consistency if recommended fiber intake of 25 to 35 g daily is not tolerated.
     c. Encourage fluids to prevent bloating that may accompany a high-fiber diet.
     d. Avoid alcohol, which has an irritant effect on the bowel.
     e. Do not exceed a fat intake of 30% of the total daily caloric intake.
  2. Avoid all fiber when symptoms of diverticulitis are present, because high-fiber foods are then irritating. As inflammation resolves, gradually add fiber back into the diet.
  3. Monitor for signs and symptoms of diverticulitis (e.g., fever, abdominal pain, and bloody stools).
  4. Avoid enemas and irritant or stimulant laxatives.

DUCTAL ECTASIA

- Ductal ectasia is a benign breast problem characterized by breast duct dilation and thickened wall, particularly in women approaching menopause.
- The ducts become blocked, distended, and filled with cellular debris, activating an inflammatory response.
- Manifestations are a hard and tender mass with irregular borders; greenish brown nipple discharge; enlarged axillary nodes; and redness and edema over the mass.
- Ductal ectasia does not increase breast cancer risk, but the mass may be difficult to distinguish from breast cancer. Nipple discharge is examined microscopically for any atypical or malignant cells.
- Warm compresses and antibiotics may be helpful in relieving symptoms and improving drainage. The affected area may be excised.

- Nursing interventions focus on reducing the anxiety and providing support through the diagnostic and treatment procedures.

DYSRHYTHMIAS, CARDIAC
OVERVIEW

- Cardiac dysrhythmias are abnormal rhythms of the heart's electrical system that are caused by disturbances of cardiac electrical impulse formation or conduction, or both.
- Many cardiac diseases cause dysrhythmia, including congenital heart disease, myocardial injury or infarction, cardiomyopathy, and left or right ventricular dysfunction.
- Contributing factors can also cause and worsen dysrhythmias. Electrolyte imbalance, hypoxemia, serum acidosis and alkalosis, and drug toxicity are the most common contributing factors.
- *Tachydysrhythmias* are heart rates greater than 100 beats/min.
  1. Signs and symptoms include palpitations; chest discomfort; pressure or pain from myocardial ischemia or infarction; restlessness; anxiety; pale, cool skin; and syncope from hypotension.
  2. They may cause heart failure as indicated by dyspnea, orthopnea, pulmonary crackles, distended neck veins, fatigue, and weakness.
- *Bradydysrhythmias* are characterized by a HR less than 60 beats/min.
  1. The patient may tolerate a low HR if BP is adequate.
  2. Symptomatic bradydysrhythmias lead to hypotension, myocardial ischemia or infarction, other dysrhythmias, and heart failure.
- *Premature complexes* are early complexes that occur when a cardiac cell or group of cells other than the sinoatrial (SA) node becomes irritable and fires an impulse before the next sinus impulse is generated.
  1. *Bigeminy* occurs when normal complexes and premature complexes occur alternately in a repetitive two-beat pattern, with a pause occurring after each premature complex so that complexes occur in pairs.
  2. *Trigeminy* is a repetitive three-beat pattern, usually occurring as two sequential normal complexes followed by a premature complex and a pause, with the same pattern repeating itself in triplets.
  3. *Quadrigeminy* is a repetitive four-beat pattern, usually occurring as three sequential normal complexes followed by a premature complex and a pause, with the same pattern repeating itself in a four-beat pattern.

- Dysrhythmias are further classified according to their site of origin.
- Sinus dysrhythmias include:
  1. *Sinus tachycardia,* which occurs when the SA node discharge exceeds 100 beats/min. Treatment is based on identifying the underlying cause (e.g., angina, fever, hypovolemia, pain); beta-adrenergic blocking agents may be prescribed.
  2. *Sinus bradycardia,* a decreased rate of SA node discharge of less than 60 beats/min. If the patient is symptomatic, treatment includes atropine, a pacemaker, and avoidance of parasympathetic stimulations such as prolonged suctioning.
- Atrial dysrhythmias
  1. *Premature atrial complex* (PAC) occurs when atrial tissue becomes irritable. This ectopic focus fires an impulse before the next sinus impulse is due.
     a. No intervention is generally needed except to treat the cause, such as heart failure or valvular disease.
  2. *Supraventricular tachycardia* (SVT) involves the rapid stimulation of atrial tissue at a rate of 100 to 280 beats/min.
     a. No intervention is generally needed except to treat the cause.
     b. Sustained SVT may need to be treated with radiofrequency catheter ablation.
     c. Oxygen therapy, antidysrhythmic drugs, or synchronized cardioversion may also be needed.
     d. *Atrial flutter* is a rapid arterial depolarization occurring at a rate of 250 to 350 times/min.
     e. Drug treatment includes ibutilide (Corvert), amiodarone (Cordarone), and diltiazem (Cardizem).
     f. Synchronized cardioversion is done if the patient is hemodynamically compromised.
     g. Rapid atrial overdrive pacing or radiofrequency catheter ablation may be needed if none of these treatments are successful.
  3. *Atrial fibrillation* (AF) consists of rapid atrial impulses at a rate of 350 to 600 times/min.
     a. Treatment is the same as for atrial flutter.
     b. Anticoagulants are given, because this rhythm places the patient at high risk for emboli formation in the atrial appendage. The clot can break off and travel through major arteries causing stroke, MI, pulmonary emboli, deep vein thrombosis, and other thrombotic disease.
- Junctional dysrhythmias may occur when the cells in the atrioventricular (AV) junctional node generate an impulse. Junctional

rhythms usually do not persist beyond the acute disease that caused slowing or absence of SA pacemaker function.

1. If treatment is needed, generally atropine is used to speed up the junctional rhythm (Advanced Cardiac Life Support [ACLS] bradycardia algorithm).
2. A pacemaker is used for definitive treatment.

- Ventricular dysrhythmias
   1. *Idioventricular rhythm* occurs when the ventricular cells become the pacemakers of the heart, usually in the absence of pacemakers above the bundle of His.
      a. This bradycardia rhythm is often symptomatic, with hypotension or decreased or absent peripheral pulses.
      b. With symptoms, initiate the ACLS bradycardia algorithm.
   2. *Premature ventricular complexes* (PVCs) result from increased irritability of the ventricular cells. PVCs are early ventricular complexes followed by a pause and often occur in repetitive rhythms.
      a. The patient may be asymptomatic or may experience palpitations, chest discomfort, or diminished or absent peripheral pulses.
      b. If there is no underlying heart disease, PVCs are not treated other than by eliminating any contributing cause.
      c. In the presence of myocardial ischemia or infarction, symptomatic PVCs are treated with oxygen and amiodarone (Cordarone); other drugs are prescribed if an MI occurs.
   3. *Ventricular tachycardia* (VT), or "V tach," occurs with repetitive firing of an irritable ventricular ectopic focus, usually at a rate of 140 to 180 beats/min.
      a. Symptoms depend on ventricular rate; the patient may be hemodynamically compromised and in cardiac arrest.
      b. Medications used to treat VT are oxygen, amiodarone, lidocaine, or magnesium sulfate.
      c. Unstable VT is treated with emergency defibrillation followed by oxygen and antidysrhythmic therapy.
      d. With pulseless VT, immediately begin cardiopulmonary resuscitation (CPR) and defibrillate as soon as possible. If the patient remains pulseless, continue CPR and other resuscitative measures.
      e. After the patient has been successfully defibrillated, attention is given to treating the reversible causes of VT.
   4. *Ventricular fibrillation* (VF), sometimes called "V-fib," is the result of electrical chaos in the ventricles.
      a. The patient immediately loses consciousness, becoming pulseless and apneic. Within minutes, death occurs unless there is prompt restoration of an organized rhythm.

      b. Immediate defibrillation is performed and the ACLS algorithm is followed.

  5. *Ventricular asystole* is the complete absence of any ventricular rhythm. The patient is in full cardiac arrest and is treated with CPR and by following the ACLS algorithm.

- *Atrioventricular* (AV) *conduction blocks* exist when supraventricular impulses are excessively delayed or totally blocked in the AV node or intraventricular conduction system.

  1. *First-degree AV block:* All sinus impulses eventually reach the ventricles; conduction is slowed.

      a. The patient usually has no symptoms, and no treatment is needed.

      b. If caused by drug therapy, the offending drug is withheld and the health care provider notified.

      c. If associated with symptomatic bradycardia, oxygen is administered.

  2. *Second-degree AV block type I (AV Wenckebach or Mobitz type I):* Each successive sinus impulse takes a little longer to conduct through the AV node, until one impulse is completely blocked and fails to depolarize the ventricles. The symptomatic patient is treated with oxygen and atropine; a pacemaker may be needed.

  3. *Second-degree AV block type II (Mobitz type II):* The block is infranodal, occurring below the bundle of His, and involves a constant block in one of the bundle branches; the impulse fails to reach the ventricle.

      a. Symptoms depend on the frequency of the dropped rate.

      b. If the patient is symptomatic, he or she is treated with prophylactic pacing to avert the threat of sudden third-degree heart block.

      c. A permanent pacemaker may be required.

  4. *Third-degree heart block (complete heart block):* None of the sinus impulses conducts to the ventricles.

      a. Clinical manifestations depend on the overall ventricular rate and cardiac output and may have hemodynamic consequences such as light-headedness, confusion, syncope, seizures, hypotension, or cardiac arrest.

      b. Oxygen and atropine are given to the patient who is symptomatic; prophylactic pacing may be initiated.

  5. *Bundle branch block:* A conduction delay or block occurs within one of the two main bundle branches below the bifurcation of the bundle of His.

      a. There are no clinical manifestations and no specific interventions.

      b. A new bundle branch block may be an indicator of a recent MI; be alert to symptoms of acute coronary syndrome.

D

PATIENT-CENTERED COLLABORATIVE CARE

Interventions

DECREASED CARDIAC OUTPUT AND INEFFECTIVE
TISSUE PERFUSION

- The major interventions are to assess for complications and monitor the patient for response to treatment.
  1. Monitor the patient's ECG and assess for signs and symptoms of dysrhythmias.
  2. Assess apical and radial pulses for a full minute for any irregularity.
  3. Management includes:
     a. Drug therapy
     b. Vagal maneuvers such as carotid sinus massage and Valsalva maneuvers
     c. Cardioversion
     d. Temporary or permanent pacing
     e. CPR or ACLS
     f. Defibrillation
     g. Radiofrequency catheter ablation
     h. Aneurysmectomy
     i. Coronary artery bypass grafting
     j. Insertion of an implantable cardiac defibrillator (ICD)

! NURSING SAFETY PRIORITY: Critical Rescue

Call the Rapid Response Team for an increase or onset in irregular pulses or rhythm when it is associated with a deterioration in consciousness or BP. It may be an early sign of electrolyte disturbance, drug toxicity, or new myocardial injury.

Community-Based Care

- Discharge planning and health care resources:
  1. Provide information on lifestyle modifications including activity restrictions.
  2. Teach the patient and family the name, dosage, schedule, and side effects of drugs.
  3. Teach and observe the patient and family taking a pulse.
  4. Stress the importance of reporting chest discomfort, shortness of breath, and change in heart rhythm and rate to the health care provider.
  5. Post emergency numbers.
  6. Encourage the patient to adhere to diet instructions.
  7. Instruct the patient to keep all appointments with the health care provider.
  8. Encourage family members to learn CPR.

- Refer to a care coordinator or case manager for home health care if needed.
- Give the following special instructions to a patient with a pacemaker or ICD device:
  1. Give instructions on how to care for the pacemaker or ICD and how it functions (if appropriate) and the importance of reporting any fever or any redness, swelling, or drainage at the pacemaker or ICD insertion site.
  2. Keep the ICD identification card in a wallet and consider wearing a medical alert bracelet.
  3. Do not wear tight clothing or belts that could cause irritation over the site.
  4. Avoid sources of strong electromagnet fields such as large electrical generators and radio or television transmitters and radar.
  5. If a patient feels symptoms when he or she is near any device, he or she should move 5 to 10 feet away from it and check his or her pulse.
  6. Notify all health care providers, including dentists, that a pacemaker or ICD device is in use.
  7. Notify airport security personnel before passing through a metal detector (screening device) that a pacemaker or ICD is in use, and show them the ICD identification card.
  8. Inform the MRI technician about pacemaker or prosthetic placement; an MRI is generally contraindicated.
- Give the following special instructions to a patient with a pacemaker:
  1. Take your pulse for 1 minute at the same time each day, and record the rate in your pacemaker diary.
  2. Take your pulse any time you feel symptoms of possible pacemaker failure, and report your HR and symptoms to your health care provider.
  3. Know the rate at which your pacemaker is set, and know the rate changes to report to your physician.
  4. Know the indications of battery failure, and report these findings to your health care provider.
  5. Report any of the following symptoms to your health care provider: difficulty breathing, dizziness, fainting, chest pain, weight gain, and prolonged hiccupping.
  6. Do not operate electrical appliances directly over your pacemaker site, because they may cause it to malfunction. Be sure electrical appliances are properly grounded.
  7. Do not lean over electrical or gasoline engines or motors.
- Give the following special instructions to a patient with an ICD:
  1. Sit or lie down immediately if you feel dizzy, faint, or light-headed.

D

2. Avoid activities that involve rough contact with the ICD implantation site.
3. Avoid sources of strong electromagnet fields such as large electrical generators and radio or television transmitters because they may inhibit tachydysrhythmia detection and therapy or alter pacing or shock settings. If beeping tones are heard coming from the device, move away from the electromagnetic field immediately before the inactivation sequence is completed, and notify the health care provider.
4. Report symptoms such as fainting, nausea, weakness, blackout, and rapid pulse to your health care provider.
5. Know how to perform cough CPR as instructed.
6. Notify your health care provider if your ICD device discharges.
7. Avoid strenuous activities that may cause your HR to meet or exceed the rate cutoff of your ICD device, because this causes the device to discharge inappropriately.

! NURSING SAFETY PRIORITY: Action Alert

Teach the patient to keep all appointments to assess the function of the ICD device. Many of these devices also maintain records that can be accessed remotely over a landline or at the cardiology visit. The device is "interrogated" to provide a record of the type, frequency, and duration of dysrhythmias and firings so that therapeutic adjustments to the device or medications can be made.

! NURSING SAFETY PRIORITY: Drug Alert

Many antidysrhythmic drugs have a narrow safety range, dangerous side effects, and interact with other medications. Avoid adding OTC or prescribed drugs to the patient's regimen without first ensuring that the prescriber is aware of the antidysrhythmic drug used.

E

ENCEPHALITIS

OVERVIEW

- Encephalitis, an inflammation of the brain tissue and often the meninges, is most frequently caused by infective organisms:
  1. Arboviruses transmitted through the bite of an infected tick or mosquito such as West Nile virus
  2. Enteroviruses associated with mumps, chickenpox, herpes zoster, and herpes simplex
  3. Amoebae such as *Naegleria* and *Acanthamoeba,* found in warm freshwater

- Encephalitis can be life-threatening or lead to persistent neurologic problems, such as learning disabilities, epilepsy, memory, or fine motor deficits.

PATIENT-CENTERED COLLABORATIVE CARE
Assessment
- Assessment findings include:
    1. Fever
    2. Nausea and vomiting
    3. Stiff neck, meningitis symptoms
    4. Decreased level of consciousness and impaired cognition
    5. Motor dysfunction
    6. Focal neurologic deficits
    7. Symptoms of increased intracranial pressure
    8. Cranial nerve weakness: ocular palsies, facial weaknesses
    9. Abnormal cerebrospinal fluid analysis
    10. Elevated WBC count

E

> **!** **NURSING SAFETY PRIORITY: Critical Rescue**
>
> Level of consciousness is the most sensitive indicator of neurologic status. Inform the physician of worsening cognition or decreased arousal, because this may mean worsening of acute neurologic disease.

Interventions
- The treatment for encephalitis is similar to that for meningitis.
    1. Maintain a patent airway; avoid aspiration.
    2. Monitor vital signs and neurologic signs, such as level of consciousness, orientation, pupil responses, and motor movement.
    3. Administer acyclovir (Zovirax) for herpes encephalitis; no specific drug therapy is available for infection by arboviruses or enteroviruses.
    4. If there are neurologic disabilities, the patient may be discharged to a rehabilitation setting or a long-term care facility.

ENDOCARDITIS, INFECTIVE
OVERVIEW
- Infective endocarditis refers to a microbial infection (virus, bacterium, or fungus) involving the endocardium.
- Infective endocarditis occurs primarily in patients who are IV drug abusers, have had cardiac valve replacements, have experienced systemic infection, or have structural cardiac defects.
- Sources for infecting organisms include:
    1. Oral cavity, especially if dental procedures have been performed
    2. Skin rashes, lesions, or abscesses

3. Infections (cutaneous, genitourinary, gastrointestinal, or systemic)
4. Surgical or invasive procedures, including IV line placement

PATIENT-CENTERED COLLABORATIVE CARE
Assessment
* Assessment findings include:
    1. Signs of infection, including fever, chills, malaise, and night sweats; older adults may remain afebrile
    2. Positive blood cultures or symptoms of sepsis
    3. Heart murmurs, usually regurgitant in nature
    4. Right- or left-sided heart failure, evidenced by:
        a. Peripheral or pulmonary edema
        b. Weight gain
        c. Fatigue
        d. Dyspnea
    5. Evidence of arterial embolization from fragments of vegetation on valve leaflets, which may travel to other organs and compromise function. Manifestations of acute embolization include:
        a. Splenic emboli, evidenced by sudden abdominal pain and radiation to the left shoulder
        b. Kidney infarction, evidenced by flank pain that radiates to the groin and is accompanied by hematuria or pyuria
        c. Mesenteric emboli, evidenced by diffuse abdominal pain often after eating and abdominal distention
        d. Brain emboli, in which the patient shows signs of stroke, confusion, reduced concentration, and difficulty speaking
        e. Pulmonary emboli, evidenced by pleuritic chest pain, dyspnea, and cough
    6. Petechiae of the neck, shoulders, wrists, ankles, mucous membranes, or conjunctivae
    7. Splinter hemorrhages, or black longitudinal lines or small red streaks in the nail bed
    8. Osler's nodes (reddish, tender lesions with a white center on the pads of the fingers, hands, and toes)
    9. Janeway's lesion (nontender hemorrhagic lesion found on the fingers, toes, nose, and earlobes)
    10. Abnormal transesophageal echocardiogram
Interventions
* Interventions include:
    1. Administering IV antimicrobial therapy
    2. Monitoring the patient's tolerance for activity; anticipating pacing activities more slowly or clustering activities to increase duration of rest if patient tires

3. Informing the Rapid Response Team if there are symptoms of embolization; collaborating and communicating to prevent complications from embolization, particularly decreased oxygenation, brain injury, and acute coronary syndromes
- Surgical intervention includes removal of the infected valve, repair or removal of congenital shunts, repair of injured valves and chordae tendineae, and draining abscesses in the heart or elsewhere.
- Perioperative care for the patient having surgery for the management of complications from infective carditis is similar to that described for patients undergoing a coronary artery bypass grafting or valve replacement.

Community-Based Care
- Educate the patient and family about:
  1. Information on the cause of the disease and its course, signs and symptoms of infection, and practices to prevent future infections, including oral hygiene and dental care
  2. Self-management of drugs, including the potential for several weeks of intravenous antibiotic therapy

ENDOMETRIOSIS
OVERVIEW
- Endometriosis occurs when the endometrial (inner uterine) tissue implants outside the uterine cavity, most commonly on the ovaries and the cul-de-sac (posterior rectovaginal wall) and less commonly on other pelvic organs and structures.
- This tissue responds to cyclic hormonal stimulation just as if it were in the uterus.
- Monthly cyclic bleeding occurs at the site of implantation, where it is trapped, causing pain, irritation, scarring, and adhesion formation in the surrounding tissue.
- When endometriosis is on an ovary, a brown swelling known as a "chocolate cyst" can form.
- The cause of endometriosis is unknown.
- The disorder is most often found in women during their reproductive years and can lead to infertility.

PATIENT-CENTERED COLLABORATIVE CARE
Assessment
- Obtain patient information about:
  1. Menstrual history, sexual history, and bleeding characteristics
  2. Pain, which is the most common symptom of endometriosis, peaking just before menstrual flow
  3. Dyspareunia (painful sexual intercourse)
  4. Painful defecation
  5. Low backache

    6. Infertility

    7. GI disturbances

- Assess for and document:
  1. Pelvic tenderness
  2. Anxiety, because of uncertainty about the diagnosis and potential infertility
- Diagnostic studies may include tests to rule out other diagnoses such as:
  1. PID caused by chlamydia or gonorrhea
  2. Ovarian cancer detected by serum cancer antigen CA-125
  3. Vaginal nodules or pelvic masses detected by palpation or transvaginal ultrasound
  4. Laparoscopy and biopsy to determine endometrial tissue typing

Interventions

Nonsurgical Management

- Hormonal contraceptives for cycle control
- Heat packs, relaxation techniques, yoga, and biofeedback to improve blood flow to painful areas
- Calcium and magnesium, which may relieve muscle cramping for some patients

Surgical Management

- Surgical management of endometriosis with laser therapy through laparoscopy removes the implants and adhesions, allowing the woman to remain fertile.
- In women with intractable pain, severing a pelvic nerve may provide relief.
- If the patient does not wish to have children, the uterus and ovaries may be removed.
- Nursing care is similar to that for a woman undergoing a vaginal hysterectomy (see *Surgical Management* under *Uterine Fibroids [Leiomyomas]*).

EPIDIDYMITIS

OVERVIEW

- Epididymitis is an inflammation of the epididymis, which may result from an infectious (most common) or noninfectious source such as trauma.
- Main manifestations include pain along the inguinal canal and along the vas deferens, followed by pain and swelling in the scrotum and the groin.
- It can be a complication of an STD, such as gonorrhea or chlamydia.
- If untreated, the infection can spread and an abscess may form, requiring an orchiectomy (removal of one or both testes). If both testes are affected, sterility may result.

• Less often, it can be a complication of long-term use of an indwelling urinary catheter, prostatic surgery, or a cystoscopy examination.

PATIENT-CENTERED COLLABORATIVE CARE
Assessment
• Obtain patient information about:
  1. Pain along the inguinal canal
  2. Pain and swelling of the scrotum and groin
• Assess for and document:
  1. Pyuria, bacteria
  2. Regional lymph node swelling
  3. Signs of infection such as fever, chills, and elevated WBC count
• Diagnosis is made on the basis of manifestations and a smear or culture of the urine or prostate secretions to identify the causative organism.

Interventions
• Interventions include:
  1. Drug therapy
     a. Antibiotics
     b. NSAIDs to decrease inflammation and promote comfort
  2. Comfort measures, including:
     a. Elevating or supporting the swollen scrotum (use a jock strap)
     b. Applying cold compresses or ice to the scrotum intermittently
     c. Taking sitz baths
     d. Avoiding lifting, straining, or sexual activity until the infection is under control (which may take as long as 4 weeks)
• The sexual partner should be treated if the infection is caused by an STD.
• An epididymectomy (excision of the epididymis from the testicle) may be needed if the problem is recurrent or chronic.
• An ultrasound study can rule out an abscess or tumor.

ERECTILE DYSFUNCTION
OVERVIEW
• *Erectile dysfunction* (ED) is the inability to achieve or maintain an erection for sexual intercourse. There are two major types of ED, organic and functional.
• *Organic ED* is a gradual deterioration of function. The man first notices diminishing firmness and a decrease in frequency of erections. Causes include:
  1. Inflammation of the prostate, urethra, or seminal vesicles
  2. Surgical procedures such as prostatectomy

3. Pelvic fractures
4. Lumbosacral injuries
5. Vascular disease, including hypertension
6. Chronic neurologic conditions, such as Parkinson's disease or multiple sclerosis
7. Endocrine disorders, such as diabetes mellitus or thyroid disorders
8. Smoking and alcohol consumption
9. Drugs
10. Poor overall health that prevents sexual intercourse

- *Functional ED* usually has a psychological cause. Men with functional ED have normal nocturnal (nighttime) and morning erections. Onset is usually sudden and preceded by a period of high stress.

PATIENT-CENTERED COLLABORATIVE CARE

- Assess the medical, social, and sexual history to help determine the cause of ED.
- Hormone testing is used for patients who have a poor libido, small testicles, or sparse beard growth.
- Doppler ultrasonography may be performed to determine the adequacy of arterial and venous blood flow to the penis.
  Nonsurgical Management
- Functional ED is managed by sexual counseling and drugs that increase penile blood flow.
- Nonsurgical management of organic ED may include:
  1. Drug therapy to improve penile blood flow, phosphodiesterase-5 (PDE-5) inhibitors such as:
     a. Sildenafil (Viagra)
     b. Vardenafil (Levitra)
     c. Tadalafil (Cialis)

! NURSING SAFETY PRIORITY: Drug Alert

Instruct patients taking PDE-5 inhibitors to abstain from alcohol before sexual intercourse, because it may impair the ability to have an erection. Common side effects of these drugs include dyspepsia (heartburn), headaches, facial flushing, and stuffy nose. If more than one pill a day is being taken, leg and back cramps, nausea, and vomiting also may occur. Teach men who take nitrates to avoid these drugs, because the vasodilation effects can cause a profound hypotension and reduce blood flow to vital organs. For patients who cannot take these drugs or do not respond to them, other methods are available to achieve an erection.

2. Vacuum devices:
   a. A vacuum device is a cylinder that fits over the penis, and a vacuum is created with a pump. The vacuum draws blood into the penis to maintain an erection.
   b. The device is easy and safe to use regardless of what drugs the patient may be taking.
3. Intracorporal injections:
   a. Vasoconstrictive drugs can be injected directly into the penis to reduce blood outflow and make the penis erect.
   b. Common agents are papaverine, phentolamine (Regitine), and alprostadil.
   c. Adverse effects include priapism (prolonged erection), penile scarring, fibrosis, bleeding, bruising at the injection site, pain, infection, and vasovagal responses.

Surgical Management

- Penile implants can be surgically placed when other modalities fail. Devices include semi-rigid, malleable, or hydraulic inflatable and multicomponent or one-piece instruments.
- Advantages include the man's ability to control his erections.
- The major disadvantages include device failure and infection.

F

FATIGUE SYNDROME, CHRONIC

- Chronic fatigue syndrome (CFS), also known as *chronic fatigue and immune dysfunction syndrome* (CFIDS), is characterized by severe fatigue for 6 months or longer, usually following flu-like symptoms.
- For a diagnosis of CFS, four or more of the following criteria must be met:
  1. Sore throat
  2. Substantial impairment in short-term memory or concentration
  3. Tender lymph nodes
  4. Muscle pain
  5. Multiple joint pain with redness or swelling
  6. Headaches of a new type, pattern, or severity (not familiar to the patient)
  7. Unrefreshing sleep
  8. Postexertional malaise lasting more than 24 hours
- There is no test to confirm the disorder, and the cause is unknown.

- Management is supportive and focuses on alleviation or reduction of symptoms.
  1. Nonsteroidal anti-inflammatories (NSAIDs) for body aches and pain
  2. Low-dose antidepressants for alleviating symptoms and promoting sleep
  3. Teaching the patient to follow healthy practices
     a. Adequate sleep
     b. Proper nutrition
     c. Regular exercise (but not excessive enough to increase fatigue)
     d. Stress management
     e. Energy conservation
  4. Use of complementary and alternative therapies that include acupuncture, tai chi, massage, and herbal supplements
- Refer the patient to support groups and reputable Internet sites for information and web-based support.

FIBROMYALGIA SYNDROME
OVERVIEW
- Fibromyalgia syndrome (FMS) is a chronic, noninflammatory syndrome manifested by pain and tenderness at specific sites in the back of the neck, upper chest, trunk, low back, and extremities.
- Severe fatigue and sleep disturbances are also common symptoms.
- The tender points (trigger points) can be palpated to elicit pain in a predictable, reproducible pattern. Other sensations of numbness and tingling also occur.
- Secondary FMS can accompany any connective tissue disease, particularly lupus and rheumatoid disease.
- Other symptoms include:
  1. Gastrointestinal (GI) disturbances, including abdominal pain, diarrhea and constipation, and heartburn
  2. Genitourinary manifestations, including dysuria, urinary frequency, urgency, and pelvic pain
  3. Cardiovascular symptoms, including dyspnea, chest pain, and dysrhythmias
  4. Visual disturbances, including blurred vision and dry eyes
  5. Neurologic symptoms, including forgetfulness and concentration problems
- Interventions include:
  1. Antidepressant drugs approved for fibromyalgia nerve pain (e.g., pregabalin [Lyrica] and duloxetine [Cymbalta])
  2. Tricyclic antidepressive agents to promote sleep and reduce pain or muscle spasms (amitriptyline [Elavil, Apo-Amitriptyline ✦], trazodone [Desyrel], or nortriptyline [Pamelor])

3. NSAIDs
4. Physical therapy and regular exercise, which includes stretching, strengthening, and low-impact aerobic exercise
5. Complementary and alternative therapies, such as tai chi, acupuncture, hypnosis, and stress management, may help some patients with symptom relief

FLAIL CHEST
OVERVIEW
- Flail chest is the inward movement of the thorax during inspiration, with outward movement during expiration, usually involving only one side of the chest.
- It results from multiple rib fractures or ribs fractured in more than one place caused by blunt chest trauma, leaving a segment of the chest wall loose.
- Flail chest often occurs in high-speed vehicular crashes. Another cause is bilateral separations of the ribs from their cartilage connections without an actual rib fracture during cardiopulmonary resuscitation (CPR).
- Gas exchange, the ability to cough, and the ability to clear secretions are impaired.

PATIENT-CENTERED COLLABORATIVE CARE
Assessment
- Assess the patient for and document:
  1. Paradoxical chest movement ("sucking inward" of the loose chest area during inspiration and a "puffing out" of the same area during expiration)
  2. Pain
  3. Dyspnea
  4. Cyanosis
  5. Tachycardia
  6. Hypotension
Interventions
- Interventions include:
  1. Humidified oxygen
  2. Pain management
  3. Promotion of lung expansion through deep breathing and positioning
  4. Secretion clearance by coughing and tracheal aspiration
  5. Psychosocial support
  6. Intubation with mechanical ventilation and positive end-expiratory pressure (PEEP)
  7. Surgical stabilization (only in extreme cases of flail chest)

- Monitor the patient's:
  1. Vital signs, oxygen saturation, and arterial blood gases
  2. Fluid and electrolyte balance
  3. Central venous pressure

FLUID OVERLOAD

OVERVIEW

- Fluid overload, also called *overhydration,* is an excess of body fluid, not a disease. It is a clinical sign of a problem in which fluid intake or retention is greater than the body's fluid needs.
- The most common type of fluid overload is hypervolemia, because the problems result from excessive fluid in the extracellular fluid (ECF) space.
- Most problems caused by fluid overload are related to fluid volume excess in the vascular space or to dilution of specific electrolytes and blood components.
- Causes of fluid overload are related to excessive intake or inadequate excretion of fluid and include:
  1. Excessive fluid replacement
  2. Kidney failure (late phase)
  3. Heart failure
  4. Long-term corticosteroid therapy
  5. Syndrome of inappropriate antidiuretic hormone (SIADH)
  6. Psychiatric disorders with polydipsia
  7. Water intoxication

PATIENT-CENTERED COLLABORATIVE CARE
Assessment
- Assess for and document:
  1. Cardiovascular changes
     a. Bounding pulse quality
     b. Peripheral pulses full
     c. Elevated blood pressure
     d. Decreased pulse pressure
     e. Elevated central venous pressure
     f. Distended neck and hand veins
     g. Engorged varicose veins
     h. Weight gain
  2. Respiratory changes
     a. Respiratory rate increased
     b. Shallow respirations
     c. Dyspnea increases with exertion or in the supine position
     d. Moist crackles present on auscultation
     e. Decreased peripheral oxygenation (SpO_2)

3. Skin and mucous membrane changes
   a. Pitting edema occurs in dependent areas and joints and skin around bony prominences (ankles, elbows, metacarpals, metatarsals)
   b. Skin is pale and cool to touch. Skin and puncture sites from needle sticks may "weep" as fluid tries to escape through the skin.
4. Neuromuscular changes
   a. Altered level of consciousness
   b. Headache
   c. Visual disturbances
   d. Skeletal muscle weakness
   e. Paresthesias
5. GI changes
   a. Increased motility
   b. Enlarged liver
- Diagnosis of fluid overload is based on assessment findings and the results of laboratory tests. Usually, serum electrolyte values are normal, but decreased hemoglobin, hematocrit, and serum protein levels may result from excessive water in the vascular space (hemodilution).

Interventions
- Management of patients with fluid overload aims to ensure patient safety, restore normal fluid balance, provide supportive care until the imbalance is resolved, and prevent future fluid overload.
  1. Monitor patients to prevent fluid overload or prevent worsening of fluid overload.
     a. Assess particularly for symptoms of pulmonary edema and heart failure.
     b. Evaluate for the presence of bounding pulses, engorged neck veins, unbalanced intake and output, and daily weight.
     c. Collaborate with health care team members to set a daily output goal and inform the physician when goals are at risk for not being met.

❗ NURSING SAFETY PRIORITY: Critical Rescue

Pulmonary edema can occur very quickly and can lead to death. Notify the health care provider of any change that indicates the fluid overload is not responding to therapy or is becoming worse.

d. Reduce the risk for pressure ulcers in patients with edema by using a pressure-reducing or pressure-relieving overlay on the mattress and over bony prominences (e.g., heel

delivery devices in place).
 e. Assess skin pressure areas, especially the coccyx, elbows, hips, and heels, daily for signs of redness or open areas and document findings.
 f. Assist the patient to change positions at least every 2 hours.
2. Drug therapy focuses on removing the excess fluid, including loop diuretics like furosemide (Lasix) or an inhibitor of antidiuretic hormone like conivaptan (Vaprisol).
 a. Monitor the patient's response to drug therapy.
  (1) A weight gain or loss of 1 kg in less than 24 hours is a gain or loss of 1 L of fluid.
  (2) Compute intake/output balance every 8 hours and set goals such as "negative 500 mL," indicating a desired urine output 500 mL greater than intake. Notify the health care provider when reduced urine output occurs.
 b. Observe for manifestations of electrolyte imbalance.
  (1) Changes in electrocardiographic patterns
  (2) Changes in sodium and potassium values
3. Nutritional therapy
 a. Sodium restriction
 b. Fluid restriction

FOOD POISONING

- Food poisoning is caused by ingestion of infectious organisms in food. Unlike gastroenteritis, food poisoning is not directly communicable from person to person and incubation periods are shorter.
- Prevention occurs with good handwashing and properly handling and processing food. Food poisoning is caused by over 250 pathogens.
- Examples of food poisoning are:
  1. Staphylococcal food poisoning
     a. *Staphylococcus* grows in meats and dairy products and can be transmitted by human carriers.
     b. Symptoms of staphylococcal infection include abrupt onset of vomiting, diarrhea, and abdominal cramping, usually 2 to 4 hours after the ingestion of contaminated food.
     c. The diagnosis is made when stool culture yields 100,000 enterotoxin-producing staphylococci.
     d. Treatment includes oral or IV fluids if the fluid volume is grossly depleted.
  2. *Escherichia coli* infection
     a. Some strains cause disease by making a substance called *Shiga toxin*. The bacteria that make these substances are

called *Shiga toxin-producing E. coli,* or STEC for short. Enterohemorrhagic strains of *E. coli* (EHEC) and STEC can cause serious complications, such as hemorrhagic colitis and hemolytic-uremic syndrome.

b. Symptoms include vomiting, diarrhea, abdominal cramping, and fever.

c. Treatment includes IV fluids.

3. Botulism

a. Botulism is a severe, life-threatening food poisoning associated with a high mortality rate; it is most commonly acquired from improperly processed canned foods.

b. The incubation period is 18 to 36 hours, and the illness may be mild or severe.

c. *Clostridium botulinum* enters the bloodstream from the intestines and causes symptoms of diplopia, dysphagia, dysphonia, respiratory muscle paralysis, nausea, vomiting, and diarrhea or constipation.

d. The diagnosis is made by the history and stool culture revealing *C. botulinum;* the serum may be positive for toxins.

e. Treatment of botulism includes trivalent botulism antitoxin (types A, B, and E), stomach lavage, IV fluids, and tracheostomy with mechanical ventilation if respiratory paralysis occurs.

❗ NURSING SAFETY PRIORITY: Action Alert

To prevent botulism, teach patients the importance of discarding cans of food that are punctured or swollen or with defective seals. Remind them to check for expiration dates and to not use any canned food that has expired. Containers for home-canned foods must be sterilized by boiling for 20 minutes to destroy *C. botulinum* spores before canning.

4. *Salmonellosis*

a. *Salmonellosis* is a bacterial infection; its incubation is 8 to 48 hours after ingestion of contaminated food or drink.

b. Symptoms last 3 to 5 days and include fever, nausea, vomiting, cramping abdominal pain, and severe diarrhea, which may be bloody.

c. Diagnosis is made by stool culture.

d. Treatment is based on symptoms; antibiotics are used if the patient becomes bacteremic.

e. *Salmonellosis* can be transmitted by the *five Fs: F*lies, *F*ingers, *F*ood, *F*eces, and *F*omites; strict handwashing is essential to avoid transmission.

FRACTURES

OVERVIEW

- A fracture is a break or disruption in the continuity of a bone.
- Fractures are classified as complete or incomplete
  1. *Complete fracture:* The break is across the entire width of the bone in such a way that the bone is divided into two distinct sections.
  2. *Incomplete fracture:* The fracture does not divide the bone into two portions, because the break is through only part of the bone.
- Fractures can also be described by the extent of associated soft-tissue damage
  1. A *simple fracture* does not extend through the skin and therefore has no visible wound.
  2. An *open (compound) fracture* has a disrupted skin surface that causes an external wound.
- Fractures are also defined by their cause
  1. *Pathologic (spontaneous) fractures* occur after minimal trauma to a bone that has been weakened by disease.
  2. *Fatigue (stress) fractures* result from excessive strain and stress on the bone.
  3. *Compression fractures* are produced by a loading force applied to the long axis of cancellous bone.
- Bone healing occurs in five stages
  1. Stage 1 occurs within 24 to 72 hours after the injury, with hematoma formation at the site of the fracture.
  2. Stage 2 occurs in 3 days to 2 weeks, when granulation tissue begins to invade the hematoma, stimulating the formation of fibrocartilage.
  3. Stage 3 of bone healing usually occurs within 2 to 6 weeks as a result of vascular and cellular proliferation. The fracture site is surrounded by new vascular tissue known as a *callus* that begins the nonbony union.
  4. Stage 4 usually takes 3 to 8 weeks as the callus is gradually resorbed and transformed into bone.
  5. Stage 5 consists of bone consolidation and remodeling. This stage can continue for up to 1 year.
- Bone healing requires adequate nutrition, especially calcium, phosphorus, vitamin D, and protein.
- Acute complications of fractures:
  1. *Acute compartment syndrome* (ACS) is a serious condition in which increased pressure within one or more tissue compartments causes massive compromise of circulation to the area. The most common sites for the problem in patients

Considerations for Older Adults

- For women, the loss of estrogen after menopause is detrimental to the body's ability to form new bone tissue.
- Chronic diseases affect the rate of healing. For example, arteriosclerosis reduces arterial circulation to bone and when bone receives less oxygen and reduced nutrients, repair is delayed.

experiencing musculoskeletal trauma are the compartments in the lower leg and forearm. Edema fluid forms and is trapped within the compartment pressing on nerves (causing pain) and blood vessels, preventing adequate tissue perfusion and oxygenation. Without treatment, ACS can lead to infection, loss of motor function, contracture formation, and release of myoglobin, leading to renal failure. Treatment is by surgical fasciotomy.

! NURSING SAFETY PRIORITY: Critical Rescue

Acute kidney injury from muscle breakdown (rhabdomyolysis) is a potentially fatal complication of compartment syndrome. It occurs when large or multiple compartments are involved. Injured muscle tissues release myoglobin (muscle protein) into the circulation, where it can clog the renal tubules. Report oliguria and discolored urine; both are signs of rhabdomyolysis and acute kidney injury.

2. *Crush syndrome* (CS) results from an external crush injury that compresses one or more compartments in the leg, arm, or pelvis. It is a potentially life-threatening, systemic complication that results from hemorrhage and edema after a severe fracture injury. Management involves early recognition and IV fluids.

3. *Hypovolemic shock* may occur with a fracture as a result of damage to bone blood vessels or the severing of nearby arteries.

4. *Fat embolism syndrome* (FES) is a serious complication in which fat globules are released from the yellow bone marrow into the bloodstream within 12 to 48 hours after an injury. These emboli clog small blood vessels that supply vital organs, most commonly the lungs, and impair organ perfusion. FES usually results from long bone fractures and pelvic bone or fracture repair, but it is occasionally seen in patients who have a total joint replacement. Manifestations include decreased

level of consciousness, anxiety, respiratory distress, tachycardia, tachypnea, fever, hemoptysis, and petechiae, a macular, measles-like rash that may appear over the neck, upper arms, or chest and abdomen.

5. *Venous thromboembolism* (VTE) includes deep vein thrombosis (DVT) and its major complication, pulmonary embolism (PE). It is the most common complication of lower extremity surgery or trauma and the most common fatal complication of musculoskeletal surgery.

6. Infection is possible with fractures, because the trauma disrupts the body's defense system. Wound infections may range from superficial skin infections to deep wound abscesses. Bone infection, or osteomyelitis, is most common with open fractures in which skin integrity is lost and after surgical repair of a fracture.

- Chronic complications of fractures
  1. *Ischemic necrosis,* sometimes referred to as *aseptic* or *avascular necrosis* (AVN) or *osteonecrosis,* can occur when the blood supply to the bone is disrupted and bone death follows.
  2. *Delayed union* is a fracture that has not healed within 6 months of injury. Some fractures never achieve union; that is, they never completely heal (nonunion). Others heal incorrectly (malunion).

PATIENT-CENTERED COLLABORATIVE CARE
Assessment
- Obtain patient information about:
  1. Cause of the fracture
  2. Events leading to the fracture and immediate postinjury care
  3. Drug history, including substance abuse (recreational drug use) and alcohol abuse
  4. Medical history
  5. Occupation and recreational activities
  6. Nutritional history
- Assess for and document:
  1. Life-threatening complications of the respiratory, cardiovascular, and neurologic systems (priority assessment)
  2. Fracture site:
     a. Change in bone alignment
     b. Neurovascular status (pulse, warmth, movement, and sensation) distal to fracture
  3. Degree of soft-tissue damage
  4. Amount of overt bleeding
  5. Muscle spasm

! NURSING SAFETY PRIORITY: Action Alert

Swelling at the fracture site is rapid and can result in marked neurovascular compromise due to decreased arterial perfusion. Gently perform a thorough neurovascular assessment and compare extremities. Checking for capillary refill is not as reliable as other indicators of perfusion.

- Special assessment considerations include:
  1. Fractures of the shoulder and upper arm are assessed with the patient in a sitting or standing position, if possible, so that shoulder drooping or other abnormal positioning can be seen.
  2. More distal areas of the arm are assessed with the patient in a supine position so that the extremity can be elevated to reduce swelling.
  3. Place the patient in a supine position for assessment of the lower extremities and pelvis.
  4. Pelvic fractures can cause internal organ damage resulting in hemorrhage. When a pelvic fracture is suspected, assess vital signs, skin color, and the level of consciousness for indications of shock. Check the urine for blood, which indicates damage to the urinary system, often the bladder.
- Psychosocial assessment depends on the extent of the injury and other complications.
- Stresses that result from a chronic condition affect relationships between the patient and family members or friends, body image, sexuality, and financial resources.
- Diagnostic tests for fractures may include:
  1. X-rays
  2. Computed tomography (CT) scanning
  3. Magnetic resonance imaging (MRI)

Planning and Implementation
- Manage pain related to fracture, soft-tissue damage, muscle spasm, and edema.
- Evaluate physiologic stability; provide cardiac monitoring for patients who are older than 50 years because of increased risk for acute coronary events.

! NURSING SAFETY PRIORITY: Action Alert

Patients with one or more fractured ribs have severe pain when they take deep breaths. Monitor respiratory status, which may be severely compromised from pain or pneumothorax (air in the pleural cavity). Assess the patient's pain level and manage pain before continuing the physical assessment.

- Immobilize the fracture with a splint; maintain the splint to prevent further tissue damage, reduce pain, and increase circulation.
- Place sterile gauze loosely over open areas to prevent further contamination of the wound.
- Plan for fracture reduction/realignment; premedicate with opioid drug.

! NURSING SAFETY PRIORITY: Critical Rescue

For any patient who experiences trauma in the community, first call 911 and assess for airway, breathing, and circulation (ABCs, or primary survey). Then provide lifesaving care if needed before being concerned about the fracture. In the community setting, provide emergency interventions until medical treatment in a hospital is available, or call 911 for the emergency team (first responders).

Nonsurgical Management

- Fracture management begins with reduction (realignment of the bone ends for proper healing) and immobilization of the fracture.
  1. *Closed reduction* is the manipulation of the bone ends for realignment while applying a manual pull, or traction, on the bone.
  2. *Splints and orthopedic boots/shoes* may be used to immobilize certain areas of the body, such as the scapula and clavicle.
  3. *Casts* are rigid devices that immobilize the affected body part while allowing other body parts to move. They are used to hold bone fragments in place after reduction for more complex fractures or fractures of the lower extremity. A cast allows early mobility, correction of deformity, prevention of deformity, and reduction of pain.
     a. The most common cast material is fiberglass. When plaster is used, it is applied over a well-fitted stockinette.
     b. Special considerations for casts include:
        (1) Arm cast
           i. When a patient is in bed, elevate the arm above the heart to reduce swelling; the hand should be higher than the elbow.
           ii. When the patient is out of bed, support the arm with a sling placed around the neck so that the weight is distributed over a large area of the shoulders and trunk, not just the neck.
        (2) A leg cast may require the patient to use an ambulatory aid
           i. A cast shoe, sandal, or boot that attaches to the foot or sole of the cast assists in ambulation (if weight bearing is allowed) and helps prevent damage to the cast.

       ii. Elevate the affected leg on pillows when the patient is in bed or in a chair to reduce swelling.
4. Cast brace:
   a. This device enables the patient to bend unaffected joints while the fracture is healing. The fracture must show signs of healing and minimal tissue edema before application of this cast.
   b. As healing occurs, the cast may be removed and replaced with a soft brace.
5. Body and spica cast:
   a. A body cast encircles the trunk of the body, whereas a spica cast encases a portion of the trunk and one or two extremities.
   b. The patient is at risk for skin breakdown, pneumonia or atelectasis, constipation, and joint contractures.
   c. *Cast syndrome* (superior mesenteric artery syndrome) is a serious complication in which partial or complete upper intestinal obstruction can occur and cause abdominal distention, epigastric pain, nausea, and vomiting. Placing a window in the abdominal portion of the cast or bivalving the cast may be sufficient to relieve pressure on the duodenum.

- Cast care involves:
  1. Cutting a window (done by the health care provider, orthopedic technician, or specially trained nurse) into the cast over an open wound for observation and care of the wound
  2. Ensuring that the cast is not too tight by inserting a finger between the cast and the skin
  3. Notifying the health care provider when the cast is too tight so that it can be cut with a cast cutter to relieve pressure or allow tissue swelling; the cast may be bivalved (cut lengthwise into two equal pieces) if bone healing is almost complete. Either half of the cast can be removed for inspection or for provision of care. The two halves are then held in place by an elastic bandage wrap.
  4. Protecting the cast in the perineal area from becoming contaminated with urine or feces by encasing the area in plastic before the patient uses the urinal or bedpan
  5. Inspecting the cast daily (after it is dry) for drainage, alignment, and fit:
     a. Describing and documenting any drainage on the cast in the medical record
     b. Notifying the health care provider immediately about any sudden increases in the amount of drainage or change in the integrity of the cast
  6. Smelling the cast for foul odor and palpating it for hot areas every shift

7. Assessing for and reporting complications from injury, casting, or immobility:
   a. Infection
   b. Circulation impairment
   c. Peripheral nerve damage
   d. Skin breakdown
   e. Pneumonia or atelectasis
   f. Thromboembolism
- *Traction* is the application of a pulling force to a part of the body to provide reduction, alignment, and rest. It is also used to decrease muscle spasm and prevent or correct deformity and tissue damage.
   1. Categories of traction:
      a. *Running traction* provides a pulling force in one direction, and the patient's body acts as countertraction. Moving the body or bed position can alter the countertraction force.
      b. *Balanced suspension* provides the countertraction so that the pulling force of the traction is not altered when the bed or patient is moved. This allows for increased movement and facilitates care.
   2. Types of traction
      a. *Skin traction* involves the use of a Velcro boot (Buck's traction), belt, or halter securely placed around a body part to decrease painful muscle spasms. Weight is limited to 5 to 10 pounds (2.3 to 4.5 kg) to prevent injury to the skin.
      b. *Skeletal traction* uses pins, wires, tongs, or screws that are surgically inserted directly into bone to allow the use of longer traction time and heavier weights, usually 15 to 30 pounds (6.8 to 13.6 kg). It aids in bone realignment.
   3. Care for the patient in traction includes:
      a. Inspecting the skin at least every 8 hours for signs of irritation or inflammation
      b. Removing (when possible) the belt or boot that is used for skin traction every 8 hours to inspect under the device
      c. Inspecting the points of entry of pins and wires or pin sites for signs of inflammation or infection at least every 8 hours
      d. Following agency policy for pin site care
      e. Checking traction equipment to ensure its proper functioning and inspecting all ropes, knots, and pulleys at least every 8 to 12 hours for loosening, fraying, and positioning
      f. Checking the weight for consistency with the health care provider's prescription
      g. Reporting patient complaints of severe pain from muscle spasm to the health care provider when body realignment fails to reduce the discomfort

> ### ❗ NURSING SAFETY PRIORITY: Action Alert
>
> When patients are in traction, weights usually are not removed without a prescription. They should not be lifted manually or allowed to rest on the floor. Weights should be freely hanging at all times. Teach this important point to unlicensed assistive personnel (UAP) on the unit, to other personnel such as those in the radiology department, and to visitors.

     h. Assessing neurovascular status of the affected body part at least every 4 hours and more often if indicated

Surgical Management

- *Open reduction with internal fixation* (ORIF) permits early mobilization. Open reduction allows direct visualization of the fracture site, and internal fixation uses metal pins, screws, rods, plates, or prostheses to immobilize the fracture during healing. An incision is made to gain access to the broken bone and allow implanting one or more devices into bone tissue.
- *External fixation* involves fracture reduction and the percutaneous implantation of pins into the bone. The pins are then held in place by an external metal frame to prevent bone movement but allow patient mobility. A disadvantage of external fixation is the increased risk for pin site infection and osteomyelitis.
- Provide preoperative care as described in Part One and explain if a device or cast will be used after surgery to maintain alignment.
- Provide postoperative care as described in Part One and:
  1. Routine postoperative care, as described in Part One
  2. Monitor neurovascular status at least every hour for the first 24 hours after surgery and then as often as agency policy, surgeon preference, and patient condition indicate
  3. Communicate neurovascular compromise or other complications urgently to the provider
  4. Promote self-management and mobility
- Additional procedures may be needed when surgical repairs are not successful and the bone does not heal (nonunion).
  1. *Electrical bone stimulation* may be noninvasive or invasive. It involves using electrical current stimulators near or into a fracture site. This procedure, when used for about 6 months, has resulted in bone healing for some patients.
  2. *Bone grafting* is the use of bone chips from the patient, a cadaver donor, or a living donor and packing or wiring the chips between the bone ends to facilitate union.
  3. *Low-intensity pulsed ultrasound (Exogen therapy)* involves the application of ultrasound treatments for about 20 minutes each day to the fracture site.

F

Community-Based Care

• Collaborate with the case manager or the discharge planner in the hospital to plan care for the patient with a fracture who is being discharged.

QSEN TEAMWORK AND COLLABORATION; INFORMATICS

Be sure to communicate current status and the plan of care to the health care agency receiving the patient. Ensure all drugs are current and accurate in the record.

• Assess the patient's ability to safely use a wheelchair or ambulatory aid.
• Arrange for a home health care nurse to make one or two visits to check that the home is safe and that the patient and family are able to follow the interdisciplinary plan of care.
• Provide verbal and written instructions on the care of bandages, splints, casts, or external fixators.
• Emphasize the importance of follow-up visits with the health care provider and other therapists.
• Teach the patient and family about:
  1. Care of the extremity after removal of the cast
     a. Remove scaly, dead skin carefully by soaking; do not scrub.
     b. Move the extremity carefully. Expect discomfort, weakness, and decreased range of motion (ROM).
     c. Support the extremity with pillows or an orthotic device until strength and movement return.
     d. Exercise as instructed by the physical therapist.
  2. Wound assessment and dressing
  3. Recognition of complications and when and where to seek professional health care if complications occur

FRACTURES OF SPECIFIC SITES

• *Nasal:* Bone or cartilage displacement typically associated with falling, sports, air bag deployment in a car crash, or physical assault. Management is usually a closed reduction within 6 hours of injury.
• *Clavicular, self-healing:* A splint or bandage is used for immobilization.
• *Scapular:* A commercial immobilizer is used until the fracture heals, usually in 2 to 4 weeks.
• *Proximal humerus:* When impacted, the injury is usually treated with a sling for immobilization; when displaced, the fracture often requires ORIF with pins or prosthesis.

- *Humeral shaft:* Correction is achieved by closed reduction and application of a hanging-arm cast or splint.
- *Elbow (olecranon):* Correction by closed reduction and application of a cast. ORIF is performed for displaced fractures, and a splint is worn during the healing phase.
- *Forearm:* The ulna without accompanying injury is corrected with closed reduction and casting. If it is displaced, ORIF with intramedullary rods or plates and screws is required.
- *Wrist and hand:* Injury is most commonly to the carpal scaphoid bone, which is corrected by closed reduction and casting for 6 to 12 weeks. If the bone does not heal, ORIF with bone grafting is performed.
- *Distal radius (wrist; Colles' fracture):* Fracture of the distal radius is managed by closed reduction followed by splinting or a cast although complex fractures may require ORIF.
- *Metacarpals and phalanges (fingers):* Metacarpal fractures are immobilized for 3 to 4 weeks. Phalangeal fractures are immobilized in finger splints for 10 to 14 days.
- *Hip (intracapsular):* This fracture involves the upper third of the femur within the joint capsule. Injury is managed with surgical repair.
- *Hip (extracapsular):* This fracture involves the upper third of the femur outside of the joint capsule. Injury is managed by surgical repair, depending on the exact location of the fracture; ORIF may include an intramedullary rod, pins, prostheses (for femoral head or neck fractures), or a compression screw. Buck's traction may be applied before surgery to reduce muscle spasm.

Considerations for Older Adults

- Older adults are at risk for hip fracture because of physiologic aging changes, reduced vision, disease processes, drug therapy, and environmental hazards.
- These fractures occur most often in older adults with osteoporosis.
- Other disease processes, such as foot disorders and changes in cardiac function, increase the risk for hip fracture.
- Drugs such as diuretics, cardiac drugs, antidepressants, sedatives, opioids, and alcohol are factors that increase the risks for falling in older adults. Use of three or more drugs at the same time drastically increases the risk for falls.
- The older adult is more likely to have complications from the fracture and its management.

- *Lower two thirds of the femur:* This is usually managed surgically by ORIF with nails, rods, or a compression screw. When extensive

bone fragmentation or severe tissue trauma is found, external fixation may be employed.
- *Patellar (knee cap) fracture:* This is usually repaired by closed reduction and casting or internal fixation with screws

! NURSING SAFETY PRIORITY: Critical Rescue

CSF drainage from nares or ear canals may indicate a skull fracture. When CSF is present in drainage, yellow halo will surrounds spot of blood on filter paper. Immediately report positive findings to the health care provider.

- *Tibia and fibula:* These are corrected with closed reduction with casting for 8 to 10 weeks; internal fixation with nails or a plate and screws, followed by a long leg cast for 4 to 6 weeks; or external fixation for 6 to 10 weeks followed by application of a cast.
- *Ankle:* Closed, open, and combined closed and open techniques may be used, depending on the severity and extent of the fracture. An arthrodesis (fusion) is a surgical procedure used when the bone does not heal.
- *Foot or phalanges:* These are managed with closed or open reduction. Crutches are used for ambulation.
- *Ribs and sternum:* These fractures have the potential to puncture the lungs, heart, or arteries by bone fragments or ends. Fractures of the lower ribs may damage underlying organs, such as the liver, spleen, or kidneys. These fractures tend to heal spontaneously without surgical intervention. Some clinicians may advise splinting or wrapping the chest, but this intervention is somewhat controversial because it also limits chest excursion.
- *Pelvis:* Pelvic fractures are the second most common cause of death from trauma. The major concern related to pelvic injury is venous oozing or arterial bleeding. Loss of blood volume leads to hypovolemic shock. When a non–weight-bearing part of the pelvis is fractured, management can be as minimal as bedrest on a firm mattress or bed board. A weight-bearing pelvis fracture requires external fixation with multiple pins, ORIF, or both. Progression to weight bearing depends on the stability of the fracture after fixation. Some patients can fully bear weight within days of surgery, whereas others who are managed with traction may not be able to bear weight for as long as 12 weeks.
- *Compression fractures of the vertebrae (spine):* These fractures are associated with severe pain, deformity (kyphosis), and possible neurologic compromise. Nonsurgical management includes bedrest, analgesics, nerve blocks, and physical therapy to maintain muscle strength. Compression fractures that remain painful and

impair mobility may be surgically treated with vertebroplasty or kyphoplasty, in which bone cement is injected through the skin (percutaneously) directly into the fracture site to provide stability and immediate pain relief. Kyphoplasty also includes the insertion of a small balloon into the fracture site and inflating it to contain the cement and to restore height to the vertebra.

FROSTBITE
OVERVIEW
- Frostbite is a significant cold-related injury that occurs as a result of inadequate insulation against cold weather.
- Contributors to frostbite include wearing wet clothing, fatigue, dehydration, poor nutrition, smoking, alcohol consumption, and impaired peripheral circulation.

PATIENT-CENTERED COLLABORATIVE CARE
Assessment
- Severity of frostbite is related to the degree of tissue freezing and the resultant damage it produces.
  1. *Frostnip* is a superficial cold injury with initial pain, numbness, and pallor of the affected area. It is easily remedied with application of warmth and does not induce tissue damage.
  2. *First-degree frostbite* is the least severe type of frostbite, with hyperemia of the involved area and edema formation.
  3. *Second-degree frostbite* has large, fluid-filled blisters that develop with partial-thickness skin necrosis.
  4. *Third-degree frostbite* is a full-thickness injury that appears as small blisters containing dark fluid and an affected body part that is cool, numb, blue, or red and does not blanch.
  5. *Fourth-degree frostbite* is severe, with no blisters or edema; the part is numb, cold, and bloodless. Full-thickness necrosis extends into the muscle and bone.
Interventions: First Aid
- Recognize frostbite by observing for a white, waxy appearance of exposed skin, especially on the nose, cheeks, and ears.
- Seek shelter from the wind and cold.
- Use body heat to warm up superficial frostbite-affected areas by placing warm hands over the affected areas on the face or placing cold hands under the arms in the axillary region.
Interventions: Hospital Care
- Rapidly rewarm in a water bath at a temperature range of 104° to 108°F (40° to 42°C) or by using hot towels.
- Provide analgesic agents, especially IV opiates, and IV rehydration.

❗ NURSING SAFETY PRIORITY: Action Alert

Dry heat should never be applied, nor should the frostbitten areas be rubbed or massaged as part of the warming process. These actions produce further tissue injury.

- Handle the injured areas gently, and elevate them above heart level if possible to decrease tissue edema.
- Use splints to immobilize extremities during the healing process.
- Assess the patient at least hourly for the development of compartment syndrome.
- Immunize the patient for tetanus prophylaxis.
- Apply only loose, nonadherent, sterile dressings to the damaged areas.
- Avoid compression of the injured tissues.
- Topical and systemic antibiotics may be prescribed.
- Management of severe, deep frostbite requires the same types of surgical intervention as deep or severe burns.

G

GASTRITIS
OVERVIEW
- Gastritis is inflammation of the gastric mucosa.
- Gastritis can be erosive (causing ulcers) or nonerosive.
- Prostaglandins provide a protective mucosal barrier. If there is a break in the barrier, mucosal injury occurs, allowing hydrochloric acid to diffuse into the mucosa and injure small vessels, resulting in edema, bleeding, and erosion of the gastric lining.
- Gastritis can be classified as acute or chronic:
  1. *Acute gastritis,* the inflammation of gastric mucosa or submucosa, may result from food poisoning; the onset of infection *(Helicobacter pylori, Escherichia coli)*; after exposure to local irritants such as alcohol, aspirin, NSAIDs, or bacterial endotoxins; after ingestion of corrosive substances; or from the lack of stimulation of normal gastric secretions.
     a. Gastritis related to food poisoning often occurs within 5 hours of eating contaminated food.
     b. Complete regeneration and healing usually occurs within a few days without any residual damage.

2. *Chronic gastritis* is a diffuse chronic inflammatory process involving the mucosal lining, which becomes thin and atrophies. Prolonged exposures to gastric irritants are linked to chronic gastritis. As gastric atrophy progresses, the amount and concentration of acid diminishes and production of intrinsic factor for absorption of vitamin B_{12} can stop.

   a. Bleeding (GI hemorrhage) and ulcer formation can occur. Of patients with gastric ulcers, 50% have associated chronic gastritis.

   b. Chronic gastritis is associated with an increased risk for stomach cancer.

   c. Three subtypes of chronic gastritis are:

      (1) Type A is associated with the inflammation of the glands and the fundus and body of the stomach. It is associated with autoantibodies to parietal cells and intrinsic factor.

      (2) Type B usually affects the glands of the antrum but may involve the entire stomach.

      (3) Chronic atrophic gastritis affects all layer of the stomach and includes intestinal metaplasia (abnormal tissue development).

PATIENT-CENTERED COLLABORATIVE CARE

Assessment

- Document onset and duration of symptoms
  1. Epigastric discomfort, pain, or cramping
  2. Anorexia, dyspepsia, nausea, and vomiting
  3. Hematemesis, melena
- Presence of risk factors or conditions associated with gastric inflammation
  1. Gastric infection, particularly *H. pylori*
  2. Chronic or excessive use of steroidal or nonsteroidal anti-inflammatory drugs
  3. Anorexia
  4. Autoimmune disease
  5. Occupational exposure to benzene, lead, or nickel
  6. Chronic local irritants like alcohol, radiation therapy, and smoking
  7. Chronic comorbidities including kidney disease (uremia) or systemic inflammatory disease like Crohn's

Interventions

- Acute gastritis is treated symptomatically and supportively. If the patient experienced bleeding with symptomatic blood loss, blood transfusion may be needed. Fluid replacement is indicated for less severe blood loss or symptoms of hypovolemia from low oral intake.

- Drug therapy
  1. Proton pump inhibitors are used to reduce gastric acid secretion.
  2. H_2 histamine blockers may be used instead of proton pump inhibitors.
  3. Antacids are used as buffering agents.
  4. Antibiotics with a proton pump inhibitor and possibly bismuth subsalicylates may be used if the cause is *H. pylori* or other bacterial infection.
  5. Instruct the patient to avoid using drugs associated with gastric irritation, including steroids and NSAIDs, or provide gastroprotective agents when irritants are used therapeutically.
- Diet and lifestyle therapy to avoid tobacco, alcohol, and foods that contribute to gastric irritation, such as those with caffeine, high levels of acid (e.g., tomatoes, citrus fruits), "hot" spices, and large volumes during a meal.
- Teach techniques to reduce stress and discomfort, such as progressive relaxation, cutaneous stimulation, guided imagery, and distraction.

GASTROENTERITIS
OVERVIEW
- Gastroenteritis is an increase in the frequency and water content of stools and vomiting as a result of inflammation of the mucous membranes of the stomach and intestines, primarily affecting the small bowel.
- The inflammation of gastroenteritis is caused by a viral or bacterial infection.
- Norwalk virus is the leading cause of foodborne disease causing gastroenteritis.
- Common microbes causing bacterial gastroenteritis are *Campylobacter, Escherichia coli,* and *Shigellosis.*

PATIENT-CENTERED COLLABORATIVE CARE
Assessment
- Patient's history can provide information about potential cause
  1. Recent travel outside the United States or a recent meal at a restaurant associated with an outbreak of gastroenteritis
  2. Nausea and vomiting
  3. The time of onset of bloody, mucus-filled, watery, or foul-smelling stool or diarrhea with accompanying abdominal cramping or pain
  4. Fever with associated malaise, myalgia, or headache

5. Dehydration exhibited by poor skin turgor, dry mucous membranes, orthostatic blood pressure changes, hypotension, changes in mentation, and oliguria
6. Positive result of a stool culture

Interventions

- Provide fluid replacement therapy
  1. Administer oral rehydration therapy with commercial products such as Gatorade.
  2. Administer IV fluids and electrolytes for severe dehydration.
  3. Check vital signs and orthostatic blood pressure as clinically indicated.
  4. Record intake and output and daily weight.
- Depending on the type of gastroenteritis, notify the local health department.
- Provide drug therapy as ordered
  1. Drugs that suppress intestinal motility, such as antiemetics or anticholinergics, are not routinely given.
  2. Antibacterials are given for bacterial causes of gastroenteritis caused by an organism susceptible to therapy. Viral gastroenteritis, characterized by a shorter duration of illness (less than 72 hours) is treated symptomatically.
  3. Diarrhea that continues for 10 days is probably not caused by gastroenteritis, and an investigation for other causes is done.
- Promote skin protection from stool. Teach the patient to:
  1. Avoid toilet paper and harsh soaps and to gently clean the area with warm water and absorbent material, followed by thorough, gentle drying.
  2. Apply cream, oil, or gel to a damp, warm washcloth or flushable wipe for removing excrement adhering to excoriated skin.
  3. Use protective barrier cream between stools and sitz baths to relieve discomfort.
- Teach the patient to avoid transmission of the infecting microbe
  1. Wash hands after each bowel movement for at least 30 seconds.
  2. Do not share eating utensils, glasses, and dishes.
  3. Do not prepare or handle food that will be consumed by others; the public health department can advise about return to employment if it includes food handling.
  4. Maintain clean bathroom facilities to avoid exposure to stool.
  5. Inform the health care provider if symptoms persist beyond 3 days.
  6. Follow written instructions for antibiotics, if ordered, including the dose, schedule of administration, and side effects.

G

GASTROESOPHAGEAL REFLUX DISEASE

OVERVIEW

* Gastroesophageal reflux disease (GERD) occurs as the result of the backward flow (reflux) of stomach contents into the esophagus.
* Reflux produces symptoms by exposing the esophageal mucosa to the irritating effects of gastric or duodenal contents, resulting in inflammation.
* A person with acute symptoms of inflammation is often described as having *reflux esophagitis,* which may be mild or severe.
* The degree of inflammation is related to the acid concentration of the refluxed material, the number of reflux episodes, and the length of time that the esophagus is exposed to the irritant.
* *Dyspepsia* (also called *heartburn* or *pyrosis*), the primary symptom, is described as a substernal or retrosternal burning sensation that tends to move up and down the chest in a wavelike fashion; severe heartburn may radiate to the neck or jaw or may be felt in the back. It can resemble angina, the pain associated with *acute coronary syndromes* (ACS).

PATIENT-CENTERED COLLABORATIVE CARE

Assessment

* Record patient information related to heartburn or esophageal pain
  1. Location, quality, onset, and duration of dyspepsia or esophageal pain
  2. Pain aggravated by bending over, straining, or lying in a recumbent position
* Ask whether he or she has been newly diagnosed with asthma or has experienced dysphagia, chronic cough, morning hoarseness, or pneumonia. These symptoms suggest severe reflux reaching the pharynx or mouth or pulmonary aspiration.
* Access results of upper endoscopy, 48-hour esophageal pH monitoring, or esophageal manometry (motility testing).

Interventions

Nonsurgical Management

* Explore the patient's meal plan and food preferences, and in collaboration with the dietitian, meet with the patient and family to plan diet modifications to reduce GERD symptoms by limiting or eliminating food that decreases the pressure of the lower esophageal sphincter (LES) and irritates inflamed tissue. Patient should:
  1. Avoid chocolate, peppermint, fatty (especially fried) foods, and carbonated beverages.
  2. Eat small meals that are not spicy or acidic.
  3. Avoid eating for 3 hours (or more) before bedtime.

    4. Limit or eliminate alcohol and tobacco.

    5. Remain upright after meals for 1 to 2 hours.

- Encourage lifestyle changes
  1. If the patient is obese, examine approaches to weight reduction with the patient.
  2. Promote smoking cessation and reduced alcohol intake.
  3. Instruct the patient to elevate the head of the bed by 6 inches to prevent nighttime reflux.
  4. Instruct the patient to sleep in the right lateral decubitus (side-lying) position.
  5. Encourage the patient to avoid wearing tight-fitting clothing and working in a bent-over or stooped position.
- Drug therapy:
  1. Proton pump inhibitors are the main treatment for GERD and provide effective, long-acting inhibition of gastric acid secretion.

! NURSING SAFETY PRIORITY: Drug Alert

Long-term use of proton pump inhibitors (PPIs) may increase the risk for hip fracture, especially in older adults. PPIs can interfere with calcium absorption and protein digestion and therefore reduce available calcium to bone tissue. Decreased calcium makes bones more brittle and likely to fracture.

    2. H_2 histamine receptor blockers are sometimes used instead of proton pump inhibitors to reduce gastric acid production, provide symptom improvement, and support healing of the inflamed esophageal tissue.

    3. Antacids are used to neutralize gastric acids.

    4. Prokinetic drugs are used to accelerate gastric emptying and improve LES pressure and esophageal peristalsis.

- Identify whether the patient uses drugs that may lower LES pressure and cause reflux, such as oral contraceptives, anticholinergic agents, beta-adrenergic agonists, nitrates, and calcium channel blockers.

  ### Surgical Management
- Laparoscopic Nissen fundoplication is a minimally invasive surgery that can be used to manage severe GERD.

GENDER REASSIGNMENT

- Discomfort with one's natal sex is gender dysphoria.
- *Transgender* describes patients who self-identify as the opposite gender or a gender that does not match their natal sex. Transgender individuals feel a mismatch between their gender identity and natal sex, often extending back into early childhood.

- Transgender individuals (also referred to as trans-people) encounter frequent discrimination and face numerous stressful situations related to their identity. Sources of stress such as job discrimination and harassment have an impact on patients' physical and psychological health.
- Assess:
  1. How he or she prefers to be addressed during the nursing history and physical assessment
  2. How care may affect sexual identity or treatment for transgender transition; it may be that the nurse will have to discuss this topic with a provider expert before delivering care in order to maintain trust and provide sensitive, individualized interventions
  3. Level and sources of stress that may affect health care or can be reduced with health promotion interventions
- Interventions for transgender individuals who experience gender dysphoria include one or more of these options:
  1. Changes in gender expression that may involve living part-time or full-time in another gender role
  2. Psychotherapy to explore gender identity and expression, improving body image, or strengthening coping mechanisms
  3. Hormone therapy to feminize or masculinize the body
  4. Surgery to change primary and/or secondary sex characteristics such as the breasts/chest, facial features, internal and/or external genitalia

Gender Health Considerations

- Unique needs regarding sexual health and prevention and treatment of sexually related infections of lesbian, gay, bisexual, and transgender (LGBT) patients should be identified and addressed by the nurse.
- Because of discrimination, health care inequities, and health care provider lack of understanding, the overall health status of individuals in these populations may be poor. LGBT individuals may have difficulty finding health care that identifies and addresses their particular risks and concerns.
- Taking a health history that provides opportunity for the patient to identify his or her sexual orientation, sexual identity, and sexual activity is essential to care. Especially among transgender individuals, opportunities for physical examination are avoided or missed by both the patient and care provider because of fears of being misunderstood or inadequately prepared to give or receive appropriate care.

GLAUCOMA
OVERVIEW
- Glaucoma is a group of ocular diseases resulting in increased intraocular pressure (IOP).
- The normal pressure of fluid in the eye is an IOP of 10 to 21 mm Hg, maintained when there is a balance between production and outflow of aqueous humor.
- If the IOP becomes too high, pressure on blood vessels in the eye prevents blood flow, resulting in poorly oxygenated photoreceptors and nerve fibers that then become ischemic and die. With necrosis, sight is lost and the person is permanently blind.
- In most types of glaucoma, vision is lost gradually and painlessly from the periphery to the central area.
- Types of glaucoma:
  1. *Primary:* The structures involved in circulation and reabsorption of the aqueous humor undergo direct pathologic changes from aging, heredity, and central retinal vessel occlusion.
     a. *Primary open-angle glaucoma* (POAG) has reduced outflow of aqueous humor through the chamber angle. Because the fluid cannot leave the eye at the same rate it is produced, IOP gradually increases.
     b. *Primary angle-closure glaucoma* (PACG, also called *acute glaucoma*) has a sudden onset and is an emergency.
  2. *Secondary:* Glaucoma results from other problems within the eye, such as uveitis, iritis, trauma, and ocular surgeries.
  3. *Associated:* Glaucoma results from systemic disease, such as diabetes mellitus and hypertension.

PATIENT-CENTERED COLLABORATIVE CARE
Assessment
- Assess for manifestations of early glaucoma
  1. Increased ocular pressure measured by tonometry
  2. Reduced accommodation
- Assess for late manifestations of glaucoma
  1. Peripheral visual field losses
  2. Decreased visual acuity not correctable with glasses
  3. Appearance of halos around lights
- Drug therapy for glaucoma focuses on reducing IOP with eyedrops
  1. Prostaglandin agonists dilate blood vessels to drain aqueous fluid and include bimatoprost (Lumigan), latanoprost (Xalatan), and travoprost (Travatan).
  2. Adrenergic agonists block production of aqueous humor and include apraclonidine (Iopidine), brimonidine (Alphagan), and dipivefrin (Propine).

3. Beta-adrenergic blockers block production of aqueous fluid and include betaxolol (Betoptic), carteolol (Cartrol, Ocupress), levobunolol (Betagan), and timolol (Betimol, Timoptic, Timoptic GFS for extended release).

4. Cholinergic agonists increase the outflow of fluid and slow aqueous fluid production; products include carbachol (Carboptic, Isopto Carbachol, Miostat), echothiophate (Phospholine Iodide), and pilocarpine (Adsorbocarpine, Akarpine, Isopto Carpine, Ocu-Carpine, Ocusert, Piloptic, Pilopine, Pilostat).

5. Carbonic anhydrase inhibitors directly and strongly reduce aqueous fluid production and include brinzolamide (Azopt) and dorzolamide (Trusopt).

6. There are also combination agents that use drugs from more than one of the above categories such as brimonidine tartrate and timolol maleate (Combigan).

• Teach the patient:

1. The importance of instilling the drops on time and not skipping doses

2. To wait 5 to 15 minutes between drug instillations when more than one drug is prescribed to prevent one drug from "washing out" or diluting another drug

3. The technique of punctal occlusion (placing pressure on the corner of the eye near the nose) immediately after eyedrop instillation to prevent systemic absorption of the drug

4. About the need for good handwashing, keeping the eyedrop container tip clean, and avoiding touching the tip to any part of the eye

• Surgery is used when drugs for the patient with open-angle glaucoma are not effective in controlling IOP. The two most common procedures are laser trabeculoplasty and trabeculectomy to improve the outflow of aqueous fluid.

GLOMERULONEPHRITIS, ACUTE

OVERVIEW

• Acute glomerulonephritis results from injury to the glomeruli. *Rapidly progressive glomerulonephritis,* a subtype of this condition, develops over several days and causes a rapid and significant loss of kidney function.

• Glomerular injury is the result of immune complexes deposited in kidney tissue; an immune complex is made up of antigens and antibodies.

• Immune complexes trigger inflammation, which can further damage kidney tissue, ultimately leading to chronic kidney disease (CKD) and failure.

PATIENT-CENTERED COLLABORATIVE CARE
Assessment
- Record patient information
  1. History of recent infections, particularly skin and upper respiratory infections
  2. Recent travel or activities with exposure to viruses, bacteria, fungi, or parasites
  3. Known systemic diseases, especially those associated with inflammation or autoimmunity such as systemic lupus erythematosus
- Assessment findings include:
  1. Skin lesions or incisions, including piercings that could be the source of infection
  2. Presence of symptoms indicating systemic volume overload: extra heart sound (i.e., S_3 gallop), neck vein engorgement, edema, and crackles in the lungs with tachypnea and dyspnea or orthopnea
  3. Changes in urine color (typically smoky, reddish brown, or tea-colored urine), clarity, or odor; and altered patterns of urination such as dysuria, urgency, and incontinence
  4. Decreased urine output
  5. Mild to moderate hypertension
  6. Changes in weight
  7. Fatigue, malaise, and activity intolerance
  8. Abnormal urinalysis including leukocyte esterase, nitrogen, red blood cells (RBCs), white blood cells (WBCs), and protein
  9. Increased blood urea nitrogen (BUN) and serum creatinine levels
  10. Decreased urine creatinine clearance
  11. Positive cultures from urine, blood, sputum, skin, or throat
  12. Serologic testing for antistreptolysin O titers, C3 complement levels, immunoglobulin G, antinuclear bodies, and circulating immune complexes
- A percutaneous needle biopsy of the kidney provides a precise diagnosis and helps outline treatment.

Interventions
- Appropriate anti-infective agents are given to treat infection.
- Sodium and water restriction, along with diuretics, may be needed for the patient with hypertension, circulatory overload, and edema. Fluid intake may be restricted to the previous 24-hour urinary output plus 500 to 600 mL for insensible fluid loss.
- Potassium and protein intake may be restricted to prevent hyperkalemia and reduce uremia.
- Management may include dialysis or plasmapheresis to filter out antigen-antibody complexes and manage uremia or fluid and electrolyte imbalances.

G

- Health teaching includes:
  1. Reviewing prescribed drug instructions, including purpose, timing, frequency, duration, and side effects
  2. Ensuring that the patient and family understand dietary and fluid modifications. Offer assistance with coping with fluid restrictions, such as a mouth moisturizer or mouth swabs. In some situations ice chips or hard candy may be used to offer relief from a dry mouth.
  3. Advising the patient to measure weight and blood pressure daily and to notify the health care provider of any sudden changes
  4. Instructing the patient about peritoneal or vascular access care if short-term dialysis is required to control excess fluid volume or uremic symptoms

GLOMERULONEPHRITIS, CHRONIC
OVERVIEW

- Chronic glomerulonephritis, or *chronic nephritic syndrome,* is the diagnostic name given to known and unknown causes of kidney deterioration or kidney failure that develop over 20 to 30 years.
- The exact cause is unknown. Changes are thought to result from the effects of hypertension, intermittent or recurrent infections and inflammation, and poor blood flow to the kidneys.
- Kidney tissue atrophies, and the functional mass of nephrons decreases, which alters glomerular filtration.
- Glomerular injury results in proteinuria because of increased permeability of the glomerular basement membrane.
- The process eventually results in CKD and uremia, requiring dialysis or transplantation.

PATIENT-CENTERED COLLABORATIVE CARE
Assessment

- Record the patient's history
  1. Health problems, including systemic disease, kidney or urologic problems, and infectious diseases, especially streptococcal infections and recent exposure to infection
  2. Presence of symptoms indicating systemic volume overload: the cardiac extra sound of an S_3 gallop, neck vein engorgement, edema, and crackles in the lungs with tachypnea
  3. Changes in urine and elimination, including amount, frequency of voiding, and changes in urine color, clarity, and odor
  4. Changes in activity tolerance and comfort
  5. Changes in mental concentration or memory associated with uremia

6. Abnormal urinalysis, especially proteinuria
7. Decreased creatinine clearance (glomerular filtration rate [GFR])
8. Abnormal serum kidney function and electrolyte values
9. Radiographic findings of kidney size (usually small)
- Perform a physical assessment:
  1. Inspect the skin for color, ecchymosis, and rashes.
  2. Inspect for symptoms of fluid overload and electrolyte imbalance.
  3. Measure blood pressure and weight.
  4. Assess for uremic symptoms, such as slurred speech, ataxia, tremors, or asterixis (flapping tremor of the fingers or the inability to maintain a fixed posture with the arms extended and wrists hyperextended).

Interventions
- Management of chronic glomerulonephritis is similar to management for CKD, including dialysis when kidneys fail to adequately filter the blood.
- Treatment consists of dietary modification, fluid intake sufficient to prevent reduced blood flow volume to the kidneys, and drug therapy to temporarily control the symptoms of uremia.

GONORRHEA

G

OVERVIEW
- Gonorrhea is a sexually transmitted bacterial infection caused by *Neisseria gonorrhoeae,* a gram-negative intracellular diplococcus.
- It is transmitted by direct sexual contact with mucosal surfaces (vaginal intercourse, orogenital contact, or anogenital contact).
- The first symptoms of gonorrhea may appear 3 to 10 days after sexual contact with an infected person or the disease can be present without symptoms and can be transmitted or progress without warning.
- In women, ascending spread of the organism can cause pelvic infection (pelvic inflammatory disease [PID]), endometritis (endometrial infection), salpingitis (fallopian tube infection), and pelvic peritonitis.
- *Neisseria gonorrhoeae* is a multidrug-resistant organism (MDRO) in the United States.

PATIENT-CENTERED COLLABORATIVE CARE
Assessment
- Obtain patient information about:
  1. Sexual history that includes sexual orientation and sites of intercourse
  2. Allergies to antibiotics

   3. Symptoms in men
      a. Dysuria
      b. Penile discharge (profuse, yellowish-green fluid or scant, clear fluid)
      c. Urethritis
      d. Pain or discomfort in the prostate, seminal vesicles, or epididymal regions
   4. Symptoms in women
      a. Vaginal discharge (yellow, green, profuse, odorous)
      b. Urinary frequency
      c. Dysuria and urethral discharge
   5. Anal manifestations (in men or women)
      a. Itching and irritation
      b. Rectal discharge or bleeding
      c. Diarrhea
      d. Painful defecation
- Assess for and document:
   1. Oral cavity manifestations
      a. Reddened throat
      b. Ulcerated lips
      c. Tender gingivae
      d. Blisters in the throat
   2. Tenderness of the lower abdomen
   3. Manifestations of disseminated *gonococci* infection (DGI)
      a. Fever
      b. Chills
      c. Skin lesions on hands and feet
      d. Joint pain, with or without swelling, heat, or redness
- Diagnostic testing may include:
   1. Nucleic acid amplification test (NAAT) using samples from vagina or male urethra
   2. Gram staining and cultures from a smear from penile discharge or from a vaginal swab

❗ NURSING SAFETY PRIORITY: Critical Rescue

All patients with gonorrhea should be tested for syphilis, chlamydia, hepatitis B and C, and HIV infection, because they may have been exposed to multiple sexually transmitted diseases (STDs). Sexual partners who have been exposed in the past 30 days should be examined and specimens for culture should be obtained.

Interventions
- Drug therapy for uncomplicated gonorrhea is ceftriaxone plus azithromycin.

- Disseminated gonorrhea infection requires hospitalization and IV antibiotics, typically for 48 hours, followed by 7 days of oral antibiotics.
- Sexual partners also must be treated.
- A test of cure is not required but the patient should be advised to return for a follow-up examination if symptoms persist after treatment.
- This condition must be reported to the local health department by the health care provider.
- Teach the patient about:
  1. Transmission and treatment of gonorrhea
  2. Prevention of re-infection
  3. Complications of chronic gonorrhea
     a. PID
     b. Ectopic pregnancy
     c. Infertility
     d. Chronic pelvic pain
  4. Avoiding sexual activity until the antibiotic therapy is completed
  5. Condom use if abstinence is not possible
  6. The need for all sexual contacts to be examined for STDs
- Encourage patients to express their feelings during assessments and teaching sessions.
- Provide privacy for teaching and maintain confidentiality of medical records.

GOUT

OVERVIEW

- Gout, or *gouty arthritis,* is a systemic disease in which urate crystals deposit in the joints and other body tissues, causing inflammation.
- There are two major types of gout:
  1. *Primary gout* results from one of several inborn errors of purine metabolism that allows the production of uric acid to exceed the excretion capability of the kidneys. Urate is deposited in synovium and other tissues, resulting in inflammation. A number of patients have a family history of gout. It is most common in middle-aged and older men and postmenopausal women.
  2. *Secondary gout* results from excessive uric acid crystals that are present in the blood (hyperuricemia) as a result of another disease, condition, or treatment. Causes include renal insufficiency, diuretic therapy, "crash" diets, certain chemotherapeutic agents, and diseases such as multiple myeloma and certain carcinomas. Treatment for secondary gout focuses on management of the underlying disorder.

- There are three clinical stages of primary gout:
  1. *Asymptomatic hyperuricemic stage,* in which there are no symptoms but the serum uric acid level is elevated
  2. *Acute stage,* in which the patient experiences excruciating pain and inflammation in one or more small joints, usually the metatarsophalangeal joint of the great toe, called *podagra*
  3. *Chronic tophaceous stage,* which occurs after repeated episodes of acute gout have caused deposits of urate crystals under the skin and within the major organs, particularly in the kidney system; this stage can begin between 3 and 40 years after the initial gout symptoms occur

PATIENT-CENTERED COLLABORATIVE CARE
Assessment
- Obtain patient information about:
  1. Age
  2. Gender
  3. Family history of gout
  4. Medical history and drug history to determine whether gout has been caused by another problem
- For acute gout, assess for and document joint inflammation and pain.
- For chronic gout, assess for and document:
  1. Presence of tophi (skin deposits of urate crystals):
     a. Outer ear
     b. Arms and fingers near the joints
  2. Infected skin areas
  3. Manifestations of kidney (stones) or kidney dysfunction
     a. Severe pain
     b. Changes in urine output
- Diagnostic assessment may include:
  1. Serum uric acid level
  2. Urinary uric acid levels
  3. Kidney function tests (in chronic gout)
  4. Synovial fluid aspiration (arthrocentesis)
Interventions
- Drug therapy during acute attacks
  1. Colchicine (Colsalide, Novocolchicine ✿)
  2. NSAIDs, such as indomethacin (Indocin, Novomethacin ✿) or ibuprofen (Motrin, Amersol ✿)
- Drug therapy for chronic gout
  1. Allopurinol (Zyloprim) or febuxostat (Uloric)
  2. Probenecid (Benemid, Benuryl ✿)
  3. Pegloticase (Krystexxa)

> ### ❗ NURSING SAFETY PRIORITY: Action Alert
>
> Aspirin should be avoided, because it inactivates the effects of the drug therapy.

- Nutritional therapy with a low-purine diet and teaching patient to avoid foods that precipitate attacks
  1. Organ meats
  2. Red meats
  3. Shellfish
  4. Oily fish with bones (e.g., sardines)
- Other restrictions include:
  1. All forms of aspirin
  2. Diuretics
  3. Excessive physical or emotional stress, which can exacerbate the disease
- Teach the patient to drink plenty of fluids, especially:
  1. Water
  2. Citrus juices
  3. Milk

GUILLAIN-BARRÉ SYNDROME

OVERVIEW

- Guillain-Barré syndrome (GBS) is an *acute inflammatory demyelinating polyneuropathy* (also called *polyradiculoneuropathy*) that affects the peripheral nervous system axons and myelin, causing motor weakness and sensory abnormalities.
- GBS is the result of immune-mediated pathologic processes that include antibody damage to the myelin sheath.
- Three stages make up the acute course:
  1. *Acute phase,* which begins with the onset of the first definitive symptoms and ends when no further deterioration is noted (usually 1 to 4 weeks)
  2. *Plateau phase,* which is a time of little change and lasts several days to 2 weeks
  3. *Recovery phase,* which is thought to coincide with re-myelination and axonal regeneration and occurs gradually over 4 to 6 months (sometimes up to 2 years)
- *Chronic inflammatory demyelinating polyneuropathy* (CIDP) is an unusual type of GBS that progresses over a longer period; complete recovery rarely occurs.
- The patient often relates a history of acute infection, illness, trauma, surgery, or immunization 1 to 8 weeks before the onset of neurologic signs and symptoms.

G

PATIENT-CENTERED COLLABORATIVE CARE

Assessment

- Record the patient's medical and surgical history, including:
  1. Occurrence of antecedent illness 1 to 8 weeks before the onset of GBS
  2. Description of symptoms (in chronologic order)
- Assessment findings include:
  1. Paresthesia (numbness or tingling) and pain
  2. Cranial nerve dysfunction resulting in facial weakness, dysphagia, and/or diplopia
  3. Muscle weakness or flaccid paralysis without muscle wasting in an ascending, distal-to-proximal progression
  4. Respiratory compromise or failure:
     a. Decreased peripheral oxygenation (SpO_2)
     b. Dyspnea, tachypnea, or paradoxical breathing
     c. Decreased breath sounds from reduced tidal volume or vital capacity
     d. Increased oral secretions, inability to swallow, or compromised airway patency
  5. Bowel and bladder incontinence
  6. Autonomic dysfunction evidenced by:
     a. Labile blood pressure
     b. Cardiac dysrhythmias, including tachycardia
  7. Altered coping manifested by anxiety, fear, anger, or depression
  8. Protein in cerebrospinal fluid without leukocytosis
  9. Electrophysiologic studies (EPSs) demonstrating demyelinating neuropathy

Planning and Implementation

- Treat with plasma exchange or immunoglobulin. There is no benefit to using both therapies.
  1. *Plasmapheresis* removes the circulating antibodies thought to be responsible for the disease. Nursing interventions for the patient undergoing plasmapheresis include:
     a. Providing information and reassurance
     b. Monitoring for complications of plasmapheresis: hypovolemia, hypokalemia, hypocalcemia, temporary circumoral and distal extremity paresthesia, muscle twitching, nausea, and vomiting
     c. Monitoring intake and output and weighing the patient after the procedure to detect dehydration or overhydration as a result of treatment
     d. Administering shunt care to maintain patency and prevent infections

! NURSING SAFETY PRIORITY: Critical Rescue

If a shunt is used, use these interventions to avoid infection and harm from clotting or bleeding:

- Check shunt patency by palpating a thrill or auscultating a bruit every 2 to 4 hours.
- Keep double bulldog clamps at the bedside to prevent high-volume blood loss if shunt is dislodged.
- Observe the puncture site for bleeding or ecchymosis (bruising).
- Maintain sterile, occlusive dressing at the insertion site.

2. *Intravenous immunoglobulin therapy* (IVIG) is equally effective as plasmapheresis but is safer and immediately available.
3. Side effects of immunoglobulin therapy range from minor annoyances (e.g., chills, mild fever, myalgia, and headache) to major complications (e.g., anaphylaxis, aseptic meningitis, retinal necrosis, and acute kidney injury and failure).

MANAGE THE AIRWAY AND MONITOR RESPIRATORY STATUS

- Evaluate for dysphagia and implement aspiration precautions if needed.
- Monitor the color, consistency, and amount of secretions obtained.
- Auscultate breath sounds, respiratory rate, rhythm, depth, and chest excursion every 1 to 4 hours.
- Observe for dyspnea, air hunger, adventitious breath sounds, cyanosis, and confusion.
- Administer humidified air or oxygen, as appropriate.
- Administer bronchodilator treatments, as appropriate.
- Keep equipment for suctioning available and equipment for intubation nearby.
- Elevate the head of the bed.
- Encourage the patient to use the incentive spirometer and cough and breathe deeply.
- Monitor peripheral oxygen saturation (SpO_2) and ABG results for hypoxemia, hypercarbia, or disturbances in pH.

PREVENT IMMOBILITY AND ADDRESS DEFICITS IN SELF-CARE

- Assess motor function with vital signs.
- Assist the patient's hygiene, toileting, and other activity as needed.
- Collaborate with physical therapy and occupational therapy to determine the type and duration of daily exercises or activity, such as transfer to chair, re-positioning in bed, ambulation, and activities of daily living (ADLs).
- Monitor the patient's response to activity, provide rest between activities, and reduce the frequency or duration of activity if intolerant.

G

- Collaborate with the dietitian to optimize nutritional intake and assist with meals as needed.
- Monitor intake and output for balance, and assess the patient for urinary retention every shift.
- Monitor for complications of immobility: atelectasis, pneumonia, pressure ulcers, and venothromboembolism.

QSEN EVIDENCE-BASED PRACTICE

Assess and periodically re-assess each patient's risk for developing a pressure ulcer, and take action to address any identified risks. Prevention of hospital-acquired pressure ulcers is a priority for all patients.

MANAGE PAIN
- Assess the severity and nature of the patient's pain, which is typically worse at night.
- Pain is best treated with opiates, which can be administered by a patient-controlled analgesia (PCA) pump or continuous IV drip. Document the patient's response to pain drugs.
- Other interventions include frequent positioning, massage, ice, heat, relaxation techniques, guided imagery, and distractions.

PROMOTE COMMUNICATION
- Assist the patient in developing a communication system in collaboration with the speech-language pathologist.
- Develop a communication board that lists common requests.

PROVIDE PSYCHOSOCIAL SUPPORT
- Encourage the patient to verbalize feelings concerning the illness and its effects.
- Provide information regarding the disease process.
- Encourage the patient to participate in his or her care and to make as many choices as possible.
- Provide encouragement and positive reinforcement.
- Identify factors that increase coping abilities by asking the patient and family to describe situations that they have successfully coped with in the past.
- Keep necessary items (call light, radio, or television control) within the patient's reach.
- Use the patient's own personal items, when feasible.

Community-Based Care
- Discharge planning includes:
  1. Providing a detailed plan of care at the time of discharge for patients to be transferred to a long-term care or rehabilitation facility (rehabilitation may be lengthy)

2. Assessing the patient's and family's knowledge and understanding of the disease
3. Ensuring that patient and family members understand how to use positioning and assistive or adaptive devices to enhance recovery
4. Referring the patient to local agencies or national neurological organizations such as the Guillain-Barré Foundation for assistance in the home setting and educational materials

H

HEADACHE, CLUSTER
OVERVIEW

- Cluster headaches (also referred to as *trigeminal autonomic cephalalgia*) are manifested by intense throbbing unilateral pain that may last 15 minutes to 3 hours. The headache usually occurs with:
  1. Ipsilateral (same side) tearing of the eye
  2. Rhinorrhea ("runny nose") or congestion
  3. Ptosis (drooping eyelid)
  4. Eyelid edema
  5. Facial sweating
  6. Miosis (constriction of pupils)
- The cause and mechanism of cluster headaches are not known but have been attributed to vasoreactivity and neurogenic inflammation.
- The headaches usually occur at about the same time of day (and may occur several times a day) for about 4 to 12 weeks (hence the term *cluster*), followed by a period of remission for 9 months to a year.
- Management includes:
  1. Administering drugs to treat pain, similar to migraine therapy: triptans, ergotamine preparations, and antiepileptic drugs (AEDs); additional drugs include calcium channel blockers, lithium, and corticosteroids.
  2. During an attack, administering 100% oxygen by mask for 15 to 30 minutes with the patient in a sitting position during cluster headache pain
  3. Instructing the patient to wear sunglasses and avoid bright light while the headache is occurring
  4. Helping the patient identify precipitating factors such as bursts of anger, excessive physical activity, and excitement
  5. Teaching the patient the importance of a consistent sleep-wake cycle

H

6. Surgical interventions for drug-resistant cluster headaches, such as percutaneous stereotactic rhizotomy and deep brain electrical stimulation at the posterior hypothalamus

HEADACHE, MIGRAINE

OVERVIEW

- A migraine headache is a syndrome of recurrent episodic head pain that can last 4 to 72 hours.
- It is characterized by an intense pain in one side of the head (unilateral), worsening with movement. Associated symptoms of nausea and sensitivity to light, sound, and head movement can occur.
- The cause of migraine headaches is likely a combination of neuronal hyper-excitability and vascular, genetic, hormonal, and environmental factors.
- Three categories of migraine headache are migraine with aura (classic migraine), migraine without aura, and atypical migraine.
- The priority of care is pain management
  1. Prevention includes interventions and education to reduce migraine episodes.
     a. Drugs may be used when migraine occurs more than twice per week, interferes with ADLs, or is not relieved with acute treatment.
     b. Migraine-preventive drugs include NSAIDs, beta-adrenergic blockers, calcium channel blockers, onabotulinumtoxinA (Botox), and AEDs.
  2. Abortive therapy is the administration of drugs to alleviate headache during the aura phase or shortly after the migraine starts. Examples of migraine abortive drugs are:
     a. Nonspecific analgesics and NSAIDs to reduce mild pain, such as acetaminophen, isometheptene, butalbital, ibuprofen, and naproxen; the addition of caffeine to these drugs results in vasoconstriction and symptom relief
     b. Ergotamine preparations for severe pain with or without caffeine that can be taken orally sublingually, inhaled, or as a suppository (e.g., Cafergot, Migergot, Ergomar SL, and Medihaler ergotamine)
     c. Beta blockers like propranolol or timolol
     d. Calcium channel blockers like verapamil (Calan)
     e. Triptan preparations to activate serotonin receptors in cranial arteries, such as almotriptan (Axert), eletriptan (Relpax), rizatriptan (Maxalt), zolmitriptan (Zomig), sumatriptan (Imitrex), and frovatriptan (Frova)
     f. OnabotulinumtoxinA (Botox) is used to prevent chronic (not episodic) migraines by decreasing nerve conduction.

3. Trigger management is a strategy to reduce the frequency or severity of migraines by identifying and stopping exposure to dietary and environmental factors that contribute to migraines.
   a. The patient should avoid tyramine-containing products, such as pickled products, caffeine, beer, and wine.
   b. Preservatives and artificial sweeteners are also common triggers.
   c. Instruct the patient to keep a diary to link exposures to migraine symptoms.
4. Complementary and alternative therapies associated with symptom relief include acupressure and acupuncture, yoga, meditation, massage, exercise, and biofeedback. Vitamin B_2 (riboflavin), coenzyme Q_{10}, and magnesium supplement to maintain normal serum values have a role in migraine prevention.

HEARING LOSS

OVERVIEW

- Hearing loss, a common handicap worldwide, may be conductive, sensorineural, or a combination of the two.
  1. *Conductive hearing loss* is a result of obstruction of sound wave transmission such as a foreign body in the external canal, a retracted or bulging tympanic membrane, or fused bony ossicles.
  2. *Sensorineural hearing loss* is a result of a defect in the cochlea, the eighth cranial nerve, or the brain. Also, exposure to loud noise or music damages the cochlear hair and this type of hearing loss. *Presbycusis* is a sensorineural hearing loss that occurs as a result of aging.
  3. *Combined* or *mixed hearing loss* has components of both conductive and sensorineural loss.
- About one third of people between the ages of 65 and 75 years have a hearing loss. As many as one half of people older than 85 years have some degree of hearing loss.
- The type and cause of hearing loss determine the degree to which loss can be corrected and the amount of hearing that can return.

PATIENT-CENTERED COLLABORATIVE CARE

Assessment

- Obtain patient information about:
  1. Any differences in his or her ears or hearing and whether the changes occurred suddenly or gradually, including:
     a. Feeling of ear fullness or congestion
     b. Dizziness or vertigo

✖ Genetic/Genomic Considerations

- One type of hearing loss among adults has a genetic basis with a mutation in gene *GJB2*. This mutation causes poor production of the protein connexin-26, which has a role in the function of cochlear hair cells.
- Other genetic variations in some of the drug metabolizing genes (cytochrome P450 family) slow the metabolism and excretion of drugs, including ototoxic drugs. This allows ototoxic drugs to remain in the body longer, thus increasing the risk for hearing loss.

    c. Tinnitus
    d. Difficulty hearing sounds or understanding conversations, especially in a noisy room
  2. Age
  3. Occupational or leisure exposure to loud or continuous noises
  4. Current or previous use of ototoxic drugs
  5. History of external ear or middle ear infection and whether eardrum perforation occurred with the infection
  6. History of ear trauma
  7. Whether any family members are hearing impaired
  8. Recent upper respiratory infection and allergies affecting the nose and sinuses
- Assess for and document:
  1. External ear features (pinna) including size and position
  2. Abnormal otoscopic and Rinne or Weber (tuning fork) test findings by the provider
  3. Psychosocial issues
    a. Social isolation
    b. Depression, fear, and despair
- Diagnostic studies include audiometry to determine the type and extent of hearing loss and imaging to determine possible causes.

Planning and Implementation
DIFFICULTY HEARING
- Related to obstruction, infection, damage to the middle ear, or damage to the auditory nerve.

Nonsurgical Management
- Early detection can help correct reversible problems causing the hearing loss.
  1. Drug therapy is used to correct an underlying pathologic change or to reduce side effects of problems occurring with hearing loss, including antibiotic therapy for infection.
  2. Antivertiginous drugs are used to decrease dizziness when this symptom accompanies hearing loss.

- Hearing-assistive devices
  1. Telephone amplifiers
  2. Therapy dogs
  3. Portable audio amplifiers
  4. Collaborate with the audiologist to promote safe, effective use of a hearing aid
     a. Remind the patient that background noise will be amplified along with voices and that a new hearing aid requires a period of adjustment.
     b. Teach him or her to care for the hearing aid by:
        (1) Cleaning the ear mold with mild soap and water while avoiding excessive wetting
        (2) Cleaning debris from the hole in the middle of the part that goes into the ear with a toothpick or a pipe cleaner
        (3) Turning off the hearing aid and removing the battery when not in use
        (4) Keeping extra batteries on hand and replacing the battery often
        (5) Avoiding dropping the hearing aid or exposing it to temperature extremes
        (6) Adjusting the volume to the lowest setting that allows hearing to prevent feedback squeaking
        (7) Avoiding use of hair and face products that may damage the receiver

Surgical Management

- The type of operative procedure selected depends on the cause of the hearing loss.
  1. *Tympanoplasty reconstruction* of the middle ear can improve conductive hearing loss. The procedures vary from simple reconstruction of the eardrum (myringoplasty or type I tympanoplasty) to replacement of the ossicles within the middle ear (type II tympanoplasty).
  2. *Stapedectomy* is the removal of the head and neck of the stapes and, less often, the footplate. After removal of the bone, a small hole is drilled or made with a laser in the footplate, and a prosthesis in the shape of a piston is connected between the incus and the footplate.
  3. A totally implanted device is placed to treat bilateral moderate to severe sensorineural hearing loss.
- Provide preoperative care, including:
  1. Adhering to routine preoperative care, as described in Part One
  2. Assuring the patient that hearing loss immediately after surgery is normal because of canal packing
  3. Reinforcing the information provided by the surgeon

- Provide postoperative care, including:
    1. Adhering to routine postoperative care, as described in Part One
    2. Keeping the dressing clean and dry, using sterile technique for changes
    3. Keeping the patient flat, with the head turned to the side and the operative ear facing up for at least 12 hours after surgery
    4. Using communication techniques for the hearing impaired
    5. Giving prescribed antibiotics to prevent infection
    6. Giving prescribed analgesics
    7. Giving prescribed antivertiginous drugs
    8. Assessing for and reporting complications (stapedectomy, implanted devices)
        a. Asymmetric appearance or drooping of features on the affected side of the face
        b. Changes in facial perception of touch and in taste, as reported by patient
    9. Assisting the patient with ambulating
    10. Reminding the patient to move his or her head slowly when changing position to avoid vertigo
    11. Teaching the patient about care and activity restrictions
        a. Not using small objects, such as cotton-tipped applicators, matches, toothpicks, or hairpins, to clean the external ear canal
        b. Washing the external ear and canal daily in the shower or while washing the hair
        c. Blowing the nose gently
        d. Not occluding one nostril while blowing the nose
        e. Sneezing with the mouth open
        f. Wearing sound protection around loud or continuous noises
        g. Avoiding activities with high risk for head or ear trauma, such as wrestling, boxing, motorcycle riding, and skateboarding; wearing head and ear protection when engaging in these activities
        h. Keeping the volume on head receivers at the lowest setting that allows hearing
        i. Frequently cleaning objects that come into contact with the ear (e.g., headphones, telephone receivers)
        j. Avoiding environmental conditions with rapid changes in air pressure

POTENTIAL FOR REDUCED COMMUNICATION RELATED TO HEARING DIFFICULTY

- Use best practices for communicating with a hearing-impaired patient, including:

1. Positioning yourself directly in front of the patient
2. Making sure that the room is well lighted
3. Getting the patient's attention before you begin to speak
4. Moving closer to the better hearing ear
5. Speaking clearly and slowly
6. Keeping hands and other objects away from your mouth when talking to the patient
7. Attempting to have conversations in a quiet room with minimal distractions
8. Having the patient repeat your statements rather than just indicating assent
9. Rephrasing sentences and repeating information to aid in understanding
10. Using appropriate hand motions
11. Writing messages on paper if the patient is able to read

❗ NURSING SAFETY PRIORITY: Action Alert

Do not shout to the patient, because the sound may be projected at a higher frequency, making him or her less able to understand.

- Have the patient use hearing-assistive devices described earlier.
- Manage anxiety and promote social interaction by:
  1. Enhancing communication, as described earlier
  2. Working with the patient to identify his or her most satisfying activities and social interactions and determine the amount of effort necessary to continue them
  3. Suggesting the use of closed captioning for television programming

Community-Based Care

- Teach patients who have persistent vertigo and their families to determine the best ways to maintain adequate self-care abilities, maintain a safe environment, decide about assistance needs, and provide needed care.
- Give patients written instructions about how to take drugs and when to return for follow-up care.
- Teach patients how to instill eardrops and irrigate the ears, and obtain a return demonstration.
- Support patients by listening to their concerns and recognizing the emotional response to hearing loss.
  - Provide information about public and private agencies that offer hearing evaluations, education, information, and counseling for patients with hearing disorders.

H

HEART FAILURE
OVERVIEW
- Heart failure (HF), sometimes called *pump failure,* is the chronic inability of the heart to work effectively as a pump.
- HF causes insufficient perfusion of body tissue with vital nutrients and oxygen.
- Basic cardiac physiologic mechanisms such as ejection fraction, stroke volume, cardiac output, and contractility are altered in HF.
- The American College of Cardiology (ACC) and American Heart Association (AHA) have evidence-based guidelines for staging and managing HF as a chronic progressive disease. These guidelines are combined with the New York Heart Association (NYHA) functional classification system that is used to describe symptoms exhibited by the patient to aid in determining response to interventions and prognostication.
- The major types of HF are:
  1. *Left HF,* characterized by decreased tissue perfusion from poor cardiac output and pulmonary congestion from increased pressure in the pulmonary vessels, and further subdivided into systolic HF and diastolic HF:
     a. *Systolic HF* (sometimes still referred to as *congestive heart failure* or *forward failure*) results when the heart is unable to contract forcefully enough during systole to eject adequate amounts of blood into the circulation.
        (1) Preload increases with decreased contractility, and afterload increases as a result of increased peripheral resistance.
        (2) The ejection fraction drops from a normal of 50% to 70% to below 40%.
        (3) Systemic organ and tissue perfusion diminishes; pulmonary edema is common.
     b. *Diastolic HF* occurs when the left ventricle is unable to relax adequately during diastole, which prevents the ventricle from filling with sufficient blood to ensure an adequate cardiac output.
        (1) The ejection fraction may remain near normal.
  2. *Right HF* occurs when the right ventricle is unable to empty completely. Right HF in the absence of left HF is most often the result of pulmonary problems. Increased volume and pressure develop in the systemic veins, and systemic venous congestion develops with peripheral edema.
  3. *High-output failure* can occur when cardiac output remains normal or above normal and is caused by increased metabolic needs or hyperkinetic conditions such as septicemia, anemia, and hyperthyroidism.

- When cardiac output is insufficient to meet the demands of the body, compensatory mechanisms operate to improve cardiac output. Although these mechanisms may initially increase cardiac output, they eventually have a damaging effect on pump function. Compensatory mechanisms contribute to increased myocardial oxygen consumption, leading to worsening signs and symptoms of HF. Compensatory mechanisms include:
    1. Sympathetic nervous system stimulation: increased heart rate, increased force of contraction, and arterial vasoconstriction that increases afterload
    2. Renin-angiotensin-aldosterone system (RAAS) activation: When perfusion to the kidney decreases during HF, these hormones are released to increase water and sodium reabsorption; angiotensin also increases arterial constriction or afterload
    3. Synthesis and release of B-type natriuretic peptide (BNP) from the overstretched atrium; BNP acts on kidneys to promote diuresis and decrease preload
    4. Inflammatory and growth factors are also released, contributing to myocardial hypertrophy; however, capillary or collateral vessel development may not be sufficient for adequate blood supply to the enlarged muscle, contributing to HF worsening

Considerations for Older Adults

Thyroxine (T_4) and thyroid-stimulating hormone (TSH) levels should be assessed in patients who are older than 65 years, have atrial fibrillation, or have evidence of thyroid disease. Heart failure (HF) may be caused or aggravated by hypothyroidism or hyperthyroidism.

H

PATIENT-CENTERED COLLABORATIVE CARE
Assessment
- Assessment findings include:
    1. History of hypertension, acute coronary syndrome, heart valve disease, or other myocardial disease such as myocarditis
    2. Dyspnea, orthopnea, breathlessness
    3. Decreased oxygen saturation (Spo_2) or Pao_2
    4. Increased respiratory rate and work of breathing including use of accessory muscles
    5. Crackles or rhonchi on auscultation
    6. Cough with or without frothy sputum
    7. Dysrhythmias, especially tachycardia
    8. Weak, thready peripheral pulses
    9. Weight gain, with more than 1 pound per day or 3 pounds per week indicating potential fluid retention (e.g., edema)

and a need for consultation with a physician or advanced practice nurse

! NURSING SAFETY PRIORITY: Action Alert

Edema is an extremely unreliable sign of HF. Be sure that accurate daily weights are taken every morning to document fluid retention. Weight is the most reliable indicator of fluid gain and loss! Use weight gain and loss as well as intake and output to establish goals of care.

10. Decreased mentation, restlessness, or anxiety
11. Increased heart size and vascular or interstitial fluid on chest radiograph
12. S_3 or S_4 heart sounds
13. Cardiomegaly by palpation, electrocardiograph (ECG), or chest radiograph
14. Increased serum B-type natriuretic peptide (BNP)
15. Peripheral edema
16. Jugular venous distention
17. Enlarged liver and spleen, especially with right-sided HF
18. Reduced kidney function including oliguria and increased BUN and serum creatinine
19. Anxiety and depression or other markers of psychological distress

Interventions
NONSURGICAL MANAGEMENT
Impaired Gas Exchange Related to Ventilation/Perfusion Imbalance
* Interventions include:
  1. Monitoring for improving or worsening pulmonary edema by assessing respiratory rate, rhythm, and character every 1 to 4 hours including auscultating breath sounds
  2. Titrating the amount of supplemental oxygen delivered to maintain oxygen saturation at 92% or greater
  3. Placing the patient experiencing respiratory difficulty in a high Fowler's position with pillows under each arm to maximize chest expansion and improve oxygenation
  4. Encouraging the patient to deep breathe and re-position himself or herself every 2 hours while awake and in bed

Decreased Cardiac Output Related to Altered Contractility, Preload, and Afterload
* Drug therapy to improve myocardial function
  1. Angiotensin-converting enzyme (ACE) inhibitors are used to prevent conversion of angiotensin I to angiotensin II, resulting

in reduction of arterial constriction. ACE inhibitors also block aldosterone, which prevents sodium and water retention, decreasing fluid overload. Monitor blood pressure, especially orthostatic pressure in older adults. Monitor serum potassium level for hyperkalemia, serum creatinine level for kidney dysfunction, and the patient for development of a cough. Monitor blood pressure to determine the patient's response to effective doses.

2. Beta blockers reduce the heart rate and interfere with the sympathetic nervous system compensatory mechanisms that promote adverse myocyte remodeling. Monitor for heart rates below 60 beats/min that cause the patient to exhibit symptomatic bradycardia.

3. Diuretics reduce intravascular volume, especially during an episode of exacerbation of HF. Monitor intake, output, and daily weights to determine fluid balance.

4. Oxygen therapy can be used to maintain or increase SpO_2 above 92%.

5. Digoxin (Lanoxin) increases contractility, reduces the heart rate, slows conduction through the arteriovenous node, and inhibits sympathetic activity while enhancing parasympathetic activity. Older patients, particularly those who are hypokalemic, are susceptible to digoxin toxicity.

! NURSING SAFETY PRIORITY: Drug Alert

H

Heart failure is managed with polypharmacy; typically, three or more drugs are used. The potential for drug interactions increases when three or more drugs are used regularly. Advise your patient and assist him or her in identifying potential drug interactions, including the use of NSAIDs, which can further cause significant acute kidney injury in the presence of low cardiac output.

- Diet therapy to reduce sodium and promote ideal body weight
  1. Collaborate with the dietitian and patient to select foods that meet a heart-healthy, sodium-restricted diet and to understand the importance of eliminating table salt and salt used in cooking. Increase the patient's intake of potassium-rich foods if using a loop or thiazide diuretic.
- Fluid restriction and monitoring
  1. Limit the patients in AHA class 3 or 4 to 2 L/day of fluids, including IV fluids; other HF patients may be restricted to 2.5 to 3 L/day. Weigh the patient every morning before breakfast using the same scale; this is the most reliable indicator of fluid

gain or loss (1 kg of weight gain or loss equals 1 L of fluid retained or lost).
2. Monitor and record intake and output and report or intervene when intake exceeds output by more than 500 mL.
3. Monitor for and prevent potassium deficiency from diuretic therapy. If the patient's potassium level is below 4 mEq/L, a potassium supplement may be prescribed.
4. Recognize that patients with kidney problems may develop hyperkalemia, especially with the use of potassium supplements, ACE inhibitors, or potassium-sparing diuretics. Kidney problems are indicated by a creatinine level higher than 1.8 mg/dL.

- Other options to treat HF:
  1. Continuous positive airway pressure (CPAP) improves sleep apnea (oxygen desaturation) and supports cardiac output and ejection fraction.
  2. Cardiac resynchronization therapy (CRT) uses a permanent pacemaker alone or in combination with an implantable cardioverter-defibrillator to provide biventricular pacing.
  3. Investigative stem cell and gene therapy replaces damaged myocytes or genes by a series of injections into the left ventricle.

Fatigue and Weakness Related to Hypoxia
- The most common symptom reported by patients with HF is fatigue. The purpose of collaborative care is to regulate energy, prevent fatigue, and optimize function:
  1. Provide periods of uninterrupted rest.
  2. Assess the patient's response to increased activity. Check for changes in blood pressure, pulse, and oxygen saturation before and after an episode of new or increased activity.

! NURSING SAFETY PRIORITY: Action Alert

An increase in the heart rate of more than 20 beats/min, a change (increase or decrease) in systolic blood pressure of more than 20 mm Hg, or a decrease in the SpO_2 of more than 5% indicates activity intolerance. The physician should be informed about these findings in case it is necessary to alter drug therapy or initiate a physical therapy consultation to promote rehabilitation.

SURGICAL MANAGEMENT
- Heart transplantation is the ultimate choice for end-stage HF. Procedures that include ventricular assist devices can improve cardiac output in patients who are not candidates for heart transplant or are awaiting transplantation.

- Surgical therapies to reshape the left ventricle in patients with HF include:
  1. Partial left ventriculectomy
  2. Endoventricular circular patch
  3. Acorn cardiac support device
  4. Myosplint cardiac support device perioperatively
- Care for the HF patient who is receiving a surgical intervention to improve pump failure is similar to patients receiving coronary revascularization or other open heart surgery. Specific monitoring and interventions include:
  1. Assessing the patient with HF for acute pulmonary edema. Clinical manifestations include decreased peripheral oxygenation (Spo_2); dyspnea; extreme anxiety; tachycardia; moist cough productive of frothy sputum; cold, clammy, cyanotic skin; crackles in lung bases; disorientation; and confusion.
  2. Administering rapid-acting diuretics, as prescribed
  3. Providing oxygen and maintaining the patient in a high Fowler's position
  4. Administering morphine sulfate intravenously to reduce venous return (preload), decrease anxiety, and reduce the work of breathing
  5. Administering other drugs such as bronchodilators and vasodilators
  6. Monitoring vital signs closely including pulse oximetry
  7. Monitoring intake and output; weighing daily

Community-Based Care

- Collaborate with the case manager or social worker to assess the patient's needs for health care resources (e.g., home care nurse) and social support (family and friends to help with care if needed), and facilitate appropriate placement.
- Discharge preparation includes:
  1. Encouraging the patient to stay as active as possible and developing a regular exercise program; investigating the possibility of a rehabilitation program referral
     a. If the patient experiences chest pain or pronounced dyspnea while exercising or experiences excessive fatigue, he or she is probably advancing the activity too quickly and should be returned to the previous level for 24 to 48 hours.
  2. Instructing the patient to watch for and report to the physician:
     a. Weight gain of more than 3 pounds in 1 week or 1 to 2 pounds overnight
     b. Decrease in exercise tolerance lasting 2 to 3 days
     c. Cold symptoms (cough) lasting more than 3 to 5 days
     d. Frequent urination at night

H

    e. Development of dyspnea or angina at rest, or worsening angina

    f. Increased swelling in the feet, ankles, and hands

3. Providing oral and written instructions concerning drugs
4. Teaching the patient and caregiver how to take and record the pulse rate and blood pressure to help monitor response to drug and exercise regimens
5. Instructing the patient to weigh himself or herself each day in the morning
6. Reviewing the signs and symptoms of dehydration and hypokalemia for patients on diuretics and providing information on foods high in potassium
7. Recommending that the patient restrict dietary sodium, providing written instructions on low-salt diets, and identifying food flavorings to use as a substitute for salt, such as lemon, garlic, and herbs
8. Discussing the importance of advance directives with the patient or family; if resuscitation is desired, the family should know how to activate the Emergency Medical System and how to provide CPR until an ambulance arrives. If CPR is not desired, the patient and family should be given resources on what to do and how to respond.

HEMOPHILIA

OVERVIEW

- Hemophilia is an inherited clotting disorder that leads to excessive bleeding.
- Two different clotting factor deficiencies result in hemophilia:
  1. *Hemophilia A (classic hemophilia)* is a deficiency of factor VIII and accounts for 80% of cases of hemophilia.
  2. *Hemophilia B (Christmas disease)* is a deficiency of factor IX and accounts for 20% of cases.

🧬 Genetic/Genomic Considerations

- Hemophilia is an X-linked recessive trait. Women who are carriers (able to pass on the gene without actually having the disorder) have a 50% chance of passing the hemophilia gene to their daughters (who then are carriers) and to their sons (who then have hemophilia). Affected men will pass the gene onto daughters, all of whom will be carriers, but not to their sons.
- About 30% of hemophilia arises from a new gene mutation and has no family history.

PATIENT-CENTERED COLLABORATIVE CARE

- Assess for and document:
  1. Excessive bleeding from minor cuts, bruises, or abrasions
  2. Joint and muscle hemorrhages that lead to disabling long-term problems
  3. A tendency to bruise easily or experience prolonged nosebleeds
  4. Prolonged and potentially fatal hemorrhage after surgery
  5. Prolonged partial thromboplastin time (PTT), a normal bleeding time, and a normal prothrombin time (PT)
- The bleeding problems of hemophilia A are managed by scheduled or intermittent infusions of factor VIII.
- Similarly, hemophilia B is managed with infusions of factor IX.

HEMORRHOIDS
OVERVIEW
- Hemorrhoids are unnaturally swollen or distended veins in the anorectal region that are common and not significant unless they cause pain or bleeding.
- Internal hemorrhoids cannot be seen on inspection of the perianal area and lie above the anal sphincter.
- External hemorrhoids can be seen on inspection and lie below the anal sphincter.
- Prolapsed hemorrhoids can become thrombosed or inflamed, or they can bleed.
- Common causes are increased abdominal pressure associated with pregnancy, constipation with straining, obesity, heart failure, prolonged sitting or standing, strenuous exercise, and weight lifting.

H

PATIENT-CENTERED COLLABORATIVE CARE
Assessment
- Assessment findings include:
  1. Bleeding, which is characteristically bright red and found on toilet tissue or outside the stool
  2. Pain associated with thrombosis
  3. Itching
  4. Mucous discharge
- Diagnosis is made by inspection, digital examination, and proctoscopy, if needed.

Interventions
Nonsurgical Management
- Conservative management focuses on reducing symptoms and includes:
  1. Application of cold packs to the anorectal area
  2. Tepid sitz baths 3 to 4 times daily

3. Topical anesthetics such as lidocaine (Xylocaine) or steroid cream to be used for short-term relief of pain and itching
4. Treatment for constipation: fluids, high-fiber diet, fiber supplements, stool softeners, and bowel stimulants
5. Teaching the patient to cleanse the anal area with moistened cleaning tissues and to gently dab the area rather than wipe

Surgical Management

- Ultrasound, laser removal, or other outpatient procedures may be indicated for prolapsed or thrombosed hemorrhoids. Monitor for bleeding and pain postoperatively. Warm compresses can promote comfort during recovery.

HEMOTHORAX

OVERVIEW

- Hemothorax is blood loss into the thoracic cavity and is a common result of blunt chest trauma or penetrating injuries.
  1. A simple hemothorax is a blood loss of less than 1500 mL.
  2. A massive hemothorax is a blood loss of more than 1500 mL, usually from heart, great vessels, or intercostal arteries.
- Bleeding can occur with rib and sternal fractures causing lung contusions and lacerations in addition to the hemothorax.
- Physical assessment findings depend on the size of the hemothorax.
  1. A small hemothorax may cause no symptoms.
  2. Symptoms of a hemothorax may include:
     a. Respiratory distress
     b. Reduced breath sounds
     c. Blood in the pleural space (seen on a chest x-ray and confirmed by diagnostic thoracentesis)
- Interventions, aimed at removing the blood in the pleural space to normalize pulmonary function and to prevent infection, include front and back chest tube insertion.
- A hemothorax may require an open thoracotomy to repair torn vessels and to evacuate the chest cavity.
- Nursing interventions include:
  1. Monitoring vital signs and reporting when signs of hypoperfusion or hypotension occur
  2. Carefully monitoring chest tube drainage for excessive blood loss
  3. Measuring intake and output
  4. Assessing the patient's response to the chest tubes
  5. Infusing IV fluids and blood as prescribed
- The blood lost through chest drainage can be autotransfused back into the patient if needed.

HEPATITIS

OVERVIEW

- Hepatitis is the widespread inflammation of liver cells, resulting in enlargement of the liver and congestion with inflammatory cells.
- Viral hepatitis is the most prevalent type and is caused by one of five common viruses. Many patients have multiple infections, especially the combination of hepatitis B virus with hepatitis C virus, hepatitis D, or human immunodeficiency virus infection.

1. Hepatitis A virus (HAV):
   a. HAV is an RNA virus of the enterovirus family. It is a hardy virus and survives on human hands. HAV is spread by the fecal-oral route, consuming contaminated food, or by person-to-person contact (e.g., oral-anal sexual activity). Unsanitary water, shellfish caught in contaminated water, and food contaminated by food handlers infected with HAV are all potential sources of infection.
   b. It is characterized by a mild course and often goes unrecognized. HAV is the most common type of viral hepatitis.
   c. The incubation period is usually 15 to 50 days.

2. Hepatitis B virus (HBV):
   a. HBV is a double-shelled particle containing DNA composed of a core antigen (HBcAg), a surface antigen (HBsAg), and another antigen found within the core (HBeAg) that circulates in the blood.
   b. HBV is transmitted through broken skin or mucous membranes by infected blood and serous fluids. Lower concentrations of HBV are also found in semen, vaginal fluid, and saliva.
   c. HBV is spread by sexual contact, shared needles, accidental needle sticks or injuries from sharp instruments, blood transfusion, hemodialysis, acupuncture, tattooing, ear or body piercing, mother-fetal route, and close person-to-person contact by open cuts and sores.
   d. The clinical course is varied, with an insidious onset and mild symptoms (such as anorexia, nausea, vomiting, fever, fatigue, and dark urine with light stool).
   e. The incubation period is generally between 25 and 180 days.

3. Hepatitis C virus (HCV):
   a. The causative virus is an enveloped, single-strand RNA virus that is transmitted blood to blood.
   b. HCV is spread by contaminated items such as illicit IV drug needles, blood and blood products and transplanted

H

organs received before 1992, needle stick injury with HCV-contaminated blood, tattoos, and sharing of intranasal cocaine paraphernalia.
  c. It is not transmitted by casual contact or intimate household contacts. However, those infected should not share razors, toothbrushes, or pierced earrings, because there may be microscopic blood on these items.
  d. The average incubation period is 7 weeks.
  e. Chronic liver disease occurs in 85% of those infected. HCV cirrhosis is the leading indicator for liver transplantation.
4. Hepatitis D (delta hepatitis or HDV):
  a. HDV is a defective RNA virus that needs the helper function of HBV for viral replication. HDV co-infects with HBV.
  b. Incubation period is 14 to 56 days.
  c. HDV is transmitted primarily by parenteral routes.
5. Hepatitis E virus (HEV):
  a. HEV is caused by fecal contamination of food or water.
  b. The incubation period is 15 to 64 days.

- Toxic and drug-induced forms of hepatitis result from exposure to hepatotoxins such as industrial toxins, alcohol, or drugs. Treatment is supportive.
- Hepatitis may occur as a secondary infection during the course of other viral infections, such as cytomegalovirus, Epstein-Barr virus, herpes simplex virus, and varicella-zoster virus.
- Fulminant hepatitis is a failure of the liver cells to regenerate, with progression of the necrotic process that is often fatal.
- Liver inflammation persisting longer than 6 months is considered *chronic hepatitis.*

PATIENT-CENTERED COLLABORATIVE CARE
Assessment
- Record patient information:
  1. Known exposure to persons with hepatitis infection or a contaminated water source:
    a. Crowded living conditions increase transmission occurrence
    b. Health care work increases exposure to hepatitis
    c. Travel to another country
    d. Unprotected sexual activity (with someone with a hepatic infection)
  2. Blood transfusions or organ transplantation
  3. History of hemodialysis
  4. Injectable drug use
  5. Recent ear or body piercing or tattooing

6. Recent ingestion of shellfish
7. HIV infection
8. History of alcohol abuse or illicit intravenous or intranasal drug use
- Assessment findings for viral hepatitis include:
  1. Abdominal pain
  2. Changes in skin or sclera (icterus)
  3. Fever, arthralgia (joint pain) or myalgia (muscle pain), and lethargy or malaise
  4. Diarrhea or constipation, clay-colored stools
  5. Dark or amber-colored urine
  6. Nausea and vomiting
  7. Pruritus (itching)
  8. Liver tenderness in the right upper quadrant
  9. Elevated serum liver enzymes
  10. Elevated total bilirubin (serum and urine)
  11. Serologic markers for hepatitis A, B, C, or D
- The clinical manifestations of toxic and drug-induced hepatitis depend on the causative agent.
- Patients may be angry about being sick and being fatigued; may feel guilty about having exposed others to the disease; may be embarrassed by the isolation and hygiene precautions that are necessary; and may be worried about the loss of wages, cost of hospitalization, and general financial issues.
- Family members may be afraid of contracting the disease and therefore distance themselves from the patient. Counsel about the value of hepatitis vaccination.

Planning and Implementation
- Promote rest.
  1. Maintain physical rest alternating with periods of activity to promote liver cell regeneration by reducing the liver's metabolic needs.
  2. Individualize the patient's plan of care and change it to reflect the severity of symptoms, fatigue, and the results of liver function tests and enzyme determinations.
- Provide diet therapy. A special diet is not needed, but diet should be high in carbohydrates and calories with moderate amounts of fat and protein.
  1. Determine food preferences.
  2. Provide small, frequent meals and high-calorie snacks as needed.
- Drug therapy includes immunomodulators and antiviral drugs:
  1. Interferon
  2. Tenofovir (Viread), adefovir (Hepsera) or lamivudine (Epivir-HBV), entecavir (Baraclude), and others

H

3. Simeprevir (Olysio) and sofosbuvir (Sovaldi) for patients with hepatitis C

- Liver transplantation may be performed for patients with end-stage liver disease from chronic hepatitis.

Community-Based Care

- Provide health teaching, including:
  1. Give patients information about modes of viral transmission.
  2. Maintain adequate sanitation and personal hygiene. Wash your hands before eating and after using the toilet.
  3. If traveling in underdeveloped or nonindustrialized countries, drink only bottled water. Avoid food washed or prepared with tap water, such as raw vegetables, fruits, and soups. Avoid ice.
  4. Use adequate sanitation practices to prevent the spread of the disease among family members. Do not share bed linens, towels, eating utensils, or drinking glasses.
  5. Do not share needles for injection, body piercing, or tattooing.
  6. Do not share razors, nail clippers, toothbrushes, or Waterpiks.
  7. Use a condom during sexual intercourse, or abstain from this activity.
  8. Cover cuts or sores with bandages.
  9. If ever infected with hepatitis, never donate blood, body organs, or other body tissue.

HERNIA

OVERVIEW

- A hernia is a weakness in the abdominal muscle wall through which a segment of bowel or other abdominal structure protrudes. Increased intra-abdominal pressure can contribute to hernia formation.
- Hernias are labeled by anatomic location, combined with the severity of protrusion:
  1. An *indirect inguinal hernia* is a sac formed from the peritoneum that contains a portion of the intestine or omentum; in men, indirect hernias can become large and descend into the scrotum.
  2. A *direct inguinal hernia* passes through a weak point in the abdominal wall.
  3. A *femoral hernia* occurs through the femoral ring as a plug of fat in the femoral canal that enlarges and pulls the peritoneum and the bladder into the sac.
  4. An *umbilical hernia* is congenital (infancy) or acquired as a result of increased intra-abdominal pressure, most often in obese persons.

5. An *incisional (ventral) hernia* occurs at the site of a previous surgical incision as a result of inadequate healing, postoperative wound infection, inadequate nutrition, or obesity.

6. A *reducible hernia* allows the contents of the hernia sac to be reduced or placed back into the abdominal cavity.

7. An *irreducible,* or *incarcerated, hernia* cannot be reduced or placed back into the abdominal cavity. It requires immediate surgical evaluation.

8. A *strangulated hernia* results when the blood supply to the herniated segment of the bowel is cut off by pressure from the hernia ring, causing ischemia and obstruction of the bowel loop; this can lead to bowel necrosis and perforation, which are surgical emergencies.

PATIENT-CENTERED COLLABORATIVE CARE
Assessment
- Assess for a hernia when the patient is lying down and again when the patient is standing. If a hernia is reducible, it may disappear when the patient is lying flat.
- Listen for bowel sounds (absence may indicate GI obstruction).

Interventions
Nonsurgical Management
- A truss (a pad with firm support) may be used for patients who are poor surgical risks.

Surgical Management
- Herniorrhaphy, the surgical treatment of choice, involves replacing the contents of the hernia sac into the abdominal cavity and closing the opening.
- Hernioplasty reinforces the weakened muscular wall with a mesh patch.
- Provide preoperative and postoperative care described in Part One and instruct the patient to:
  1. Avoid coughing but encourage deep breathing.
  2. For inguinal hernia repair, wear a scrotal support and elevate the scrotum with a soft pillow when in bed.
  3. Avoid bladder and bowel distention by:
     a. Using techniques to stimulate voiding, such as assisting a man to stand
     b. Avoiding constipation and teaching the patient to avoid straining with stool during healing

Community-Based Care
- Teach the patient:
  1. How to care for the incision if surgery corrects the muscle defect

H

   2. To limit activity, including avoiding lifting and straining, for several weeks after surgery
      3. To report to the health care provider symptoms such as fever and chills, wound drainage, redness or separation of the incision, and increasing incisional pain

HERNIA, HIATAL

OVERVIEW

- Hiatal hernias, also called *diaphragmatic hernias,* involve the protrusion of the stomach through the esophageal hiatus (opening) of the diaphragm into the chest.
- There are two major types of hiatal hernias:
  1. *Sliding hernia,* which occurs when the esophagogastric junction and a portion of the fundus of the stomach slide upward through the esophageal hiatus into the thorax, with the hernia moving freely and sliding into and out of the thorax with changes in position or increases in intra-abdominal pressure
  2. *Paraesophageal,* or *rolling, hernia,* which occurs when the gastroesophageal junction stays below the diaphragm but the fundus and portions of the greater curvature of the stomach roll through the esophageal hiatus and into the thorax beside the esophagus; risk for volvulus, obstruction, and strangulation are high

PATIENT-CENTERED COLLABORATIVE CARE

Assessment

- Assessment findings include:
  1. Symptoms of gastroesophageal reflux disease (GERD), dysphagia, heartburn, chest or esophageal pain, belching
  2. A feeling of fullness after eating or a feeling of breathlessness or suffocation
  3. Increased symptoms when the patient is in a supine position
  4. Confirmation via a barium swallow study with fluoroscopy is the most specific diagnostic test

Interventions

Nonsurgical Management

- Drug therapy includes the use of a proton pump inhibitor to control esophageal reflux and its symptoms.
- Teach the patient to avoid fatty foods, caffeine, carbonation, chocolate, alcohol, spicy foods, and acidic foods such as orange juice.
- Encourage the patient to eat small-volume meals and consume liquids between meals to avoid abdominal distention.
- Encourage weight reduction, because obesity increases intra-abdominal pressure.
- Elevate the head of the bed 6 or more inches.

- Instruct the patient to avoid lying down for several hours after eating, and to avoid straining or excessively vigorous exercise and wearing tight or constrictive clothing.

Surgical Management

- Elective surgery is indicated when the risk of complications such as aspiration are high and damage from chronic reflux is severe.
- Surgical approaches for sliding hernias involve reinforcement of the LES to restore sphincter competence and prevent reflux through some degree of fundoplication, or the wrapping of a portion of the stomach fundus around the distal esophagus to anchor it and reinforce the LES.
- Provide preoperative and postoperative care as described in Part One and:
    1. Provide safe and effective care for the patient with a chest tube if a transthoracic approach was used.
    2. Assess for complications of surgery, such as temporary dysphagia after oral feeding begins, gas bloat syndrome, atelectasis or pneumonia, and obstruction of the NG tube.
    3. Prevent aspiration and respiratory complications with positioning, early ambulation, and use of incentive spirometry while providing adequate pain relief.
    4. Elevate the head of the bed at least 30 degrees.
    5. Teach the patient to support the incisional area during coughing and deep breathing.
    6. Ensure correct placement and patency of the NG tube.
    7. Reinforce dietary restrictions and nutritional goals.

Community-Based Care

- Advise the patient:
    1. To avoid lifting and restrict stair climbing for 3 to 6 weeks after surgical repair
    2. To inspect the surgical wound daily and report the incidence of swelling, redness, tenderness, or discharge to the physician
    3. About the importance of reporting fever or other signs of infection to the surgeon
    4. To avoid people with respiratory infection because prolonged coughing can cause the incision to break open (dehisce)
    5. To stop smoking; inform about strategies for smoking cessation
    6. About diet modifications, including weight loss goals if needed, eating small portions, avoiding irritating foods and liquids, and reporting recurrence of reflux symptoms to the physician
    7. To avoid straining and prevent constipation; stool softeners or bulk laxatives may be needed

HERPES, GENITAL
OVERVIEW
- Genital herpes (GH) is an acute, recurring, incurable viral disease.
- The two types of herpes simplex virus (HSV) are diagnosed and treated with the same interventions. The two types are:
  1. Type 1 (HSV-1), which causes most nongenital lesions such as cold sores and about one third of genital herpes infections
  2. Type 2 (HSV-2), which causes most of the genital lesions

! NURSING SAFETY PRIORITY: Action Alert

Either type of virus can produce oral or genital lesions through oral-genital contact with an infected person.

- The incubation period is 2 to 20 days, with the average period being 1 week; many people do not have symptoms during this time.
- Recurrences are not caused by re-infection but by reactivation of dormant virus. Recurrent episodes are usually less severe and of shorter duration than the primary infection. However, there is viral shedding and the patient is infectious with each outbreak of vesicles.
- Long-term complications of GH include the risk of neonatal transmission and an increased risk for acquiring HIV infection.

PATIENT-CENTERED COLLABORATIVE CARE
Assessment
- Obtain patient information about:
  1. The sensation of itching or tingling felt in the skin 1 to 2 days before the outbreak
  2. Whether he or she has had headaches or general malaise
  3. Presence of painful urination or urinary retention
  4. Factors that can trigger virus re-activation such as stress, fever, sunburn, poor nutrition, menses, and sexual activity
- Assess for and document:
  1. The presence of *vesicles* (blisters) in a typical cluster on the penis, scrotum, vulva, vagina, cervix, or perianal region
  2. The presence of painful erosions
  3. Swelling of inguinal lymph nodes
- Diagnostic tests for GH include:
  1. Viral culture
  2. Polymerase chain reaction (PCR) assay of the lesions from blister fluid
  3. Serology testing to identify the HSV type, including type-specific rapid assays

Interventions

- GH is treated with antiviral medications such as acyclovir (Zovirax, Avirax ❧), famciclovir (Famvir), or valacyclovir (Valtrex).

> **! NURSING SAFETY PRIORITY: Drug Alert**
>
> The drugs do not cure the infection, but while they are being used they do decrease the severity, promote healing, and decrease the frequency of recurrent outbreaks.

- Emphasize the risk for neonatal infection to all patients, both male and female.
- Teach patients to avoid transmission by:
  1. Adhering to suppressive therapy
  2. Abstaining from sexual activity while lesions are present
  3. Using condoms during all sexual exposures

> **! NURSING SAFETY PRIORITY: Action Alert**
>
> Remind patients to abstain from sexual activity while lesions are present. Urge condom use during all sexual exposures because of the increased risk for HSV transmission. Viral shedding can occur even when lesions are not present. Teach the patient about how and when to use condoms.

  4. Keeping the skin in the genital region clean and dry
  5. Washing hands thoroughly after contact with lesions and laundering towels that have had direct contact with lesions
  6. Wearing gloves when applying ointments
- Help patients and their partners cope with the diagnosis by assessing the patient's and partner's emotional responses to the diagnosis of genital herpes

HIV DISEASE (HIV/AIDS)

OVERVIEW

- Human immunodeficiency virus (HIV) disease is the most common immunodeficiency disease worldwide.
- From the onset of HIV infection through progression to acquired immunodeficiency syndrome (AIDS), the late and final stage, HIV disease represents a continuing battle between the virus and the patient's immune system.
- HIV is a retrovirus, with proteins on its surface that allow it to dock onto T4 (CD4+) cells. The virus has *reverse transcriptase* (RT) and *integrase,* which allow it to incorporate its genetic material into the host cell. These features give HIV major advantages for infecting humans by reproducing sufficient viruses to pass the infection along.

- HIV is transmitted in three ways:
  1. *Sexual:* genital, anal, or oral sexual contact with exposure of mucous membranes to infected semen or vaginal secretions
  2. *Parenteral:* sharing of needles or equipment contaminated with infected blood or receiving contaminated blood products
     a. Needle stick or "sharps" injuries are the main means of occupation-related HIV infection for health care workers.
     b. Health care workers also can be infected through exposure of nonintact skin and mucous membranes to blood and body fluids.
  3. *Perinatal:* from the placenta, from contact with maternal blood and body fluids during birth, or from breast milk from an infected mother to child
- *A person with HIV infection can transmit the virus to others at all stages of disease.*
- As a result of immune abnormalities, the patient who is HIV positive is at risk for bacterial, fungal, and viral infections, and for some opportunistic cancers.
- *Opportunistic infections* are those caused by organisms that are present as part of the normal environment and are kept in check by normal immune function.
- The Centers for Disease Control defines HIV in stages:
  1. Stage 1: A patient with a CD4+ T-cell count greater than 500 cells/mm^3 or a percentage of 29% or greater; a person at this stage has no AIDS-defining illnesses.
  2. Stage 2: A patient with a CD4+ T-cell count between 200 and 499 cells/mm^3 or a percentage between 14% and 28%; a person at this stage has no AIDS-defining illnesses.
  3. Stage 3: Any patient with a CD4+ T-cell count less than 200 cells/mm^3 or a percentage of less than 14%; a person who has higher CD4+ T-cell counts or percentages but who also has an AIDS-defining illness meets the Stage 3 CDC case definition.
  4. Stage 4: This stage describes any patient with a confirmed HIV infection but no information regarding CD4+ T-cell counts, CD4+ T-cell percentages, and AIDS-defining illnesses is available.
- Everyone who has AIDS has HIV infection; however, not everyone who has HIV infection has AIDS.
- A diagnosis of AIDS requires that the person is HIV positive and has one of the following:
  1. A CD4+ T-cell count of less than 200 cells/mm^3
  2. An opportunistic infection
- Immune system abnormalities resulting from HIV disease include:
  1. Lymphocytopenia (decreased numbers of lymphocytes, especially CD4+ T-cell levels)

    2. Increased production of incomplete and nonfunctional antibodies

    3. Abnormally functioning macrophages

- Once AIDS is diagnosed, even if the patient's cell count goes higher than 200 cells/mm³ or if the infection is successfully treated, the AIDS diagnosis remains and the patient never reverts to being just HIV positive.

- The time from the beginning of HIV infection to development of AIDS ranges from months to years, depending on:

    1. How HIV was acquired

    2. Personal factors, such as frequency of re-exposure to HIV, presence of other STDs, nutritional status, and stress

    3. Interventions used

Genetic/Genomic Considerations

- About 1% of people with HIV infection are long-term nonprogressors (LTNPs). These people have been infected with HIV for at least 10 years and have remained asymptomatic, with CD4+ T-cell counts within the normal range and a viral load that is either undetectable or very low.

- A genetic difference for this population is that their CCR5/CXCR4 co-receptors on the CD4+ T-cells are abnormal and nonfunctional as a result of gene mutations for these co-receptors. The mutation creates defective co-receptors that do not bind to the HIV docking proteins. Cells with this defective co-receptor successfully resist the entrance of HIV.

H

Cultural Considerations

- Most new HIV infections reported in the United States occur in racial and ethnic minority groups, particularly among African Americans and Hispanics. These two groups show an increasing trend in HIV infection compared with a leveling off among white people.

Considerations for Older Adults

- Infection with HIV can occur at any age, and older patients should be assessed for risk behaviors, including a sexual and drug use history. Age-related decline in immune function increases the likelihood that the older adult will develop the infection after an HIV exposure.

Gender Health Considerations

- About 25% of newly diagnosed cases are women. In less affluent countries, 50% of cases occur in women. The largest risk factor is sexual exposure. Strategies specifically targeted to reducing sexual exposures of HIV to women may help prevent an increase in HIV infection in that group. Women with HIV infection have a poorer outcome with shorter mean survival time than that of men. This outcome may be the result of late diagnosis and social or economic factors that reduce access to medical care.
- Gynecologic problems, especially persistent or recurrent vaginal candidiasis, may be the first signs of HIV infection in women. Other problems include pelvic inflammatory disease, genital herpes, other STDs, and cervical dysplasia or cancer.
- The effect of HIV on pregnancy outcomes includes higher incidence of premature delivery, low-birth-weight infants, and transmission of the disease to the infant. Appropriate antiretroviral drug therapy during pregnancy reduces the risk for transmitting the infection to the infant.

PATIENT-CENTERED COLLABORATIVE CARE

Assessment
- Obtain patient information about:
  1. Age and gender
  2. Occupation
  3. Current illness
     a. Nature of the illness
     b. When it started
     c. Severity of symptoms
     d. Associated problems
     e. Interventions to date
  4. When HIV infection was diagnosed
  5. Chronologic history of infections and clinical problems since the diagnosis
  6. Health history, including transfusion history
  7. Sexual practices
  8. Any infectious diseases, including STDs, tuberculosis, and hepatitis
  9. Injection drug use, including needle exposure and needle sharing
  10. Level of knowledge regarding the diagnosis, symptom management, diagnostic tests, treatments, community resources, and modes of HIV transmission
  11. Understanding and use of safer sex practices

- Assess for and document:
  1. Immune system changes
     a. WBC count and differential
     b. Hypergammaglobulinemia
     c. Opportunistic infections
     d. Lymphadenopathy
     e. Fatigue
  2. Skin changes
     a. Dry, itchy, irritated skin
     b. Rashes
     c. Folliculitis
     d. Eczema
     e. Psoriasis
     f. Poor wound healing
     g. Purple lesions
  3. Respiratory changes
     a. Shortness of breath
     b. Cough
  4. Central nervous system (CNS) changes
     a. Confusion and memory loss
     b. AIDS dementia complex
     c. Fever
     d. Headache
     e. Visual changes
     f. Personality changes
     g. Pain
     h. Peripheral neuropathies
     i. Gait changes, ataxia
     j. Seizures
  5. GI changes
     a. Diarrhea
     b. Nausea
     c. Weight loss
  6. Opportunistic infections
     a. Protozoal infections
        (1) *Pneumocystis jiroveci* pneumonia
        (2) *Toxoplasma gondii*
        (3) *Cryptosporidium*
     b. Fungal infections
        (1) *Candida albicans*
        (2) *Cryptococcus neoformans*
        (3) *Histoplasma capsulatum*
     c. Bacterial infections
        (1) *Mycobacterium avium*
        (2) *Mycobacterium intracellulare*
        (3) *Mycobacterium tuberculosis*

H

      d. Viral infection
        (1) Cytomegalovirus (CMV)
        (2) Herpes simplex virus (HSV)
        (3) Varicella-zoster virus (VZV)
   7. Malignancies
      a. Kaposi's sarcoma (KS)
      b. Hodgkin's lymphoma
      c. Non-Hodgkin's lymphoma
      d. Invasive cervical cancer
   8. Endocrine changes
      a. Gonadal dysfunction
      b. Adrenal insufficiency
      c. Diabetes mellitus
      d. Hyperlipidemia
   9. Abnormal laboratory findings
      a. WBC count of less than 3500 cells/mm^3
      b. CD4+ T-cell numbers decreased
      c. Low ratio of CD4+ to CD8+ T-cells

- Assess psychosocial issues, such as:
  1. The availability of a support system, such as family and significant others:
     a. Learn who in this support system is aware of the patient's diagnosis.
     b. Identify whether a health care proxy or durable power-of-attorney document has been signed.
  2. Employment status and occupation
  3. Changes in performance of ADLs
  4. Living arrangements
  5. Financial resources, including health insurance
  6. Alcohol or recreational drug use
  7. Anxiety level, mood, cognitive ability, and level of energy
  8. Self-esteem and changes in body image
  9. Suicidal ideation, depression
  10. Use of support groups or other community resources
  11. Energy level

- Diagnostic testing includes:
  1. Antibody tests
     a. Enzyme-linked immunosorbent assay (ELISA)
     b. Western blot analysis
     c. Genomic viral testing
     d. Transmucosal exudate (not saliva) collected from cheek and gums: solution turns positive with presence of HIV antibodies
  2. Viral load testing (also called viral burden testing) by quantitative RNA assays

3. Other laboratory tests to monitor for abnormal values or changes that affect the overall health of the patient
   a. Blood chemistries
   b. Complete blood count (CBC) with differential
   c. Toxoplasmosis antibody titer
   d. Liver function tests
   e. Cervical and anal Papanicolaou (Pap); serologic test for syphilis (STS)
   f. Antigens to hepatitis A, hepatitis B, and hepatitis C
   g. Purified protein derivative (PPD) for tuberculosis
   h. Lipid profile

Planning and Implementation
RISK FOR INFECTION RELATED TO IMMUNE DEFICIENCY

- Patients with AIDS are at high risk for opportunistic infections.
- Drug therapy for HIV/AIDS prolongs immune function and prevents opportunistic infections.
- Antiretroviral therapy only inhibits viral replication and does not kill the virus.
- Multiple drugs are used together in regimens popularly called *cocktails,* consisting of combinations of different types of antiretroviral agents, an approach called *highly active antiretroviral therapy* (HAART).

> **! NURSING SAFETY PRIORITY: Critical Rescue**
>
> Ensure that HAART drugs are not missed, delayed, or administered in doses lower than prescribed in the inpatient setting to prevent the development of drug resistance in the virus.

1. *Nucleoside analogue reverse transcriptase inhibitors* (NRTI) suppress production of reverse transcriptase (RT) and inhibit viral DNA synthesis and replication. Drugs in this class include abacavir (Ziagen), didanosine (Videx), emtricitabine (Emtriva), lamivudine (Epivir), stavudine (Zerit), tenofovir (Viread), and zidovudine (Retrovir).
2. *Non-nucleoside reverse transcriptase inhibitors* (NNRTI) inhibit synthesis of reverse transcriptase to suppress viral replication. These drugs include delavirdine (Rescriptor), efavirenz (Sustiva), and etravirine (Intelence), nevirapine (Viramune, others), and rilpivirine (Edurant).
3. *Protease inhibitors* block the HIV protease enzyme, preventing release of viral particles from the infected CD4+ cell to infect other cells. These drugs include atazanavir (Reyataz), darunavir (Prezista), fosamprenavir (Lexiva), indinavir (Crixivan), lopinavir/ritonavir (Kaletra), nelfinavir (Viracept), saquinavir (Invirase), and tipranavir (Aptivus).

4. *Integrase inhibitors* work to prevent infection by inhibiting the enzyme integrase, which is needed to insert the viral DNA into the host cell's human DNA. These drugs include dolutegravir (DTG), elvitegravir (EVG), and raltegravir (Isentress).
5. *Fusion inhibitors* work by blocking the fusion of HIV with a host cell; without fusion, infection of new cells does not occur. The major drug in this category is enfuvirtide (Fuzeon).
6. *Entry inhibitors* work to prevent infection by blocking the CCR5 receptor on CD4+ T-cells. Because this drug prevents only one type of receptor-virus interaction, the HIV virus must be tested to be sure it uses this receptor before adopting this drug. The major drug in this category is maraviroc (Selzentry).
7. Combination products have multiple agents; each ingredient has the same mechanism of action as the parent drug. The combination products reduce pill burden. These drugs include Atripla (emtricitabine, tenofovir, and efavirenz), Combivir (lamivudine and zidovudine), Complera (emtricitabine, rilpivirine, and tenofovir), Epzicom (lamivudine and abacavir), Stribild (elvitegravir, cobicistat, emtricitabine, and tenofovir), Truvada (emtricitabine and tenofovir), and Trizivir (lamivudine, zidovudine, and abacavir).

- Nursing measures to prevent infection in the patient with HIV/AIDS include:
  1. Following Standard Precautions and good handwashing techniques
  2. Using best practices for IV site care and wound care
  3. Using best practices to prevent hospital-acquired infections, particularly related to indwelling urinary catheters, central venous lines, and peripheral intravenous lines
  4. Minimizing exposure to crowds and other patients with infection
- Nursing measures to promote oxygenation and maintain adequate gas exchange include:
  1. Monitoring the rate and depth of respiration and informing the provider of deterioration
  2. Assessing pulse oximetry (Spo_2) every 8 hours and with a change in respiratory status
  3. Assessing breath sounds and determining presence of cyanosis or pallor indicating inadequate oxygenation
  4. Ensuring oxygen therapy, if ordered, maintains Spo_2 of greater than 92%
  5. Elevating the head of bed 30 to 45 degrees to minimize the risk for aspiration in intubated adults
  6. Ensuring administration of drug therapy for gas exchange problems resulting from *Pneumocystis carinii* pneumonia (PCP);

these drugs include trimethoprim/sulfamethoxazole (Apo-Sulfatrim ♣, Bactrim, Cotrim, Septra), pentamidine (Pentacarinat ♣, Pentam), dapsone (Avlosulfon), and atovaquone (Mepron)

7. Pacing activities to avoid dyspnea

MANAGING PAIN

- Pain with HIV/AIDS has many origins, including enlarged organs stretching the viscera or compressing nerves, tumor invasion of bone and other tissues, peripheral neuropathy, and generalized joint and muscle pain.
- Drug therapy with different classes of drugs is used to manage pain from different causes:
  1. Arthralgia and myalgia respond to NSAIDs
  2. Neuropathic pain of peripheral neuropathy
     a. Tricyclic antidepressants, such as amitriptyline (Elavil)
     b. Anticonvulsant drugs, such as phenytoin (Dilantin) or carbamazepine (Tegretol)
  3. General pain can be managed with opioids
     a. Weaker opioids, such as oxycodone or codeine
     b. Stronger opioids, such as morphine, hydromorphone (Dilaudid), or transdermal fentanyl (Duragesic)
- Comfort measures
  1. Pressure-relieving mattress pads
  2. Warm baths or other forms of hydrotherapy
  3. Massage
  4. Application of heat or cold to painful areas
  5. Use of lift sheets to avoid pulling or grasping the patient with joint pain
  6. Frequent position changes
- Complementary and alternative therapies
  1. Acupuncture
  2. Guided imagery
  3. Distraction
  4. Progressive relaxation
  5. Body-talk
  6. Biofeedback
- Poor nutrition has many causes and requires an interdisciplinary team to determine the exact cause or causes.
  1. Medications
     a. Drug therapy to treat underlying causes includes antifungal agents for esophagitis, such as ketoconazole (Nizoral) or fluconazole (Diflucan)
     b. Antiemetics for nausea and vomiting can improve oral intake
  2. Comfort measures
     a. Providing frequent mouth care
     b. Keeping the environment pleasant and free from offensive odors

H

   3. Nutritional therapy
      a. Assessing food preferences and any dietary cultural or religious practices
      b. Monitoring weight, intake and output, and calorie count to detect weight gain/loss
      c. Teaching the patient about a high-calorie, high-protein, nutritionally sound diet
      d. Encouraging him or her to avoid dietary fat
      e. Collaborating with the dietitian
      f. Providing small, frequent meals
      g. Administering prescribed supplemental vitamins, fluid, or supplements
      h. Providing prescribed tube feedings or total parenteral nutrition

MINIMIZING DIARRHEA AND ITS COMPLICATIONS

- Nursing interventions include:
   1. Administering antidiarrheals, such as diphenoxylate (Diarsed ✚, Lomotil) or loperamide (Imodium), as prescribed
   2. Consulting with the dietitian to identify food with low fiber; provide less fatty, spicy, and sweet food; and no alcohol or caffeine
   3. Assessing the perineal skin every 8 to 12 hours
   4. Providing a bedside commode or a bedpan if needed

RESTORING SKIN INTEGRITY

- Kaposi's sarcoma (KS) is the most common skin lesion
   1. Lesions may be localized or widespread; monitor for progression.
   2. Lesions are managed with local radiation, intralesional chemotherapy, or cryotherapy.
      a. Lesions respond well to antiretroviral therapy. For rapidly progressive disease or with major involvement of the intestinal tract, lungs, or other organs, therapy may include antineoplastic agents (chemotherapy) or interferon-alpha.
   3. Clean and dress open, weeping KS lesions.
   4. To disguise the lesions, teach patients to:
      a. Use makeup over intact lesions
      b. Wear long-sleeved shirts
      c. Wear hats
- HSV lesions or shingles may occur and form abscesses.
   1. Provide good skin care to keep the area clean and dry.
   2. Clean abscesses at least once per shift with normal saline and allow them to air-dry.
   3. Provide aluminum acetate (Burow's solution, Domeboro) soaks.
   4. Administer prescribed antiviral drugs, including acyclovir (Zovirax) or valacyclovir (Valtrex).

Minimizing Confusion
- Nursing interventions include:
  1. Assessing baseline neurologic and mental status
  2. Evaluating the patient for subtle changes in memory, ability to concentrate, affect, and behavior
  3. Re-orienting the confused patient to person, time, and place
  4. Reminding the patient of your identity and explaining what is to be done at any given time
  5. Giving information and directions in short, uncomplicated sentences
  6. Involving the patient in planning the daily schedule
  7. Asking relatives or significant others to bring in familiar items from home
  8. Making the environment safe and comfortable
  9. Administering prescribed psychotropic drugs, antidepressants, or anxiolytics
  10. Assessing the patient with neurologic manifestations for increased intracranial pressure

! NURSING SAFETY PRIORITY: Critical Rescue

Immediately report to the physician changes in level of consciousness or seizure activity, vital signs, pupil size or reactivity, and limb strength for appropriate intervention.

SUPPORTING SELF-ESTEEM

H

- Self-esteem is affected by dramatic changes in appearance that alter the person's body image; abrupt, significant changes in his or her relationships with others; and changes in day-to-day activities, employment, or other productive activities.
- Nursing interventions include:
  1. Providing a climate of acceptance for patients with AIDS by promoting a trusting relationship
  2. Helping patients to express feelings and identify their positive aspects
  3. Allowing for privacy, but not avoiding or isolating the patient
  4. Encouraging self-care, independence, control, and decision making by helping him or her set short-term, attainable goals and offering praise when goals are achieved
  5. Maintaining social contact and helping him or her identify support systems, including those already in place and those that need to be arranged

Community-Based Care
- *Teaching about HIV transmission is the most important aspect for prevention of HIV.* All people, regardless of age, gender, ethnicity,

or sexual orientation, are susceptible to HIV infection. HIV infection is preventable because of the mode of viral transmission and the fragile nature of the virus.

- Collaborate with the health care team members, patient, and family to plan for self-management
  1. Assess the patient's status, ability to perform self-care activities, and identify the potential need for care, such as:
     a. Assistance with ADLs
     b. Around-the-clock nursing care
     c. Drug administration
     d. Nutritional support
  2. Assess available resources, including family members and significant others willing and able to be caregivers.
  3. Help the family make arrangements for outside caregivers or respite care, if needed.
  4. Refer the patient to support groups, a financial counselor, a social worker, legal services, and a spiritual counselor.
  5. Determine the need for assistance with end of life decisions.
- Teach the patient, family, and significant others about:
  1. Modes of HIV transmission and preventive behaviors
  2. Guidelines for safer sex
  3. Not sharing toothbrushes, razors, and other potentially blood-contaminated articles
  4. Manifestations of infection
     a. Temperature higher than 100° F (38° C)
     b. Persistent cough (with or without sputum)
     c. Pus or foul-smelling drainage from any open skin area or normal body opening
     d. Presence of a boil or abscess
     e. Urine that is cloudy or foul-smelling or that causes burning on urination
  5. Good infection control practices, such as:
     a. Avoiding crowds and other large gatherings of people where someone may be ill
     b. Not sharing personal toilet articles, such as toothbrushes, toothpaste, washcloths, or deodorant sticks, with others
     c. Bathing daily, using an antimicrobial soap; if total bathing is not possible, washing the armpits, groin, genitals, and anal area twice daily with an antimicrobial soap
     d. Cleaning the toothbrush daily by running it through the dishwasher or rinsing it in liquid laundry bleach
     e. Washing hands thoroughly with an antimicrobial soap before eating or drinking, after touching a pet, after shaking hands with anyone, returning home from any outing, and after using the toilet

   f. Washing dishes between uses with hot sudsy water or using a dishwasher
   g. Not drinking water, milk, juice, or other cold liquids that have been standing for longer than an hour
   h. Not reusing cups and glasses without washing
   i. Not changing pet litter boxes; if unavoidable, using gloves and washing hands immediately
   j. Avoiding turtles and reptiles as pets
   k. Not feeding pets raw or undercooked meat
6. Good dietary habits, including:
   a. Establishing protein and calorie goals
   b. Eating a low-bacteria diet and avoiding undercooked meat, fish, or eggs
   c. Thoroughly washing fruit and vegetables
   d. Refrigerating perishable foods
7. Psychosocial health:
   a. Helping identify ways to avoid problems with social stigma and rejection
   b. Identifying coping strategies for difficult situations
   c. Supporting family members and friends in efforts to help the patient and provide protection from discrimination
   d. Encouraging patients to continue as many usual activities as possible
   e. Supporting patients in their selection of friends and relatives with whom to discuss the diagnosis
   f. Reminding the patient that sexual partners and care providers should be informed of the diagnosis
   g. Making referrals to community resources, mental health professionals, behavioral health professionals, and support groups

HUNTINGTON'S DISEASE

OVERVIEW

- Huntington's disease is a hereditary disorder transmitted as an autosomal dominant trait at the time of conception.
- It is most prevalent in people of western European ancestry.
- The two main symptoms of the disease are progressive mental status changes leading to dementia and choreiform involuntary movements.
- Other clinical manifestations of Huntington's disease include poor balance, hesitant or explosive speech, dysphagia, impaired respirations, and bowel and bladder incontinence. Mental status changes include decreased attention span, poor judgment, memory loss, personality changes, and later, dementia.
- The first drug to be approved to decrease chorea associated with Huntington's disease is tetrabenazine (Xenazine). It is thought to

work by depleting the monoamines (e.g., dopamine, serotonin) from nerve terminals.

- There is no known cure for the disease.
- Genetic testing can determine risk for Huntington's disease; it is an autosomal dominant trait with high penetrance on chromosome 4. This means that a person who inherits just one mutated allele has nearly a 100% chance of developing the disease.
- Management of the disease is symptomatic. Physical and occupational therapy and social support can promote function and engagement.

HYDROCELE

OVERVIEW

- A hydrocele usually is a painless cystic mass filled with a straw-colored fluid that forms around the testis.
- It is caused by impaired lymphatic drainage of the scrotum, leading to swelling of the tissue surrounding the testes.
- Unless the swelling becomes large and uncomfortable or begins to impair blood flow to the testis, no treatment is necessary.
- When a hydrocele is large, uncomfortable, or cosmetically unacceptable, intervention is done by one of the following two methods:
  1. Drainage through a needle and syringe
  2. Surgical removal
- Provide postoperative care, including:
  1. Explaining the importance of wearing a scrotal support (jock strap) for the first 24 to 48 hours after surgery to keep the dressing in place and to prevent edema
  2. Assessing for pain and wound complications (infection or bleeding)
  3. Instructing the patient to schedule a follow-up visit with the surgeon
  4. Instructing the patient to stay off his feet for several days and to limit physical activity for a week
  5. Reassuring him that this swelling is normal and eventually subsides

HYDRONEPHROSIS, HYDROURETER, AND URETHRAL STRICTURE

OVERVIEW

- Several disorders obstruct the outflow of urine.
- In *hydronephrosis*, the kidney becomes enlarged as urine accumulates in the renal pelvis and the calyces. Obstruction within the pelvis or ureteropelvic junction results in renal pelvic distention,

and extensive damage to the vasculature and renal tubules can result.

- *Hydroureter* is the obstruction of the ureter and obstruction of urine outflow to the bladder.
- A *urethral stricture* is the most distal point of obstruction, with bladder distention occurring before hydroureter and hydronephrosis.
- Urinary tract obstruction causes structural damage to the urinary tract with potential for subsequent infection and kidney failure.
- Causes of hydronephrosis and hydroureter include tumors, stones, trauma, congenital structural defects, and retroperitoneal fibrosis.
- Urethral stricture occurs from chronic inflammation.
- Management includes:
  1. Recording history of kidney or urologic disorders, including pelvic radiation or surgery
  2. Documenting pattern of urination, including amount and frequency, and communicating decreases in urine flow
  3. Describing urine, including color, clarity, and odor
  4. Reporting new symptoms, including flank or abdominal pain, chills, fever, and malaise
  5. Re-establishing urine flow with irrigation of drainage device
  6. Managing flank, abdominal, or ureteral pain
  7. Monitoring urinalysis for protein, bacteria, or WBCs
  8. Anticipating an enlarged ureter or kidney on ultrasound, x-ray, or CT
  9. Preparing the patient and managing recovery if a urologic procedure to restore urine flow, such as a stent placement, or a nephrostomy drain to divert urine flow is performed

HYPERALDOSTERONISM

OVERVIEW

- Hyperaldosteronism is increased secretion of aldosterone by the adrenal glands that results in mineralocorticoid excess.
- Primary hyperaldosteronism (Conn's syndrome) results from excessive secretion of aldosterone from one or both adrenal glands and is most often caused by a benign adrenal tumor (adrenal adenoma).
- Secondary hyperaldosteronism is excessive secretion of aldosterone from high levels of angiotensin II stimulated by high plasma renin levels. Causes include kidney hypoxemia, diabetic nephropathy, and excessive use of some diuretics.
- Regardless of the cause, hyperaldosteronism is manifested by hypernatremia, hypokalemia, metabolic alkalosis, hypervolemia, and hypertension.

PATIENT-CENTERED COLLABORATIVE CARE
Assessment
- Obtain patient information about:
  1. Headache
  2. Fatigue
  3. Muscle weakness or paresthesia from hyperkalemia
- Assess for and document:
  1. Hypertension
  2. Elevated serum levels of sodium
  3. Low serum levels of potassium
- Diagnostic assessment includes:
  1. Serum electrolyte levels
  2. Serum renin levels (low)
  3. Serum aldosterone levels (high)
  4. Imaging with CT scans or MRI

Interventions
- Adrenalectomy of one or both adrenal glands is the most common treatment for early-stage hyperaldosteronism.
  1. Provide preoperative care as described in Part One and:
     a. Correct the serum fluid and electrolyte imbalances by administering prescribed potassium supplements, potassium-sparing diuretics, or aldosterone antagonists
     b. Manage preoperative hypertension
  2. Provide postoperative care as described in Part One and:
     a. Teach the patient about glucocorticoid replacement (replacement is lifelong if both adrenal glands are removed)
     b. Instruct the patient to wear a medical alert bracelet while he or she is taking glucocorticoids
- For patients who do not have surgery and must remain on spironolactone therapy to control hypokalemia and hypertension, teach them about:
  1. Avoiding potassium supplements and foods rich in potassium
  2. Reporting symptoms of hyponatremia
     a. Mouth dryness
     b. Thirst
     c. Lethargy or drowsiness
  3. Side effects of spironolactone therapy
     a. Gynecomastia
     b. Diarrhea
     c. Drowsiness
     d. Headache
     e. Rash, urticaria (hives)
     f. Confusion

g. Erectile dysfunction
h. Hirsutism
i. Amenorrhea

HYPERCALCEMIA

OVERVIEW

- Hypercalcemia is a total serum calcium level above 10.5 mg/dL or 2.75 mmol/L.
- Because the normal range for serum calcium is so narrow, even small increases have severe effects.
- The effects of hypercalcemia occur first in excitable tissues.
- Common causes of hypercalcemia include:
  1. Actual calcium excesses
     a. Excessive oral intake of calcium
     b. Excessive oral intake of vitamin D
     c. Kidney failure
     d. Use of thiazide diuretics
  2. Relative calcium excesses
     a. Hyperparathyroidism
     b. Malignancy
     c. Hyperthyroidism
     d. Immobility
     e. Use of glucocorticoids
     f. Dehydration

PATIENT-CENTERED COLLABORATIVE CARE

Assessment

- Assess for and document:
  1. Cardiovascular changes, which are the most serious and life threatening
     a. Irregular or increased heart rate and blood pressure (early)
     b. Slow heart rate (late or severe)
     c. Cyanosis and pallor from impaired blood flow and hypercoagulation
        (1) Assess hand and foot temperature, color, and capillary refill
  2. Neuromuscular changes, which include:
     a. Severe muscle weakness
     b. Decreased deep tendon reflexes without paresthesia
     c. Altered level of consciousness (confusion, lethargy, coma)
  3. Intestinal changes, which include:
     a. Constipation, anorexia, nausea, vomiting, and abdominal pain
     b. Hypoactive or absent bowel sounds
     c. Increased abdominal size

H

Interventions

- Prevent additional increases in calcium by:
  1. Discontinuing IV solutions containing calcium (lactated Ringer's solution)
  2. Discontinuing oral drugs containing calcium or vitamin D (e.g., calcium-based antacids, over-the-counter [OTC] vitamin supplements)
  3. Discontinuing thiazide diuretics that increase kidney calcium resorption
- Administer drug therapy to reduce circulating calcium and monitor effects
  1. IV normal saline (0.9% sodium chloride) to dilute serum levels and promote elimination
  2. Diuretics that enhance calcium excretion, such as furosemide (Lasix, Furoside ♣)
  3. Calcium chelators (calcium binders)
     a. Plicamycin (Mithracin)
     b. Penicillamine (Cuprimine, Pendramine ♣)
  4. Drugs that inhibit calcium resorption from bone
     a. Calcitonin (Calcimar)
     b. Bisphosphonates (etidronate)
     c. Prostaglandin synthesis inhibitors (aspirin, NSAIDs)
- Anticipate hemodialysis or blood ultrafiltration for rapid calcium reduction when levels are life threatening.
  1. Consider cardiac monitoring to evaluate changes in the T waves, QT interval, and heart rate and rhythm.
- Additional nursing actions include:
  1. Monitoring intake and output and reporting imbalances in a timely manner
  2. Assessing for fluid overload
  3. Encouraging weight-bearing exercise to slow bone resorption in chronic conditions of hypercalcemia

HYPERCORTISOLISM (CUSHING'S SYNDROME; ADRENAL GLAND HYPERFUNCTION)

OVERVIEW

- Excess cortisol (i.e., hypercortisolism) results in *Cushing's syndrome.*
- Excess cortisol secretion can be a result of a problem in the:
  1. Anterior pituitary gland (excess adrenocorticotropin hormone [ACTH])
  2. Hypothalamus (excess corticotrophin hormone [CRH])
  3. Adrenal cortex
- Glucocorticoid (corticosteroid) therapy also can lead to hypercortisolism.

- *Adrenal hyperfunction* can also result in hyperaldosteronism, excessive androgen production, and *pheochromocytoma* or excess catecholamines.
- Regardless of cause, excess cortisol or cortisol-like drugs affect metabolism and all body systems to some degree and these effects include:
  1. Immune dysfunction with reduced lymphocytes and lymph tissue and inactive forms of WBCs
  2. Altered fat metabolism leading to central obesity
  3. Hyperglycemia from insulin resistance
  4. Osteoporosis from excessive bone resorption
  5. Hypertension from hypervolemia, hypernatremia, and vascular endothelial changes (vasoconstriction)
  6. Thrombocytopenia (reduced platelets) and bleeding
  7. Reduced mucosal protection and increased gastric acidity; peptic ulcer disease
  8. Skeletal muscle wasting leading to thin extremities and decreased activity
  9. Changes in skin (thinning) and impaired wound healing

PATIENT-CENTERED COLLABORATIVE CARE
Assessment
- Obtain patient information about:
  1. History of all health problems and drug therapies
  2. Age, gender, and usual weight
  3. Changes in weight, diet, or eating behaviors
  4. Change in activity or sleep patterns, fatigue, and muscle weakness
  5. Bone pain or a history of fractures
  6. Frequent infections
  7. Easy bruising
  8. Cessation of menses
  9. GI ulcers
- Assess for and document:
  1. General appearance
     a. Buffalo hump on shoulder; central fat; moon face
     b. Thin arms and legs; generalized muscle wasting and weakness
  2. Skin changes
     a. Bruises
     b. Thin, translucent skin
     c. Wounds that have not healed
     d. Reddish purple striae ("stretch marks") on the abdomen, thighs, and upper arms
     e. Acne
     f. Fine coating of hair over the face and body

H

    3. Cardiac changes
       a. Tachycardia
       b. Hypertension
       c. Edema and evidence of hypervolemia
    4. Emotional lability, mood swings, irritability, confusion, depression
    5. Hyperglycemia
    6. Hypernatremia
- Diagnostic assessment includes:
    1. Elevated blood, salivary, and urine cortisol levels
    2. Dexamethasone suppression testing
    3. Abnormal serum electrolyte values (increased sodium, decreased calcium, decreased potassium)
    4. X-rays, CT scans, or MRI to identify tumors of the adrenal or pituitary glands, lung, GI tract, or pancreas

Planning and Implementation

FLUID OVERLOAD

Nonsurgical Management

- Restore fluid volume balance. Prevent fluid overload leading to pulmonary edema and heart failure:
    1. Monitor for indicators of increased fluid overload (increased pulse quality, increasing neck vein distention, presence of crackles in lungs, increasing peripheral edema, reduced urine output) at least every 2 hours.

> **❗ NURSING SAFETY PRIORITY: Critical Rescue**
>
> Notify the health care provider of any change that indicates the fluid overload is not responding to therapy or is becoming worse.

RISK FOR INJURY

- Injury is related to skin thinning, poor wound healing, and bone density loss
- Prevent skin injury by:
    1. Assessing the patient's skin for reddened areas, excoriation, breakdown, and edema
    2. Using pressure-relieving intervention during bedrest, including re-positioning or assisting with turns every 2 hours
    3. Teaching the patient activities to avoid trauma
       a. Use a soft toothbrush.
       b. Use an electric shaver.
       c. Keep the skin clean and dry it thoroughly after washing.
       d. Use a moisturizing lotion.
       e. Use tape sparingly and take care when removing it.
- Prevent pathologic fractures by:
    1. Using a lift sheet to move the patient instead of grasping him or her

2. Reminding the patient to call for help when ambulating
3. Reviewing the use of ambulatory aids (walkers or canes), if needed
4. Keeping rooms free of extraneous objects that may cause a fall
5. Teaching UAP to use a gait belt when ambulating the patient
6. Teaching the patient about safety issues and dietary support for bone health

- Prevent GI bleeding by:
    1. Implementing prescribed drug therapy
        a. Antacids
            (1) H_2 histamine receptor blockers like ranitidine (Zantac, Apo-Ranitidine ✿), famotidine (Pepcid), or nizatidine (Axid)
            (2) Proton pump inhibitors like Omeprazole (Losec ✿, Prilosec) or esomeprazole (Nexium)
        b. Encourage the patient to reduce or eliminate habits that contribute to gastric irritation, such as:
            (1) Consuming alcohol or caffeine
            (2) Smoking
            (3) Using NSAIDs

REDUCE RISK FOR INFECTION RELATED TO IMMUNE DYSFUNCTION

- Ensure that anyone with an upper respiratory tract infection who must enter the patient's room wears a mask.
- Continually assess the patient for the presence of infection.
    1. Monitor the daily CBC with differential WBC count and absolute neutrophil count (ANC) to detect and report abnormal values
    2. Inspect the mouth during every shift for mucosal integrity
    3. Assess the lungs every 8 hours for crackles, wheezes, or reduced breath sounds
    4. Assess all urine for odor and cloudiness
    5. Ask the patient about any urgency, burning, or pain present on urination
    6. Take vital signs at least every 4 hours to assess for fever
- Urge the patient to cough and deep breathe or to perform sustained maximal inhalations every 1 to 2 hours while awake.
- Administer drug therapy
    1. Administer prescribed drugs to interfere with ACTH production or adrenal hormone synthesis
        a. Aminoglutethimide (Elipten, Cytadren)
        b. Metyrapone (Metopirone)
        c. Cyproheptadine (Periactin)
        d. Mitotane (Lysodren)

H

    2. Monitor the patient for response to drug therapy
      a. Weight loss
      b. Increased urine output
    3. Assess laboratory findings, especially sodium and potassium values.
- Teach the patient about radiation therapy for hypercortisolism caused by pituitary adenomas as described in Part One and:
    1. Observe for any changes in the patient's neurologic status, such as headache, elevated blood pressure or pulse, disorientation, or changes in pupil size or reaction.
    2. Assess for skin dryness, redness, flushing, or alopecia at the radiation site.

Surgical Management

- When adrenal hyperfunction results from increased pituitary secretion of ACTH, removal of a pituitary adenoma may be done.
- When hypercortisolism is caused by adrenal tumors, a partial or complete adrenalectomy (removal of the adrenal gland) may be performed by open abdominal procedures or laparoscopic procedures.
- Provide preoperative care as described in Part One and:
    1. Implement prescribed drug and diet therapy to correct electrolyte imbalances
    2. Monitor blood potassium, sodium, and chloride levels for abnormal values
    3. Monitor ECG for dysrhythmias
    4. Monitor blood glucose levels and managing hyperglycemia
    5. Prevent infection with handwashing and aseptic technique
    6. Implement fall prevention measures with changes in mental status
    7. Teach the patient about the care needs after surgery and the need for long-term drug therapy
- Provide postoperative care as described in Part One and:
    1. Assess the patient every 15 minutes for shock (e.g., hypotension, a rapid and weak pulse, decreasing urine output) during the first 6 hours
    2. Monitor vital signs and other hemodynamic variables to detect hypervolemia/hypovolemia:
      a. Central venous pressure
      b. Intake and output
      c. Daily weights
      d. Serum electrolyte levels

Community-Based Care

- Teach the patient who must take glucocorticoids to:
    1. Take the drug in divided doses, with the first dose in the morning and the second dose between 4 and 6 PM.

2. Take the drug with meals or snacks.
3. Weigh himself or herself daily, record it, and compare it with previous weights.
   a. Call the health care provider if more than 3 pounds are gained in a week or more than 1 to 2 pounds is gained within 24 hours.
4. Increase the dosage as directed for increased physical stress or severe emotional stress, including surgery, dental work, influenza, fever, pregnancy, and family problems.
5. *Never skip a dose of the drug.* If the patient has persistent vomiting or severe diarrhea and cannot take the drug by mouth for 24 to 36 hours, he or she must call the physician. If the patient cannot reach the physician, he or she must go to the nearest emergency department, because an injection may be needed in place of the usual oral drug.
6. Always wear his or her medical alert bracelet or necklace.
7. Make regular visits for health care follow-up.
8. Urge attention to handwashing and personal hygiene to reduce exposure to transmissible disease.
9. Avoid crowds or others with infections
10. Encourage the patient and all people living in the same home to maintain recommended vaccine schedule, including annual influenza vaccinations.

HYPERKALEMIA

OVERVIEW

- Hyperkalemia is a serum potassium level greater than 5 mEq/L (5 mmol/L).
- The normal range for serum potassium values is narrow, so even slight increases above normal values can affect excitable tissues, especially the heart.
- The consequences of hyperkalemia can be life threatening, and the imbalance usually is not seen in people with normally functioning kidneys.
- Causes include:
  1. Intake of potassium-containing foods or drugs:
     a. Salt substitutes
     b. Potassium chloride
     c. Potassium-sparing diuretics
  2. Rapid infusion of potassium-containing IV solution
  3. Transfusions of whole blood or packed cells
  4. Adrenal insufficiency (Addison's disease, adrenalectomy)
  5. Tissue damage (crushing injuries, burns)
  6. Acidosis

7. Hyperuricemia
8. Chronic or acute kidney disease
- The problems that occur with hyperkalemia are related to how rapidly ECF potassium levels increase. Sudden rises in serum potassium cause severe problems at potassium levels between 6 and 7 mEq/L. When serum potassium rises slowly, problems may not occur until potassium levels reach 8 mEq/L or higher.

PATIENT-CENTERED COLLABORATIVE CARE
Assessment
- Obtain patient information about:
  1. Age
  2. Chronic illnesses (particularly kidney disease and diabetes mellitus)
  3. Recent medical or surgical treatment
  4. Urine output, including the frequency and amount of voiding
  5. Drug use, particularly potassium-sparing diuretics and ACE inhibitors
  6. Nutrition history to determine the intake of potassium-rich foods or the use of salt substitutes that contain potassium
  7. Palpitations, skipped heartbeats, and other cardiac irregularities
  8. Muscle twitching and weakness in the leg muscles
  9. Unusual tingling or numbness in the hands, feet, or face
  10. Recent changes in bowel habits, especially diarrhea
- Assess for and document:
  1. Cardiovascular changes
     a. Bradycardia
     b. Hypotension
     c. ECG changes
        (1) Tall, peaked T waves
        (2) Prolonged PR intervals
        (3) Flat or absent P waves
        (4) Wide QRS complexes
  2. Neuromuscular changes, early
     a. Skeletal muscle twitches
     b. Tingling and burning sensations followed by numbness in the hands and feet and around the mouth
  3. Neuromuscular changes, late
     a. Muscle weakness
     b. Flaccid paralysis first in hands and feet, then moving higher
  4. Intestinal changes
     a. Increased motility
     b. Hyperactive bowel sounds
     c. Frequent watery bowel movements
  5. Laboratory data: serum potassium level greater than 5 mEq/L

Interventions
- Interventions for hyperkalemia are aimed at rapidly reducing the serum potassium level, preventing recurrences, and ensuring patient safety during the electrolyte imbalance.
- Drug therapy
  1. IV therapy
     a. Discontinuing potassium-containing infusions
     b. Keeping the IV catheter open
     c. Administering IV preparation of 100 mL of 10% to 20% glucose with 10 to 20 units of regular insulin
  2. Withholding oral potassium supplements
  3. Potassium-excreting diuretics, such as furosemide
  4. Sodium polystyrene sulfonate (Kayexalate) exchange resins
- Hemodialysis or ultrafiltration
- Nursing care priorities include:
  1. Cardiac monitoring for early recognition of dysrhythmias and other manifestations of hyperkalemia on cardiac function

> ## ❗ NURSING SAFETY PRIORITY: Critical Rescue
>
> Notify the health care provider or Rapid Response Team if the patient's heart rate falls below 60 beats/min or if the T waves become spiked.

  2. Collaborating with the dietitian to reduce dietary potassium intake by reading product packages and avoiding foods high in potassium including many salt substitute products, preserved meats, dried fruit, and large volumes of dark green vegetables or beans

HYPERLIPIDEMIA

OVERVIEW
- Hyperlipidemia is a condition of elevated serum lipid levels, including total cholesterol, low density lipoproteins (LDL), and triglycerides.
- High density lipoproteins (HDL) reduce hyperlipidemia; these cholesterol particles act as scavengers moving LDL out of the blood and into the liver for metabolism.
- Hyperlipidemia contributes to the formation of atherosclerotic plaque.
- Patients with metabolic syndrome and diabetes experience increased total cholesterol, LDL, and triglycerides, contributing to early atherosclerosis and cardiovascular events like heart attack or stroke.
- Hyperlipidemia is treated with lifestyle interventions (e.g., diet and exercise) and drugs, typically statins (e.g., atorvastatin

[Lipitor], fluvastatin [Mevacor], lovastatin [Pravachol], and simvastatin [Zocor]).

HYPERNATREMIA

OVERVIEW

- Hypernatremia is a serum sodium level greater than 145 mEq/L and is often accompanied by changes in fluid volumes.
- It makes excitable tissues more easily excited, a condition known as irritability, and leads to cellular dehydration.
- Common causes include:
  1. Actual sodium excesses
     a. Hyperaldosteronism
     b. Kidney failure
     c. Corticosteroids
     d. Cushing's syndrome or disease
     e. Excessive oral sodium ingestion
     f. Excessive administration of sodium-containing IV fluids
  2. Relative sodium excesses
     a. Nothing by mouth
     b. Increased rate of metabolism
     c. Fever
     d. Hyperventilation
     e. Infection
     f. Excessive diaphoresis
     g. Watery diarrhea
     h. Dehydration

PATIENT-CENTERED COLLABORATIVE CARE

Assessment

- Assess for and document:
  1. Nervous system changes
     a. Altered cognition such as decreased attention span and recall of recent events
     b. Agitation or confusion
     c. Lethargy, drowsiness, stupor, or coma (when accompanied by fluid overload)
  2. Skeletal muscles changes
     a. Muscle twitching and irregular muscle contractions (mild hypernatremia)
     b. Muscle weakness and reduced hand grip strength
  3. Cardiovascular changes that differ with fluid status
     a. Hypovolemia leads to increased pulse rate, hypotension, and reduced quality of peripheral pulses
     b. Hypervolemia leads to slow to normal bounding pulses, full peripheral pulses, neck vein distention, and elevated diastolic blood pressure

4. Respiratory changes occur with hypervolemia
   a. Pulmonary edema
   b. Decreased oxygen saturation

Interventions

- Increase fluid intake when hypernatremia is caused by fluid loss.
- Restrict fluid intake when hypervolemic hypernatremia occurs.
- Drug therapy includes diuretics that promote sodium loss, such as furosemide (Lasix, Furoside ✦) or bumetanide (Bumex).
- Measure fluid intake and output and communicate goals of therapy with health care team.
- Dietary sodium restriction may be needed to prevent sodium excess.
- Priorities for nursing care of the patient with hypernatremia include monitoring the patient's response to therapy and preventing hyponatremia and dehydration.
  1. Prevent fluid overload, leading to pulmonary edema and heart failure.
     a. Monitor for indicators of increased fluid overload at least every 2 hours.

> **! NURSING SAFETY PRIORITY: Critical Rescue**
>
> Pulmonary edema can occur very quickly and can lead to death. Notify the health care provider about decrease in peripheral oxygen saturation or increased work of breathing (rate and depth of respirations) or ineffective breathing (hypoventilation) that can occur with fluid overload.

  2. Prevent skin and tissue injury from edema or reduced mobility.
  3. Monitor for patient response to drug therapy:
     a. Weigh the patient daily.
     b. Document intake and output.
     c. Establish intake and output goals with health care provider.
  4. Observe for manifestations of sodium imbalance
     a. Changes in nerve, muscles, or cardiac excitability
     b. Changes in serum and urine sodium levels
  5. Promote nutrition therapy by teaching patients and families about:
     a. Sodium restriction
     b. Fluid restriction

HYPERPARATHYROIDISM

OVERVIEW

- Hyperparathyroidism results from increased levels of parathyroid hormone (PTH) that act directly on the kidney, causing increased kidney resorption of calcium and increased phosphate excretion. These processes cause hypercalcemia (excessive calcium) and hypophosphatemia (inadequate phosphate).

- Primary hyperparathyroidism results when one or more parathyroid glands do not respond to the normal feedback mechanisms for serum calcium levels. The most common cause is a benign tumor in one parathyroid gland.
- Secondary hyperparathyroidism is a response to the hypocalcemia associated with CKD and vitamin D deficiency, which leads to hyperplasia of the parathyroid glands.

PATIENT-CENTERED COLLABORATIVE CARE
Assessment

- Obtain patient information about:
  1. Bone fractures
  2. Recent weight loss
  3. Arthritis
  4. Psychological distress
  5. History of radiation treatment to the head or neck
  6. History of kidney stones
- Assess for and document:
  1. Waxy pallor of the skin
  2. Bone deformities in the extremities and back
  3. GI manifestations
     a. Anorexia, nausea, vomiting
     b. Epigastric pain
     c. Constipation
  4. Fatigue and lethargy
  5. Confusion, coma (severe hyperparathyroidism)
  6. Laboratory values
     a. High serum calcium levels
     b. High serum PTH levels
     c. Low serum phosphorus levels
- Diagnostic studies include:
  1. Serum electrolyte levels
  2. Serum PTH and urine cyclic adenosine monophosphate (cAMP) levels
  3. X-rays that show calcium deposits, renal stones, or bone lesions and loss of bone density
  4. CT with or without arteriography

Interventions
Nonsurgical Management

- Intravenous fluids followed by a loop diuretic (furosemide [Lasix]) are used most often for reducing serum calcium levels in patients who are not candidates for surgery.

- When hydration and furosemide (Lasix) do not correct hypercalcemia, drug therapy includes:
  1. Cinacalcet (Sensipar) to decrease serum calcium
  2. Oral phosphates to interfere with dietary calcium absorption
- Nursing management includes:
  1. Evaluating cardiac rate, rhythm, and waveforms with continuous ECG monitoring
  2. Measuring intake and output 2 to 4 hours during hydration therapy
  3. Closely monitoring serum calcium levels for return to safe range
  4. Assessing for tingling and numbness in the hands, feet, and around the mouth
  5. Preventing injury by:
     a. Teaching all members of the health care team to handle the patient carefully
     b. Using a lift sheet to re-position the patient rather than pulling him or her
     c. Implementing fall precaution

QSEN SAFETY, EVIDENCE-BASED PRACTICE

Ensure patients are evaluated for fall risk on admission, with any change in health status, and when cognition or balance decrease. Use a standard, reliable, and valid risk assessment tool.

H

Surgical Management

- Surgical management of hyperparathyroidism is parathyroidectomy. It involves a transverse incision in the lower neck. All four parathyroid glands are examined for enlargement. If a tumor is present on one side but the other side is normal, the surgeon removes the glands containing tumor and leaves the remaining glands on the opposite side intact. If all four glands are diseased, they are all removed.
  1. Provide preoperative care as described in Part One and teaching about neck support by having the patient place both hands behind his or her neck to assist in elevating the head.
  2. Provide postoperative care as described in Part One and:
     a. Closely observe the patient for respiratory distress, which may occur from calcium gluconate, compression of the trachea by hemorrhage, or swelling of neck tissues
     b. Ensure that emergency equipment, including suction, oxygen, and tracheostomy equipment, is at the bedside

> ## ❗ NURSING SAFETY PRIORITY: Critical Rescue
>
> If severe swelling occurs and the airway begins to be obstructed, notify the Rapid Response Team to remove the clips from the incision to preserve the airway.

3. Check serum calcium levels immediately after surgery and every 4 hours thereafter until calcium levels stabilize.
4. Monitor for manifestations of hypocalcemia
   a. Tingling and twitching in the extremities and face
   b. Positive Trousseau's sign
   c. Positive Chvostek's sign (see *Hypocalcemia*)
5. Assess for damage to the recurrent laryngeal nerve
   a. Changes in voice patterns
   b. Hoarseness
- If all four parathyroid glands are removed, the patient will need lifelong treatment with calcium and vitamin D, because the resulting hypoparathyroidism is permanent.

HYPERPITUITARISM

OVERVIEW

- Hyperpituitarism is hormone oversecretion that occurs with pituitary tumors or hyperplasia.
- Tumors occur most often in the anterior pituitary cells that produce growth hormone (GH), prolactin (PRL), and ACTH.
  1. Overproduction of GH results in acromegaly, manifested by increased skeletal thickness, hypertrophy of the skin, and enlargement of all visceral organs.
  2. Excessive PRL inhibits secretion of sex hormones in men and women and results in galactorrhea, amenorrhea, and infertility.
  3. Excess ACTH overstimulates the adrenal cortex, resulting in excessive production of glucocorticoids, mineralocorticoids, and androgens, which leads to the development of Cushing's disease.

🧬 Genetic/Genomic Considerations

- An uncommon cause of hyperpituitarism is type 1 multiple endocrine neoplasia (MEN1), in which there is inactivation of a suppressor gene leading to excessive GH and acromegaly. This problem has an autosomal dominant inheritance pattern and is usually expressed as a benign tumor that affects the pituitary gland, parathyroid glands, and pancreas.

PATIENT-CENTERED COLLABORATIVE CARE
Assessment
- Obtain patient information about:
  1. Age and gender
  2. Family history of endocrine problems
  3. Change in appearance: lip or nose size, gain or change in hat, glove, ring, or shoe size
  4. Fatigue and lethargy
  5. Backache
  6. Arthralgias (joint pain)
  7. Headaches and changes in vision
  8. Menstrual changes (e.g., amenorrhea, irregular menses, difficulty in becoming pregnant)
  9. Changes in sexual functioning (e.g., decreased libido, painful intercourse, impotence)
  10. Loss of or change in secondary sexual characteristics
  11. Weight gain or loss (unplanned)
- Assess for and document:
  1. Changes in the facial features (e.g., increases in lip and nose sizes; prominent brow ridge; increases in head, hand, and foot sizes); moon face
  2. Extremity muscle wasting
  3. Acne
  4. Hirsutism
  5. Striae
  6. Hypertension
  7. Areas of uneven pigmentation or hyperpigmentation
  8. Dysrhythmias, including tachycardia or bradycardia
- Diagnostic testing may include:
  1. Blood test for hormone levels (any or all may be elevated)
  2. CT
  3. MRI
  4. Hormone suppression tests

Interventions
Surgical Management
- Surgical removal of the pituitary gland and tumor (hypophysectomy) is the most common treatment for hyperpituitarism.
- A minimally invasive trans-nasal or a trans-sphenoidal hypophysectomy is the most commonly used surgical approach. With a trans-sphenoidal approach, the surgeon makes an incision just above the upper lip and reaches the pituitary gland through the sphenoid sinus.
- A craniotomy may be needed if the tumor cannot be reached by a trans-sphenoidal approach.

H

- Provide preoperative care as described in Part One and:
    1. Explain that hypophysectomy decreases hormone levels, relieves headaches, and may reverse changes in sexual functioning
    2. Remind the patient that body changes, organ enlargement, and visual changes are not usually reversible
    3. Explain that because nasal packing is present for 2 to 3 days after surgery, it will be necessary to breathe through the mouth, and a "mustache dressing" ("drip pad") will be placed under the nose
    4. Instruct the patient not to brush teeth, cough, sneeze, blow the nose, or bend forward after surgery
- Provide postoperative care as described in Part One and:
    1. Monitor neurologic responses hourly for the first 24 hours and then every 4 hours and document any changes in vision, mental status, altered level of consciousness, or decreased strength of the extremities.
    2. Observe for complications such as transient diabetes insipidus, cerebrospinal fluid (CSF) leakage, infection, and increased intracranial pressure (ICP).
        a. Excess urine output may indicate onset of diabetes insipidus.
        b. Any postnasal drip may indicate leakage of CSF.
        c. Assess nasal drainage for quantity, quality, and odor; send a sample to the laboratory for testing because the presence of glucose may confirm CSF drainage.
    3. Keep the head of the bed elevated.
    4. Instruct the patient to avoid coughing early after surgery and remind him or her to perform deep-breathing exercises hourly while awake.
    5. Instruct the patient to avoid bending at the waist for any reason, because this position increases ICP.
    6. Perform frequent oral rinses and apply water-soluble jelly to dry lips.
    7. Assess for manifestations of meningitis.
        a. Headache
        b. Fever
        c. Nuchal (neck) rigidity
    8. Teach the patient self-administration of the prescribed hormones.

Nonsurgical Management

- The goals of therapy for the patient who has hyperpituitarism are to return hormone levels to normal or near normal, reduce or eliminate headache and visual disturbances, prevent complications, and reverse as many of the body changes as possible.

- Encourage the patient to express concerns and fears about his or her altered physical appearance.
- Help him or her identify personal strengths and positive characteristics.
- Drug therapy may be used alone or in combination with surgery or radiation.
  1. Dopamine agonists to stimulate dopamine receptors in the brain and inhibit the release of many pituitary hormones, especially prolactin and GH
     a. Bromocriptine (Parlodel)
     b. Cabergoline (Dostinex)
     c. Pergolide (Permax)
  2. Somatostatin analogs and GH receptor blockers (for GH-secreting tumors)
     a. Octreotide (Sandostatin)
     b. Pegvisomant (Somavert)
- Radiation therapy regimens take a long time to complete, and several years may pass before a therapeutic effect can be seen. Side effects of radiation therapy include hypopituitarism, optic nerve damage, and other eye and vision problems.

HYPERTENSION

OVERVIEW

- Hypertension is a blood pressure (BP) above 140/90. In adults aged 60 years or older, hypertension is above 150/90. Patients with diabetes and heart disease should have a blood pressure (BP) below 130/90.
- Hypertension is the major risk factor for coronary, cerebral, kidney, retinal (vision), and peripheral vascular disease.
- There are two major classifications of hypertension:
  1. Primary, with no known cause and associated with risk factors such as a family history of hypertension, age older than 60 years, hyperlipidemia, stress, and smoking
  2. Secondary hypertension, which results from specific diseases such as kidney vascular and kidney disease, primary aldosteronism, Cushing's disease, coarctation of the aorta, brain tumors

🌐 Cultural Considerations

The prevalence of hypertension in African Americans in the United States is among the highest in the world and is constantly increasing. When compared with Euro-Americans, they develop high BP earlier in life, making them much more likely to die from strokes, heart disease, and kidney disease. The reason for these differences is not known, but genetics and environmental factors may play a role.

and encephalitis, psychiatric disorders, and some drugs, such as estrogen-containing oral contraceptives, glucocorticoids, mineralocorticoids, cyclosporine, and erythropoietin

PATIENT-CENTERED COLLABORATIVE CARE
Assessment
- Record patient information
  1. Blood pressures in both arms while sitting
  2. Age
  3. Race or ethnic origin
  4. Family history of hypertension
  5. Dietary intake pattern, including alcohol
  6. Smoking
  7. Exercise habits
  8. Past and present history of cardiovascular, kidney or chronic disease, and diabetes
  9. Drug use (prescribed, OTC, and illicit)
  10. Peripheral pulse rate, rhythm, and force
  11. Psychosocial stressors

QSEN INFORMATICS

Accurately and completely record medications from home used to treat hypertension so that home drugs can be continued in the hospital.

- Assess for hypertensive symptoms
  1. Headache, dizziness, facial flushing, or fainting
  2. Edema
  3. Nosebleeds
  4. Vision changes or retinal changes on funduscopic examination
  5. Signs of kidney injury, such as elevated BUN or creatinine levels or low urine output
  6. Physical findings related to vascular damage, including atherosclerosis, acute coronary syndrome, and heart failure
     a. Abdominal, carotid, or femoral bruits
     b. Dysrhythmias, tachycardia, sweating, and pallor
     c. Decreased or absent peripheral pulses
     d. Cardiomegaly or left ventricular hypertrophy
  7. Diagnostic tests that indicate the severity of primary or secondary causes of hypertension
     a. Kidney disease can be diagnosed by the presence of protein, red blood cells, pus cells, and casts in the urine; elevated levels of BUN; and elevated serum creatinine levels.
     b. Urinary test results are positive for the presence of catecholamines in patients with a pheochromocytoma (tumor of the adrenal medulla).

    c. An elevation in levels of serum corticoids and 17-ketosteroids in the urine is diagnostic of Cushing's disease.

    d. An ECG can determine atrial and ventricular hypertrophy, although echocardiography is a more sensitive and specific diagnostic test for myocardial derangements from hypertension.

Planning and Implementation

- Assist with planning and implementing lifestyle changes, including the regular evaluation of BP outside of office visits.

  1. In collaboration with the dietitian:

    a. Advise the patient to restrict daily sodium intake to less than 2 grams.

    b. Suggest that the patient use spices, herbs, fruits, and other non–salt-containing substances such as powdered garlic and onion or a salt substitute to enhance the flavor of food.

    c. Advise the patient to consider strategies to promote ideal body weight.

    d. Develop a plan to reduce saturated fat and cholesterol in the diet.

  2. Advise the patient to restrict alcohol intake and stop smoking.

  3. Assist the patient in developing a regular exercise program.

  4. Teach or refer the patient to physical therapy and stress management programs to improve activity and reduce stress. Yoga, massage, biofeedback, and hypnosis programs may help reduce hypertension.

  5. Administer drug therapy as prescribed and support adherence to prescribed drugs at home.

    a. The most common drugs to control hypertension are:

      (1) Diuretics

        i. Thiazide diuretics prevent sodium and water resorption in the distal tubules of the kidneys and may improve endothelial health.

        ii. Loop diuretics depress sodium resorption in the ascending loop of Henle and promote potassium excretion.

      (2) Potassium-sparing diuretics act on the distal tubules of the kidneys to inhibit resorption of sodium in exchange for potassium ions, retaining potassium. Aldosterone inhibitors also interfere with the renin-angiotensin-aldosterone system, promoting vascular health.

    b. Angiotensin blockers

      (1) ACE inhibitors convert angiotensin I to angiotensin II, resulting in vasorelaxation.

H

Considerations for Older Adults

Loop diuretics are not used commonly for older adults as initial antihypertensive therapy because they can cause dehydration and orthostatic hypotension. These complications increase the patient's risk for falls. Teach families to monitor for and report patient dizziness, falls, or confusion to the health care provider as soon as possible and discontinue the medication.

　　　(2) Angiotensin receptor blockers (ARBs) selectively block the binding of angiotensin II in the vascular and adrenal tissue.
　　c. Other drugs that are used to manage hypertension
　　　(1) Beta-adrenergic blockers lower blood pressure by blocking beta receptors in the heart and kidneys, reducing the cardiac rate and blocking renin release.
　　　(2) Central alpha agonists act on the central nervous system, preventing reuptake of norepinephrine, resulting in lower peripheral vascular resistance and blood pressure.
　　　(3) Calcium channel blockers lower blood pressure by interfering with transmembrane influx of calcium ions, resulting in vasoconstriction.
　　　(4) Renin inhibitors are used for mild to moderate hypertension.
　　　(5) Alpha-adrenergic antagonists such as prazosin (Minipress), doxazosin (Cardura), and terazosin (Hytrin) dilate the arterioles and veins. These drugs can lower blood pressure quickly, but their use is limited because of frequent and bothersome side effects.

! NURSING SAFETY PRIORITY: Drug Safety

Monitor the patient's serum potassium level for abnormal values when administering a diuretic, ACE inhibitor (ACEI), or ARB. The most frequent side effect associated with thiazide and loop diuretics is hypokalemia (low potassium level). Assess for hyperkalemia (high potassium level) for patients taking potassium-sparing diuretics, such as spironolactone and ACEI or ARB.

- Monitor kidney function, cardiac function, and vascular perfusion to the brain and periphery to detect and manage end-organ damage from hypertension.
- Evaluate for self-management related to knowledge and behaviors for adherence to prescribed medications, lifestyle changes, and self-monitoring of BP.

Community-Based Care
- Provide educational information for hypertension control, especially:
  1. Salt/sodium restriction
  2. Weight maintenance or reduction
  3. Self-awareness for healthy food selections
  4. Stress reduction or coping strategies
  5. Alcohol restriction
  6. Exercise program
  7. Taking prescribed antihypertensive drugs even in the absence of symptoms
  8. Regular ongoing follow-up with health care provider
- Give oral and written information on drug therapy, including:
  1. Rationale for use, dose, and time of administration
  2. Side effects and vigilance for drug interactions
  3. The value of blood pressure control to avoid serious adverse health consequences like stroke
- Instruct the patient and family members in the technique of blood pressure monitoring at home and record values to share with scheduled provider interactions.
- Refer the patient to home care agency if necessary.

HYPERTHYROIDISM

OVERVIEW
- Hyperthyroidism is excessive thyroid hormone secretion from the thyroid gland.
- The manifestations of hyperthyroidism are called *thyrotoxicosis.*
- Thyroid hormones affect metabolism in all body organs and excesses produce many different manifestations.
- The most common form of this condition is Graves' disease, an autoimmune disorder in which antibodies are made and attach to the TSH receptor sites on the thyroid tissue. The thyroid-stimulating immunoglobulins (TSIs) bind to the thyroid gland, increasing its size and overproducing thyroid hormones.

Genetic/Genomic Considerations

- Susceptibility to Graves' disease is associated with mutations in several genes, including GRD1, GRD2, GRDX1, and GRDX2. The pattern of inheritance appears to be autosomal recessive with sex limitation to females and reduced penetrance. Graves' disease also has a strong association with other autoimmune disorders, such as diabetes mellitus, vitiligo, and rheumatoid arthritis.

- Other causes include benign or malignant tumors and excessive use of thyroid replacement drugs.
- *Thyroid storm,* or *thyroid crisis,* is a life-threatening condition of an extreme hyperthyroidism that occurs when the condition is uncontrolled or triggered by stressors such as trauma, infection, diabetic ketoacidosis, and pregnancy. Key manifestations include fever, tachycardia, and systolic hypertension.

PATIENT-CENTERED COLLABORATIVE CARE
Assessment
- Obtain patient information about:
  1. Age and gender
  2. Usual weight and any unplanned weight loss
  3. Increased appetite
  4. Increased number of daily bowel movements
  5. Heat intolerance with diaphoresis (increased sweating)
  6. Palpitations or chest pain
  7. Dyspnea (with or without exertion)
  8. Changes in eye or vision, especially exophthalmos (specific to Graves' disease)
  9. Fatigue, weakness
  10. Insomnia (common)
  11. Irritability, depression
  12. Amenorrhea or a decreased menstrual flow (common)
  13. Changes in libido
  14. Previous thyroid surgery or radiation therapy to the neck
  15. Past and current drugs, especially the use of thyroid hormone replacement or antithyroid drugs
- Assess for and document:
  1. Exophthalmos (Graves' disease)
  2. Photophobia, double vision, blurring
  3. General appearance:
     a. Eyelid retraction (Graves' disease)
     b. Eyeball lag (the upper eyelid pulls back faster than the eyeball when the patient gazes upward) (Graves' disease)
  4. Presence or absence of a goiter (enlarged thyroid gland)
  5. Hypertension
  6. Dysrhythmias and tachycardia
  7. Fine, soft, silky hair
  8. Warm, moist skin
  9. Tremor
- Psychosocial issues or changes may include:
  1. Wide mood swings
  2. Irritability

   3. Decreased attention span
   4. Mild to severe hyperactivity
- Diagnostic assessment may include:
   1. Blood tests for:
      a. Triiodothyronine (T_3)
      b. Thyroxine (T_4)
      c. TSH
      d. Antibodies to TSH (TSH-rAb) (Graves' disease)
   2. Thyroid scan (radionuclide)
   3. Ultrasonography of the thyroid gland
   4. ECG with tachycardia, atrial fibrillation, T-wave changes

Interventions

- Interventions are described for Graves' disease because it is the most common form of hyperthyroidism. The goals of management are to decrease the effect of thyroid hormone on cardiac function and to reduce thyroid hormone secretion.

Nonsurgical Management

- Monitoring, including:
   1. Measuring apical pulse and blood pressure at least every 4 hours and reporting status changes in a timely manner
   2. Instructing the patient to report palpitations or chest pain immediately
   3. Checking temperature at least every 4 hours and reporting fever in a timely manner

> ❗ **NURSING SAFETY PRIORITY: Critical Rescue**
>
> Immediately report a temperature increase of even 1° F (0.3° C) because it may indicate impending thyroid crisis.

- Immediately report hyperthermia and hypertension to the provider because thyroid storm is preceded by these signs.
- Drug therapy
   1. Antithyroid drugs
      a. Methimazole (Tapazole)
      b. Propylthiouracil (PTU)

> ❗ **NURSING SAFETY PRIORITY: Drug Alert**
>
> Methimazole can cause birth defects and should not be used during pregnancy, especially during the first trimester. Instruct women to notify their health care provider if pregnancy occurs.

   2. Supportive drug therapy with propranolol (Inderal, Detensol ♣) to relieve diaphoresis, anxiety, tachycardia, and palpitations

- Radioactive iodine (RAI) therapy
  1. Is not used in pregnant women because ^{131}I crosses the placenta and can damage the fetal thyroid gland
  2. Can be delivered as an oral drug or IV
  3. Is dependent on the thyroid gland's size and sensitivity to radiation for dosage
  4. Destroys some of the cells that produce thyroid hormone
  5. Is performed on an outpatient basis
  6. May take 4 to 8 weeks for results
  7. May cause some patients to experience hypothyroidism as a result of the treatment

Surgical Management

- Surgery to remove all (total thyroidectomy) or part of the thyroid gland (subtotal thyroidectomy) may be needed for patients who have a large goiter-causing tracheal or esophageal compression or who do not have a good response to antithyroid drugs.
- A thyroidectomy is performed with the patient under general anesthesia. The surgeon makes a "collar incision" just above the clavicle.
- After a total thyroidectomy, patients must take lifelong thyroid hormone replacement.
- Provide preoperative care as described in Part One and:
  1. Administer antithyroid drugs and iodine preparations to decrease the secretion of thyroid hormones and reduce thyroid size and vascularity
  2. Ensure that hypertension, dysrhythmias, and tachycardia are controlled before surgery
  3. Teach the patient to support the neck when coughing or moving by placing both hands behind the neck when moving
- Providing postoperative care as described in Part One and:
  1. Use sandbags or pillows to support the head and neck
  2. Place the patient, while he or she is awake, in a semi-Fowler's position
  3. Decrease tension on the suture line by avoiding neck extension
  4. Prevent complications from airway obstruction or respiratory distress by:
     a. Listening for laryngeal stridor (harsh, high-pitched respiratory sounds)
     b. Keeping emergency tracheostomy equipment in the patient's room
     c. Ensuring that oxygen and suctioning equipment are nearby and in working order
  5. Monitor for hemorrhage
     a. Inspect the neck dressing and behind the patient's neck for blood at least every 2 hours for the first 24 hours
     b. Assess drainage for amount, color, and character

! NURSING SAFETY PRIORITY: Critical Rescue

If symptoms of airway obstruction such as stridor, dyspnea, or decreased oxygenation occur, notify the Rapid Response Team.

6. Avoid injury from concurrent parathyroid removal and hypocalcemia and tetany
   a. Ask the patient hourly about any tingling around the mouth or of the toes and fingers
   b. Assess for muscle twitching
   c. Ensure calcium gluconate or calcium chloride is available
7. Evaluate intraoperative and postoperative laryngeal nerve damage
   a. Assess the patient's voice at 2-hour intervals
   b. Reassure the patient that hoarseness is usually temporary
- Emergency management of thyroid storm or thyroid crisis
  1. Thyroid storm or crisis is a life-threatening event that occurs in patients with uncontrolled hyperthyroidism and occurs most often with Graves' disease.
  2. Key manifestations include fever, tachycardia, and systolic hypertension.
  3. Even with treatment, thyroid storm may lead to death.
     a. Maintain a patent airway and adequate ventilation.
     b. Give antithyroid drugs as prescribed: propylthiouracil (PTU, Propyl-Thyracil ✦), 300 to 900 mg daily, and methimazole (Tapazole), up to 60 mg daily.
     c. Administer sodium iodide solution, 2 g IV daily, as prescribed.
     d. Give propranolol (Inderal, Detensol ✦), 1 to 3 mg IV, as prescribed. Give slowly over 3 minutes; the patient should be connected to a cardiac monitor, and a central venous pressure catheter should be in place.
     e. Give glucocorticoids as prescribed: hydrocortisone, 100 to 500 mg IV daily; prednisone, 4 to 60 mg orally daily; or dexamethasone, 2 mg IM or IV every 6 hours.
     f. Monitor continually for cardiac dysrhythmias.
     g. Monitor vital signs every 30 minutes for early detection of status change.
     h. Provide comfort measures, including a cooling blanket.
     i. Give antipyretics, as prescribed.
     j. Correct dehydration with normal saline infusions.
     k. Apply cooling blanket or ice packs to reduce fever.

H

Community-Based Care
- Teach the patient and family about:
  1. The manifestations of hyperthyroidism and instruct them to report an increase or recurrence of symptoms
  2. The manifestations of hypothyroidism and the need for thyroid hormone replacement
  3. The need for regular follow-up, because hypothyroidism can occur several years after RAI therapy
  4. Prescribed drugs, including side effects
  5. Inspecting the incision area and reporting redness, tenderness, drainage, or swelling to the surgeon
  6. Possible continued mood changes, reassuring the patient and family that these effects will decrease with continued treatment

HYPOCALCEMIA

OVERVIEW

- Hypocalcemia is a total serum calcium (Ca^{2+}) level less than 9 mg/dL or 2.25 mmol/L.
- Because the normal blood level of calcium is so low, any change in calcium levels has major effects on function.
- Common causes of hypocalcemia include:
  1. Decreased vitamin D intake
  2. Complication of chemotherapy
  3. Hypoparathyroidism
  4. Certain types of leukemia or blood disorders
  5. Chronic renal failure
  6. Alcoholism
  7. Certain drugs such as diuretics and estrogen replacement therapy
  8. Excessive laxative use
  9. Consuming excess phosphate
- Low serum calcium levels increase sodium movement across excitable membranes, allowing depolarization to occur more easily and at inappropriate times.
- The more rapidly hypocalcemia occurs and the more severe it is, the more likely life-threatening manifestations will occur.

Gender Health Considerations

Postmenopausal women are at risk for chronic calcium loss. This problem is related to reduced weight-bearing activities and a decrease in estrogen levels. As they age, many women decrease weight-bearing activities such as running and walking, which allows osteoporosis to occur at a more rapid rate. Also the estrogen secretion that protects against osteoporosis diminishes.

PATIENT-CENTERED COLLABORATIVE CARE

Assessment

- Assess for and document dietary intake of calcium or calcium supplement and:
  1. Neuromuscular changes (most common)
     a. Paresthesias with sensations of tingling and numbness
     b. Muscle twitches, painful cramps, and spasms
     c. Anxiety, irritability
     d. Positive Trousseau's sign: Place a blood pressure cuff around the upper arm, inflate the cuff to greater than the patient's systolic pressure, and keep the cuff inflated for 1 to 4 minutes. Under these hypoxic conditions, a positive Trousseau's sign occurs when the hand and fingers go into spasm in palmar flexion.
     e. Positive Chvostek's sign: Tap the face just below and in front of the ear (over the facial nerve) to trigger facial twitching of one side of the mouth, nose, and cheek.
  2. Cardiovascular changes
     a. Bradycardia or tachycardia
     b. Weak, thready pulse
     c. Hypotension (severe hypocalcemia)
     d. ECG changes (prolonged ST interval, prolonged QT interval)
  3. GI changes
     a. Hyperactive bowel sounds
     b. Abdominal cramping
     c. Diarrhea
  4. Skeletal changes (thin, brittle, and fragile bones)
     a. Overall loss of height
     b. Unexplained bone pain

Interventions

- Drug therapy with:
  1. Direct calcium replacement (oral and IV)
  2. Drugs that enhance the absorption of calcium, such as vitamin D
- Nutrition therapy with a high-calcium diet (collaborate with a dietitian to teach patients about foods high in calcium)
- Additional interventions include:
  1. Managing the environment to reduce stimulation, such as keeping the room quiet or adjusting lighting
  2. Instituting seizure precautions including placing emergency equipment (e.g., oxygen, suction) at the bedside
  3. Preventing injury especially for the patient with fragile bones
     a. Use a lift sheet when lifting or moving a patient with fragile bones.

H

b. Observe for normal range of joint motion and for any unusual surface bumps or depressions over bony areas because both may indicate a new fracture.

HYPOKALEMIA

OVERVIEW

- Hypokalemia is a serum potassium level less than 3.5 mEq/L (3.5 mmol/L).
- It can be life threatening, because every body system is affected.
- With hypokalemia, the cell membranes of all excitable tissues, such as nerve and muscle, are less responsive to normal stimuli.
- Rapid reduction of serum potassium levels results in dramatic changes in function, whereas gradual reductions may not show changes in function until the level is very low.
- Older adults are more vulnerable to hypokalemia because of risk factors of chronic conditions and drug therapy that contribute to this electrolyte imbalance.
- Common causes include:
  1. Actual potassium deficits
     a. Inappropriate or excessive use of drugs
        (1) Diuretics
        (2) Digitalis
        (3) Corticosteroids
     b. Increased secretion of aldosterone
     c. Cushing's syndrome
     d. Diarrhea
     e. Vomiting
     f. Wound drainage (especially gastrointestinal)
     g. Prolonged nasogastric suction
     h. Heat-induced excessive diaphoresis
     i. Kidney disease impairing reabsorption of potassium
     j. Nothing by mouth status
  2. Relative potassium deficits
     a. Alkalosis
     b. Hyperinsulinism
     c. Hyperalimentation
     d. Total parenteral nutrition
     e. Water intoxication

PATIENT-CENTERED COLLABORATIVE CARE
Assessment

- Obtain patient information about:
  1. Drugs, especially diuretics, corticosteroids, digoxin, beta-adrenergic agonists or antagonists, and potassium supplements

2. Presence of acute or chronic disease
3. Diet history
- Assess for and document:
1. Respiratory changes:

! NURSING SAFETY PRIORITY: Critical Rescue

Assess the respiratory status of a patient who has hypokalemia at least every 3 hours because respiratory insufficiency is a major cause of death for these patients.

    a. Breath sounds
    b. Respiratory effort including rate and depth of respiration
    c. Oxygen saturation
    d. Color of nail beds and mucous membranes
2. Musculoskeletal changes that indicate weakness
    a. Weak hand grasps
    b. Lethargy, inability to complete ADLs
    c. Flaccid paralysis
3. Cardiovascular changes
    a. Rapid, thready pulse that is difficult to palpate
    b. Dysrhythmias and ECG changes
      (1) ST-segment depression
      (2) Flat or inverted T waves
      (3) Increased U waves
    c. Orthostatic hypotension

! NURSING SAFETY PRIORITY: Critical Rescue

Dysrhythmias can lead to death, particularly in older adults. Report new onset dysrhythmias and all ECG changes consistent with hypokalemia to the physician or Rapid Response Team.

4. Neurologic changes
    a. Altered mental status
    b. Irritability and anxiety
    c. Lethargy, acute confusion, coma
5. GI changes of reduced peristalsis leading to:
    a. Hypoactive or absent bowel sounds
    b. Abdominal distension
    c. Nausea, vomiting
    d. Constipation

Interventions
- Interventions for hypokalemia aim to prevent potassium loss, increase serum potassium levels, and provide a safe environment for the patient.

- Medical interventions include:
  1. Drug therapy
     a. Oral and IV potassium replacement therapy
     b. In the presence of persistent hypokalemia despite replacement therapy, evaluate and consider replacing magnesium.

QSEN SAFETY

Potassium carries a high alert warning as a concentrated intravenous electrolyte solution. Vials of concentrated potassium are no longer available in patient care areas. Before infusing any IV solution containing potassium chloride (KCl), check and recheck the dilution of the drug in the IV solution container.

! NURSING SAFETY PRIORITY: Drug Alert

A dilution of at least 1 mEq of potassium to 10 mL of solution is recommended for IV administration. The maximum recommended infusion rate is 5 to 10 mEq/hr; this rate is never to exceed 20 mEq/hr under any circumstances. Potassium is a severe tissue irritant and is never given by IM or subcutaneous injection.

     c. Potassium-sparing diuretics
        (1) Spironolactone (Aldactone, Novo-Spiroton ♣)
        (2) Triamterene (Dyrenium)
        (3) Amiloride (Midamor)
  2. Nutrition therapy to increase dietary potassium intake
- The priorities for nursing care of the patient with hypokalemia are ensuring adequate oxygenation, preventing patient falls, preventing injury from potassium administration, and monitoring the patient's response to therapy.
  1. Instituting fall precautions as a safety measure
  2. Performing respiratory monitoring at least hourly for severe hypokalemia
     a. Respiratory effort including rate and depth (checking for increasing rate and decreasing depth)
     b. Oxygen saturation by pulse oximetry
  3. Monitoring patient response to potassium replacement therapy including cardiac and neurological derangements from too rapid or delayed replacement therapy
  4. Collaborating with the dietician to teach the patient about dietary sources of potassium

HYPONATREMIA

OVERVIEW

- Hyponatremia is a serum sodium (Na^+) level less than 136 mEq/L (136 mmol/L), and it often occurs with fluid volume imbalances.

- The problems caused by hyponatremia involve reduced excitable membrane depolarization and cellular swelling.
- The cells especially affected are those involved in cerebral, neuromuscular, intestinal smooth muscle, and cardiovascular functions.
- Common causes of hyponatremia include:
    1. Actual sodium deficits
        a. Excessive diaphoresis
        b. Diuretics (high-ceiling diuretics)
        c. Wound drainage (especially gastrointestinal)
        d. Decreased secretion of aldosterone
        e. Hyperlipidemia
        f. Kidney disease (scarred distal convoluted tubule)
        g. Nothing by mouth
        h. Low-salt diet
        i. Cerebral salt-wasting syndrome
        j. Hyperglycemia
    2. Relative sodium deficits (dilution)
        a. Excessive ingestion of hypotonic fluids
        b. Psychogenic polydipsia
        c. Freshwater submersion accident
        d. Kidney failure (nephrotic syndrome)
        e. Irrigation with hypotonic fluids
        f. Syndrome of inappropriate antidiuretic hormone secretion
        g. Heart failure

PATIENT-CENTERED COLLABORATIVE CARE
Assessment
- Assess for and document:
    1. Cerebral changes
        a. Acute confusion
        b. Reduced level of cognition
        c. Seizure activity
    2. Neuromuscular changes
        a. General muscle weakness, especially in arms and legs
        b. Diminished deep tendon reflexes

! NURSING SAFETY PRIORITY: Critical Rescue

If the patient has muscle weakness, immediately check respiratory effectiveness such as SpO2 and consciousness or cognition. Ventilation depends on adequate strength of respiratory muscles.

    3. GI changes
        a. Increased motility
        b. Diarrhea

   c. Abdominal cramping
   d. Hyperactive bowel sounds
4. Cardiovascular changes
   a. Hyponatremia with hypovolemia
      (1) Rapid, weak, thready pulse
      (2) Reduced peripheral pulses
      (3) Hypotension
   b. Hyponatremia with hypervolemia
      (1) Full, bounding pulse
      (2) Normal or high blood pressure
      (3) Edema

Interventions

- Drug therapy
  1. Discontinuing or reducing drugs that increase sodium loss, such as loop diuretics and thiazide diuretics
  2. Hyponatremia with a fluid deficit: prescribing IV saline infusion to restore both sodium and fluid volume; severe hyponatremia may be treated with small-volume infusions of hypertonic (2% to 3%) saline
  3. Hyponatremia with fluid excess: using osmotic diuretics that promote the excretion of water rather than sodium, such as mannitol (Osmitrol) or conivaptan (Vaprisol)
  4. Hyponatremia caused by inappropriate secretion of antidiuretic hormone (ADH): therapy that includes agents that antagonize ADH, such as lithium and demeclocycline (Declomycin)
- Nutrition therapy
  1. Increased oral sodium intake
  2. Fluid restriction when hyponatremia occurs with fluid excess
- Priorities for nursing care of the patient with hyponatremia include monitoring the patient's response to therapy and preventing hypernatremia and fluid overload
  1. Prevent fluid overload leading to pulmonary edema and heart failure
     a. Monitor for indicators of increased fluid overload at least every 2 hours.
  2. Monitor for patient response to drug therapy
     a. Evaluate serum and urine lab results
     b. Weigh daily
     c. Monitor the amount and quality of oral and IV intake and urine output
  3. Observe for manifestations and complications of electrolyte imbalance
     a. Changes in neurologic, muscular, GI, and cardiovascular health, including ECG patterns

b. Changes in serum and urine sodium values
c. Provide skin protection interventions if the patient with hyponatremia has decreased consciousness, muscle weakness leading to reducing mobility, or edema
4. Nutritional therapy; teach patients and families about:
   a. Sodium intake
   b. Fluid restriction

HYPOPARATHYROIDISM

OVERVIEW

- Hypoparathyroidism is a rare endocrine disorder in which parathyroid function is decreased, resulting in a deficiency of circulating PTH levels.
- The main result is hypocalcemia.
- There are two forms:
  1. *Iatrogenic hypoparathyroidism,* the most common form, which is caused by the removal of all parathyroid tissue during total thyroidectomy or by deliberate surgical removal of the parathyroid glands
  2. *Idiopathic hypoparathyroidism,* which is rare and probably caused by an autoimmune problem

PATIENT-CENTERED COLLABORATIVE CARE

Assessment

- Obtain patient information about:
  1. Any head or neck surgery
  2. History of head or neck radiation therapy
  3. History of serious neck injury from a car crash or strangulation
  4. Presence of mild tingling and numbness around the mouth or in the hands and feet
  5. Presence of muscle cramps and spasms of the hands and feet
- Assess for and document hypocalcemia signs or symptoms:
  1. Irritability or psychosis
  2. Tetany: excessive or inappropriate muscle contractions that cause finger, hand, and elbow flexion
     a. Positive Chvostek's sign (see *Hypocalcemia*)
     b. Positive Trousseau's sign (see *Hypocalcemia*)
  3. Bands or pits encircling the crowns of the teeth
- Diagnostic tests for hypoparathyroidism include:
  1. Serum electrolyte tests, vitamin D and PTH levels
  2. CT scan of the brain (may show calcium deposits) and neck
  3. Urine cyclic adenosine monophosphate (cAMP) levels

H

Interventions

- Medical management focuses on correcting hypocalcemia, vitamin D deficiency, and hypomagnesemia.
    1. For severe hypocalcemia, IV calcium is given as a 10% solution of calcium chloride or calcium gluconate over 10 to 15 minutes
    2. Calcitriol (Rocaltrol), 0.5 to 2 mg daily for vitamin D deficiency
    3. For hypomagnesemia, magnesium sulfate is typically given orally at 3 g/dose to a maximum of 12 g/24 hr, or IV as 1 g/100 mL over 2 or more hours, repeated as needed to a maximum of 5 g/24 hr
    4. Long-term oral therapy of calcium, 0.5 to 2 g daily, in divided doses
    5. Long-term therapy for vitamin D deficiency
- Nursing care includes:
    1. Teaching about the drug regimen and interventions to reduce anxiety
    2. Teaching the patient to eat foods high in calcium but low in phosphorus (milk, yogurt, and processed cheeses are avoided because of their high phosphorus content)
    3. Stressing that therapy for hypocalcemia is lifelong
    4. Advising the patient to wear a medical alert bracelet

HYPOPITUITARISM

OVERVIEW

- Hypopituitarism is a deficiency of one or more anterior pituitary hormones, resulting in metabolic problems and sexual dysfunctions that vary depending on the undersecreted hormones.
- Decreased production of all anterior pituitary hormones is a rare condition known as *panhypopituitarism.*
- Usually, there is a decrease in the secretion of one hormone and a lesser decrease in the other hormones.
- Deficiencies of ACTH and TSH are the most life threatening, because they result in a corresponding decrease in the secretion of vital hormones from the adrenal and thyroid glands.
- Causes of hypopituitarism include pituitary tumors, severe malnutrition or rapid loss of body fat, shock or severe hypotension, head trauma, brain tumors or infection, radiation or surgery of the head and brain, and acquired immune deficiency syndrome (AIDS).

PATIENT-CENTERED COLLABORATIVE CARE

Assessment

- Assess for and document:
    1. Loss of secondary sexual characteristics (men)
        a. Facial and body hair loss
        b. Impotence
        c. Decreased libido

2. Loss of secondary sexual characteristics (women)
   a. Absence of menstrual periods
   b. Painful intercourse
   c. Infertility
   d. Decreased libido
   e. Breast atrophy
   f. Decreased amount or absence of auxiliary and pubic hair
3. Neurologic changes
   a. Loss of visual acuity, especially peripheral vision
   b. Temporal headaches
   c. Diplopia (double vision)
   d. Ocular muscle paralysis, limiting eye movement
- Diagnostic assessment may include:
  1. Blood levels of pituitary hormones
  2. Hormone stimulation testing
  3. CT scan of the head
  4. MRI of the head
  5. Angiography (brain)

Interventions

- Management of the patient with hypopituitarism focuses on replacement of deficient hormones.
- Instruct the patient about the hormone replacement method and regimen.
  1. Men with gonadotropin deficiency receive sex steroid replacement therapy with androgens (testosterone) parenterally or with transdermal testosterone patches.
     a. High doses are used until virilization (presence of male secondary sex characteristics) occurs, and then maintenance doses are used.
     b. Side effects may include gynecomastia (development of breast tissue in men), acne, baldness, and prostate enlargement.
     c. Fertility is difficult to achieve and requires additional therapy.
  2. Women who have gonadotropin deficiency receive hormone replacement with a combination of estrogen and progesterone.
     a. Combined estrogen and progestin are used, usually orally or by transdermal patch.
     b. Complications include hypertension and deep vein thrombosis.
     c. Additional therapy is needed for fertility.
  3. Adult patients with growth hormone (GH) deficiency may be treated with injections of GH.
  4. ACTH and TSH are not replaced; instead thyroid hormone and cortisol are given.

H

HYPOTHYROIDISM

OVERVIEW

- Hypothyroidism is the underproduction of thyroid hormones by the thyroid gland, resulting in decreased whole-body metabolism.
- Most cases of hypothyroidism in the United States occur as a result of thyroid surgery and RAI treatment of hyperthyroidism.
- Worldwide, hypothyroidism is common in areas where the soil and water have little natural iodide, causing endemic goiter.
- Other causes of hypothyroidism include autoimmune thyroid destruction; infection of thyroid tissue; congenital absence or hypoplasia of thyroid tissues; neck surgery, irradiation, or trauma; and a wide variety of drugs.
- Women are affected much more often than men.
- Myxedema coma is a rare, serious complication of untreated or poorly treated hypothyroidism.

PATIENT-CENTERED COLLABORATIVE CARE

Assessment

- Obtain patient information about:
    1. Activity levels now compared with the previous year
    2. Amount of time spent sleeping
    3. Generalized weakness, anorexia, muscle aches, and paresthesias
    4. Constipation
    5. Cold intolerance (use of more blankets at night or sweaters and extra clothing, even in warm weather)
    6. Change in libido
    7. Heavy, prolonged menses or amenorrhea
    8. Impotence and infertility
    9. Current or previous use of drugs known to interfere with thyroid function, such as lithium, amiodarone, aminoglutethimide, sodium or potassium perchlorate, thiocyanates, or cobalt
    10. Medical history, including whether the patient has ever been treated for hyperthyroidism and what specific treatment was used
    11. Recent weight gain
- Assess for and document:
    1. Overall appearance
        a. Coarse features
        b. Edema around the eyes and face
        c. Blank expression
        d. Thick tongue
    2. Slow muscle movement
    3. Slurred or unclear speech
    4. Slow response to questions

  5. Bradycardia
  6. Hypotension
  7. Slow respiratory rate
  8. Low core body temperature
  9. Presence or absence of a goiter
- Psychosocial assessment and issues may include:
  1. Depression
  2. Lethargy, apathy, drowsiness
  3. Reduced attention span and memory
- Diagnostic assessment may include blood tests for:
  1. Triiodothyronine (T_3)
  2. Thyroxine (T_4)
  3. TSH levels

Interventions

- Drug therapy is the mainstay of management for hypothyroidism.
- The patient requires lifelong thyroid hormone replacement; the most commonly used drug is levothyroxine (Synthroid, Levothroid, Levoxyl, Unithroid, generic).
  1. Therapy is started with a low dose that is gradually increased over a period of weeks.
  2. The patient with more severe symptoms of hypothyroidism is started on the lowest dose of thyroid hormone replacement, because starting at too high a dose or increasing the dose too rapidly can cause severe hypertension, heart failure, and myocardial infarction.
     a. Teach patients and the families of patients who are beginning thyroid replacement hormone therapy to take the drug exactly as prescribed and not to change the dose or schedule without consulting the health care provider.
     b. Assess the patient for chest pain and dyspnea during initiation of therapy.
  3. Dosage is determined by blood levels of TSH and the patient's physical responses.
  4. Monitor for and teach the patient and family about the manifestations of hyperthyroidism/excess treatment, including:
     a. Tachycardia
     b. Intolerance to heat
     c. Difficulty sleeping
     d. Diarrhea
     e. Excessive weight loss
     f. Fine tremors of the hands
- Management of myxedema coma
  1. *Myxedema coma* is a severe and life-threatening form of hypothyroidism in which the patient's overall metabolism slows to the point that cardiac and respiratory arrest can occur.

H

2. Factors leading to myxedema coma include acute illness, surgery, chemotherapy, discontinuing thyroid replacement therapy, and the use of sedatives or opioids.
3. Manifestations include:
   a. Coma
   b. Respiratory failure
   c. Hypotension
   d. Hyponatremia
   e. Hypothermia
   f. Hypoglycemia
4. Untreated myxedema coma leads to shock, organ damage, and death.
5. Treatment is instituted quickly according to the patient's manifestations and without waiting for laboratory confirmation.
6. Best practices for emergency care of the patient with myxedema coma are:
   a. Maintaining a patent airway and instituting aspiration precautions
   b. Replacing fluids with IV normal or hypertonic saline
   c. Giving levothyroxine IV as prescribed
   d. Giving glucose IV as prescribed
   e. Giving corticosteroids as prescribed
   f. Monitoring vital signs hourly and reporting significant or symptomatic changes
   g. Managing hypothermia with warm blankets or a warming device
   h. Monitoring for changes in mental status, reporting decreased consciousness in a timely manner

Community-Based Care

- Hypothyroidism is usually a chronic condition and the patient may live in any type of environment. Ensure that whoever is responsible for overseeing the patient's daily care is aware of the condition and understands its treatment.
- The patient who has a decreased attention span may need help from family, friends, or a home care aide with the drug regimen.
- Develop a plan for drug therapy, and be sure that one person is clearly designated as responsible for drug preparation and delivery so that doses are neither missed nor duplicated.
- Teach the patient and family about hormone replacement therapy and its side effects.
  1. Emphasize the need for lifelong drugs.
  2. Review the manifestations of both hyperthyroidism and hypothyroidism.
  3. Teach the patient to wear a medical alert bracelet.

   4. Instruct the patient to carefully evaluate OTC drugs and fiber
      preparations, because thyroid hormone preparations interact
      with many other drugs.
- Teach the family to orient the patient often and to explain every-
  thing clearly, simply, and as often as needed.
- Teach the patient to monitor himself or herself for therapy effectiveness by assessing the need for sleep and the frequency of bowel
  elimination.
   1. When the patient requires more sleep and is constipated, the
      dose of replacement hormone may need to be increased.
   2. When the patient has difficulty getting to sleep and has more
      bowel movements than normal for him or her, the dose may
      need to be decreased.

I

IMMUNODEFICIENCIES
OVERVIEW
- Immunodeficiency is a failure of the immune system to recognize
  infectious agents or foreign proteins as a result of a missing or
  damaged immune component.
- A *primary (congenital) immunodeficiency* is a condition in which
  one or more parts of the system are not functioning properly from
  birth.
- A *secondary immunodeficiency* is acquired after birth as the result
  of viral infection, contact with a toxin, drug therapy, or radiation
  therapy.
- The immunodeficient patient is at increased risk for infection,
  cancer, and other diseases.
- Types of congenital or primary antibody-mediated immunodeficiencies that adults may have include:
   1. Bruton's agammaglobulinemia
      a. This is a classic congenital antibody-mediated immune
         deficiency that has an X-linked pattern of inheritance.
      b. Boys born with this disease usually start to have problems
         at about age 6 months with manifestations of recurrent
         otitis, sinusitis, pneumonia, furunculosis, meningitis, and
         septicemia.
      c. Laboratory assessment shows an absence of circulating
         immunoglobulin (antibodies).
      d. The overall prognosis is good if antibody replacement is
         started early.
      e. Antibiotics are used for specific infections, and long-term
         prophylactic antibiotic therapy may also be used.

    2. Common variable immune deficiency
       a. Common variable immune deficiency affects men and women.
       b. Patients have low levels of circulating antibodies (immunoglobulins) of all classes.
       c. It usually first appears later (in adolescence or young adulthood), and the infections are less severe than those seen in patients with Bruton's agammaglobulinemia.
       d. Common problems include giardiasis (intestinal infection with *Giardia lamblia*), pneumonia, sinusitis, gastric cancer, bronchiectasis, and gallstones.
       e. Management requires regular infusions of immune serum globulin and regular or intermittent use of antibiotics to protect the affected person against infection.
    3. Selective immunoglobulin A (IgA) deficiency
       a. This is the most common congenital immunodeficiency seen in adults.
       b. The person may be asymptomatic or have chronic or recurrent upper respiratory tract infections, skin infections, urinary tract infections, vaginal infections, and diarrhea.
       c. It does not reduce the person's life span.
       d. Management is limited to vigorous treatment of infections.

❗ NURSING SAFETY PRIORITY: Action Alert

Unlike other immunoglobulin deficiencies, IgA deficiency should never be treated with exogenous immune globulin. Because patients with IgA deficiency make normal amounts of all other antibodies, they are at high risk for severe allergic reactions to exogenous immune globulin.

- Types of iatrogenic or therapy-induced immunodeficiencies include:
    1. Drug-induced immune deficiencies caused by:
       a. Cytotoxic drugs used in the treatment of cancer and autoimmune disorders
       b. Corticosteroids used to treat many autoimmune diseases, neoplasms, and endocrine disorders
       c. Cyclosporine (Sandimmune, Neoral), a specific immunosuppressant that is used to prevent organ transplant rejection and graft-versus-host disease and is occasionally used for other disorders, such as uveitis, rheumatoid arthritis, and other autoimmune disorders
       d. Biologics or disease-modifying immune suppressive drugs specifically slow the damage caused by a variety of autoimmune diseases.

   2. Radiation-induced immunodeficiency when the iliac and femur in adults are exposed to high doses of radiation (these are the blood cell-producing sites of adults)

- Management of treatment-induced immune deficiency aims to improve immune function and protect the patient from infection.
- Usually, treatment-related immunodeficiencies resolve after the suppressive drug or radiation therapy is stopped and the hematopoietic cells recover.
- Teach the patient how to protect himself or herself from infection by:
  1. Avoiding crowds and other large gatherings of people where someone might be ill
  2. Not sharing personal toilet articles, such as toothbrushes, toothpaste, washcloths, or deodorant sticks, with others
  3. Bathing daily, using an antimicrobial soap, and, if total bathing is not possible, washing the armpits, groin, genitals, and anal area twice daily with an antimicrobial soap
  4. Cleaning the toothbrush daily by running it through the dishwasher or rinsing it in liquid laundry bleach
  5. Cleaning hands thoroughly with an antimicrobial soap or solution before eating or drinking, after touching a pet, after shaking hands with anyone, returning home from any outing, and after using the toilet
  6. Washing dishes between uses with hot, sudsy water, or using a dishwasher
  7. Not drinking water, milk, juice, or other cold liquids that have been standing for longer than an hour
  8. Not reusing cups and glasses without washing
  9. Not changing pet litter boxes or, if unavoidable, using gloves and washing hands immediately
  10. Avoiding birds, turtles, and other reptiles as pets
  11. Avoiding raw or undercooked meat, fish, and eggs (even if served as pet food)
  12. Thoroughly washing fruit and vegetables

INFLUENZA, SEASONAL AND PANDEMIC
OVERVIEW
- Influenza, or "flu," is a highly contagious, acute viral respiratory infection that can occur at any age.
- Epidemics are common and lead to complications of pneumonia or death, especially in older adults or debilitated or immunocompromised patients.

- Influenza may be caused by one of several virus families, referred to as A, B, and C.
- Pandemic influenza refers to respiratory viral infections that have the potential to spread globally.
- While most viral infections among animals are not transmitted to humans, when these viruses mutate and become infectious to humans, these new viral infections have great potential to cause pandemics.
  1. The H1N1 strain, also known as swine flu, mutated and became highly infectious to humans in 2009, infecting an estimated 61 million people, resulting in more than 12,000 deaths.

PATIENT-CENTERED COLLABORATIVE CARE

- The prioritized care reduces risk of infection through vaccination, handwashing, and community and personal quarantine to avoid droplet spread of the virus. Adults are contagious from 24 hours before symptoms occur and up to 5 days after they begin.
- Supportive care for the patient infected with influenza includes early identification through symptom manifestation.
  1. Cough, sore throat
  2. Fever, fatigue, weakness
  3. Rapid progression to shortness of breath and pneumonia

Interventions

- Vaccination for everyone older than 3 months of age
  1. Seasonal vaccination, usually in late fall with a vaccine containing three antigens for the three expected viral strains (trivalent influenza vaccine [TIV])
  2. Influenza vaccinations can be taken as an IM injection (Fluvirin, Fluzone) or as a live attenuated influenza vaccine (LAIV) by intranasal spray (FluMist)
- For infected patients:
  1. Promote social distance or quarantine/isolation to decrease the spread of the virus.
  2. Provide fluids and rest to promote recovery.
  3. Consider administration of antiviral agents given within 12 to 24 hours of symptom onset to reduce the severity or duration of influenza; these agents include amantadine (Symmetrel) and rimantadine (Flumadine) for influenza A strains and zanamivir (Relenza), which is used as an oral inhalant, and oseltamivir (Tamiflu) for any strain of influenza.
- Anticipate hospitalization for frail or immunocompromised patients, infants, and older adults, who require respiratory support or close monitoring to prevent complications.

IRRITABLE BOWEL SYNDROME
OVERVIEW
- Irritable bowel syndrome (IBS) is a functional GI disorder that causes chronic or recurrent diarrhea, constipation, and/or abdominal pain and bloating.
- Increased or decreased bowel transit times result in changes in the normal *bowel elimination* pattern to one of these classifications: diarrhea (IBS-D), constipation (IBS-C), or alternating diarrhea and constipation.
- The etiology is unclear and a combination of environmental, immunologic, genetic, hormonal, and stress factors have a role in the development and course of IBS.

PATIENT-CENTERED COLLABORATIVE CARE
Assessment
- Assess for and document:
  1. Weight change (weight loss is uncommon)
  2. Fatigue, malaise
  3. Abdominal pain, cramps, particularly pain in the left lower quadrant
  4. Changes in the bowel pattern (constipation, diarrhea, or an alternating pattern of both) or consistency of stools and the passage of mucus
  5. Food intolerance
  6. Serum albumin, CBC, erythrocyte sedimentation rate, and *H. Pylori* testing to detect infection and nutritional deficits
  7. Occult blood or melena

Interventions
- Diet therapy includes:
  1. Suggesting a symptom diary to help identify triggers and bowel habits
  2. Helping the patient identify and eliminate foods associated with exacerbations
  3. Consulting with the dietitian to promote intake of fiber and fluid
     a. Teaching the patient to ingest 30 to 40 g of fiber daily
     b. Teaching the patient to drink 8 to 10 cups of liquid per day
- Drug therapy includes:
  1. Bulk-forming laxatives, such as psyllium hydrophilic mucilloid (Metamucil), may be taken at mealtimes with a glass of water to prevent dry, hard, or liquid stools.
  2. Lubiprostone (Amitiza) or linaclotide (Linzess) can be used to increase intestinal fluid and promote bowel elimination in IBS-C.

3. Antidiarrheal agents such as loperamide (Imodium) may be used to decrease cramping and frequency of stools.
4. Alosetron (Lotronex), a serotonin-selective ($5\text{-}HT_3$) drug, may be used with caution for women with diarrhea-predominant IBS-D.
5. Patients with IBS who have bloating and abdominal distention without constipation may be prescribed rifaximin (Xifaxan), an antibiotic with little systemic absorption.
6. For IBS in which pain is the predominant symptom, tricyclic antidepressants such as amitriptyline (Elavil) have also been used successfully.
7. Holistic, complementary, and alternative therapy includes:
   a. Probiotics to reduce bacteria and alleviate GI symptoms of IBS
   b. Peppermint oil capsules to reduce GI symptoms
   c. Stress management such as meditation, imagery, and/or yoga to decrease GI symptoms

K

KIDNEY DISEASE, CHRONIC
OVERVIEW
- Chronic kidney disease (CKD) is a progressive, irreversible kidney injury; kidney function does not recover.
- The progression toward CKD occurs in five stages.
  1. *Stage 1:* At risk for CKD. Normal kidney function with a GFR greater than 90 mL/min. Kidney function is normal, but the patient has sufficient risk factors to require screening and ongoing monitoring of kidney function.
  2. *Stage 2:* Mild CKD. GFR is reduced to 60 to 89 mL/min. The focus of care is to be vigilant about reducing risk factors for kidney disease.
  3. *Stage 3:* Moderate CKD. GFR 30 to 59 mL/min. The focus of care is to slow progression of the disease through diet and increase vigilance to avoid hypoperfusion, toxins, and other risk factors.
  4. *Stage 4:* Severe CKD. GFR 15 to 29 mL/min. The intensity of the care is increased to manage complications (anemia, hypertension) and prepare for eventual renal replacement therapy.
  5. *Stage 5:* End-stage kidney disease (ESKD); renal replacement therapy is started. Alternatively, kidney transplantation is performed.
- As kidney disease progresses pathologic alterations include abnormal urine production, poor water excretion, electrolyte imbalance, and metabolic anomalies (e.g., loss of erythropoietin synthesis).

- When less than 20% of nephrons are functional, hyposthenuria (loss of urine concentrating ability) and polyuria occur; left untreated, severe dehydration occurs.
- Urea is the primary product of protein metabolism and is normally excreted by the kidney; BUN varies with dietary intake of protein.
- Creatinine is derived from creatine and phosphocreatine; the normal rate of excretion depends on muscle mass, physical activity, and diet.
- Azotemia is the increased accumulation of nitrogenous waste (BUN) in the blood and is a classic indicator of kidney failure.
- Variations in sodium excretion occur and depend on the stage of CKD.
    1. There is an increased risk for hyponatremia, or sodium depletion, in early CKD.
    2. Hyponatremia occurs because the reduced number of functional nephrons is insufficient to reabsorb sodium, and sodium is lost in the urine.
- Hyperkalemia results from an increase in potassium load, including ingestion of potassium in drugs, failure to restrict potassium in the diet, blood transfusions, and excess bleeding.
- Other metabolic derangements in CKD include changes in pH (metabolic acidosis), calcium (hypocalcemia) and phosphorus (hyperphosphatemia) imbalances, and vitamin D insufficiency.
    1. Renal osteodystrophy caused by hypocalcemia and phosphorus retention results in skeletal demineralization manifested by bone pain, pseudofractures, sclerosis of the spine, skull demineralization, osteomalacia, reabsorption of bone, and loss of tooth lamina.
- Cardiovascular alterations include anemia, hypertension, hyperlipidemia, heart failure, and pericarditis.
- GI alterations include uremic stomatitis, anorexia, peptic ulcer disease, nausea, and vomiting.

PATIENT-CENTERED COLLABORATIVE CARE
Assessment
- Obtain patient information about:
    1. Age (because a reduction in the number and function of nephrons occurs with age)
    2. Height and weight, including recent weight gain or loss
    3. Current and past medical conditions
    4. Drugs, prescription and OTC
    5. Family history of kidney disease
    6. Dietary and nutritional habits, including food preferences
    7. History of GI problems, such as nausea, vomiting, anorexia, diarrhea, or constipation

K

    8. Recent injuries and abnormal bruising or bleeding
    9. Activity intolerance, weakness and fatigue
  10. Detailed urinary elimination history
- Assess for and document:
  1. Neurologic manifestations
     a. Changes in mentation or new lethargy
     b. Changes in sensation or weakness in extremities indicating uremic neuropathy
  2. Cardiovascular manifestations of CKD from fluid overload, hypertension, or cardiac disease
     a. Systolic blood pressure (SBP) higher than 130 mm Hg or diastolic blood pressure (DBP) higher than 80 mm Hg (lower tolerance for elevations in blood pressure with CKD)
     b. Cardiomyopathy
     c. Uremic pericarditis
     d. Peripheral edema
     e. Heart failure
     f. Pericardial friction rub or effusion
  3. Respiratory manifestations
     a. Breath that smells like urine (uremic fetor or halitosis)
     b. Deep sighing or yawning
     c. Tachypnea or shortness of breath
     d. Pulmonary edema or pleural effusion
     e. Kussmaul respiration with acidemia
     f. Uremic lung or hilar pneumonitis
  4. Hematologic manifestations
     a. Anemia
     b. Abnormal bleeding: bruising petechiae, abnormal vaginal bleeding, GI bleeding
  5. GI complications
     a. Mouth ulceration
     b. Abdominal pain or cramping
     c. Nausea or vomiting
  6. Urinary findings
     a. Change in urinary amount, frequency, and appearance of urine
     b. Proteinuria or hematuria
  7. Integumentary or dermatologic manifestations
     a. Yellow coloration from pigment deposition; darkening of skin for some African Americans
     b. Severe itching (pruritus)
     c. Uremic frost, a layer of uremic crystals from evaporated sweat on the face, eyebrows, axilla, and groin (rare)
     d. Bruises or purple patches and rashes

8. Immunologic considerations
    a. Increased susceptibility to infections
- Diagnostic testing may include:
    1. Serum creatinine, BUN, sodium, potassium, calcium, phosphorus, bicarbonate, hemoglobin, and hematocrit
    2. Urinalysis
    3. A 24-hour urinalysis for creatinine and creatine clearance
    4. Ultrasound, CT scan, or x-ray to observe progression, which manifests as small and fibrotic kidneys

Planning and Implementation

- Priority problems for patients with CKD are:

FLUID OVERLOAD

- Fluid overload is related to the inability of diseased kidneys to maintain body fluid balance.
- The goal is to achieve and maintain acceptable fluid balance. Indicators include:
    1. Blood pressure
    2. Heart rate
    3. Body weight
    4. Central venous pressure
    5. Serum electrolytes
- Diuretic drugs may be used in patients with CKD in stages 1 through 4.

POTENTIAL FOR PULMONARY EDEMA

- Potential for pulmonary edema is related to fluid overload.
- The goal is to remain free of pulmonary edema and maintain optimal fluid balance.
- Interventions include:
    1. Assessing for early signs of pulmonary edema, such as restlessness, dyspnea, and crackles
    2. If the patient is dyspneic, placing the patient in a high Fowler's position and giving oxygen to maximize lung expansion and improve gas exchange
    3. Measuring and recording intake and output
    4. Assessing cardiovascular system for fluid overload: S_3 heart sounds, peripheral edema, jugular venous distention, tachycardia, hypotension, or hypertension
    5. Monitoring serum chemistry results for electrolyte imbalance
    6. Monitoring peripheral oxygenation (Spo_2) to detect hypoxemia
    7. Providing drug therapy
        a. Diuretics for stages 1 through 4 CKD; monitor for ototoxicity with loop diuretics
        b. Morphine to reduce myocardial oxygen demands; monitor for respiratory depression
        c. Vasodilators such as nitroglycerin

K

ALTERED CARDIAC OUTPUT
- Cardiac output is related to hypovolemia or hypervolemia, dysrhythmias, and peripheral vascular resistance influenced by CKD.
- The goal is to attain and maintain adequate cardiac output. Indicators include:
  1. Systolic and diastolic blood pressures
  2. Ejection fraction
  3. Peripheral pulses
  4. Cognitive status
- Interventions include:
  1. Administering calcium channel blockers, ACE inhibitors, alpha- and beta-adrenergic blockers, and vasodilators
  2. Teaching the family to measure the patient's blood pressure and weight daily and to bring these records when visiting the physician, nurse, or nutritionist
  3. Monitoring the patient for decreased cardiac output, heart failure, congestive heart failure, and dysrhythmias

INADEQUATE NUTRITION
- Nutrition is related to inability to ingest and digest food or to absorb nutrients as a result of physiologic factors. Provide food and fluids to prevent malnutrition.
- The nutritional need and diet restrictions for the patient with CKD vary according to the degree of remaining kidney function and the type of renal replacement therapy used.
- Common changes include control of protein intake; fluid intake limitation; restriction of potassium, sodium, and phosphorus intake; taking vitamin and mineral supplements; and eating enough calories to meet metabolic demand.
- Consult with the nutritionist to provide nutritional teaching and planning and to assist the patient in adapting the diet to food preferences, ethnic background, and budget.

POTENTIAL FOR INFECTION
- Infection is related to skin breakdown, immunomodulation from uremia, exposure to bloodborne pathogens during hemodialysis treatment, and malnutrition.
- The goals are to prevent infection and detect infection early by monitoring for:
  1. Fever
  2. Lymph node enlargement
  3. Positive culture or serum markers (e.g., markers for hepatitis)
  4. Tenderness, redness, or drainage at dialysis access site
  5. Abnormal WBC count and differential
  6. Skin integrity

POTENTIAL FOR INJURY
- Potential for injury is related to effects of kidney disease on bone density, blood clotting, and drug elimination.

- The goals are to prevent the following problems: falls, pathologic fractures, bleeding, and toxic effects of prescribed drugs. Interventions include:
  1. Monitoring the patient closely for drug-related complications
  2. Teaching the patient to avoid certain drugs that can increase kidney damage, such as NSAIDs, antibiotics, antihypertensives, and diuretics in the presence of hypovolemia
  3. Anticipating dosage adjustment as kidney function decreases
  4. Administering agents to control phosphorus excess, such as calcium acetate, calcium carbonate, and aluminum hydroxide
  5. Instructing the patient to avoid compounds containing magnesium
  6. Administering opioid analgesics cautiously, because the effects may last longer and uremic patients are sensitive to the respiratory depressant effects

FATIGUE
- Fatigue is related to kidney disease, anemia, and reduced energy production.
- The goal is to conserve energy and preserve the ability to perform self-care, retain interest in surroundings, and sustain mental concentration. Interventions include:
  1. Providing vitamin and mineral supplementation
  2. Administering erythropoietin to maintain hemoglobin 7 to 9 g/dL3; administer iron supplements to maintain safe levels of hemoglobin and hematocrit (hematocrit goal is usually 27% to 28%)
  3. Monitoring dietary intake (improved appetite challenges patients in their attempts to maintain protein and potassium) and fluid restriction

ANXIETY
- Anxiety is related to threat to or change in health status, economic status, relationships, role function, systems, or self-concept; situational crisis; threat of death; lack of knowledge about diagnostic tests, disease process, treatment; loss of control; or disrupted family life.
- The goal is to reduce feelings of apprehension and tension. Interventions include:
  1. Observing the patient's behavior for signs of anxiety
  2. Evaluating the patient's support system
  3. Explaining all procedures, tests, and treatments
  4. Providing instruction on kidney function and kidney failure
  5. Encouraging the patient to discuss current problems, fears, or concerns and to ask questions
  6. Facilitating discussion with family members concerning the patient's prognosis and potential impacts on the patient's lifestyle

K

RENAL REPLACEMENT THERAPY
- Renal replacement therapy is required when the clinical and laboratory manifestations of kidney failure present complications that are potentially life threatening or that pose continuing discomfort to the patient.
- *Hemodialysis* removes excess fluid and waste products and restores chemical and electrolyte balance. It is based on the principle of diffusion, in which the patient's blood is circulated through a semipermeable membrane that acts as an artificial kidney.
    1. Dialysis settings include the acute care facility, free-standing centers, and the home.
    2. Total dialysis time is usually 12 hours per week, which usually is divided into three 4-hour treatments.
    3. A vascular access route is needed to perform hemodialysis.
        a. Long-term vascular access for hemodialysis is accomplished by arteriovenous (AV) fistula or graft
        b. Temporary vascular access for hemodialysis is accomplished by a specially designed catheter inserted into the subclavian, internal jugular, or femoral vein.
        c. Complications of vascular access include:
            (1) Thrombosis or stenosis
            (2) Infection
            (3) Ischemia, loss of patency
- Nurses are specially trained to perform hemodialysis.
- Post-dialysis care includes:
    1. Closely monitoring for side effects: hypoglycemia, hypotension, headache, nausea, malaise, vomiting, dizziness, and muscle cramps
    2. Obtaining the patient's weight and vital signs
    3. Avoiding invasive procedures for 4 to 6 hours because of heparinization of the dialysate
    4. Monitoring for signs of bleeding
    5. Monitoring laboratory results for abnormal values
- Complications of hemodialysis include:
    1. Dialysis disequilibrium
    2. Infectious disease
    3. Hepatitis infection
    4. Human immunodeficiency virus (HIV) infection
- Peritoneal dialysis (PD), an alternative and slower dialysis method, is accomplished by the surgical insertion of a silicone rubber catheter (Tenckhoff catheter) into the abdominal cavity to instill dialysis solution into the abdominal cavity.
- Candidates for PD include:
    1. Patients who are unable to tolerate anticoagulation
    2. Patients who lack vascular access

Considerations for Older Adults

- Stage 5 CKD or CKD requiring dialysis occurs most often in people between 65 and 69 years of age.
- Patients older than 65 years who are receiving dialysis have a greater risk than younger patients for dialysis-induced hypotension. Older adults require more frequent monitoring of vital signs and level of consciousness during and after dialysis.

   3. Patients without peritoneal adhesions and without extensive abdominal surgery
- The PD process occurs by means of a transfer of fluid and solutes from the bloodstream through the peritoneum.
- The types of PD include intermittent, continuous ambulatory (CAPD), automated, and others; the type is selected based on patient ability and lifestyle.
- Complications of PD include:
  1. Peritonitis
  2. Pain
  3. Poor dialysate flow
  4. Leakage of the dialysate
  5. Exit site and tunnel infection
- Nursing interventions include:
  1. Implementing and monitoring PD therapy and instilling, dwelling, and draining the solution, as ordered
  2. Maintaining PD flow data and monitoring for negative or positive fluid balances
  3. Obtaining baseline and daily weights
  4. Monitoring laboratory results to measure the effectiveness of the treatment
  5. Maintaining accurate intake and output records
  6. Taking vital signs every 15 to 30 minutes during initiation of PD
  7. Performing an ongoing assessment for signs of respiratory distress or pain
- Kidney transplantation is appropriate for selected patients with ESKD.

Community-Based Care
- Case managers can plan, coordinate, and evaluate care.
  1. The physical and occupational therapist collaborates with the patient and family to evaluate the home environment and to obtain needed equipment before discharge.
  2. Refer the patient to home health nursing as needed.

K

- Provide in-depth health teaching about diet and pathophysiology of kidney disease and drug therapy:
    1. Provide information and emotional support to assist the patient with decisions about treatment course, personal lifestyle, support systems, and coping.
    2. Teach the patient about the hemodialysis treatment.
    3. Teach the patient about care of the vascular access.
    4. Provide patients with home-based renal replacement therapy with extensive teaching and assist the patient to obtain the needed equipment and supplies. Emphasize the importance of strict sterile technique and of reporting manifestations of infection at any dialysis access site.
    5. Assist the patient and family to identify coping strategies to adjust to the diagnosis and treatment regimen.
    6. Instruct patients and family members in all aspects of diet therapy, drug therapy, and complications. Assist patients to schedule drugs so that drugs will not be unintentionally eliminated by dialysis.
    7. Teach patients and family members to report complications, such as fluid overload, bleeding, and infection.
    8. Stress that although uremic symptoms are reduced as a result of dialysis procedures, the patient will not return completely to his or her previous state of well-being.
    9. Instruct the family to monitor the patient for any behaviors that may contribute to nonadherence to the treatment plan and to report such to the health care provider.
    10. Refer the patient to a home health nurse and to local and state support groups and agencies such as the National Kidney Foundation.

KIDNEY DISEASE, POLYCYSTIC

OVERVIEW

- Polycystic kidney disease (PKD) is an inherited kidney disorder in which fluid-filled cysts develop in nephrons.
- Growing cysts damage the nephron (i.e., glomerular and tubular membranes), reducing kidney function.
- Kidney tissue is eventually replaced by nonfunctioning cysts; each cystic kidney may enlarge to two to three times its normal size, causing discomfort and abdominal organ displacement. The fluid-filled cysts are at increased risk for infection, rupture, and bleeding.
- Most patients with PKD have high blood pressure and heart problems.
- Cysts may occur in other tissues, such as the liver or blood vessels.

PATIENT-CENTERED COLLABORATIVE CARE
Assessment
- Obtain patient information about:
  1. Family history and genetic testing, because PKD can be autosomal dominant (most common form of PKD with several different subtypes) or autosomal recessive (which is more severe, with death typically occurring in early childhood)
  2. Current health status
  3. Changes in urine or pattern of urination
     a. Hypertension
- Assess for and document:
  1. Pain (flank or abdominal)
  2. Distended abdomen
  3. Enlarged, tender kidney on palpation
  4. Changes in urine including hematuria, clarity, odor
  5. Changes in pattern of urination including nocturia
  6. Dysuria
  7. Hypertension
  8. Edema
  9. Uremic symptoms: nausea, vomiting, pruritus, and fatigue
  10. Emotional responses such as anger, resentment, futility, sadness, or anxiety related to chronicity or inheritable condition
- Diagnostic studies may include:
  1. Urinalysis with findings of proteinuria and hematuria
  2. Urine culture and sensitivity if infection is suspected
  3. Serum creatinine and BUN to assess kidney function
  4. Renal sonography, CT scan, or MRI to assess the presence and size of cysts

Interventions
- Manage pain.
  1. Provide drug therapy.
     a. Administer analgesics for comfort; use NSAIDs cautiously, and avoid aspirin-containing products.
     b. Administer antibiotics such as trimethoprim/sulfamethoxazole (Bactrim, Septra) or ciprofloxacin (Cipro) if a cyst infection is causing discomfort.
  2. Provide other interventions.
     a. Apply dry heat to the abdomen or flank.
     b. Teach relaxation or distraction techniques to self-manage pain and discomfort.
- Provide hypertension and fluid management.
  1. Administer antihypertensive agents, including ACE inhibitors, vasodilators, beta blockers, and calcium channel blockers, as ordered.

K

2. Administer diuretics, as ordered, to eliminate fluid overload.
3. Monitor daily weight to detect fluid-related weight gain.
- Implement diet therapy with dietitian consultation to slow progression of kidney injury with salt and protein restriction.
- Prevent constipation associated with fluid restriction and intestinal tract displacement from cysts.
- Provide counseling, support, and teaching about health maintenance to promote self-management.
- Teach the patient and family:
   1. How to measure and monitor blood pressure and weight
   2. Diet considerations to promote health; salt, protein, and fiber intake may need dietitian consultation
   3. Self-administration of drugs and potential adverse effects of prescribed drugs, including antihypertensive drugs and diuretics

KIDNEY INJURY, ACUTE

OVERVIEW

- Acute kidney injury (AKI), formerly known as acute renal failure, is a rapid decrease in kidney function resulting in failure to maintain fluid, electrolyte, and acid-base balance, along with accumulation of metabolic wastes in the body.
- AKI can result from conditions that reduce blood flow or oxygen to the kidneys (prerenal failure); damage to the glomeruli, interstitial tissue, or tubules (intrarenal or intrinsic renal failure); or obstruction of urine flow (postrenal failure).
- AKI is associated with acute and severe illnesses and with increased mortality in acute and critical illnesses.
- AKI is classified by the extent of changes in serum creatinine and urine output. One strategy is the Kidney Disease, Improving Global Outcomes System (KDIGO):

KDIGO Staging

Stage 1	Serum creatinine increased × 1.5-1.9 baseline or by≥26.2 μmol/L	<0.5 mL/kg/hr for 6 to 12 hours
Stage 2	Serum creatinine increased × 2-2.9 baseline	<0.5 mL/kg/hr for≥12 hours
Stage 3	Serum creatinine increased >× 3 baseline or serum creatinine ≥354 μmol/L with an acute rise ≥44 μmol/L or initiation of renal replacement therapy	<0.3 mL/kg/hr for≥24 hours or anuria for ≥12 hours

PATIENT-CENTERED COLLABORATIVE CARE

Assessment

- Obtain patient information about:
  1. Exposure to nephrotoxins, including:
     a. Dye used in imaging procedures
     b. Drugs, especially antibiotics, ACE inhibitors, and NSAIDs
  2. History of diseases that contribute to impaired kidney function such as diabetes mellitus, systemic lupus erythematosus, and hypertension
  3. History of acute infections, including influenza, colds, gastroenteritis, and sore throat or pharyngitis that contribute to glomerulonephritis
  4. History of intravascular volume depletion (from surgery or trauma) or the need for transfusion
  5. History of urinary obstructive disease, such as prostatic hypertrophy or kidney stones
- Assess for and document:
  1. Symptoms of low tissue perfusion and hypovolemia before AKI occurs or progresses

---

! NURSING SAFETY PRIORITY: Critical Rescue

In any acute care setting, preventing volume depletion and providing intervention early when volume depletion occurs is a nursing priority. Reduced perfusion from volume depletion is a common cause of AKI. Recognize the manifestations of volume depletion (low urine output, decreased systolic blood pressure, decreased pulse pressure, orthostatic hypotension, thirst, rising blood osmolarity, sodium, BUN, and creatinine). Intervene early with oral fluids, or if the patient is unable to take or tolerate oral fluid request an increase in IV fluid rate from the provider to prevent permanent kidney damage.

K

  2. Urine output less than 0.5 ml/kg or absent urine output
  3. Abnormal or sharply increasing values for BUN and serum creatinine
  4. Serum electrolytes and reduced estimated or measured creatinine clearance (glomerular filtration rate [GFR])
  5. Protein in urine or signs of a urinary tract infection
  6. Symptoms of fluid overload including pulmonary edema (dyspnea, crackles, reduced SpO_2) and peripheral edema

7. ECG changes indicating electrolyte abnormalities
8. Symptoms of electrolyte derangements including nausea and vomiting, anorexia, impaired cognitions, and acute abnormalities in neuromuscular function
9. Flank pain
- Diagnostic studies may include:
  1. Urinalysis
  2. Urine and serum electrolytes, creatinine, and BUN
  3. Abdominal or pelvic ultrasound to assess the size of the kidneys and CT without contrast dye to identify obstruction
  4. Renal biopsy to determine uncertain cause of AKI or if immunologic disease is suspected

Interventions

- Monitor fluid and electrolyte status to detect imbalance and abnormal values. The patient may move from an oliguric phase (fluids and electrolytes are retained) to a diuretic phase, in which hypovolemia and electrolyte loss are the main problems.
- Assess the patient's response to renoprotective and other drugs to manage fluid and electrolytes.
  1. As kidney function changes, drug dosages are modified.
  2. Monitor for drug side effects and interactions.
- Fluid challenges and diuretics are commonly used to promote fluid balance and kidney perfusion.
  1. Monitor for fluid overload and dehydration.
- Hypercatabolism during illness, surgery, or trauma results in the breakdown of muscle for protein, which leads to increased azotemia. Patients require increased calories.
- Indications for hemodialysis or peritoneal dialysis in patients with AKI are symptomatic uremia, persistent hyperkalemia, uncompensated metabolic acidosis, fluid overload, uremic pericarditis, and uremic encephalopathy (see *Kidney Disease, Chronic*, for a discussion of dialysis).
- Continuous hemofiltration, an alternative to dialysis, may be used in the intensive care unit (ICU).

Community-Based Care

- The needs of the patient depend on the status of the disease on discharge (see *Community-Based Care* under *Kidney Disease, Chronic*).
- Follow-up care may include medical visits, laboratory tests, consultation with a nutritionist, temporary dialysis, home nursing care, and social work assistance.

L

LABYRINTHITIS

- Labyrinthitis is usually an infection of the labyrinth of the inner ear.
- Other causes include cholesteatoma (benign squamous cell overgrowth), complications of middle ear or inner ear surgery, and aftermath of a viral upper respiratory infection or mononucleosis.
- Manifestations include hearing loss, tinnitus, nystagmus on the affected side, and vertigo with nausea and vomiting.
- Management includes supportive care with rest in a darkened room, antiemetics, and antivertiginous drugs.

LACERATIONS, EYE

- Lacerations are wounds caused by sharp objects and projectiles.
- The most commonly injured areas involved in eye lacerations are the eyelids and the cornea.
  1. Eyelid lacerations:
     a. Bleed heavily and look more severe than they are
     b. Are managed by closing the eye and applying a small icepack, checking visual acuity, and cleaning and suturing the eyelid
     c. Should be managed by an ophthalmologist if they involve the eyelid margin, affect the lacrimal system, involve a large area, or have jagged edges
  2. Corneal lacerations:
     a. Are an emergency because eye contents may prolapse through the laceration
     b. Are manifested by severe eye pain, photophobia, tearing, decreased visual acuity, and inability to open the eyelid

---

! NURSING SAFETY PRIORITY: Action Alert

If an object is seen protruding from the eye, do not remove it. The object should be removed only by the ophthalmologist, because it may be holding eye structures in place.

L

     c. Are managed with surgical repair and antibiotic therapy
     d. May require a corneal transplant if scarring alters vision
     e. May need *enucleation* (surgical eye removal) if the eye contents have prolapsed through the laceration or if the injury is severe

LEIOMYOMAS (UTERINE FIBROIDS)
OVERVIEW
- Uterine leiomyomas, also called *fibroids* or *myomas,* are benign, slow-growing solid tumors of the uterine myometrium (muscle layer).
- These tumors are classified according to their position in the layers of the uterus and anatomic position. The most common types are:
  1. *Intramural tumors,* contained in the uterine wall in the myometrium
  2. *Submucosal tumors* that protrude into the cavity of the uterus
  3. *Subserosal tumors* that protrude through the outer uterine surface and may extend into the broad ligament

PATIENT-CENTERED COLLABORATIVE CARE
Assessment
- Assessment findings include:
  1. No symptoms
  2. Abnormal uterine bleeding
  3. Reports of a feeling of pelvic pressure
  4. Constipation
  5. Urinary frequency or retention
  6. Increased abdominal size
  7. Dyspareunia (painful intercourse)
  8. Infertility
  9. Abdominal pain occurring with torsion of the fibroid around a connecting stalk or pedicle
  10. Uterine enlargement on abdominal, vaginal, or rectal examination

Planning and Implementation
POTENTIAL FOR HEMORRHAGE
Nonsurgical Management
- The patient who has no symptoms or who desires childbearing should be observed and examined for changes in the size of the leiomyoma every 4 to 6 months.
- Many fibroids spontaneously shrink after menopause and require no treatment.
- Mild leiomyoma symptoms can be managed with nonsteroidal anti-inflammatories (NSAIDs), hormonal contraceptives, or a levonorgestrel intrauterine device (IUD).
- Artificial menopause and fibroid shrinkage can be induced with agonists to gonadotropin-releasing hormone (GnRH).
- Magnetic resonance imaging (MRI)–focused ultrasound pulsed into the uterus can destroy the fibroid.

- Uterine artery embolization or uterine fibroid embolization (UFE) involves the injection of embolic particles into the blood supply of the tumors, occluding the blood supply to the tumor and thereby causing its shrinkage and resorption.

Surgical Management

- Surgical management depends on whether future childbearing is desired, the age of the woman, the size of the fibroid, and the degree of symptoms.
- A *myomectomy* (removal of the leiomyomas with preservation of the uterus) is performed to preserve childbearing capabilities and relieve the symptoms.
- A *transcervical endometrial resection* (TCER) involves destroying the endometrium with a diathermy rectoscope or with radioablation. This procedure manages submucosal fibroids and menorrhagia.

! NURSING SAFETY PRIORITY: Critical Rescue

Monitor for rare but potential complications of hysteroscopic surgery, which include:

- Fluid overload (fluid used to distend the uterine cavity can be absorbed)
- Embolism
- Hemorrhage
- Perforation of the uterus, bowel, or bladder and ureter injury
- Persistent increased menstrual bleeding
- Incomplete suppression of menstruation

Monitor for any indications of these problems, and report signs and symptoms such as severe pain and heavy bleeding to the surgeon immediately. Scarring may cause a small risk for complications in future pregnancies.

- *Hysterectomy,* surgical removal of the uterine body, is the usual surgical management in the older woman who has multiple leiomyomas and unacceptable symptoms. One of three approaches may be used: vaginal, abdominal, or laparoscopic.
  1. *Total abdominal hysterectomy* (TAH) includes the removal of the uterus, ovaries, and fallopian tubes.
  2. A *radical hysterectomy* involves removal of the uterus, lymph nodes, upper one third of the vagina, and the surrounding tissues.
- Provide preoperative nursing care outlined in Part One and:
  1. Listen to the patient's concerns about her sexuality
  2. Identify the patient's support system

L

- Provide postoperative care for the patient described in Part One and:
  1. Assess and document vital signs with vaginal bleeding (more than one saturated perineal pad in 4 hours is concerning and needs to be reported to the health care provider; anticipate fluid or blood replacement therapy)
  2. Pay specific attention to:
     a. Abdominal bleeding at the incision site(s) (a small amount is normal)
     b. Urine output from urinary catheter for 24 hours or less (for open surgery) with a goal of > 0.5mL/kg/hour urine output

Considerations for Older Adults

- Older women are more at risk for all complications, especially pulmonary complications, than are younger women.
- Obese women are more at risk for all complications than are women who are not obese.

LEUKEMIA
OVERVIEW

- Leukemia is cancer with uncontrolled production of immature white blood cells (WBCs) in the bone marrow. The bone marrow is overcrowded with immature, nonfunctional cells ("blast" cells) and production of normal blood cells is greatly decreased.
- Leukemia may be *acute,* with a sudden onset, or *chronic,* with a slow onset and symptoms that persist for years.
- There are two major types of leukemia.
  1. *Lymphocytic (lymphoblastic) leukemias* have cells from lymphoid pathways.
  2. *Myelocytic (myelogenous) leukemias* have abnormal cells originating in myeloid pathways and have several subtypes classed by cell characteristics; identifying the subtype determines treatment options.
- The basic problem causing leukemia involves damage to genes controlling cell growth. This damage then changes cells from a normal to a malignant (cancer) state. Analysis of the bone marrow of a patient with acute leukemia shows abnormal chromosomes about 50% of the time.
  1. Environmental, genetic, and immunity factors influence leukemia development. For example, previous treatment for cancer poses risks for leukemia development from exposure

to radiation, some chemotherapy drugs, or ongoing immune deficiencies.
2. The risk for adult-onset leukemia increases with age.
- Leukemic cells can invade all tissues and organs and lead to infection or hemorrhage when untreated.

PATIENT-CENTERED COLLABORATIVE CARE
Assessment
- Obtain patient information about:
  1. Age
  2. Exposure to agents or ionizing radiation that increase the risk for leukemia
  3. Recent history of frequent or severe infections (e.g., influenza, pneumonia, bronchitis) or unexplained fevers
  4. A tendency to bruise or bleed easily or for a long period; platelet function is often decreased with leukemic disorders
  5. Weakness and fatigue
  6. Associated symptoms (headaches, behavior changes, increased somnolence, decreased attention span, lethargy, muscle weakness, loss of appetite, or weight loss)
- Assess for and document:
  1. Anemia and anemia-related symptoms
  2. Neutropenia
  3. Signs of infection, particularly in the respiratory, skin, and urinary systems
     a. Increased respiratory rate or dyspnea
     b. Abnormal breath sounds with cough
     c. Skin ulcer formation
     d. Urgent, frequent, or painful urination
  4. Skin changes from reduced perfusion
     a. Pallor and coolness to the touch
     b. Pale conjunctiva and palmar creases
     c. Bruising or petechiae
     d. Mouth sores that do not heal
  5. GI changes from bleeding or decreased perfusion
     a. Nausea and anorexia
     b. Weight loss
     c. Rectal fissures
     d. Bloody stools
     e. Reduced bowel sounds, constipation
     f. Enlarged liver or spleen
     g. Abdominal distension or tenderness
  6. Central nervous system (CNS) changes from bleeding or reduced perfusion
     a. Cranial nerve dysfunction

L

      b. Papilledema

      c. Seizures or coma

  7. Miscellaneous changes

      a. Bone and joint tenderness

      b. Lymph node enlargement

  8. Psychosocial issues and concerns, especially anxiety and fear about the diagnosis, treatment, and outcome

  9. Abnormal complete blood count (CBC), including:

      a. Decreased hemoglobin and hematocrit levels

      b. Low platelet count

      c. WBC count (low, normal, or elevated) and differential

- Diagnosis of leukemia is based on findings from a bone marrow biopsy. The leukemia type is diagnosed by cell surface antigens and chromosomal or gene markers.

Planning and Implementation

DRUG THERAPY FOR ACUTE LEUKEMIA

- *Induction therapy* consists of combination chemotherapy started at the time of diagnosis.
  1. Neutropenia is a common side effect of induction therapy. Prolonged hospitalizations of 2 to 3 weeks are common until recovery of bone marrow function occurs.
  2. Other side effects from drugs used for induction therapy include nausea, vomiting, diarrhea, alopecia (hair loss), stomatitis (mouth sores), kidney toxicity, liver toxicity, and cardiac toxicity.
- *Consolidation therapy* consists of another course of either the same drugs used for induction at a different dosage or a different combination of chemotherapy drugs.
- Consolidation therapy may be either a single course of chemotherapy or repeated courses.
- *Hematopoietic stem cell transplantation* also may be considered, depending on the disease subtype and the patient's response to induction therapy.
- *Maintenance therapy* may be prescribed for months to years after successful induction and consolidation therapies for acute lymphocytic leukemia (ALL) and acute promyelocytic leukemia (APL).
- The purpose is to maintain the remission. Not all types of leukemia respond to maintenance therapy.

DRUG THERAPY FOR CHRONIC LEUKEMIA

- The decision to initiate therapy is based on cytogenetic testing, disease stage, manifestations, and disease activity.
- *Imatinib mesylate* (Gleevec) is used for *chronic myelogenous leukemia* (CML) that is Philadelphia chromosome positive.
- For patients with resistant CML or who are intolerant to imatinib, dasatinib (Sprycel) or rituximab (Rituxan) are used.

- Rituximab is often combined with standard chemotherapy drugs or used as a single agent for patients with *chronic lymphocytic leukemia* (CLL).
- Hematopoietic stem cell transplantation is an option for patients with CLL.

REDUCING RISK FOR INFECTION

- Potential for infection is related to decreased immune response and chemotherapy.
- Infection is a major cause of death in the patient with leukemia because the WBCs are immature and cannot function or the cells are depleted from chemotherapy.
- Infection occurs through *autocontamination* (normal flora over-grows and penetrates the internal environment) and *cross-contamination* (organisms from another person or the environment are transmitted to the patient).
- The three most common sites of infection are the skin, respiratory tract, and intestinal tract.
- Implement infection control and patient protection measures listed under *Cancer Treatment* in Part One and:
  1. Wear a mask when entering the patient's room if there is a chance of transmitting an upper respiratory tract infection.
  2. Observe strict aseptic procedures when performing dressing changes.
  3. Place the patient in a private room, if possible.
  4. Reduce environmental sources of contamination.
     a. Do not leave standing collections of water in vases, denture cups, or humidifiers in the patient's room.
     b. Use a minimal bacteria diet (no raw fruits and vegetables, undercooked meat, pepper, or paprika).
     c. Use high-efficiency particulate air (HEPA) filtration or laminar airflow systems.
  5. Monitor for infection.
     a. Monitor the daily CBC with differential WBC count and absolute neutrophil count (ANC).
     b. Inspect the skin and mouth during every shift for lesions and breakdown.
     c. Assess the lungs every 8 hours for crackles, wheezes, or reduced breath sounds.
     d. Assess all urine for odor and cloudiness and ask the patient about any urgency, burning, or pain present with urination.
     e. Take vital signs, including temperature, at least every 4 hours.
     f. Provide interventions to maintain skin integrity.
     g. Implement agency neutropenia protocols when infection is suspected.

L

> **⚠ NURSING SAFETY PRIORITY: Critical Rescue**
>
> A temperature elevation of even 1°F (or 0.5°C) above baseline is significant for a patient with leukopenia and indicates infection until it has been proved otherwise.

    h. Drug therapy for infection may include antibiotic, antiviral, or antifungal drugs.

REDUCING RISK FOR INJURY

- Potential for injury is related to bleeding and adverse drug reactions from chemotherapy.
- Thrombocytopenia increases the risk for excessive bleeding and occurs from both leukemia and chemotherapy.
- Institute precautions for patients with thrombocytopenia described in *Cancer Treatment* in Part One.
- Administer chemotherapy using best practices and monitor patient response as listed under *Cancer Treatment* in Part One.

DECREASING FATIGUE

- Fatigue is related to decreased tissue oxygenation and increased energy demands.
- Production of red blood cells (RBCs) is limited in leukemia, causing anemia that contributes to fatigue.
  1. Collaborate with a nutritionist to provide small, frequent meals high in protein and carbohydrates.
  2. Administer transfusion therapy (e.g., packed RBCs, platelets, or clotting factors).
  3. Evaluate the patient's response to drug therapy with hematopoietic growth factors such as:
     a. Darbepoetin alfa (Aranesp) and epoetin alfa (Epogen and Procrit) to increase RBCs
     b. Oprelvekin (Neumega) to increase the production of platelets
  4. Eliminate or postpone activities that do not have a direct positive effect on the patient's condition.

Community-Based Care

- Teach the patient and family about:
  1. Measures to prevent infection
  2. The importance of continuing therapy and medical follow-up
  3. The need to report manifestations of infection or bleeding immediately to the health care provider
  4. Assessing for petechiae, avoiding trauma and sharp objects, applying pressure to wounds for 10 minutes, and reporting blood in the stool or urine or headache that does not respond to acetaminophen

  5. Resources for psychological and financial support and for role and self-esteem adjustment
  6. Care of the central catheter if in place at discharge
- Assess the patient's need for a home care nurse, aide, or equipment.

LIVER, FATTY

- Fatty liver is caused by the accumulation of fats in and around hepatic cells.
- Causes include chronic alcohol abuse, diabetes, obesity, and elevated lipid profile.
- The patient usually has no symptoms; the typical finding is elevated serum liver enzymes.
- Assess for signs of cirrhosis (see *Cirrhosis*).
- MRI, ultrasound, or liver biopsy confirms the diagnosis.
- Interventions are aimed at removing the underlying cause of the infiltration and include administration of lipid-lowering drugs and dietary restriction of fats.
- Monitoring liver function tests regularly evaluates treatment effectiveness or progression of disease.

LYME DISEASE

- Lyme disease is a reportable systemic infection transmitted by infected deer ticks.
- The disease can be prevented by avoiding heavily wooded areas or areas with thick underbrush; by wearing long-sleeved tops, long pants, and socks; and by using an insect repellent on skin and clothing when in an area where infected ticks are likely to be found.
- Symptoms appear in three stages:
  1. Stage I symptoms appear in 3 to 32 days after the tick bite.
     a. Fever and chills
     b. Swollen glands
     c. Headache
     d. Joint and muscle aches
     e. Spreading, oval or circular rash (erythema migrans)
  2. Stage II symptoms appear 2 to 12 weeks after the tick bite.
     a. Cardiac symptoms (dysrhythmia, dizziness, palpitations, dyspnea)
     b. Neurologic symptoms (meningitis, cranial neuropathy, peripheral neuritis)
  3. Stage III, chronic persistent Lyme disease, occurs weeks to years after the tick bite and may lead to chronic complications.
     a. Arthralgia and arthritis (may be the only symptom of Lyme disease)

L

   b. Memory and thinking problems
   c. Fatigue
   d. Enlarged lymph nodes
- Testing for Lyme disease is not accurate until 4 to 6 weeks after the initial tick bite.
- Management consists of antibiotic therapy, typically doxycycline, amoxicillin, or cefuroxime for stage I; ceftriaxone or cefotaxime for stage II; and oral tetracycline or an IV cephalosporin for stage III disease.
- Vaccination against Lyme disease is available and should be encouraged for adults living in high-risk areas.

LYMPHOMA, HODGKIN'S AND NON-HODGKIN'S

OVERVIEW

Lymphomas are cancers of the lymphoid tissues with abnormal over-growth of lymphocytes. Lymphomas are cancers of committed lymphocytes rather than stem cell precursors (as in leukemia). The two major adult forms of lymphoma are Hodgkin's lymphoma (HL) and non-Hodgkin's lymphoma (NHL).

- *Hodgkin's lymphoma* (HL) is a cancer of the lymphoid tissues with abnormal overgrowth of one type of leukocyte, the lymphocyte. It usually starts in a single lymph node or a single chain of nodes and contains a specific cancer cell type, the Reed-Sternberg cell. HL usually spreads from one group of lymph nodes to the next in an orderly fashion.
- *Non-Hodgkin's lymphoma* (NHL) includes all lymphoid cancers that do not have the Reed-Sternberg cell. There are more than 602 subtypes of NHL, and they usually spread through the lymphatic system in a less orderly way than HL.
- HL affects any age group, but it is most common among teens and young adults and among adults in their 50s and 60s. NHL is more common in older white men.
- The most common manifestation of either lymphoma type is lymphadenopathy, large but painless lymph node or nodes.
- Other manifestations of either type may include fever, drenching night sweats, and unexplained weight loss.
- Diagnosis is made based on findings from lymph node biopsy. After diagnosis, lymphoma is classified by subtype and staged to determine the extent of the disease (which determines exact therapy).

PATIENT-CENTERED COLLABORATIVE CARE

- HL is one of the most treatable types of cancer. Generally for stage I and stage II disease the treatment is external irradiation of involved lymph node regions. With more extensive disease, irradiation and combination chemotherapy are used to achieve remission.

- Treatment options for patients with NHL vary based the subtype of the tumor, international prognostic index (IPI) score, stage of the disease, performance status, and overall tumor burden. Options include combinations of chemotherapy drugs, targeted therapies, localized radiation therapy, radiolabeled antibodies, hematopoietic stem cell transplantation, and newer investigational agents.
- Nursing management of the patient undergoing chemotherapy treatment for HL or NHL focuses on the side effects of therapy, especially:
  1. Drug-induced pancytopenia, which increases the risk for infection, anemia, and bleeding
  2. Severe nausea and vomiting
  3. Constipation or diarrhea
  4. Impaired hepatic function
  5. Additional interventions listed under *Cancer Treatment* in Part One
- Nursing management of the patient undergoing radiation therapy for HL or NHL focuses on the side effects of therapy, especially:
  1. Skin problems at the site of radiation
  2. Fatigue and taste changes
  3. Permanent sterility for men receiving radiation to the abdominopelvic region in the pattern of an inverted Y in combination with specific chemotherapy drugs
  4. Specific interventions listed under *Cancer Treatment* in Part One

M

MACULAR DEGENERATION
OVERVIEW

- Macular degeneration is the deterioration of the macula (the area of central vision). It can be age-related (atrophic) or exudative.
- Age-related macular degeneration (AMD) has two types:
  1. Dry AMD is caused by gradual blockage of retinal capillaries, which allows retinal cells in the macula to become ischemic and necrotic. Central vision declines first, but eventually the person loses all central vision.
  2. Wet AMD is caused by the growth of new blood vessels in the macula, which have thin walls and leak blood and fluid.
- Exudative macular degeneration is also wet, but it can occur at any age. The condition may occur only in one eye or in both eyes.

M

Patients have a sudden decrease in vision after a serous detachment of pigment epithelium in the macula.

PATIENT-CENTERED COLLABORATIVE CARE

* Management of dry AMD aims to slow disease progression and maximize remaining vision, because there is no cure.
* The loss of central vision reduces the ability to read, write, recognize safety hazards, and drive.
* Suggest alternative strategies (e.g., large-print books, public transportation) and referrals to community organizations that provide a wide range of adaptive equipment.
* See *Visual Impairment (Reduced Vision)* for more discussion of patients' care needs.
* Management of wet macular degeneration focuses on slowing the process and identifying further changes in visual perception.
  1. Laser therapy to seal the leaking blood vessels in or near the macula can limit the extent of the damage.
  2. Vascular endothelial growth factor inhibitors (VEGFIs) injected monthly into the vitreous can also slow disease progression.

MALABSORPTION SYNDROME

* Malabsorption syndrome is associated with a variety of disorders and intestinal surgical procedures and interferes with the ability to absorb nutrients because of altered mucosa of the small intestine.
* Physiologic mechanisms limit absorption of nutrients as a result of one or more abnormalities:
  1. Bile salt deficiencies
  2. Enzyme deficiencies
  3. Presence of bacteria
  4. Disruption of the mucosal lining of the small intestine
  5. Alteration in lymphatic or vascular circulation
  6. Decreased gastric or intestinal surface area
* Clinical manifestations of malabsorption include chronic diarrhea, steatorrhea, weight loss, fatigue, bloating and flatus, easy bruising, anemia, bone pain, and edema.
* Interventions focus on avoiding dietary substances that aggravate malabsorption, supplementing nutrients, and surgical or nonsurgical management of the primary causative disease.

MALNUTRITION

OVERVIEW

* Malnutrition, also known as *under-nutrition,* results from inadequate nutrient intake, increased nutrient loss, and increased nutrient requirements; it is a multinutrient problem.

- A weight loss of 5% or more in 30 days, a weight loss of 10% in 6 months, or a weight that is below ideal may indicate malnutrition.
- The function of the liver, heart, lungs, GI tract, and immune system decreases in the patient with malnutrition
- *Protein-energy malnutrition* (PEM), also known as *protein-calorie malnutrition,* may present in three forms.
  1. *Marasmus* is a calorie malnutrition in which body fat and protein are wasted. Serum proteins are often preserved.
  2. *Kwashiorkor* is a lack of protein quantity and quality in the presence of adequate calories. Body weight is normal, and serum levels of proteins are low.
  3. *Marasmic-kwashiorkor* is a combined protein and energy malnutrition.
- Unrecognized dysphagia is a common problem in older patients and can cause malnutrition.
- Anorexia nervosa (self-induced starvation) and bulimia nervosa (binge eating followed by purging behavior such as self-induced vomiting) also lead to malnutrition.
- Clinical manifestations include:
  1. Leanness and cachexia
  2. Decreased activity tolerance and lethargy
  3. Intolerance to cold
  4. Edema
  5. Dry, flaking skin; dermatitis; or other skin impairment
  6. Poor wound healing
  7. Infections, particularly postoperative

Considerations for Older Adults

Older adults in the community or in any health care setting are most at risk for poor nutrition, especially PEM. Risk factors include physiologic changes of aging, environmental factors, and health problems.

PATIENT-CENTERED COLLABORATIVE CARE

- Initiate safety precautions to prevent potential injury from falls due to weakness.
- Evaluate skin and initiate interventions to prevent pressure ulcer formation related to nutritional deficits.
- Treatment
  1. Identify and treat the precipitating cause.
  2. Examine and treat oral conditions (e.g., caries, pain, ill-fitting dentures) that may contribute to impaired oral intake.
  3. Determine the patient's height and weight, and calculate a BMI.
  4. Provide a high-calorie, high-protein diet and consider forti-fied nutritional supplements.

M

5. Monitor the patient's ability to eat the ordered diet and the amount eaten.
6. Obtain a dietician consultation.
7. Provide an environment conducive to eating.
8. Multivitamins and minerals may be used to supplement intake. Anabolic hormones or steroids such as megestrol (Megace) may be given to stimulate appetite.
9. Maintain a daily calorie count, and weigh the patient daily. Evaluate whether nutrients consumed are sufficient to meet basal and stress-related energy needs.
10. Monitor laboratory results for abnormal serum values, especially electrolytes, protein, albumin, prealbumin, hematocrit, hemoglobin, and WBC count.
• Ensure best practices with enteral feeding.
1. Prevent tube clogging by rinsing with at least 60 mL of water whenever feeding is interrupted (when giving a drug or stopping feeding).
2. Mark the tube at the nares or lip, and evaluate tube placement by noting migration of the mark every 4 hours.

QSEN QUALITY IMPROVEMENT

All health care facilities are required to establish and implement procedures and systems to prevent patient harm from medical complications such as tube misplacement and dislodgement.

3. Monitor intake and output to determine fluid excess or dehydration.
4. Prevent aspiration by maintaining back rest elevation greater than 30 degrees unless contraindicated by the patient's condition.
5. Prevent contamination of the enteral solution and equipment; replace every 48 hours.
• If the patient cannot meet caloric and protein goals with oral or combined oral and enteral intake, add specialized nutrition support (parenteral nutrition).
• Evaluate nutritional indices at least weekly: skin intactness, weight, serum albumin, electrolytes, renal function, hemoglobin and hematocrit, and WBC count.

❗ NURSING SAFETY PRIORITY: Action Alert

Undernutrition is a risk factor for development of iatrogenic pressure ulcers. Implement nutritional consultation and skin pressure-relieving interventions for patients with malnutrition.

MASTOIDITIS

- Mastoiditis is a progression of an infection of the middle ear (otitis media) to include temporal bone.
- Manifestations include swelling behind the ear and pain with minimal movement of the tragus, the pinna, or the head. Cellulitis develops on the skin or external scalp over the mastoid process, and the ear is pushed sideways and down.
- Otoscopic examination shows a red, dull, thick, immobile eardrum with or without perforation.
- Other manifestations include low-grade fever, malaise, ear drainage, loss of appetite, and enlarged lymph nodes.
- Hearing loss is common.
- Management involves IV antibiotics and surgical removal of the infected tissue if the infection does not respond to antibiotic therapy. A simple or modified radical mastoidectomy with tympanoplasty is the most common treatment.
- Complications of surgery include damage to cranial nerves VI and VII, decreasing the patient's ability to look sideways (cranial nerve VI) and causing a drooping of the mouth on the affected side (cranial nerve VII). Other complications include vertigo, meningitis, brain abscess, chronic purulent otitis media, and wound infection.

MELANOMA

OVERVIEW

- Melanomas are pigmented cancers arising in the melanin-producing epidermal cells.
- Melanoma is highly metastatic, and a person's survival depends on early diagnosis and treatment.
- Risk factors include genetic predisposition, excessive exposure to UV light, and the presence of one or more precursor lesions that resemble unusual moles.
- It occurs most often among light-skinned races and people older than 60 years.

PATIENT-CENTERED COLLABORATIVE CARE
Assessment
- Obtain patient information about:
  1. Age and ethnicity/race
  2. Family history of skin cancer
  3. Any past surgery for removal of skin growths
  4. Recent changes in the size, color, or sensation of any mole, birthmark, wart, or scar
  5. Sun exposure

M

6. Exposure to arsenic, coal tar, pitch, radioactive waste, or radium
- Assess for and document all lesions for:
  1. Location, size, and color
  2. Surface features (ABCDE)
     a. *A*symmetry of shape
     b. *B*order irregularity
     c. *C*olor variation within one lesion
     d. *D*iameter greater than 6 mm
     e. *E*xudate presence and quality
- Diagnosis is made based on biopsy findings.

Interventions

Surgical Management

- Surgical intervention is the management of choice for melanoma.
  1. *Excision* is used for the biopsy of small lesions, and a sentinel node biopsy can determine whether tumor spread has started.
  2. *Wide excision* for deeper melanoma often involves removing full-thickness skin in the area of the lesion. Subcutaneous tissues and lymph nodes may also be removed, and grafting may be needed for wound closure.

Nonsurgical Management

- Drug therapy may involve systemic chemotherapy, biotherapy, or targeted therapy.
  1. Systemic chemotherapy with a combination of agents; the general management issues for care of patients undergoing chemotherapy are presented in Part One under *Cancer Treatment*.
  2. Biotherapy with interferon
  3. Targeted therapy with experimental drugs such as a CTLA-4 receptor blocker
- Radiation therapy for melanoma may be helpful for patients with metastatic disease when used in combination with systemic corticosteroids. General management issues for care of patients undergoing radiation therapy are presented in Part One under *Cancer Treatment*.

MELANOMA, OCULAR

- Melanoma is the most common malignant eye tumor in adults and is associated with exposure to UV light. Because of its rich blood supply, a melanoma can spread easily into nearby tissue and the brain.
- Manifestations may not be readily apparent, and the tumor may be discovered during a routine examination.
- Manifestations vary with the exact location and may include blurred vision, reduced visual acuity, increased intraocular pressure (IOP), change in iris color, and visual field loss.
- Diagnostic tests usually include ultrasonography or MRI.

- Management depends on the tumor's size and growth rate and on the condition of the other eye.
  1. *Enucleation* (surgical removal of the entire eyeball) with insertion of a ball implant to provide a base for fitting the socket prosthesis (in about 1 month)
  2. *Radiation therapy* using an implanted radioactive disk to reduce the size and thickness of melanoma; but this is associated with complications of vitreous hemorrhage, retinopathy, glaucoma, necrosis of the sclera, and cataract formation

MÉNIÈRE'S DISEASE

- Ménière's disease has three features: tinnitus, one-sided sensorineural hearing loss, and vertigo; these occur in attacks that can last for several days
- It is caused by an excess of endolymphatic fluid that distorts the entire inner-ear canal system.
- The disease usually begins in people between the ages of 20 and 50 years and is more common in men and in white people.

  Nonsurgical Management
- Teach patients about attack prevention strategies, including:
  1. Making slow head movements to prevent worsening of the vertigo
  2. Stopping smoking, because nicotine constricts blood vessels
  3. Participating in the hydrops diet to reduce endolymphatic fluid excess; the diet includes:
     a. Distributing food and fluid intake evenly throughout the day and from day to day
     b. Avoiding foods or fluids that have a high salt content
     c. Drinking adequate amounts of fluids (low in sugar) daily
     d. Avoiding caffeine-containing fluids and foods
     e. Limiting alcohol intake to one serving daily
     f. Avoiding foods containing monosodium glutamate (MSG)
- Drug therapy to control the vertigo and vomiting and restore normal balance
  1. Mild diuretics
  2. Nicotinic acid
  3. Antihistamines (just before and during an acute attack)
     a. Diphenhydramine hydrochloride (Benadryl, Allerdryl)
     b. Dimenhydrinate (Dramamine, Gravol)
  4. Antivertiginous drugs like meclizine (Antivert, Bonamine)
  5. Antiemetics
  6. Intratympanic therapy with gentamycin and steroids
- Use of pulse pressure treatments, such as the Meniett device, to apply low-pressure micropulses to the inner ear for 5 minutes three times daily

M

Surgical Management

- Surgical treatment of Ménière's disease is a last resort, because the hearing in the affected ear is often lost from the procedure.
- A labyrinthectomy resects the vestibular nerve or removes the labyrinth.
- Endolymphatic decompression is performed with drainage and a shunt.

MENINGITIS

OVERVIEW

- Meningitis is inflammation of the meninges that surround the brain and spinal cord.
- The infecting organism produces an inflammatory response in the pia mater, the arachnoid, the cerebrospinal fluid (CSF), and the ventricles.
- Bacterial meningitis is potentially life threatening; viral meningitis is usually self-limiting; and cryptococcal meningitis is the most common fungal meningitis.
- Vaccinations can prevent meningitis from meningococcal and *Haemophilus influenzae* microorganisms.

PATIENT-CENTERED COLLABORATIVE CARE

Assessment

- Obtain patient information about:
  1. Recent viral or respiratory diseases and exposure to communicable disease
  2. Head or spine surgery or trauma or ear, nose, or sinus infection
  3. Heart disease, diabetes mellitus, cancer, immunosuppressive therapy, and neurologic procedures that increase the risk for infection or invading organisms
- Assess for and document:
  1. Fever, neck stiffness, headache, and altered mental status
  2. Rash, especially on trunk or abdomen
  3. Photophobia
  4. Kerning's and Brudzinski's signs, which are present in only a small percentage of patients with definite meningitis
  5. Seizure and focal neurologic deficits, especially with bacterial meningitis
  6. Change in level of consciousness
  7. Complications of meningitis, including syndrome of inappropriate antidiuretic hormone (SIADH) or coagulopathy resulting in emboli that compromise peripheral circulation
- Diagnostic studies may include:
  1. Lumbar puncture is performed to obtain CSF for cell count, differential, protein, and culture; although antibiotic

administration should *not* be delayed for this procedure, it is desirable to complete the spinal fluid collection before the first dose of antibiotics

2. Serum levels of WBCs and electrolytes, especially to detect low sodium levels associated with diuresis
3. Computed tomography (CT) scan to detect inflamed meninges, abscess (encapsulated pus), and intracranial hypertension

Interventions

- Assess and record the patient's neurologic status with vital signs and peripheral circulation at least every 4 hours. Level of consciousness is the most sensitive indicator of change in patient status.
- Assess and record with particular attention to cranial nerves III, IV, VI, VII, and VIII (pupillary response to light and ability to move eyes through four quadrants promotes early detection concerning deterioration of the patient's condition).
- Administer drugs such as antibiotics and analgesics as ordered.
- Maintain isolation precautions according to hospital policy.
- Implement institutional seizure precautions when indicated.
- Monitor for complications such as vascular compromise from emboli, shock, coagulation disorders, prolonged fever, and septic complications.
- Encourage vaccinations, especially if traveling or living in shared residential spaces (e.g., group homes, dormitories, or skilled nursing facilities).

METABOLIC SYNDROME

- Metabolic syndrome is the simultaneous presence of metabolic factors known to increase risk for developing type 2 diabetes and cardiovascular disease. Features of the syndrome include:
  1. Abdominal obesity: waist circumference of 40 inches (100 cm) or more for men and 35 inches (88 cm) or more for women
  2. Hyperglycemia: fasting blood glucose level of 100 mg/dL or more or on drug treatment for elevated glucose
  3. Abnormal A_{1C}: between 5.5% and 6.0%
  4. Hypertension: systolic BP of 130 mm Hg or more or diastolic BP of 85 mg Hg or more or on drug treatment for hypertension
  5. Hyperlipidemia: triglyceride level of 150 mg/dL or more or on drug treatment for elevated triglycerides; high-density lipoprotein (HDL) cholesterol less than 40 mg/dL for men or less than 50 mg/dL for women
- Management consists of addressing each of the features (e.g., drug therapy for hypertension, hyperglycemia [diabetes], and hyperlipidemia) and teaching patients about the lifestyle changes that can improve health and reduce obesity.

M

MULTIDRUG-RESISTANT ORGANISMS (MDRO)

- Multidrug-resistant organisms (MDROs) are infectious agents that are no longer responsive to antibiotics.
- The most common MDROs are methicillin-resistant *Staphylococcus aureus* (MRSA), vancomycin-resistant *enterococcus* (VRE), and carbapenem-resistant *enterococcus* (CRE) and *Neisseria gonorrhea.*
  1. MRSA is spread by direct contact and invades hospitalized patients through indwelling urinary catheters, vascular access devices, and endotracheal tubes. It is susceptible to only a few antibiotics, such as vancomycin (Lyphocin, Vancocin) and linezolid (Zyvox). A newer IV antibiotic, ceftaroline fosamil (Teflaro), is the first cephalosporin approved to treat MRSA.
  2. *Enterococci* are bacteria that live in the intestinal tract and are important for digestion. VRE can live on almost any surface for days or weeks and still be able to cause an infection. Contamination of toilet seats, door handles, and other objects is very likely for a lengthy period. The most common infections caused by VRE include wound infections, urinary tract infections (UTIs), and bloodstream infections.
  3. *Klebsiella* and *Escherichia coli (E. coli)* are types of *Enterobacteriaceae* that are located within the intestinal tract; these bacteria have become increasingly resistant to carbapenem antibiotics, which are most often given for abdominal infections.

> ### ❗ NURSING SAFETY PRIORITY: Action Alert
>
> To help prevent the transmission of an MDRO, change clothes before leaving work. Keep work clothes separate from personal clothes. Take a shower when you get home, if possible, to rid your body of any unwanted pathogens. Be careful not to contaminate equipment that is commonly used, such as your stethoscope.

- Experts suggest several strategies to decrease the incidence of this growing problem.
  1. Perform frequent hand hygiene, including using hand sanitizers.
  2. Use chlorhexidine (2% dilution) bathing to prevent CRE or decrease colonization and other types of infections from MDROs.
  3. Stop administering multiple antimicrobials when a specific effective drug is identified from culture results.
  4. Use best practices in infection control in hospital and other health care settings, including the use of personal protective

equipment (staff and visitors) and cleaning surfaces and equipment.
5. Teach patients and health care providers to avoid the use of antibiotics to treat common viral illnesses such as colds.
6. Follow guidelines or best practices to ensure selection of the most effective antibiotic, the correct dose for the condition, and the duration of treatment.

MULTIPLE SCLEROSIS

OVERVIEW
* Multiple sclerosis (MS) is a chronic inflammatory disease that affects the myelin sheath and conduction pathway of the CNS.
* Women are affected twice as often as men.
* MS often mimics other neurologic diseases, which makes the diagnosis difficult and prolonged.
* The major types of MS are:
  1. Relapsing-remitting MS (RRMS), which is characterized as mild or moderate, depending on the degree of disability; symptoms develop and resolve in a few weeks to months, after which the patient may return to baseline.
  2. Primary progressive MS (PPMS), which is characterized by a steady and gradual neurologic deterioration without remission of symptoms; the patient has progressive disability with no acute attacks. Patients with this type of MS tend to be between 40 and 60 years old at onset of the disease.
  3. Secondary progressive MS (SPMS) begins with a relapsing-remitting course that later becomes steadily progressive. About half of all people with RRMS develop SPMS within 10 years. The current addition of disease-modifying drugs as part of disease management may decrease the development of SPMS.
  4. Progressive-relapsing MS (PRMS) is characterized by frequent relapses with partial recovery, but not a return to baseline. This type of MS is seen in only a small percentage of patients. Progressive, cumulative symptoms and deterioration occur over several years.

PATIENT-CENTERED COLLABORATIVE CARE
Assessment
* Assess for and document:
  1. Progression of symptoms
  2. Factors that aggravate symptoms
     a. Stress
     b. Fatigue
     c. Overexertion

M

      d. Temperature extremes such as a hot shower or bath
   3. Motor function
      a. Fatigue
      b. Stiffness of legs
      c. Flexor spasms, clonus
      d. Increased deep tendon reflexes
      e. Positive Babinski's reflex
   4. Cerebellar function
      a. Ataxic gait
      b. Intention tremor (tremor when performing activity)
      c. Dysmetria (inability to direct or limit movement)
      d. Clumsy motor movements
   5. Cranial nerve function
      a. Hearing loss
      b. Facial weakness
      c. Swallowing difficulties (dysphagia)
      d. Tinnitus
      e. Vertigo
   6. Vision
      a. Decreased visual acuity
      b. Blurred vision
      c. Diplopia
      d. Scotoma (changes in peripheral vision)
      e. Nystagmus
   7. Sensation
      a. Hypalgesia
      b. Paresthesia
      c. Facial pain
      d. Change in bowel and bladder function
      e. Impotence, difficulty sustaining an erection
      f. Decreased vaginal secretion
   8. Cognitive changes seen late in the course of the disease
      a. Memory loss
      b. Decreased ability to perform calculations
      c. Inattention
      d. Impaired judgment
   9. Psychosocial function
      a. Apathy, emotional lability, and depression
      b. Disturbed body image
- Diagnostic testing may include:
   1. MRI to determine the presence of plaques in the CNS
   2. Lumbar puncture for analysis of CSF

Interventions
- Provide sufficient time to complete ADLs; as a result of weakness and fatigue, the patient requires more time or assistance.

- Collaborate with physical and occupational therapists and vocational rehabilitation specialists to assist the patient with:
  1. Implementing an exercise program to strengthen and stretch muscles
  2. Using assistive devices, such as a cane, walker, or electric (Amigo) cart
- Drug therapy includes:
  1. Current therapies are designed to alter the immune system responses associated with MS
     a. Interferon-beta (Avonex, Betaseron, Rebif), immunomodulators that modify the course of the disease and have antiviral effects
     b. Glatiramer acetate (Copaxone), a synthetic protein that is similar to myelin-based protein
     c. Natalizumab (Tysabri), a monoclonal antibody that binds to WBCs to prevent further damage to the myelin
     d. Fingolimod (Gilenya), teriflunomide (Aubagio), or dimethyl fumarate (Tecfidera) to modulate the immune system
     e. Mitoxantrone (Novantrone), a chemotherapy drug, during worsening symptoms
     f. A combination of cyclophosphamide (Cytoxan) and methylprednisolone (Solu-Medrol) may be used for some patients for immunosuppression during the onset and acute exacerbation of MS symptoms
  2. Adjunctive therapy to treat muscle spasticity and paresthesia
  3. Adjunctive therapy for bladder and bowel dysfunction; urine and fecal incontinence can be debilitating for this population
  4. Antispasmodics, antiepileptic drugs (AEDs), analgesics, NSAIDs, tranquilizers, or antidepressants to treat pain, paresthesia, and mood disorder
- Other interventions include:
  1. Strategies to maintain or modify mobility and independence in ADLs
  2. Managing cognitive problems in the areas of attention, memory, problem solving, visual perception, and use of speech
  3. Applying an eye patch to relieve diplopia and switching the eye patch every few hours
  4. Teaching scanning techniques to compensate for peripheral vision deficits
  5. Teaching the patient to test the temperature of the bath water at home before placing his or her hands in hot water
  6. Referring the patient to a therapist or nurse educated in issues surrounding sexuality

M

- Patients using complementary therapies of nutritional supplements, acupressure, and bee stings report improvement in their condition, but these modalities have not been scientifically tested.

Community-Based Care
- Home care management includes:
  1. Avoiding factors that may exacerbate the symptoms including overexertion, extremes of temperatures (fever, hot baths, overheating, excessive chilling), humidity, and exposure to infection
  2. Providing drug information
  3. Encouraging the patient to follow the exercise program developed by the physical therapist (PT) and to remain independent in all activities for as long as possible
  4. Encouraging the patient to engage in regular social activities, obtain adequate rest, and manage stress
  5. Teaching the family strategies to cope with personality changes
  6. Reinforcing established bowel and bladder, skin care, and nutrition programs
  7. Identify community organizations and support groups for education and to promote adaptive psychosocial coping

MYASTHENIA GRAVIS

OVERVIEW
- Myasthenia gravis (MG) is an acquired autoimmune disease characterized by muscle weakness. The thymus gland may be abnormal.
- MG is caused by an autoantibody attack on the acetylcholine receptors (AChRs) in the muscle end plate membranes. As a result, nerve impulses are reduced at the neuromuscular junction.
- There are two types of MG: ocular and generalized.
- MG may take many forms—from mild disturbances of the cranial and peripheral motor neurons to a rapidly developing, generalized weakness that may lead to death from respiratory failure.
- In *Eaton-Lambert syndrome,* a form of myasthenia often observed in combination with small cell carcinoma of the lung, the muscles of the trunk and the pelvic and shoulder girdles are most commonly affected.

PATIENT-CENTERED COLLABORATIVE CARE
Assessment
- Obtain patient information about:
  1. Muscular weakness that increases on exertion or as the day wears on and improves with rest (with a temporary increase

in weakness sometimes noted after vaccination, menstruation, and exposure to extremes in environmental temperature)
2. Rapid, temporary onset of fatigue or weakness associated with infection, pregnancy, or anesthesia and after vaccination, menstruation, and exposure to extremes in environmental temperature
3. Inability to perform ADLs
4. Ptosis, diplopia, or weakness in facial muscles
5. Difficulty swallowing (dysphagia), choking
6. Respiratory distress
7. Family history of MG or thymic disorder
8. Weakness of voice
9. Decreased sensation (paresthesia) or aching in weakened muscles
- Assess for and document:
  1. Progressive paresis of affected muscle groups that is resolved by rest, at least in part
  2. Symptoms related to involvement of the levator palpebrae or extraocular muscles
     a. Ocular palsies
     b. Ptosis
     c. Diplopia
     d. Weak or incomplete eye closure
  3. Involvement of muscles for facial expression, chewing, and speech
     a. The patient's smile may turn into a snarl.
     b. The jaw hangs.
     c. Difficulty chewing and swallowing may lead to severe nutritional deficits.
  4. Proximal limb weakness that leads to difficulty climbing stairs, lifting heavy objects, or raising arms overhead
  5. Mild or severe neck weakness
  6. Difficulty sustaining a sitting or walking posture
  7. Respiratory distress
  8. Bowel and bladder incontinence
  9. Weakness of the pelvic and shoulder girdles (seen in Eaton-Lambert syndrome)
  10. Disturbed body image
  11. Feelings of loss, fear, helplessness, and grief
  12. Usual coping methods
- Diagnostic studies may include:
  1. Serum thyroid function tests
  2. Serum protein electrophoresis tests to evaluate the presence of autoantibodies
  3. Serum AChR antibodies

M

4. Chest x-ray and CT scan to evaluate the thymus gland in the mediastinum
5. Pharmacologic tests with the cholinesterase inhibitors edrophonium (Tensilon) and neostigmine (Prostigmin); anticipate a marked improvement of muscle tone that lasts 4 to 5 minutes
6. Repetitive nerve stimulation of proximal nerves, the most common electrodiagnostic test performed to detect MG; alternatively, electromyography to test muscle contraction or single fiber contraction after electrical stimulation is used

Interventions

Nonsurgical Management

- Administer drugs to reduce the symptoms of MG without influencing the actual course of the disease (anticholinesterases or cholinergic drugs). Give these drugs for MG on time to avoid respiratory compromise and muscular weakness:
  1. Cholinesterase inhibitor drugs, also referred to as *anticholinesterase drugs* (typically pyridostigmine [Mestinon, Regonol]), prevent the breakdown of acetylcholine by enzymes in the neuromuscular junction, thereby increasing the response of muscles to nerve impulses and improving strength.
     a. The drug is given with a small amount of food to minimize GI side effects; meals are provided 45 minutes to 1 hour after taking the drug.
  2. Drugs containing magnesium, morphine or its derivatives, curare, quinine, quinidine, procainamide, hypnotics, or sedatives may increase weakness and should be avoided.
  3. Antibiotics such as neomycin, kanamycin, streptomycin, polymyxin B, and certain tetracyclines increase myasthenic symptoms by impairing transmitter release.
- Implement interventions to induce remission, such as the administration of immunosuppressive drugs or corticosteroids, plasmapheresis, and thymectomy (removal of the thymus gland).
- Observe for myasthenic crisis, an exacerbation of the myasthenic symptoms caused by underdosing with anticholinergic drugs or by infection.
  1. Maintain adequate respiratory functioning (ABCs [airway, breathing, circulation] of emergency care); intubation and mechanical ventilation may be needed.
  2. Withhold cholinesterase-inhibiting drugs, because they increase respiratory secretion and are usually ineffective for the first few days after the crisis begins.
  3. Anticipate restarting drugs gradually at lower doses.
- Observe for cholinergic crisis, an acute exacerbation of muscle weakness caused by overdosing with cholinergic (anticholinesterase) drugs.

1. Withhold cholinesterase-inhibiting drugs until symptoms resolve.
2. Anticipate administration of atropine to treat excess acetylcholine. Atropine may thicken secretions, causing more difficulty with airway clearance and possible development of mucous plugs.

- Monitor the patient's responses to and vascular access for plasmapheresis. Plasmapheresis is a method by which autoantibodies are removed from the plasma.
- Provide respiratory support and frequent assessment of airway and breathing, including:
  1. Performing a respiratory assessment at least every 4 hours
  2. Reporting respiratory distress: dyspnea, shortness of breath, air hunger, and confusion
  3. Encouraging the patient to turn, cough, and deep breathe every 2 hours
  4. Performing chest physiotherapy, including postural drainage, percussion, and vibration to aid in the removal of secretions
  5. Keeping an Ambu bag, equipment for oxygen administration, and endotracheal intubation equipment at the bedside in case of respiratory distress
- Promote mobility and in-bed positioning to maintain function.
- Enhance self-care, including:
  1. Encouraging the patient to perform activities as independently as possible
  2. Planning activities to follow the administration of drug to maximize independence and successful attempts at self-care
  3. Collaborating with physical and occupational therapists to identify the need for assistive devices
- Assist with communication.
  1. Collaborate with the speech-language pathologist to develop communication strategies when needed.
  2. Instruct the patient to speak slowly and repeat information to verify that it is correct.
- Ensure adequate nutritional support.
  1. Provide small, frequent meals and high-calorie snacks. Record calorie counts.
  2. Measure intake and output, serum albumin levels, and daily weight.
  3. Assess for the onset of dysphagia. Implement aspiration precautions as needed.
  4. Promote or provide oral hygiene.
  5. Obtain a dietitian consultation to optimize nutrition.

M

- Maintain eye protection.
  1. Apply artificial tears to keep corneas moist and free from abrasion.
  2. Consider a lubricant gel and eye shield at bedtime.
  3. To help relieve diplopia, cover alternate eyes with a patch for 2 to 3 hours at a time.

Surgical Management

- Thymectomy may be performed early in the disease. Remission may not occur even with a thymectomy or may take up to 2 years to show effect.
- Provide routine preoperative care as outlined in Part One, including:
  1. Administering pyridostigmine (Mestinon), as ordered, to keep the patient stable throughout surgery
  2. If steroids have been used, administering before surgery but tapering postoperatively
  3. Giving antibiotics before and after surgery
- Provide routine postoperative care as outlined in Part One, including:
  1. Observing for signs of pneumothorax or hemothorax such as chest pain, sudden shortness of breath, diminished or absent breath sounds, and restlessness or a change in vital signs
  2. Focusing on respiratory health, including using spirometry, coughing, deep breathing, and frequent monitoring for respiratory distress
  3. Observing for signs and symptoms of wound infection
  4. Providing chest tube care if indicated

Community-Based Care

- Emphasize specific points concerning the disease process:
  1. MG is characterized by episodic exacerbations (worsening of symptoms). If rest does not relieve symptoms or respiratory distress occurs, contacting your health care provider is indicated.
  2. Avoid factors that predispose the patient to exacerbation, such as infection, stress, surgery, and hard physical exercise.
  3. Teach the patient and family to monitor for these two types of crises:
     a. Myasthenic crisis: an exacerbation (flare-up or worsening) of the myasthenic symptoms caused by not enough anticholinesterase drugs
     b. Cholinergic crisis: an acute exacerbation of muscle weakness caused by too many anticholinesterase drugs
  4. Promote lifestyle adaptations, such as avoiding heat (sauna, sunbathing), crowds, overeating, and erratic changes in sleep habits.

- Provide information concerning the drug regimen, and include the name, effects, side effects, and the importance of taking drugs on time and not missing doses.
- Refer the patient to community agencies and support groups such as the Myasthenia Gravis Foundation.

N

NEPHROSCLEROSIS

- Nephrosclerosis is a problem of thickening in the nephron blood vessels, resulting in narrowing of the lumen, decreased renal blood flow, and chronically hypoxic kidney tissue.
- Ischemia and fibrosis of renal tubules develops over time.
- Nephrosclerosis is associated with hypertension, atherosclerosis, and diabetes mellitus.
- Prevention and reduction of kidney vessel and kidney damage includes control of hyperlipidemia, hyperglycemia, and hypertension.

NEPHROTIC SYNDROME

- Nephrotic syndrome is a condition of increased glomerular permeability that allows larger molecules to pass through the membrane into the urine and be removed from the blood.
- Nephrotic syndrome is commonly caused by changes in an immune or inflammatory process.
- The main features are severe proteinuria, hypoalbuminemia, hyperlipidemia, lipiduria, facial and periorbital edema, and derangements in blood pressure.
- Treatment depends on what is causing the disorder (identified by renal biopsy) and may include:
  1. Angiotensin-converting enzyme inhibitors to preserve kidney function in early stages
  2. Cholesterol-lowering drugs and drugs to control hypercholesterolemia
  3. Anti-inflammatory and immunosuppressive agents such as glucocorticoids
  4. Heparin to reduce clot formation and extension (clots form as part of the inflammatory response)
  5. Diuretics
  6. Diet changes, including fluid and sodium restriction
- Assess the patient's hydration status and monitor for dehydration. If the plasma volume is depleted, kidney problems worsen.
- Assess laboratory values for changes in kidney function, including serum blood urea nitrogen (BUN), creatinine, glomerular filtration rate, electrolytes, and urinalysis.

NEUROMA, ACOUSTIC

- An acoustic neuroma is a nonmalignant tumor of cranial nerve VIII (vestibulocochlear nerve, also known as the *auditory* or *acoustic* nerve). Damage to hearing, facial movements, and sensation can occur as the tumor grows.
- Manifestations begin with tinnitus and progress to gradual sensorineural hearing loss in most patients. Constant, mild vertigo occurs later.
- Diagnosis is made by CT scanning or MRI.
- Surgical removal is usually achieved by a craniotomy, and the remaining hearing is lost. For care of the patient having a craniotomy, see *Surgical Management* under *Tumors, Brain*. See *Hearing Loss* for a review of care needs for the patient whose hearing is reduced.

0

OBESITY/BARIATRIC CONDITIONS

OVERVIEW

- *Obesity* refers to an excess amount of body fat compared with lean body mass.
- An obese person weighs at least 20% above the upper limit of the normal range for ideal body weight (IBW) and has a body mass index (BMI) of 30 m/kg^2 or more.
- *Morbid obesity*, also called *extreme obesity*, refers to a weight that has a severely negative effect on health, usually more than 100% above IBW or a BMI of 40 m/kg^2 or more.
- More than one third of the U.S. population is obese and around 10% of adults are morbidly obese. This problem is the second leading cause of preventable deaths in the United States.
- Obesity involves complex interrelationships among genetic, environmental, psychological, social, cultural, pathologic, behavioral, and physiologic factors.
- Causes of obesity include high-fat and high-cholesterol diets, physical inactivity, drug treatment (corticosteroids, NSAIDs), dysregulation of hormones that affect appetite and fat metabolism, and familial or genetic factors.
- Complications of obesity include diabetes mellitus, hypertension, hyperlipidemia, cardiac disease, sleep apnea, cholelithiasis, chronic back pain, early degenerative arthritis, susceptibility to infections, and certain cancers.
- Bariatrics is a branch of medicine that manages obesity and its related diseases.

QSEN PATIENT-CENTERED CARE

The Joint Commission's Core Measures require that a nutritional screening occur within 24 hours after the patient's admission to the hospital. If indicated, an in-depth nutritional assessment should be performed. When patients are in the hospital for more than 1 week, nutritional assessment should be part of the daily plan of care.

PATIENT-CENTERED COLLABORATIVE CARE

- Obtain patient information about:
  1. Usual food intake or 24-hour diet history recall
  2. Changes in eating behaviors or appetite
  3. Cultural and economic background
  4. Attitude toward food and current weight
  5. Drugs, including prescriptive, over-the-counter (OTC), and herbal or food additives
  6. Physical activity and functional ability
  7. Height and weight
  8. Waist-to-hip ratio or waist circumference; a ratio greater than 0.95 in men or greater than 0.8 in woman or a waist greater than 40 inches indicates central obesity and high risk for cardiovascular conditions
  9. Comorbid or chronic conditions
  10. Family history of obesity
- Management includes:
  1. Diet programs managed through close interaction among the patient, dietitian, nutritionist, and health care provider
  2. Exercise programs to include aerobic activity
  3. Short-term drug therapy
     a. Anorectic drugs work to suppress appetite and reduce food intake. Lorcaserin (Belviq) acts on central serotonin receptors. Phentermine and Contrave a combination of bupropion (Wellbutrin, an antidepressant) and naltrexone (an opioid antagonist) also work centrally but on norepinephrine receptors. Qsymia is a combination of phentermine and topiramate (an antiseizure drug).
     b. Orlistat (Xenical) works in the gastrointestinal tract to inhibit lipase and leads to partial hydrolysis of triglycerides. Because fats are only partially digested, absorption is reduced and calorie intake is decreased.
  4. Behavioral treatment to change habits around eating and weight management

- Surgery is indicated for the patient who is morbidly obese or who has a BMI greater than 35 with comorbidities that contribute to poor health.
  1. Bariatric surgical procedures include three types: gastric restrictive, malabsorption, or both. *Restrictive surgeries* decrease the volume capacity of the stomach to limit the amount of food that can be eaten at one time. As the name implies, *malabsorption procedures* interfere with the absorption of food and nutrients from the GI tract.
     a. Most patients have laparoscopic adjustable gastric band (LAGB) surgery or the laparoscopic sleeve gastrectomy (LSG). Both procedures are classified as restrictive surgeries.
     b. The most common malabsorption surgery is the *Roux-en-Y gastric bypass.*
- Provide routine postoperative care after bariatric surgery and:
  1. Attend to airway management, because a thick neck may lead to compromised airway.
  2. Monitor vital signs with peripheral oxygen saturation (Spo_2).
  3. Focus on patient and staff safety, using bariatric equipment to promote mobility and reduce skin complications.
  4. Monitor the patency of the nasogastric tube (NGT) and record the amount of drainage.
  5. Monitor for manifestations of anastomotic leak if this process was part of the surgical approach. Manifestations of leak are increasing back, shoulder, or abdominal pain; restlessness; unexplained tachycardia; and oliguria (scant urine). Report any of these findings to the surgeon immediately.
  6. Apply an abdominal binder to prevent wound dehiscence.
  7. Place the patient in a semi-Fowler's position.
  8. Use continuous positive airway pressure (CPAP) ventilation at night to improve ventilation and decrease risk for sleep apnea.
  9. Implement best practices for maintaining skin integrity and observe skin folds for redness, excoriation, or breakdown.
  10. Observe for dumping syndrome, manifested by frequent, liquid stools.
  11. Provide venothromboembolism prevention including early mobility and sequential compression stockings and/or subcutaneous low molecular weight heparin.
  12. Follow the institutional protocol about starting and advancing oral intake; avoid large volumes of liquid intake to avoid discomfort and stimulating hyperperistalsis.

Community-Based Care
- Give the patient a list of community resources, such as Weight Watchers, Overeaters Anonymous, and Take Off Pounds Sensibly (TOPS).

- In collaboration with the nutritionist, provide health teaching regarding the diet and the importance of maintaining a healthy eating pattern.
- Encourage the patient to increase physical activity, decrease fat intake and reliance on drug use, establish a normal eating pattern in response to physiologic hunger, and address medical and psychological problems.
- Emphasize the necessity for follow-up after bariatric surgery to avoid complications and ensure safe weight loss.

OBSTRUCTION, INTESTINAL
OVERVIEW

- Intestinal obstruction can be partial or complete and can occur in either the small or large intestine. Obstructions are classified as mechanical or nonmechanical.
  1. *Mechanical obstruction* occurs when the bowel is physically obstructed by disorders outside the intestine (adhesions or hernias) or blockages in the lumen of the intestine (tumor, fecal impaction, fibrosis, intussusception, volvulus, and stricture).
  2. *Nonmechanical obstruction (paralytic or adynamic ileus)* occurs when peristalsis is decreased or absent, resulting in a slowing of the movement or a backup of intestinal content caused by physiologic, neurogenic, or chemical imbalances.
     a. Paralytic ileus is associated with opioids and other drugs, trauma, surgery, hypokalemia, peritonitis, and vascular insufficiency to the bowel.
- Distention, edema, and increased capillary permeability occur with obstruction. Increased intraintestinal secretions contribute to distension. Absorption of fluid and electrolytes into the vascular space is compromised and can lead to reduced circulatory blood volume and electrolyte imbalances. Hypovolemia ranges from mild to extreme.
- Strangulated obstruction results when there is obstruction with compromised blood flow. This is a surgical emergency.

PATIENT-CENTERED COLLABORATIVE CARE
Assessment

- Obtain patient information about:
  1. Medical history, including abdominal surgical procedures, radiation therapy, and bowel diseases such as Crohn's disease, ulcerative colitis, diverticular disease, gallstones, hernias, trauma, and peritonitis
  2. Diet history and drug use
  3. Bowel elimination patterns, including the presence of blood in the stool

4. Familial history of colorectal cancer
5. Nausea and vomiting, including the color of emesis
- Assess for and document:
    1. The quality of abdominal pain, onset, and aggravating and alleviating factors associated with pain
    2. Bowel sounds (borborygmi): High-pitched bowel sounds may be heard early in an obstructive process and absent bowel sounds in later stages.
    3. Abdominal distention (hallmark sign)
    4. Nausea, vomiting, and character of emesis:
        a. Obstruction above the ileum causes early and profuse vomiting of partially digested food and chyme, changing to watery contents containing bile and mucus.
        b. Obstruction in the large intestine produces vomitus with an orange-brown color and a foul odor caused by bacterial overgrowth, which may be fecal contamination.
    5. No passage of stool (obstipation), a characteristic of total small- and large-bowel mechanical obstruction
    6. Hiccups (singultus), which is common with all types of intestinal obstruction
- Diagnostic studies include:
    1. CT scan
    2. A screening abdominal ultrasound may be used to evaluate the type of obstruction.

! NURSING SAFETY PRIORITY: Critical Rescue

The sudden change in abdominal pain from dull to sharp or local to generalized may indicate a perforation. Inform the physician immediately of this change in patient pain, along with current vital signs and oxygen status. A perforation is a surgical emergency.

Interventions

Interventions are aimed at uncovering the cause and relieving the obstruction.

Nonsurgical Management

- Decompress the GI tract by inserting or maintaining a gastric tube, which can be inserted nasally or orally.
    1. Monitor and record quantity and character of nasogastric output every 4 hours.
    2. Assess the nares for integrity at the site of tube insertion.
    3. Mark the tube at the nares to provide ongoing confirmation of placement.
    4. Record the passage of flatus and the amount and character of bowel movements.

> ### ❗ NURSING SAFETY PRIORITY: Action Alert
>
> At least every 4 hours, assess the patient with an NGT for proper placement of the tube, tube patency, and output (quality and quantity). Monitor the nasal skin around the tube for irritation. Use a device that secures the tube to the nose to prevent accidental removal. Assess for peristalsis by auscultating for bowel sounds with the suction disconnected (suction masks peristaltic sounds).

    5. Inform the health care provider if gastric or intestinal outflow stops or becomes bloody.
- Obstruction caused by fecal impaction resolves after disimpaction and enema.
- Intussusception (telescoping of bowel) and volvulus may resolve with hydrostatic pressure changes with manipulation under fluoroscopy.
- Administer fluid and electrolyte replacement.
  1. Administer IV fluid because of dehydration from NPO status, lack of normal reabsorption in the intestine, increased intestinal secretions, and NG suction.
  2. Monitor fluid status with vital signs, adequacy of urine output, and daily weight.
- Provide pain management.
  1. Report uncontrolled or severe pain to the provider, including pain that significantly increases or changes from a colicky, intermittent type to constant discomfort.
  2. Administer stool softeners or stimulants with opioids unless the obstruction is complete.
  3. Provide a position of comfort, including the semi-Fowler's position, to relieve the pressure of abdominal distention and facilitate thoracic excursion and normal breathing patterns.
- Broad-spectrum antibiotics are given if surgery is anticipated.

Surgical Management
- Surgical management is required for complete mechanical obstruction and for many cases of incomplete mechanical obstruction.
- An exploratory laparotomy is performed to locate the obstruction and determine the nature of the problem.
- The specific surgical procedure performed depends on the cause and location of the obstruction. Examples of procedures include lysis of adhesions, colon resection with anastomosis for obstruction resulting from tumor or diverticulitis, and embolectomy or thrombectomy for intestinal infarction. A colon resection and colostomy may be necessary.

- Nursing care for abdominal surgery is similar to that described under *Cancer, Colorectal.*

Community-Based Care

- Patient and family education depend on the specific cause and treatment of the obstruction.
    1. Report signs that may indicate recurrent obstruction, including abdominal pain or distention, nausea, vomiting, or constipation (for nonmechanical obstruction after surgery or trauma).
    2. Develop a structured bowel regimen, such as a high-fiber diet or fiber supplements and daily exercise with sufficient oral water for prevention of recurrences of fecal impaction.
- Information about incision care (if surgery was performed), drug therapy, and activity restriction is given to the patient and family.

OBSTRUCTION, UPPER AIRWAY

OVERVIEW

- Upper airway obstruction, a life-threatening emergency, is an interruption in airflow through the nose, mouth, pharynx, or larynx.
- Causes include:
    1. Tongue edema (surgery, trauma, angioedema as an allergic response to a drug)
    2. Tongue occlusion (e.g., loss of gag reflex, loss of muscle tone, unconsciousness, and coma)
    3. Laryngeal edema
    4. Peritonsillar and pharyngeal abscess
    5. Head and neck cancer
    6. Thick secretions
    7. Stroke and cerebral edema
    8. Smoke inhalation edema
    9. Facial, tracheal, or laryngeal trauma
    10. Foreign body aspiration
    11. Burns of the head or neck area
    12. Anaphylaxis
- Partial obstruction may have only subtle or general manifestations such as diaphoresis, tachycardia, and elevated blood pressure. To rule out a tumor, foreign body, or infection, diagnostic procedures, such as a chest x-ray, neck films, laryngoscopic examination, and CT scan, are performed.
- Observe for arterial blood gases (ABG) and symptoms related to low oxygenation or carbon dioxide retention, including restlessness, increasing anxiety, sternal retractions, a "seesawing" chest, abdominal movements, or a feeling of impending doom related to actual air hunger.

- Use pulse oximetry for ongoing monitoring of oxygen saturation to maintain values above 92%. Continually assess for stridor, cyanosis, and changes in level of consciousness.

! **NURSING SAFETY PRIORITY: Action Alert**

Early recognition is essential to preventing further complications, including respiratory arrest. Unexplained or persistent recurrent symptoms warrant evaluation even if the symptoms are vague.

PATIENT-CENTERED COLLABORATIVE CARE

- Management depends on the cause of the obstruction.
  1. Prevent airway obstruction from thick, hardened oral and nasopharyngeal secretions with regular oral hygiene and adequate hydration.
  2. For tongue occlusion or excessive secretions, slightly extend the patient's head and neck and insert a nasal or oral airway, suctioning to remove secretions.
  3. For a foreign body, perform abdominal thrusts.
  4. For complete obstruction from edema, cancer, or abscesses, anticipate the need for direct visualization of the airway (laryngoscopy) by a provider or placement of an artificial airway, including:
     a. Cricoidectomy
     b. Endotracheal intubation
     c. Tracheotomy

OBSTRUCTIVE SLEEP APNEA

- Obstructive sleep apnea is a breathing disruption during sleep that lasts at least 10 seconds and occurs a minimum of five times in an hour.
- The most common cause of sleep apnea is upper airway obstruction by the soft palate or tongue. Factors that contribute to sleep apnea include obesity, a large uvula, a short neck, smoking, enlarged tonsils or adenoids, and oropharyngeal edema.
- The most accurate test for sleep apnea is an overnight sleep study in which the patient is directly observed while wearing a variety of monitoring equipment to evaluate the depth of sleep, type of sleep, respiratory effort, oxygen saturation, and muscle movement.
- A common method to prevent airway collapse is the use of noninvasive positive-pressure ventilation (NPPV) to hold open the upper airways.
- A change in sleeping position, weight loss, or devices to prevent the tongue or neck anatomy from obstructing the airways may correct mild sleep apnea.

OSTEOARTHRITIS

OVERVIEW

- Osteoarthritis (OA), sometimes called *osteoarthrosis* or *degenerative joint disease* (DJD), is the most common arthritis, with joint pain and loss of function leading to disability.
- The disease includes progressive deterioration and loss of cartilage in one or more joints (articular cartilage), especially the hips and knees, the vertebral column, and the hands.
- The major pathologic problems are thinning and deteriorating joint cartilage, narrowing of the joint space, bone spur formation, inflammation, and joint deformity leading to immobility, pain, muscle spasm, and muscle atrophy.
- Known risk factors for OA include obesity, joint trauma, and smoking.

Considerations for Older Adults

Age is the biggest risk factor for OA, because the production of proteoglycans and synovial fluid in the joint decreases with age, reducing cartilage strength and function. Repeated joint injury and use contribute to damage that accelerates OA and leads to manifestations in older adults.

Genetic/Genomic Considerations

Some patients report a family history of OA, which supports a possible genetic cause, especially for women who have hand involvement. Inheritance may contribute to cartilage destruction, osteophyte formation, or the inability of the cartilage to repair itself.

PATIENT-CENTERED COLLABORATIVE CARE

Assessment

- Obtain patient information about:
  1. The course of the disease
     a. The nature and location of joint pain, stiffness, or swelling
     b. What relieves or increases pain or stiffness
     c. Any loss of mobility or difficulty in performing ADLs
  2. Age and gender
  3. Trauma or recurrent stress to joints from occupational and recreational activity or sports
  4. Weight history
  5. Smoking history
  6. Family history of arthritis

- Assess for and document:
  1. Chronic joint pain and stiffness
  2. Aggravating and relieving factors such as activity and rest
  3. Limitations in range of motion (ROM)
  4. Crepitus (a continuous grating sensation felt or heard as the joint goes through its ROM)
  5. Joint enlarged from bony hypertrophy
  6. Joint warmth or inflammation (indicates a secondary synovitis)
  7. Hand changes with Heberden's nodes (at the distal interphalangeal [DIP] joints) and Bouchard's nodes (at the proximal interphalangeal [PIP] joints)
  8. Joint effusions (excess joint fluid), especially in the knee
  9. Atrophy of skeletal muscle from disuse
  10. Compression of spinal nerve roots that produces radiating pain, stiffness, and muscle spasms in one or both extremities with vertebral involvement
  11. Reduced mobility and function
  12. Change in role and self-esteem
  13. Depression, anger, stress
- Imaging assessment may include x-rays or MRI.

Planning and Implementation

CHRONIC PAIN

   Nonsurgical Management

- Drug therapy
  1. Analgesic drugs
     a. Acetaminophen (Tylenol, Exdol, Datril) because OA is not primarily an inflammatory process
  2. Topical drug applications
     a. Lidocaine 5% patches
     b. Topical salicylates (trolamine salicylate [Aspercreme], 1% diclofenac [Voltaren])

> **! NURSING SAFETY PRIORITY: Drug Alert**
>
> Patients are at risk for liver damage from NSAID use if they take more than 3000 mg daily of acetaminophen, have alcoholism, or have liver disease. Older adults are particularly at risk because of normal changes of aging, such as slowed excretion of drug metabolites. Remind patients to read the labels of OTC or prescription drugs that could contain acetaminophen before taking them.

  3. NSAIDs
     a. Celecoxib (Celebrex)
     b. Ibuprofen (Advil)

4. Joint injection (typically no more than three times per year)
   a. Cortisone
   b. Hyaluronan (Hyalgan)
   c. Hylan G-F 20 (Synvisc)
5. Muscle relaxants (cyclobenzaprine [Flexeril])
- Nonpharmacologic measures
  1. Joint rest, using a joint immobilizer
  2. Balancing rest and activity to promote 8 to 10 hours of night-time sleep and avoid prolonged inactivity
  3. Position joint to avoid excessive flexion of involved joint and maintain normal extension
  4. Heat or cold applications (hot showers and baths, hot packs or compresses, moist heating pads)
  5. Weight control
  6. Complementary and alternative therapies (topical capsaicin products, acupuncture, acupressure, tai chi, music therapy)
  7. Cognitive-behavioral therapies (imagery, prayer, meditation)

Surgical Management

- Surgery may be indicated when conservative measures no longer provide pain control, when mobility becomes so restricted that the patient cannot participate in enjoyable activities, or when he or she is unable to maintain the desired quality of life.
  1. *Total joint arthroplasty* (TJA) (surgical creation of a joint), also known as *total joint replacement* (TJR), is the most common type of surgery for OA. Almost any synovial joint of the body can be replaced with a prosthetic system that consists of at least two parts, one for each joint surface.
  2. An *osteotomy (bone resection)* may be performed to correct joint deformity, but this procedure is less common because of the success rate of TJR.
- *Total hip arthroplasty* (THA) with a replacement prosthesis can be done by a traditional open hip incision or, for select patients, by minimally invasive surgery (MIS) using one or two smaller 2- to 4-inch incisions with special instruments to reduce muscle cutting. The replacement joint consists of four parts, the acetabular component (this has two parts) and the femoral component (this has two parts).
  1. Provide preoperative care
     a. Assess the patient's level of understanding about the surgery.
     b. Reinforce the surgeon's explanations about the procedure and postoperative expectations.
     c. Ensure that the surgical site is correct using best practices as described in Part One.
     d. Explain about transfers, positioning, ambulation, and postoperative exercises.

  e. Demonstrate assistive-adaptive devices for ADLs.
  f. Teach patients having MIS how to perform muscle-strengthening exercises at home before the procedure.
  g. Explain the importance of having any necessary dental procedures done before the surgery to decrease the risk for oral bacterial infection resulting in prosthetic site infection.
  h. Assess the patient's risk factors for clotting problems and administering any prescribed anticoagulants.
  i. Determine whether the patient needs preoperative supplementation to treat anemia or has made an autologous blood donation or is a candidate for autotransfusion.
  j. Administer any prescribed antibiotic therapy before the initial surgical incision is made.
2. Provide postoperative care
  a. Perform routine postoperative care as described in Part One.
  b. Prevent operative joint dislocation by:
     (1) Maintaining correct positioning (supine position with the head slightly elevated)
     (2) Placing a trapezoid-shaped abduction pillow, wedge, sling, or splint (with or without straps) between the legs to prevent adduction beyond the midline of the body
     (3) Placing and supporting the affected leg in neutral rotation
     (4) Following agency policy or surgeon preference for postoperative turning
     (5) Observing for signs of possible hip dislocation (increased hip pain, shortening of the affected leg, and leg rotation)

! NURSING SAFETY PRIORITY: Critical Rescue

If manifestations of hip dislocation occur, keep the patient in bed and notify the surgeon immediately.

  c. Prevent thromboembolic complications by:
     (1) Administering prescribed anticoagulants, such as subcutaneous heparin or low–molecular-weight heparin
     (2) Assessing for manifestations of venous thromboembolism (VTE) (swelling, pain)
     (3) Teaching leg exercises (plantar flexion and dorsiflexion, circles of the feet, gluteal and quadriceps muscle setting, straight-leg raises)

      (4) Applying prescribed antiembolic stockings or devices
      (5) Collaborating with the PT to promote early ambulation
  d. Prevent infection and detect infection early by:
      (1) Keeping surgical incision clean and covered until the edges of the incision are sealed.
      (2) Observing the incision and patient for signs of infection such as discolored or odorous drainage and signs of poor healing at the incision and the presence of fever or elevated white blood cells (WBCs).

❗ NURSING SAFETY PRIORITY: Critical Rescue

An older patient may not have a fever with infection but instead may experience an altered mental state. Consider infection in any older patient with new-onset confusion or inability to rouse.

---

  e. Prevent neurovascular complications by:
      (1) Checking and documenting color, temperature, distal pulses, capillary refill, movement, and sensation
      (2) Comparing these parameters with those of the nonoperative leg
      (3) Reporting any changes to the surgeon

❗ NURSING SAFETY PRIORITY: Critical Rescue

Check and document color, temperature, distal pulses, capillary refill, movement, and sensation. Remember to compare the operative leg with the nonoperative leg. These assessments are performed at the same time the vital signs are checked. Report any changes in neurovascular assessment to the surgeon, and carefully monitor for changes. Early detection of changes in neurovascular status can prevent permanent tissue damage.

---

  f. Manage pain by:
      (1) Assessing the patient's pain level
      (2) Ensuring proper use of pain control devices such as epidural analgesia, intraspinal analgesia, patient-controlled analgesia (PCA), and IV opioid analgesia
      (3) Administering prescribed analgesics as needed
  g. Progress activity by assisting the patient with getting out of bed by:
      (1) Standing on the same side of the bed as the affected leg

      (2) Teaching the patient to stand on the unaffected leg and pivot to the chair

      (3) Assisting the patient to a sitting position

      (4) Ensuring that the patient does not flex the hips beyond 90 degrees

      (5) Preventing hyperflexion of the replaced joint with the use of raised toilet seats, straight-back chairs, and reclining wheelchairs

3. Weight bearing on the affected leg depends on the surgeon, type of prosthesis, and surgical procedure.

4. Work with the PT to teach the patient how to follow weight-bearing restrictions and progress to full weight-bearing (FWB) status.

5. The occupational therapist (OT) may recommend assistive-adaptive devices to help with ADLs, especially for patients having traditional surgery.

6. For patients who have traditional surgery, the length of stay in the acute care hospital is typically 3 days; those who have MIS procedures may be discharged on the second postoperative day or, in a few cases, on the day of surgery.

7. The interdisciplinary team provides written instructions for posthospital care and reviews them with patients and their family members.

8. Complete recovery may take 6 weeks or more.

• *Total knee arthroplasty* (TKA) can be performed by traditional open surgery or by MIS procedures for some patients.

1. Provide preoperative care.

  a. Routine preoperative care described in Part One

  b. Care as described for THA

  c. Explanation and demonstration of a continuous passive motion (CPM) machine (if prescribed)

2. Provide postoperative care.

  a. Care to prevent complications as described for THA

  b. Implement the CPM machine as prescribed for ROM and cycles per minute.

      (1) Check the cycle and ROM settings at least once every 8 hours.

      (2) Ensure that the joint being moved is properly positioned on the machine.

      (3) Place the controls to the machine out of reach of a confused patient.

      (4) Assess the patient's response to the machine.

      (5) Turn off the machine while the patient is having a meal.

      (6) Store the machine off the floor when it is not in use.

    c. Apply ice packs or a Hot/Ice device to decrease surgical site swelling.

    d. Ensure safe use of peripheral nerve blockade (PNB) for pain control.

      (1) If the nerve block is continuous, perform neurovascular assessments every 2 to 4 hours or according to hospital protocol.

      (2) Assess that the patient can plantar flex and dorsiflex the affected foot but does not feel pain in the extremity.

      (3) Check for movement, sensation, warmth, color, pulses, and capillary refill.

      (4) Monitor for symptoms of systemic infusion of the nerve-blocking drug (a metallic taste, tinnitus, restlessness, nervousness, slurred speech, bradycardia, hypotension, or decreased respirations).

    e. Maintain the knee in a neutral position, not rotated internally or externally.

    f. Ensure that the surgical knee is not hyperextended.

    g. Monitor neurovascular status frequently to check for compromise to the distal operative leg every time vital signs are taken.

- *Total shoulder arthroplasty* (TSA) can be performed either as a total joint replacement or as a hemiarthroplasty (replacement of part of the joint, typically the humeral component). These surgeries are most commonly performed using traditional open incisions, but minimally invasive shoulder arthroplasty can be used instead for some patients.

    1. Preoperative care and postoperative care are similar to those for other joint replacement surgeries.

    2. A sling is applied to immobilize the joint and prevent dislocation until therapy begins.

    3. The hospital stay for TSA is usually 1 to 2 days, until pain is controlled.

    4. Rehabilitation with an OT usually takes 2 to 3 months.

- Other joints that can be replaced include:

    1. Elbow (total elbow arthroplasty [TEA])

    2. Hand or foot joints (phalangeal joint, metacarpal, or metatarsal arthroplasty)

    3. Any bone of the wrist

    4. Ankle (total ankle arthroplasty [TAA]), which has more postoperative complications than other arthroplasties

IMPAIRED PHYSICAL MOBILITY

- Reinforce the techniques and principles of exercise, ambulation, promotion of ADLs, and use of assistive devices developed by the PT and OT to meet the goal of independent function.

- The ideal time for exercise is immediately after the application of heat.
- Teach the patient to follow these instructions:
    1. Follow the exercise instructions that have been specifically prescribed. There are no universal exercises; exercises have been specifically tailored to each individual's needs.
    2. Do exercises on both "good" and "bad" days. Consistency is important.
    3. Respect pain. If pain increases with exercise, stop and report this to the health care provider.
    4. Use active rather than active-assist or passive exercise whenever possible.
    5. Reduce the number of repetitions if the inflammation is severe and there is more pain.
    6. Do not substitute normal activities or household tasks for the prescribed exercises.
    7. Avoid resistive exercises if joints are severely inflamed.

Community-Based Care

- Collaborate with the discharge planner and the health care provider to determine the best placement for the patient with OA at discharge.
- Provide health teaching.
    1. Explain the general principles of joint protection.
        a. Use large joints instead of small ones; for example, place a purse strap over the shoulder instead of grasping the purse with a hand.
        b. Turn doorknobs toward the thumb (rather than toward the little finger) to avoid twisting the arm and promoting ulnar deviation.
        c. Use two hands instead of one to hold objects.
        d. Sit in a chair that has a high, straight back.
        e. When getting out of bed, do not push off with the fingers; use the entire palm of both hands.
        f. Do not bend at the waist; instead, bend the knees while keeping the back straight.
        g. Use long-handled devices, such as a hairbrush with an extended handle.
        h. Use assistive-adaptive devices, such as Velcro closures and built-up utensil handles, to protect joints.
        i. Do not use pillows in bed, except a small one under the head.
        j. Avoid twisting or wringing the hands.
    2. Explain the drug protocol, desired and potential side effects, and toxic effects.
    3. Emphasize the importance of reducing weight and eating a well-balanced diet to promote tissue healing.

4. Refer the patient to the Arthritis Foundation for up-to-date information about new treatments and helpful complementary and alternative practices.
5. Provide written instructions about the required care, regardless of whether the patient goes home or to another inpatient facility.
6. Refer the patient to the nutritionist, counselor, home health nurse, rehabilitation therapist, financial counselor, and local and state support groups as needed.

OSTEOMALACIA

OVERVIEW

- Osteomalacia is a softening of the bone tissue related to vitamin D deficiency, causing inadequate deposits of calcium and phosphorus in the bone matrix.
- Vitamin D deficiency can occur as a result of inadequate exposure to sunlight, poor dietary intake, abnormal metabolism, chronic use of many drugs, or the presence of chronic disease.
- Older adults are most at risk for osteomalacia.

PATIENT-CENTERED COLLABORATIVE CARE

- Obtain patient information about:
  1. Age
  2. Exposure to sunlight and skin pigmentation (darker skin reduces vitamin D activation)
  3. Dietary habits
  4. Current prescribed and OTC drug use
     a. Chronic GI inflammatory disease or gastric or intestinal bypass surgery
  5. Renal or liver dysfunction
  6. History of bone fracture
- Assess for and document:
  1. Muscle weakness (causing a waddling and unsteady gait) and cramping
  2. Bone pain (aggravated by activity and worse at night)
  3. Bone tenderness to palpation (especially tibia or rib cage)
  4. Skeletal misalignment (long-bone bowing or spinal deformity)
  5. Hypocalcemia or hypophosphatemia
  6. Presence of radiolucent bands (Looser's lines or zones) on x-ray
- The major intervention for osteomalacia is vitamin D.
  1. Teach patients to take the amount of vitamin D supplementation prescribed by their health care provider.
  2. Remind patients, especially those who are homebound, about the importance of daily sun exposure (at least 15 minutes each day) to activate the vitamin.

3. Teach patients to choose foods that are fortified with vitamin D (milk and dairy products) or are rich in vitamin D (eggs, swordfish, chicken, and liver), in addition to enriched cereals and bread products.

OSTEOMYELITIS

OVERVIEW

* Osteomyelitis is an infection in bony tissue caused by bacteria, viruses, or fungi.
* Osteomyelitis is difficult to treat and can result in chronic recurrence of infection, loss of function, amputation, and even death.
* The pathologic processes that occur in infected bone tissue include inflammation, blood vessel thromboses, and necrosis.
* Categories of osteomyelitis include:
    1. *Exogenous osteomyelitis,* in which infectious organisms enter from outside the body, as in an open fracture
    2. *Endogenous osteomyelitis,* also called *hematogenous osteomyelitis,* in which organisms are carried by the bloodstream from other areas of infection in the body
    3. *Contiguous osteomyelitis,* in which bone infection results from skin infection of adjacent tissues
* The two major types of osteomyelitis are acute and chronic.
* Common causes include bacteremia, pre-existing conditions that interfere with immune health or wound healing such as diabetes, penetrating and nonpenetrating trauma, long-term IV therapy, hemodialysis, *Salmonella* infection of the GI tract, sickle cell disease, poor dental hygiene and periodontal (gum) infection, and skin infection, particularly with MDROs like MRSA.

Considerations for Older Adults

The most common cause of contiguous spread in older adults is slow-healing foot ulcers in patients with diabetes or peripheral vascular disease.

PATIENT-CENTERED COLLABORATIVE CARE

Assessment

* Assess for and document:
    1. Bone pain described as a constant, localized, pulsating sensation that worsens with movement
    2. Fever, usually greater than 101°F (38°C) (in acute disease)
    3. Swelling, tenderness, erythema, and heat around the site of infection
    4. Ulcerations on the feet or hands (if circulation is poor)

5. Sinus tract formation and drainage (with chronic infection)
6. Elevated WBC count and erythrocyte sedimentation rate (ESR)
7. Positive blood cultures

Interventions

Nonsurgical Management

- Nonsurgical interventions include:
  1. Administering IV antibiotic therapy for several weeks, followed by oral antibiotic therapy for weeks or months

> **! NURSING SAFETY PRIORITY: Action Alert**
>
> Even if symptoms of the disease appear to be improved, the full course of IV and oral antibiotics must be completed. Teach patients the importance of completing the full course of therapy.

  2. Irrigating the wound either continuously or intermittently, with one or more antibiotic solutions
  3. Packing the wound with beads made of bone cement that have been impregnated with an antibiotic
  4. Administering drugs for pain control
  5. Covering the wound to prevent infection spread
  6. Administering hyperbaric oxygen (HBO) therapy for patients with chronic, unremitting osteomyelitis

Surgical Management

- Surgery is reserved for patients with chronic osteomyelitis and may include revascularization and:
  1. Sequestrectomy with excision of dead and infected bone to allow revascularization of tissue
  2. Application of bone grafts to repair bone defects
  3. Reconstruction with microvascular bone transfers if excision is extensive
  4. Closure of the defect with muscle flaps and skin grafts
  5. Amputation of the affected limb if the infection cannot be controlled or revascularization is not successful
- Provide postoperative care described in Part One and:
  1. Perform frequent neurovascular (NV) assessments of:
     a. Pain
     b. Movement
     c. Sensation
     d. Warmth
     e. Temperature
     f. Distal pulses
     g. Capillary refill

! NURSING SAFETY PRIORITY: Critical Rescue

Immediately report to the surgeon any of these signs of neurovascular compromise: pain that cannot be controlled, paresis or paralysis (weakness or inability to move), paresthesias (abnormal tingling sensation), pallor, and pulselessness.

2. Elevate the affected extremity to increase venous return and control swelling.

OSTEOPOROSIS

OVERVIEW

- Osteoporosis is a chronic metabolic disease in which bone loss causes decreased density and possible fracture, most often of the spine, hip, and wrist.
- The main mechanism of osteoporosis is an imbalance in the continuous bone remodeling processes such that osteoclastic (bone resorption) activity is greater than osteoblastic (bone building) activity.
- Generalized osteoporosis involves many structures in the skeleton and is further divided into two categories.
  1. *Primary osteoporosis,* which is more common and occurs in postmenopausal women and in men in their sixth or seventh decade of life
  2. *Secondary osteoporosis,* which results from other medical conditions, such as hyperparathyroidism, long-term drug therapy (such as with corticosteroids), or prolonged immobility
- Regional osteoporosis occurs when a limb is immobilized related to a fracture, injury, or paralysis for longer than 8 to 12 weeks.
- Risk factors include menopause; lean and thin body build; Euro-American or Asian ancestry; sedentary lifestyle; diet deficient in protein, calcium, and vitamin D, or malabsorption syndromes; high intake of carbonated beverages; excessive alcohol and tobacco use; genetics; and long-term use of certain drugs, especially corticosteroids.

Gender Health Considerations

Primary osteoporosis most often occurs in women after menopause as a result of decreased estrogen levels. Women lose about 2% of their bone mass every year in the first 5 years after natural or surgical (ovary removal) menopause.

Men also develop osteoporosis after the age of 50 because their testosterone levels decrease. Testosterone is the major sex hormone that builds bone tissue. Men are often underdiagnosed, even when they become older adults.

PATIENT-CENTERED COLLABORATIVE CARE
Assessment
- Obtain patient information about:
  1. Age, gender, race, body build, weight
  2. Loss of height
  3. Back pain after bending, lifting, or stooping (worse with activity, relieved with rest)
  4. Mobility or weakness
  5. Current drugs
- Assess for and document:
  1. Features of the spinal column (presence of classic "dowager's hump," or kyphosis of the dorsal spine)
  2. Location of all painful areas and signs of fracture such as swelling and misalignment
  3. Constipation, abdominal distention
  4. Respiratory compromise
  5. Body image disturbance
  6. Changes in quality of life and sexuality
- Diagnostic tests may include:
  1. Biochemical markers (commonly used to determine response to therapy)
     a. Bone-specific alkaline phosphatase (BSAP)
     b. Proteins indicating bone resorption: osteocalcin, pyridinium (PYD), N-telopeptide (NTX), and C-telopeptide (CTX)
     c. Levels of serum calcium, vitamin D, phosphorus, and protein
  2. Imaging (to determine bone density)
     a. Dual-energy x-ray absorptiometry (DXA or DEXA)
     b. Quantitative computed tomography (QCT)
     c. Quantitative ultrasound (QUS)

Interventions
Nonsurgical Management
- Nutrition therapy
  1. Coordinate health teaching and nutrition planning with the dietitian.
  2. Teach patients to eat a diet that includes:
     a. Calcium and vitamin D
     b. Low-fat protein sources
     c. Moderation in alcohol intake
     d. Low soda intake; phosphorus in soda may reduce calcium absorption
  3. Work with patients who are lactose intolerant to choose from a variety of soy and rice products, fruit juices, bread, and cereal products that are fortified with or have additional calcium and vitamin D.

- Exercise is important in both prevention and management of osteoporosis.
  1. Coordinate health teaching with the PT for exercises to improve posture, support, and pulmonary capacity; strengthen extremity muscles; and improve ROM.
     a. Abdominal muscle tightening, deep breathing, and pectoral stretching
     b. Extremity muscle tightening, resistive, and ROM exercises
     c. Walking for 30 minutes three to five times a week
  2. Teach patients to avoid high-impact recreational activities such as running, bowling, and horseback riding.
- Teach about other lifestyle changes.
  1. Smoking cessation, avoiding secondhand tobacco smoke
  2. Preventing falls
- Drug therapy for prevention and management
  1. Bisphosphonates
     a. Alendronate (Fosamax) (oral drug)
     b. Ibandronate (Boniva) (oral and IV)
     c. Risedronate (Actonel) (oral drug)
     d. Zoledronic acid (Reclast) (IV drug)
  2. Estrogen agonist/antagonist: raloxifene (Evista)
  3. Calcium and vitamin D supplementation
  4. Denosumab (Prolia, Xgeva), a monoclonal antibody against osteoclast-specific protein

! NURSING SAFETY PRIORITY: Drug Alert

Osteonecrosis of the jaw is a rare but serious complication of bisphosphonate therapy. Teach patients to have an oral assessment and preventive dentistry before beginning any bisphosphonate therapy. To promote safety, instruct them to inform any dentist who is planning invasive treatment, such as a tooth extraction or implant, that they are taking a bisphosphonate.

OTITIS MEDIA

OVERVIEW

- Otitis media is an inflammation or infection of the middle ear mucosa.
- The inflammation leads to swelling and irritation of the small bones (ossicles) within the middle ear, a purulent exudate, pain, and temporary hearing loss.
- If otitis media progresses or recurs without treatment, permanent conductive hearing loss may occur.
- Otitis media can be acute, chronic, or serous.

PATIENT-CENTERED COLLABORATIVE CARE
Assessment
* Assess for manifestations of acute or chronic otitis media.
  1. Ear pain with or without movement of the external ear (which is relieved when the eardrum ruptures)
  2. Sensation of fullness in the ear
  3. Reduced or distorted hearing
  4. Tinnitus
  5. Headaches
  6. Dizziness or vertigo
  7. Systemic symptoms of fever, malaise, or nausea and vomiting
  8. Otoscopic examination findings
     a. Dilated and red eardrum blood vessels
     b. Red, thickened, or bulging eardrum
     c. Decreased eardrum mobility
     d. Eardrum perforation with pus present in the canal

Interventions
  Nonsurgical Management
* Application of heat or cold
  1. Analgesics for mild to moderate pain such as aspirin, ibuprofen (Advil), and acetaminophen (Tylenol, Abenol)
* Antihistamines and decongestants
* Systemic antibiotics if a bacterial infection is suspected
  Surgical Management
* Surgical management with a myringotomy (surgical opening of the eardrum), often combined with tube insertion (to provide ongoing drainage), may be needed.
  1. Preoperative care, following best practices, outlined in Part One
  2. Postoperative care
     a. Teach the patient to keep the external ear and canal free of other substances.
     b. Instruct him or her to avoid washing the hair or showering for 48 hours.

OVARIAN CYSTS
* Functional ovarian cysts can occur in a woman of any age but are rare after menopause.
* Primary assessment involves pelvic examination and transvaginal ultrasound. Further testing with CT, MRI, or laparoscopic biopsy may be needed to rule out cancer.
* Laparoscopic surgery may be needed to remove the cyst or ovary.

P

PAGET'S DISEASE OF THE BONE

OVERVIEW

- Paget's disease, or osteitis deformans, is a chronic metabolic disorder in which bone is excessively broken down (osteoclastic activity) and re-formed (osteoblastic activity). The result is structurally disorganized bone that is weak with increased risk of bowing of long bones and fractures.
- There are three phases of the disorder.
  1. *Active,* in which there is a rapid increase in osteoclasts (cells that break down bone), causing massive bone destruction and deformity
  2. *Mixed,* in which the osteoblasts (bone-forming cells) react to compensate in forming new but structurally weak bone
  3. *Inactive,* in which the osteoblastic activity exceeds the osteoclastic activity, resulting in hard, sclerotic bone
- The most common areas of disease involvement are the vertebrae, femur, skull, clavicle, humerus, and pelvis.
- The risk for developing Paget's disease increases as a person ages and is particularly high for those who are age 80 or older.
- Most patients with Paget's disease are asymptomatic and have disease confined to one bone. In more severe disease, the manifestations are diverse and potentially fatal.

✇ Genetic/Genomic Considerations

- Two types of Paget's disease can occur: familial and sporadic. Possible mutation areas for the familial form include the *RANKL/RANK/OPG* gene system, the gene for the valosin-containing protein *(VCP)* that controls complement, and the gene for sequestosome 1 *(SQSTM1)*.
- Teach patients the importance of genetics in familial Paget's disease, and refer them to the appropriate genetic counseling resource.

PATIENT-CENTERED COLLABORATIVE CARE

Assessment

- Obtain patient information about:
  1. History of fracture
  2. Bone pain (mild to moderate aching, deep, worsened by pressure and weight bearing), especially of the hip and pelvis
  3. Redness and warmth at the affected sites
  4. Arthritis at the joints (cartilage) of the affected bones

   5. Nerve impingement in the lumbosacral area of the vertebral column (back pain that radiates along one or both legs)
   6. Any changes in hearing, vision, swallowing, balance, or speech
   7. Loose teeth or difficulty chewing
- Assess for and document:
   1. Posture, stance, and gait for gross bony deformities
   2. Long-bone bowing (legs and arms)
   3. Decreased height
   4. Kyphosis, scoliosis, or loss of normal spinal curvature
   5. Flexion contracture in the hip joint
   6. Soft, thick, and enlarged skull
   7. Deafness and vertigo
   8. Problems with vision, swallowing, or speech
   9. Hydrocephalus
   10. Bone fractures, especially of the femur or tibia, after minimal trauma
   11. Apathy, lethargy, and fatigue
   12. Hyperparathyroidism and gout (along with an increase in serum and urinary calcium levels and serum uric acid levels)
   13. Kidney stones (renal calculi)
   14. Cardiac complications (heart failure)
- Diagnosis is made based on physical findings, increases in serum alkaline phosphatase (ALP) and urinary hydroxyproline levels, x-ray findings, and radionuclide bone scanning.

Interventions
- Drug therapy for pain management includes:
   1. Aspirin or NSAIDs such as ibuprofen (Motrin, Apo-Ibuprofen) for mild to moderate pain
   2. More potent analgesics for severe pain
- Drug therapy to decrease bone resorption includes:
   1. Bisphosphonates
      a. Alendronate (Fosamax) (oral drug)
      b. Risedronate (Actonel) (oral drug)
      c. Etidronate (Didronel) (oral drug)
      d. Tiludronate (Skelid) (oral drug)
      e. Zoledronic acid (Reclast) (IV drug)
   2. Calcium: 1500 mg daily
   3. Vitamin D: 800 IU daily
   4. Calcitonin (subcutaneous injection or nasal spray)
   5. Denosumab (Prolia), a monoclonal antibody that bocks osteoclast formation and function
- Non-impact or strengthening exercises to maintain mobility
- Use of orthotic device to immobilize and provide support for the vertebrae or long bones
- Nutrition therapy with a diet rich in calcium

PAIN, BACK

OVERVIEW

- The areas of the back most commonly affected by back pain are the cervical and lumbar vertebrae.
- *Acute lumbosacral (low back) pain* (LBP) is typically caused by a muscle strain, spasm, ligament sprain, disk degeneration, or herniated nucleus pulposus (usually between the fourth and fifth lumbar vertebrae). Osteoporosis can cause vertebral fractures and back pain. Over time, these injuries can contribute to spinal stenosis, a narrowing of the spinal canal, nerve root canals, or intervertebral foramina.
- Back pain may also be caused by *spondylolysis,* a defect in one of the vertebrae, usually in the lumbar spine. Spondylolisthesis occurs when one vertebra slips forward on the one below it, often as a result of vertebral bony defect.
- Back pain is classified as chronic when it continues for 3 months or if more than two episodes occur annually.
- Risk factors for acute and chronic back pain include:
  1. Trauma (forceful back movement and lifting)
  2. Obesity
  3. Structural and congenital spinal problems, such as scoliosis or spondylolysis
  4. Smoking (causes premature disk degeneration)
  5. Age-related disk disease
  6. Sedentary lifestyle
  7. Prior injury to back

Considerations for Older Adults

- In older adult patients, osteoarthritis and osteoporosis contribute to back pain.
- Cervical pain is also common in patients with rheumatoid arthritis who experience cervical disk subluxation, most often at the C1 to C2 level (first and second cervical vertebrae).
- Physiologic changes associated with aging, such as spinal stenosis, vertebral malalignment, and vascular changes, contribute to back pain in the older adult.

PATIENT-CENTERED COLLABORATIVE CARE

Assessment

- Assess and document:
  1. Pain location, quality, radiation, severity, and alleviating and aggravating factors
  2. Posture and gait

3. Vertebral alignment
4. Muscle spasm
5. Tenderness or swelling of the spinal column
6. Sensory changes: paresthesia and numbness
7. Muscle tone and strength
8. Limitations in movement
9. Psychosocial reaction to illness
10. Vertebral changes seen on an x-ray, CT scan, or MRI
11. Abnormal electromyography and nerve conduction studies
12. Medication and other interventions to treat pain, including OTC drugs and homeopathic treatments

Interventions

Nonsurgical Management

- To treat acute LBP:
  1. Have the patient use the Williams position when in bed (semi-Fowler's bed position with the knees flexed). For patients with a herniated disk, a flat position may aggravate the pain. In a sidelying position, a pillow between the knees may be helpful.
  2. Collaborate with the PT to develop an individualized exercise program.
  3. Drug therapy includes NSAIDs and other drugs to manage acute pain.
  4. Epidural or local steroid injection may be helpful in some cases.
  5. Apply ice and heat therapy.
     a. Apply moist heat in the form of heat packs or hot towels for 20 to 30 minutes four times daily; hot showers or baths also are beneficial for some patients.
     b. Apply ice therapy using ice packs or ice massage over the affected area for 10 to 15 minutes every 1 to 2 hours.
     c. Some patients prefer alternating ice and heat therapy.
     d. Deep heat therapy such as ultrasound treatments and diathermy may be administered by the PT.
- Approaches for treating chronic back pain
  1. Collaborate with the dietitian to implement a weight loss program if appropriate.
  2. Facilitate evaluation and use of a custom-fitted lumbosacral brace.
  3. Collaborate with the OT for ergonomic and adaptive furniture and aids.
  4. Administer drugs such as gabapentin (Neurontin) to relieve neuropathic pain.
  5. Local electrical stimulation may provide significant pain relief.

6. Adjunctive therapy, such as spinal manipulative therapy, distraction, imagery, and music therapy, can reduce maladaptive responses to chronic pain.

Surgical Management

- Conventional open operative procedures include:
  1. *Diskectomy,* in which a portion of the disk is removed
  2. *Laminectomy,* which is the removal of one or more vertebral laminae, plus osteophytes, and the herniated nucleus pulposus through a 3 inch (7.5 cm) incision
  3. *Spinal fusion,* which stabilizes the spine if repeated laminectomies are performed
  4. *Disk prosthesis,* involving insertion of an artificial compound or a hard plastic prosthesis that replaces the patient's natural disk and is shaped to allow full spinal movement
- Minimally invasive operative procedures include *microscopic* (or *surgical*) *endoscopic diskectomy* (MED) and *percutaneous endoscopic diskectomy* (PED), a procedure that may be used with *laser thermodiskectomy* to shrink the herniated disk before removal.
- Provide preoperative care as described in Part One and:
  1. Explain to the patient that various sensations may be experienced in the affected leg or both legs (for lumbar surgery) because of manipulation of nerves and muscles during surgery.
  2. Address the need for a postoperative brace and bone grafting if the patient is having a spinal fusion.
- Provide routine postoperative care as described in Part One and:
  1. Perform neurologic assessment with vital signs every 4 hours during the first 24 hours.
  2. Check the patient's ability to void. An inability to void may indicate damage to sacral spinal nerves. Opioid analgesics have been associated with difficulty voiding and constipation.
  3. Log roll the patient if bedrest is prescribed immediately after surgery.
  4. Ensure that a brace or other type of thoracolumbar support is worn when the patient is out of bed (for spinal fusion).

Community-Based Care

- Health teaching includes:
  1. The prescribed exercise program, including daily walking in collaboration with physical therapy
  2. Restrictions on climbing stairs, lifting, bending, and activities such as driving
  3. Drug information, using best practices to ensure drug reconciliation and avoid drug-drug interactions
  4. A weight-reduction diet, if needed
  5. The importance of smoking cessation
  6. For unresolved pain, referral to a pain specialist or clinic

> **! NURSING SAFETY PRIORITY: Critical Rescue**
>
> For the patient after back surgery, inspect the surgical dressing for blood or any other type of drainage. Clear drainage may mean CSF leakage. The loss of a large amount of CSF may cause the patient to report having a sudden headache. Report signs of any drainage on the dressing to the surgeon immediately. Bulging at the incision site may be due to a CSF leak or a hematoma, both of which should also be reported to the surgeon.

PAIN, CERVICAL SPINE

OVERVIEW

- Cervical spine or neck pain is usually related to herniation of the nucleus pulposus in an intervertebral disk (ruptured disk) between the fifth and sixth vertebrae or to nerve compression caused by osteophyte formation.
- Pain also may result from muscle strain or ligament sprain, repetitive motion, poor posture, or history of trauma.

PATIENT-CENTERED COLLABORATIVE CARE

Assessment

- Assess for:
  1. Pain, numbness, and tingling that radiates to the scapula and down the arm
  2. Sleep disturbances caused by pain
  3. Headache
  4. Vertebral changes seen on CT scan or MRI

Interventions

Nonsurgical Management

- Nonsurgical management of cervical spine pain is the same as for back pain, except that the exercises focus on the neck and shoulder.
- A cervical collar may be prescribed for the patient for no more than 10 days; prolonged use can lead to increased pain and decreased muscle strength and ROM.

Surgical Management

- Depending on the causative factors, an anterior or a posterior approach may be used.
- Provide routine preoperative and postoperative care as described in Part One.
  1. Anticipate that the patient will wear some type of cervical collar for several weeks.
  2. Monitor for complications.
     a. Hoarseness resulting from laryngeal injury
     b. Dysphagia

  c. Esophageal, tracheal, or vertebral artery injury
  d. Graft extrusion and screw loosening if a fusion was performed

PANCREATITIS, ACUTE
OVERVIEW
- Acute pancreatitis is a serious and, at times, life-threatening inflammation caused by premature activation of pancreatic enzymes that destroy ductal tissue and pancreatic cells and results in autodigestion and fibrosis of the pancreas.
- The extent of the inflammation and tissue destruction ranges from mild involvement, characterized by edema and inflammation, to severe, necrotizing hemorrhagic damage leading to diffusely bleeding pancreatic tissue with fibrosis and tissue death.
- The hallmark is fat necrosis of the pancreatic cells by lipase. Many factors can cause injury to the pancreas, including:
  1. Biliary tract disease and gallstones or pancreatic obstruction
  2. Excessive alcohol ingestion or chronic alcoholism
  3. Surgical manipulation after biliary tract, pancreatic, gastric, and duodenal procedures
  4. Blunt or penetrating trauma
  5. Metabolic disturbances: hyperlipidemia, hyperparathyroidism, hypercalcemia
  6. Kidney failure or kidney transplant
  7. Drug toxicities, including opiates, sulfonamides, thiazides, steroids, and oral contraceptives
- Complications include transient hyperglycemia, hypocalcemia, jaundice, pleural effusion, acute respiratory distress syndrome (ARDS), multisystem organ dysfunction, shock, and coagulation defects.

PATIENT-CENTERED COLLABORATIVE CARE
Assessment
- Obtain patient information about:
  1. History of abdominal pain, especially if related to alcohol ingestion or high intake of fat
  2. Individual and family history of alcoholism, pancreatitis, or biliary tract disease
  3. Previous abdominal surgeries or diagnostic procedures
  4. Medical history, including kidney disease, abdominal surgery or procedures, biliary tract diseases, trauma, hyperparathyroidism, and hyperlipidemia
  5. Recent viral infection
  6. Use of prescription and OTC drugs
- Assess for and document:
  1. Abdominal pain (the most frequent symptom), particularly sudden-onset pain in a midepigastric or left upper quadrant

location with radiation to the back, aggravated by a fatty meal, ingestion of a large amount of alcohol, or lying in the recumbent position
2. Weight loss, with nausea and vomiting
3. Jaundice
4. Gray-blue discoloration of the abdomen and periumbilical area (Cullen's sign)
5. Gray-blue discoloration of the flanks (Turner's sign)
6. Absent or decreased bowel sounds
7. Abdominal tenderness, rigidity, and guarding
8. Dull sound on abdominal percussion, indicating ascites
9. Elevated temperature with tachycardia and decreased blood pressure
10. Adventitious breath sounds, dyspnea, or orthopnea
11. Elevated serum amylase and lipase levels

! NURSING SAFETY PRIORITY: Critical Rescue

Monitor for significant changes in vital signs that may indicate shock, which can be a life-threatening complication. Hypotension and tachycardia may result from pancreatic hemorrhage, excessive fluid volume shifting, or the toxic effects of abdominal sepsis. Observe the patient for changes in behavior and mental status that may be related to alcohol withdrawal, hypoxia, or impending sepsis with shock.

- Diagnostic studies may include:
  1. Serum lipase, amylase, alkaline phosphatase, alanine aminotransferase (ALT), bilirubin, WBC, hemoglobin, hematocrit, coagulation factors, basic metabolic panel (electrolytes and kidney function), calcium, magnesium, triglycerides, and albumin
  2. Imaging of the pancreas and gallbladder with ultrasound or CT scan

Planning and Implementation

- The priority for patient care is supportive care by relieving pain and other symptoms, decreasing inflammation, and anticipating or treating complications. As for any patient, continually assess for and support the ABCs (airway, breathing, and circulation).

Acute Pain

Nonsurgical Management

- Decrease pain with interventions that reduce GI activity (decrease pancreatic synthesis of enzymes).
  1. Initiate NPO status for 24 to 48 hours.
     a. Decrease gastric acid during fasting with administration of a proton pump inhibitor or H_2 (histamine-2) blocker.
  2. Consider nasogastric drainage and suction.

- Manage pain with nonopioid and opioid analgesics.
  1. Comfort measures include helping the patient assume a side-lying position to decrease abdominal pain and providing antinausea drugs and antiemetics as needed.
- Promote nutrition and evaluate diet therapy.
  1. Withhold food and fluids in the acute period; maintain hydration with IV fluids.
  2. Maintain nasogastric intubation to decrease gastric distention and suppress pancreatic secretion.
  3. Provide jejunal enteral or parenteral nutrition early, within 72 hours of admission to the hospital for treatment of pancreatitis.
  4. When food is tolerated, provide small-volume, high-carbohydrate, and high-protein feedings with limited fats.
- Administer antibiotics for patients with acute necrotizing pancreatitis.
- Patients with complications such as pancreatic pseudocyst or abscess may require surgical drainage; a procedure to remove gallstones may be needed.

Community-Based Care
- Patient and family health teaching is aimed at preventing both future episodes and disease progression to chronic pancreatitis.
  1. Encourage alcohol abstinence to prevent pain and extension of the inflammatory damage.
  2. Teach the patient to notify the physician if he or she is experiencing acute abdominal pain or symptoms of biliary tract disease such as jaundice, clay-colored stools, and dark urine.
  3. Emphasize the importance of follow-up visits with the health care provider.
  4. Refer the patient with an alcohol abuse problem to support groups such as Alcoholics Anonymous.
  5. Refer the patient to home health nursing as needed.

PANCREATITIS, CHRONIC

OVERVIEW
- Chronic pancreatitis is a progressive, destructive disease with remissions and exacerbations.
- Inflammation and fibrosis of pancreatic tissue contribute to pancreatic insufficiency and the onset of diabetes.
  1. Pancreatic insufficiency is characterized by the loss of exocrine function resulting in a decreased output of enzymes and bicarbonate and altered digestion.
  2. Diabetes results from loss of endocrine function.

PATIENT-CENTERED COLLABORATIVE CARE

Assessment

- Assess for and document:
    1. Abdominal pain (major clinical manifestation): continuous, burning, or gnawing dullness with intense and relentless exacerbations
    2. Left upper quadrant mass, indicating a pseudocyst or abscess
    3. Dullness on abdominal percussion, indicating pancreatic ascites
    4. Steatorrhea, foul-smelling stools that may increase in volume as pancreatic insufficiency progresses
    5. Family history of pancreatic disorders
    6. Weight changes
    7. Jaundice and dark urine
    8. Signs and symptoms of diabetes mellitus
    9. Elevated serum amylase, bilirubin, and alkaline phosphatase levels
    10. Identification of calcification of pancreatic tissue in biopsy specimen
    11. Fatigue and muscle wasting

Interventions

Nonsurgical Management

- Drug therapy includes:
    1. Opioid analgesia (the patient may become dependent on opioids with long-term use)
    2. Non-opioid analgesics
    3. Pancreatic-enzyme replacement therapy (PERT) is the standard of care to prevent malnutrition, malabsorption, and excessive weight loss

> **! NURSING SAFETY PRIORITY: Drug Alert**
>
> Teach the patient to take these drugs with meals and snacks and a glass of water. If needed, open the capsules and spread their contents over applesauce, mashed fruit, or rice cereal. Enzyme preparations should not be mixed with foods containing proteins, because the enzymatic action dissolves the food into a watery substance. Be sure that patients drink a full glass of water after taking the drug to ensure that none of the enzymes remain in the mouth. Advise the patient to wipe his or her lips with a wet towel to prevent the skin irritation and breakdown that residual enzymes can cause.

    4. Insulin to control diabetes
    5. H₂-blocker or proton pump inhibitor to decrease gastric acid
- Record daily weight and the number and consistency of stools per day to monitor the effectiveness of drug therapy.

- Diet therapy includes:
  1. Fasting to avoid recurrent pain exacerbated by eating
  2. Providing jejunal or total parenteral nutrition (TPN)
  3. Consult with the dietician to provide sufficient calories and protein to maintain health
- Surgical management of both complications from and precursors to pancreatitis include:
  1. Incision and drainage for abscess or pseudocyst
  2. Laparoscopic cholecystectomy or endoscopic procedures for biliary tract disease
  3. Sphincterotomy (incision of the sphincter) for fibrosis
  4. Pancreatojejunostomy (the pancreatic duct is opened and anastomosed to the jejunum, relieving obstruction) to relieve pain and preserve pancreatic tissue and function
  5. Partial pancreatectomy, which may be performed for advanced pancreatitis or disabling pain
  6. Vagotomy with gastric antrectomy to alter nerve stimulation and decrease pancreatic secretion

Community-Based Care
- Health teaching is aimed at preventing further exacerbations.
  1. Avoid known precipitating factors, such as alcohol and foods with a high-fat content.
  2. Comply with diet instructions: high protein, high carbohydrate, and a low or no fat.
  3. Follow written instructions and prescriptions for pancreatic enzyme therapy regarding:
     a. How and when to take enzymes
     b. The importance of maintaining therapy
     c. The importance of notifying the physician of increased steatorrhea, abdominal distention, cramping, and skin breakdown
  4. Comply with elevated glucose management, including oral hypoglycemic drugs or insulin injections and monitoring of blood glucose levels.
  5. Keep follow-up visits with the physicians.
- Refer the patient to case management, financial counseling, social services, vocational rehabilitation, home health services, and Alcoholics Anonymous, as needed.

PARALYSIS, FACIAL

- Facial paralysis, or Bell's palsy, is an acute paralysis of cranial nerve VII, with maximal paralysis reached within 2 to 5 days of onset.
- The disorder is characterized by an inability to close the eye, wrinkle the forehead, smile, whistle, or grimace; the face appears masklike and sags.

- This syndrome is thought to be caused by inflammation from herpes simplex virus-1 (HSV-1).
- Treatment includes:
  1. Administering antiviral agents early in the syndrome
  2. Administering mild analgesics for pain
  3. Protecting the eye from corneal abrasion or ulceration by patching and administering artificial tears
  4. Teaching the patient to use warm, moist heat, massage, and facial exercises such as whistling, grimacing, and blowing air out of the cheeks three or four times a day

PARKINSON DISEASE

OVERVIEW

- Parkinson disease is a common, debilitating neurologic disorder involving the basal ganglia and substantia nigra. Loss of dopamine in the affected CNS structures results in difficulty with initiation and coordination of voluntary movement. Loss of other neurotransmitters can contribute to mood disorders and autonomic dysfunction.
- The disease is characterized by muscle rigidity, akinesia (slow movements), postural instability, and tremors.
- The disease involves five stages.
  1. *Stage 1:* Mild disease with unilateral limb involvement
  2. *Stage 2:* Bilateral limb involvement
  3. *Stage 3:* Significant gait disturbances and moderate generalized disability
  4. *Stage 4:* Severe disability, akinesia, and muscle rigidity
  5. *Stage 5:* Complete dependency in all aspects of ADLs

PATIENT-CENTERED COLLABORATIVE CARE

Assessment

- Obtain patient information about:
  1. Time and the progression of symptoms such as resting tremors, bradykinesia, and difficulty in completing fine motor tasks such as handwriting
  2. Family history related to neurologic disorders
  3. History of head injury, which can damage CNS structures
  4. Use of drugs to treat serious mental illness; some antipsychotic medications can have Parkinson-like adverse effects
- Assess for and document:
  1. Rigidity, which is present early in the disease process and progresses over time
     a. Cogwheel rigidity, manifested by a rhythmic interruption of the muscles of movement

     b. Plastic rigidity, or mildly restrictive movements

     c. Lead-pipe rigidity, which is total resistance to movement

2. Posture
   a. Stooped posture
   b. Flexed trunk
   c. Fingers adducted and flexed at the metacarpophalangeal joint
   d. Wrists slightly dorsiflexed

3. Gait
   a. Slow and shuffling
   b. Short, hesitant steps
   c. Propulsive gait
   d. Difficulty stopping quickly

4. Speech
   a. Soft, low-pitched voice
   b. Dysarthria
   c. Echolalia, or automatic repetition of what another person says
   d. Repetition of sentences
   e. Change in voice volume, phonation, or articulation

5. Motor dysfunction
   a. Bradykinesia or difficulty completing two tasks simultaneously
   b. Akinesia
   c. Tremors, especially at rest
   d. "Pill-rolling" movement
   e. Masklike face
   f. Difficulty chewing and swallowing
   g. Uncontrolled drooling, especially at night
   h. Difficulty getting into and out of bed
   i. Little arm swinging when walking
   j. Change in handwriting, micrographia

6. Autonomic dysfunction
   a. Orthostatic hypotension
   b. Excessive perspiration and oily skin
   c. Flushing, changes in skin texture
   d. Blepharospasm

7. Psychosocial effects
   a. Emotional lability
   b. Depression
   c. Paranoia
   d. Easily upset
   e. Rapid mood swings
   f. Cognitive impairments

    g. Delayed reaction time
    h. Sleep disturbances

Interventions

- Provide drug therapy.
  1. Administer drug therapy on time to maintain continuous therapeutic drug levels.
     a. Levodopa combinations
     b. Dopamine agonists
     c. Catechol O-methyltransferase (COMT) inhibitors to interfere with the breakdown of dopamine in the CNS
     d. Anticholinergic drugs, if the patient's primary symptom is tremor
     e. Monoamine oxidase inhibitors
     f. Variety of investigational drugs
  2. Monitor the patient for drug toxicity and side effects such as delirium, cognitive impairment, decreased effectiveness of the drug, postural hypotension, and hallucination.
  3. Treatment of drug toxicity or intolerance includes:
     a. Reduction in drug dosage
     b. Change in drugs or in the frequency of administration
     c. Drug holiday (particularly with levodopa therapy) for up to 10 days with close surveillance
- Other interventions include:
  1. PT and OT consultations to plan and maintain a mobility and muscle-stretching program (e.g., traditional exercise, yoga, tai chi) and exercises for the muscles of the face and tongue to facilitate swallowing and speech
  2. Providing assistive devices for participation in ADLs; PT and OT consultation to provide training in ADLs and the use of adaptive devices
  3. Teaching the patient and family to monitor the patient's sleeping pattern and to discuss whether it is safe for the patient to operate machinery or perform other potentially dangerous tasks
  4. Monitoring the patient's ability to eat and swallow; monitoring food and fluid intake; collaborating with the registered dietitian for caloric calculation and diet planning
  5. Assessing the need for a speech-language pathologist consultation for evaluation of swallowing dysfunction and communication problems
  6. Teaching the patient to speak slowly and clearly; using alternative communication methods such as a communication board
  7. Referring the patient and family to a social worker to help with financial and health insurance agencies and to state and social agencies and support groups

8. Instructing the patient with orthostatic hypotension to wear elastic stockings and to change position slowly, especially when moving from a sitting to a standing position
9. Allowing sufficient time for the patient to complete activities; scheduling appointments and activities for late in the morning to prevent rushing the patient, or scheduling them at the time of the patient's optimal level of functioning
10. Implementing interventions to prevent complications of immobility such as constipation, pressure ulcers, contractures, and atelectasis

- Surgical interventions may be used to treat severe or early onset of Parkinson disease.
  1. Stereotactic pallidotomy can be a very effective treatment for Parkinson disease. The target area in the brain receives a mild electrical stimulation through a probe to decrease tremor and rigidity. The probe is placed in the ideal location, and a temporary lesion is made. If this is successful, a permanent lesion is made.
  2. Unilateral thalamotomy treats the tremor through thermocoagulation of brain cells.
  3. Deep brain stimulation involves placing a thin electrode in the thalamus or subthalamus and connecting it to a "pacemaker" that delivers electrical current to interfere with "tremor cells." The electrodes are connected to an implantable pulse generator that is placed underneath the skin in the patient's chest, something like a cardiac pacemaker.

PELVIC INFLAMMATORY DISEASE

OVERVIEW

- Pelvic inflammatory disease (PID) is a complex infectious process in which organisms from the lower genital tract migrate from the endocervix upward through the uterine cavity into the fallopian tubes.
- It is a major cause of infertility and ectopic pregnancies.
- It is most often caused by sexually transmitted organisms, especially *Chlamydia trachomatis* and *Neisseria gonorrhoeae.* Other organisms may include *Gardnerella vaginalis, Haemophilus influenzae, Staphylococcus, Streptococcus,* and *Escherichia coli.*
- The infection may spread to other organs and tissues. Resultant infections include:
  1. Endometritis (infection of the endometrial cavity)
  2. Salpingitis (inflammation of the fallopian tubes)
  3. Oophoritis (ovarian infection)
  4. Parametritis (infection of the parametrium)
  5. Peritonitis (infection of the peritoneal cavity)
  6. Tubal or tubo-ovarian abscess

- Sepsis and death can occur, especially if treatment is delayed or inadequate.
- Although common manifestations include tenderness in the tubes and ovaries (adnexa) and low, dull abdominal pain, some patients have only mild discomfort or menstrual irregularity, and others experience no symptoms at all. These variations can make the diagnosis of PID challenging.
- PID increases the risk of ectopic pregnancies and infertility.

PATIENT-CENTERED COLLABORATIVE CARE
Assessment
- Obtain patient information about:
  1. Menstrual history
  2. Obstetric and sexual history, including whether unprotected sex or sexual abuse occurred
  3. Results of cultures or serum analysis congruent with infection or infecting organism
  4. Results of pelvic examination, particularly the presence of purulent cervical discharge or friable cervical tissue
  5. Previous reproductive surgery
  6. Abnormal vaginal bleeding
  7. Dysuria (painful urination)
  8. Increase or change in vaginal discharge
  9. Dyspareunia (painful sexual intercourse)
  10. Risk factors, including:
      a. Age younger than 26 years
      b. Multiple sexual partners
      c. Intrauterine device (IUD) in place within the previous 3 weeks
      d. Smoking
      e. Previous episodes of sexually transmitted diseases or PID
- Assess for and document:
  1. Pain, especially lower abdominal pain
  2. Fever, chills, generalized aches
  3. Hunched-over gait
  4. Abdominal tenderness, rigidity, or rebound tenderness
- Assess for psychosocial issues, such as:
  1. Anxiety and fear
  2. Need for reassurance and support during the physical examination
  3. Embarrassment
  4. Discomfort when discussing symptoms or sexual history
- Diagnosis is made based on history, physical symptoms and signs, cervical or vaginal mucopurulent discharge, presence of WBCs on saline microscopy of vaginal secretions, and positive culture (e.g.,

laboratory documentation of cervical infection with *N. gonor-rhoeae* or *Chlamydia*). Other tests that may be helpful include ultrasonography, MRI, and endometrial biopsy.

Planning and Implementation

INFECTION

- Uncomplicated PID is usually treated on an ambulatory care basis.
- Hospitalization for PID is recommended if the patient has a complicated history, does not respond to oral antibiotic therapy, or has severe illness.
- Drug therapy includes oral and/or parenteral antibiotics for 14 days.
- Teach the patient about the need to:
  1. Abstain from sexual intercourse during treatment
  2. Check her temperature twice a day
  3. Be seen by the health care provider within 72 hours after starting the antibiotics and then at 1 and 2 weeks from the time of the initial diagnosis
- In a small number of patients, a laparotomy may be needed to remove a pelvic abscess.

PERICARDITIS

OVERVIEW

- Pericarditis is an inflammation or alteration of the pericardium, the membranous sac enclosing the heart. Alterations include fibrotic, serous, hemorrhagic, purulent, and neoplastic changes to the sac or fluid in the pericardial space.
- There are two types of pericarditis.
  1. *Acute pericarditis* is most commonly associated with infective organisms (bacteria, viruses, fungi), malignant neoplasms, post-myocardial infarction syndrome, postpericardiotomy syndrome, systemic connective tissue diseases, kidney failure, and idiopathic causes.
  2. *Chronic constrictive pericarditis* is caused by tuberculosis, radiation therapy, trauma, kidney failure, connective tissue disorders, and metastatic cancer, with the pericardium becoming rigid, preventing adequate ventricular filling and resulting in cardiac failure.

PATIENT-CENTERED COLLABORATIVE CARE

- Obtain patient information about:
  1. History of cardiac disease, cardiac surgery, chest trauma, or recent systemic infections
  2. History of chest radiation, connective tissue diseases, or cancer

- Assess for and document:
  1. Substernal precordial pain that can radiate to the left neck, shoulder, and back and is aggravated by breathing, coughing, and swallowing
  2. Pericardial friction rub
  3. Acute pericarditis
     a. Elevated WBC count
     b. Nonspecific ST-T wave elevation on electrocardiogram (ECG)
     c. Fever (infectious cause)
  4. Chronic constrictive pericarditis
     a. Right-sided heart failure, including dyspnea, exertional fatigue, and orthopnea
     b. Pericardial thickening on echocardiogram and CT scan
     c. Inverted or flat T waves on ECG
     d. Atrial fibrillation
- Treatment depends on the type of pericarditis.
- Acute pericarditis is treated by:
  1. Administering NSAIDs, corticosteroids, and antibiotics
  2. Encouraging rest
- For recurrent tamponade or effusions or adhesions resulting from chronic pericarditis, a partial or complete pericardiectomy is done to allow adequate ventricular filling and contraction.
- Complications of pericarditis include pericardial effusions and cardiac tamponade.
  1. Cardiac tamponade can occur when fluid accumulates in the pericardium. Symptoms of cardiac tamponade are:
     a. Jugular venous distention
     b. Paradoxical pulse: systolic blood pressure at least 10 mm hg higher on expiration than on inspiration
     c. Decreased cardiac output: abnormal heart rate, dyspnea and fatigue
     d. Muffled heart sounds
     e. Hypotension or signs of obstructive shock
  2. Emergent treatment of cardiac tamponade is pericardiocentesis or inserting a needle into the pericardial space to withdraw pericardial fluid. IV fluids are administered to improve cardiac output.

PERIPHERAL ARTERIAL DISEASE

OVERVIEW

- Peripheral arterial disease (PAD) is a result of atherosclerosis, a chronic condition in which partial or total arterial blockage decreases perfusion to the legs.
- The most common symptom is leg pain known as *intermittent claudication*.

- Inflow PAD obstructions involve the distal end of the aorta and the common, internal, and external iliac arteries, manifested by discomfort in the lower back, buttocks, or thighs.
- Acute peripheral vascular disease occurs when there is an acute obstruction by a thrombus or embolus, causing severe, acute pain below the level of the obstruction.

PATIENT-CENTERED COLLABORATIVE CARE
Assessment
- Assessment findings include:
  1. Abnormal ankle-brachial index (ABI): The value can be derived by dividing the ankle blood pressure by the brachial blood pressure. A value of less than 0.9 indicates outflow disease. With inflow disease, pressures taken at the thigh level indicate the severity of disease. Mild inflow disease may cause a difference of only 10 to 30 mm Hg in pressure on the affected side compared with the brachial pressure.
  2. Leg pain (burning, cramping in calves, ankles, feet, and toes with exercise or rest) or discomfort in the lower back, buttocks, or thighs
  3. Ischemic changes of the extremity
     a. Loss of hair on the lower calf, ankle, and foot
     b. Dry, scaly skin
     c. Thickened toenails
     d. Color changes (elevation pallor or dependent rubor)
     e. Mottled and cool or cold extremity
  4. Decreased or absent leg pulses: The most sensitive and specific indicator of arterial function is the quality of the posterior tibial pulse, because the pedal pulse is not palpable in a small percentage of people.
  5. Painful arterial ulcers that develop on the toes, between the toes, or on the upper aspect of the foot; PAD ulcers differ from diabetic and venous ulcers.
     a. Diabetic ulcers develop on the plantar surface of the foot, over metatarsal heads, on the heel, or on pressure areas; they may not be painful.
     b. Venous stasis ulcers occur at the ankles, with discoloration of the lower extremity at the ulcer; they cause minimal pain.
- Diagnostic assessment includes:
  1. Blood pressure and ankle-brachial index measurement
  2. Doppler/ultrasound assessment of blood flow
  3. Exercise tolerance test
  4. Plethysmography

Planning and Implementation

Nonsurgical Management

- Teach the following methods of increasing arterial blood flow in chronic arterial disease:
    1. Exercising to promote collateral circulation
    2. Positioning to promote circulation and decrease swelling
        a. Legs should be elevated at rest but not above the level of the heart.
        b. Avoid crossing legs and wearing restrictive clothing.
    3. Avoiding cold exposure to the affected extremity with warm socks and room temperature modulation
    4. Cautioning the patient not to apply direct heat to the lower limbs, which may cause burns because of decreased sensitivity
    5. Avoiding nicotine, caffeine, and emotional stress
    6. Complying with drug therapy, including antiplatelet therapy
    7. Controlling blood pressure
- Endovascular procedures may be used to restore arterial circulation. Treat the patient with typical preoperative interventions. The procedural approach is one of the following:
    1. Percutaneous transluminal angioplasty (PTA) dilates arteries that are occluded or stenosed with a balloon catheter; a stent or atherectomy may be used to reduce occlusion from atherosclerotic plaque.
    2. Laser-assisted angioplasty may be used to open an occluded artery.
- After angioplasty, care of the patient includes:
    1. Observing the puncture site for bleeding
    2. Closely monitoring vital signs for hypotension and hypertension
    3. Checking the distal pulses and sensation of both limbs
    4. Encouraging the patient to maintain bedrest for 6 to 8 hours, as ordered, with the limb straight
    5. Administering antiplatelet or anticoagulation therapy, which may continue for 3 to 6 months after the procedure

Surgical Management

- An emergency surgical embolectomy is performed on patients who experience an acute peripheral artery occlusion by an embolus.
- Acute arterial insufficiency often presents with the "6 *Ps*" of ischemia.
    1. *P*ain
    2. *P*allor
    3. *P*ulselessness
    4. *P*aresthesia
    5. *P*aralysis
    6. *P*oikilothermia (coolness)

- Arterial revascularization surgery is used to increase arterial blood flow in an affected limb and includes inflow procedures such as aortoiliac bypass, aortofemoral bypass, and axillofemoral bypass and outflow procedures, including femoropopliteal bypass and femorotibial bypass.
- Grafting materials for bypass surgeries include the autogenous saphenous vein and synthetic graft material such as polytetrafluoroethylene.
- Provide postoperative care.
  1. Monitor for the patency of the graft by checking for changes in the extremity.
     a. Color
     b. Temperature
     c. Pulse quality; mark the site of pulses for consistent evaluation
     d. Pain intensity (typical pain is described as throbbing pain, which occurs from increased blood flow to the affected limb)
  2. Monitor the patient's blood pressure, notifying the physician about increases and decreases beyond desired ranges.
  3. Avoid bending the knee and hip of the affected limb for 6 to 8 hours.
  4. Monitor for signs and symptoms of vessel reocclusion at or around the graft and incision sites, such as hardness, tenderness, redness, or coolness or warmth.
- Thrombectomy (removal of the clot) is the most common treatment for acute graft occlusion; thrombolytic therapy may be used.
- Compartment syndrome occurs when tissue pressure within a confined body space becomes elevated and restricts blood flow.
- Use sterile technique when in contact with the incision and observe for symptoms of infection.

! NURSING SAFETY PRIORITY: Critical Rescue

Immediately inform the vascular surgeon if assessment of the operative extremity includes worsening pain, swelling or tenseness, absent pulse, demarcations of color or temperature distal to revascularization, or loss of sensation.

Community-Based Care
- Patient and family education includes:
  1. Teaching the patient to monitor tissue perfusion to the affected extremity
     a. Distal circulation, sensation, and motion
     b. Presence of pain, pallor, paresthesias, pulselessness, paralysis, coolness

2. Reinforcing the need for individualized positioning and an exercise plan
    a. Teaching the patient to avoid raising the legs above the level of the heart unless he or she also has venous stasis
3. Providing written and oral foot care instructions, instructing the patient to:
    a. Keep the feet clean by washing with a mild soap in room-temperature water.
    b. Keep the feet dry, especially between the toes and ankles.
    c. Avoid injury or extended pressure to the feet and ankles.
    d. Wear comfortable, well-fitting shoes and socks; avoid constricting garments.
    e. Keep the toenails clean, and cut the nails straight across and avoid dry, cracked skin
    f. Prevent exposure to extreme heat or cold, including not using heating pads.
4. Providing dressing change and incision care instructions, if necessary
5. Providing instructions concerning discharge medications, particularly to improve safety when using antiplatelet and anticoagulant drugs
6. Encouraging healthy diet choices to reduce atherosclerotic plaque formation and growth

PERIPHERAL VENOUS DISEASE

OVERVIEW

- Peripheral venous disease (PVD) is a condition that alters the natural flow of blood through the veins of the peripheral circulation. Three health problems result in PVD:
    1. Venous blood flow may be altered by thrombus formation and defective valves.
        a. Thrombus formation is associated with bedrest of more than 3 days, pitting edema, endothelial injury, dilated superficial veins, and hypercoagulability from cancer and previous venothromboembolism (VTE).
        b. Phlebitis occurs when inflammation in superficial veins occurs, often in conjunction with thrombus (i.e., thrombophlebitis).
        c. VTE describes both *deep vein thrombosis* (DVT) and *pulmonary embolism* (PE). DVT is more serious than superficial thrombophlebitis because it presents a greater risk for PE. In PE, a dislodged blood clot travels to the pulmonary artery. DVT develops most often in the legs but can occur also in the upper arms as a result of invasive procedures like the placement of central venous catheters.

2. Venous insufficiency results from prolonged venous hypertension and phlebitis, which stretch the veins and damage valves, resulting in swelling, venous stasis ulcers, and cellulitis.
3. Reduced skeletal muscle activity
   a. Skeletal muscles help pump blood in veins.
   b. When weight bearing is limited or muscle tone decreases, PVD can develop.

PATIENT-CENTERED COLLABORATIVE CARE

- For the patient with PVD, assess for:
  1. Lower extremity pain, swelling, and perfusion
  2. Inactivity
  3. Cellulitis, the presence of open wounds, or venous stasis ulcers
- For the patient at risk for or diagnosed with VTE, assess:
  1. Calf or groin tenderness and pain
  2. Unilateral swelling, warmth of the leg
  3. Induration along the occluded vein
  4. Results of ultrasonography or Doppler flow studies identifying the location of thrombosis
  5. Serum markers of inflammation and coagulation

! NURSING SAFETY PRIORITY: Critical Rescue

The Joint Commission's VTE Core Measure Set requires that hospitals report data on six areas related to VTE prophylaxis and management. If VTE is not prevented or adequately managed, the hospital may not be paid by the third party payer (e.g., Medicare) for the patient's care. In the inpatient setting, all patients must be assessed for risk of VTE on admission. For those at moderate to high risk, initiate interventions to prevent VTE, including early progressive mobility and administration of anticoagulants like subcutaneous heparin.

- For recovery from PVD complications of thrombosis, phlebitis syndromes, and venous ulcer formation, interventions include:
  1. Positioning the lower extremities to reduce the risk for injury from venous insufficiency
  2. Informing patients of increased risk for future VTE events, to monitor for symptoms, and to follow up with their health care provider at regular intervals
  3. Having the patient wear compression stockings during the day and evening
  4. Teaching the patient to elevate his or her legs for 20 minutes four or five times a day
  5. Avoiding bedrest or prolonged periods of inactivity such as standing still or sitting

6. Treating open venous ulcers with occlusive dressings and topical agents, with or without antibiotics to chemically débride the ulcer, and using an Unna boot to promote ulcer healing by relieving pressure for ambulatory patients with venous stasis ulcers
7. Adhering to anticoagulation drug regimens for 3 to 6 months after diagnosis of VTE and monitoring serum factors to avoid unintended bleeding

! NURSING SAFETY PRIORITY: Drug Alert

Provide all patients discharged with antiplatelet and anticoagulant drug therapy with instructions that address:
- Drug compliance issues (the need to take drug as prescribed)
- Dietary advice (e.g., foods to avoid)
- Follow-up monitoring (e.g., Coumadin clinic, international normalized ratio [INR] testing)
- Information about the potential for adverse drug reactions/interactions (e.g., bleeding, bruising)

PERITONITIS
OVERVIEW
- Peritonitis is an acute inflammation of the viscera/parietal and endothelial peritoneum (the lining of the abdominal cavity).
- *Primary peritonitis* is a rare acute bacterial infection that develops as a result of contamination of the peritoneum through the vascular system.
- *Secondary peritonitis* is caused by bacterial invasion as a result of perforation or a penetrating wound, such as appendicitis, diverticulitis, peptic ulcer, ascending genital infection, or a gunshot injury to the abdomen. Chemical peritonitis is the result of leakage of bile, pancreatic enzymes, and gastric acid.
- Peritonitis is life threatening and associated with shock, respiratory problems, and paralytic ileus.

PATIENT-CENTERED COLLABORATIVE CARE
Assessment
- Obtain patient information about:
  1. History of abdominal trauma or surgery
  2. Character of abdominal pain, onset, duration, location, quality, aggravating and alleviating factors; the cardinal signs of peritonitis are abdominal pain, tenderness, and distension; often, pain is aggravated by coughing or movement and relieved by knee flexion

3. Abdominal distention and presence/absence of bowel sounds
4. Tachypnea with low peripheral saturation (decreased Spo_2)
5. Low-grade fever or recent spikes in temperature

! NURSING SAFETY PRIORITY: Action Alert

For patients with peritonitis, assess for abdominal wall rigidity, which is a classic finding that is sometimes referred to as a "board-like" abdomen. Monitor the patient for a high fever because of the infectious process. Assess for tachycardia occurring in response to the fever and decreased circulating blood volume. Observe whether he or she has dry mucous membranes and a low urine output seen with edema or third spacing. Nausea and vomiting may also be present. Hiccups may occur as a result of diaphragmatic irritation. Be sure to document all assessment findings

- Diagnostic tests may include:
  1. CBC; anticipate an elevated WBC count and neutrophilia
  2. Serum electrolytes, BUN, and creatinine
  3. Abdominal x-rays or CT scans to determine the presence of dilation, edema, and inflammation of the intestines

! NURSING SAFETY PRIORITY: Critical Rescue

A sudden worsening of abdominal pain or a change from localized to generalized abdominal pain may signal perforation or new-onset peritonitis from an abdominal condition. This symptom is a medical emergency and needs to be communicated, along with vital signs, to the health care provider immediately to avoid patient progression to vascular and respiratory compromise.

Interventions
Nonsurgical Management
- Monitor vital signs and peripheral oxygenation (Spo_2) with level of consciousness and report concerning findings (systolic blood pressure [SBP] less than 90 mm Hg, heart rate [HR] greater than 110, respiratory rate [RR] greater than 20, Spo_2 less than 92% on supplemental oxygen or decreased cognition) to the provider urgently.
- Administer IV fluids and antibiotics.
- Record intake and output and daily weight.
- Monitor and record drainage from the NGT used for gastric and intestinal decompression.
- Provide and evaluate pain management with analgesics.
- Administer oxygen to maintain Spo_2 greater than 92%.

Surgical Management
- Surgical management may be necessary to identify and repair the underlying cause of the peritonitis.
- Surgery is focused on controlling the contamination, removing foreign material from the peritoneal cavity, and draining fluid collections.
- During surgery, the peritoneum is irrigated with antibiotic solution, and drainage catheters are inserted.
- Provide routine postoperative care as described in Part One, including:
    1. Close monitoring of the patient's cardiovascular stability for early detection of shock (level of consciousness, HR, SBP, SpO$_2$, and urine output should remain within normal limits for the patient)
    2. Providing meticulous wound care; irrigating and packing the wound, as prescribed
    3. Assisting the patient in gradually increasing his or her activity level

Considerations for Older Adults

The early signs and symptoms of shock, infection, or dehydration in the older adult may consist of a subtle decrease in mental status, such as confusion or lethargy. Do not delay in communicating subtle changes in consciousness or cognition to the health care provider.

Community-Based Care
- The patient may be discharged home or to a transitional care unit to complete antibiotic therapy and recovery.
- If the patient is discharged home, collaborate with the case manager to determine the need for assistance.
- Provide written and oral postoperative instructions, including:
    1. The necessity to report any redness, swelling, tenderness, or unusual or foul-smelling drainage from the wound
    2. Care of the incision and dressing; ensuring that the patient has the necessary equipment to perform wound care (dressings, solutions, catheter-tipped syringe); and stressing the importance of handwashing
    3. The need to report fever (typically 101° F [38° C]) or abdominal pain to the physician
    4. Administration and monitoring of drugs for pain

PHEOCHROMOCYTOMA

OVERVIEW
- Pheochromocytoma is a catecholamine-producing tumor that arises in the adrenal medulla.

- These tumors are most often benign, but at least 10% are malignant.
- Pheochromocytomas produce, store, and release epinephrine and norepinephrine; these hormones stimulate adrenergic receptors and can have wide-ranging adverse effects mimicking the action of the sympathetic division of the autonomic nervous system.

PATIENT-CENTERED COLLABORATIVE CARE

Assessment

- Obtain patient information about intermittent manifestations, including:
  1. Severe headaches
  2. Palpitations
  3. Heat intolerance, flushing, profuse diaphoresis
  4. Apprehension or a sense of impending doom
  5. Pain in the chest or abdomen, with nausea and vomiting
- Assess for and document:
  1. Hypertension
  2. Tremors
  3. Weight loss

! NURSING SAFETY PRIORITY: Action Alert

Do not palpate the abdomen, because this action could cause a sudden release of catecholamines and severe hypertension.

- Diagnosis is made based on high urine levels of metanephrine and catecholamines.
- A clonidine suppression test can be used when catecholamine levels are not diagnostic.
- MRI or CT scans can precisely locate tumors.

Interventions

- Surgery is performed to remove the tumors and the adrenal gland or glands.
- Provide preoperative care as described in Part One.
  1. Monitor blood pressure regularly; place the cuff consistently on the same arm, with the patient in lying and standing positions.
  2. Avoid heat and other stressors that may lead to a hypertensive crisis.
  3. Teach the patient not to smoke, drink caffeine-containing beverages, or change position suddenly postoperatively.
  4. Ensure adequate hydration.
  5. Administer prescribed drug therapy (phenoxybenzamine [Dibenzyline]) to stabilize the patient's blood pressure (usually started days before surgery).

- Provide postoperative care as described in Part One and:
  1. Closely monitor for hypertension, hypotension, and hypovolemia.
  2. Monitor for adequate tissue perfusion.
     a. Vital signs with level of consciousness
     b. Fluid intake and output
  3. Check opioid effects on blood pressure.
- If inoperable, tumors are managed with alpha- and beta-adrenergic blocking agents and self-measurement of blood pressure with home monitoring equipment.

PHLEBITIS

- Phlebitis is an inflammation of the superficial veins caused by an irritant, commonly IV therapy.
- Phlebitis is manifested as pain with a reddened, warm, swollen area radiating up an extremity.
- Treatment involves application of warm, moist soaks, which dilate the vein and promote circulation. *Do not massage the area.*

PNEUMONIA

OVERVIEW

- Pneumonia is an excess of fluid in the lungs resulting from an inflammatory process.
- It can be caused by many infectious organisms and by inhalation of irritating agents or aspiration of stomach contents.
- Infectious pneumonias are categorized as *community-acquired pneumonia* (CAP) or *hospital-acquired pneumonia* (HAP), *health care–acquired pneumonia* (HCAP), and *ventilator-associated pneumonia* (VAP).
- Inflammation and infection in the lungs result in local capillary leak, edema, and exudate that reduce gas exchange and lead to hypoxemia, interfering with oxygenation and tissue perfusion and possibly leading to death.
- Risk factors for pneumonia include:
  1. Being an older adult
  2. The presence of a chronic health problem, particularly a respiratory problem or condition that is associated with immunosuppression
  3. Recent exposure to respiratory viral or influenza infections

PATIENT-CENTERED COLLABORATIVE CARE

Assessment

- Obtain patient information about:
  1. Age
  2. Living, work, and school environments, including exposure to droplet-based infection

3. Diet, exercise, and sleep routines
4. Swallowing problems or presence of oral or NG tubes that may result in aspiration
5. Tobacco and alcohol use
6. Past and current use of drugs, including drug addiction or injection drug use
7. Acute or chronic respiratory problems
8. Recent skin rashes, insect bites, or exposure to animals
9. Home respiratory equipment use and cleaning
10. Date of last influenza or pneumococcal vaccine

- Assess for and document:
  1. General appearance
  2. Oxygen saturation
  3. Abnormal lung sounds, particularly crackles, rhonchi, and wheezing
  4. Increased effort of breathing, especially dyspnea, tachypnea, and use of accessory muscles
  5. Chest or pleuritic pain or discomfort
  6. Fever, chills, and fatigue
  7. Cough and mucus or sputum production
  8. Tachycardia, hypotension
  9. Mental status changes (especially in an older adult)

Considerations for Older Adults

- The most common manifestation of pneumonia in the older adult patient is confusion from hypoxia rather than fever or cough.
- Diagnosis is based on manifestations, sputum Gram stain or culture, elevated WBC count, chest x-ray, peripheral oxygenation (SpO$_2$), and arterial blood gas (ABG) levels.

Planning and Implementation

- Priority nursing problems are:
  1. Hypoxemia related to decreased diffusion at the alveolar-capillary membrane and potential for airway obstruction related to excessive tracheobronchial secretions, fatigue, chest discomfort, and muscle weakness
     a. Monitor rate, rhythm, depth, and effort of ventilation.
     b. Assess pulse oximetry and administer oxygen by nasal cannula or mask as prescribed.
     c. Instruct the patient on cough and deep-breathing technique or the correct use of incentive spirometry (sustained maximal inspiration) and encourage him or her to perform 5 to 10 breaths per session every hour while awake.

   d. Assess the patient's ability to cough effectively.
   e. Monitor fluid intake and encourage the alert patient to maintain sufficient intake to provide a dilute urine output.
   f. Administer prescribed bronchodilators and corticosteroids by aerosol nebulizer or by metered dose inhaler.
   g. Monitor for complications such as hypoxemia, ventilatory failure, atelectasis, pleural effusion, and pleurisy.
2. Potential for sepsis related to the presence of microorganisms in a very vascular area
   a. Administer prescribed anti-infective therapy based on organism sensitivity.
   b. For pneumonia resulting from aspiration of food or stomach contents, steroids and NSAIDs are used with antibiotics to reduce the inflammatory response.

Community-Based Care
*   Teach the patient about:
    1. The importance of completing the full course of antibiotic therapy
    2. Notifying the health care provider if chills, fever, persistent cough, dyspnea, wheezing, hemoptysis, increased sputum production, chest discomfort, or increasing fatigue recurs or if symptoms fail to resolve
    3. The importance of getting plenty of rest and gradually increasing exercise
    4. Preventing upper respiratory tract infections and viruses by:
        a. Using handwashing
        b. Avoiding crowds and people who have a cold or flu
        c. Avoiding exposure to irritants such as smoke
        d. Obtaining an annual influenza vaccination
        e. Obtaining the pneumococcal vaccination
*   Encourage the patient to quit smoking, and provide information on smoking cessation.

QSEN EVIDENCE-BASED PRACTICE

Three care actions, known as a *ventilator bundle*, have been shown to reduce the incidence of VAP: hand hygiene, oral care to decontaminate the mouth, and elevation of the head of the bed.

*   Implement these practices for the intubated patient to reduce VAP:
    1. Wash hands before and after contact with the patient.
    2. If possible, use a disinfecting oral rinse immediately before the intubation.
    3. Provide oral care with a disinfecting mouthwash every 12 hours.

4. Remove subglottic secretions; this can be done continuously if the endotracheal tube has a separate lumen that opens directly above the tube cuff.
5. Keep the head of the bed elevated 30 to 45 degrees.
6. Use best practices to promote weaning from the mechanical ventilator as soon as feasible.

PNEUMOTHORAX

- Pneumothorax, also called a *collapsed lung,* is an accumulation of air in the pleural space. The lung collapses with the subsequent rise in chest pressure; there is a concurrent reduction in vital capacity.
- Any injury that allows air to enter the pleural space, including blunt chest trauma, can cause a pneumothorax. Injury may also cause some degree of hemothorax. Pneumothorax also may occur spontaneously.
- Assess for and document:
  1. Reduced breath sounds on auscultation
  2. Hyperresonance on percussion
  3. Prominence of the involved side of the chest, which moves poorly with respirations
  4. Deviation of the trachea away from (closed) or toward (open) the affected side
  5. Pleuritic chest pain
  6. Tachypnea
  7. Subcutaneous emphysema (air under the skin in the subcutaneous tissues)
- An ultrasound examination or a chest x-ray is used for diagnosis.
- Chest tubes may be needed to allow the air to escape and the lung to reinflate.

PNEUMOTHORAX, TENSION

- Tension pneumothorax is a rapidly developing and life-threatening complication of large amounts of air entering the pleural space from an air leak in the lung or chest wall.
- Air that enters the pleural space during inspiration does not exit during expiration, allowing air to continue to collect under pressure, collapsing the lung, compressing blood vessels, limiting venous return, and reducing cardiac output.
- Causes include blunt chest trauma, mechanical ventilation with positive end-expiratory pressure (PEEP), closed-chest drainage (chest tubes), burst alveoli blebs, and insertion of central venous access catheters.

> **! NURSING SAFETY PRIORITY: Critical Rescue**
>
> If not promptly detected and treated, tension pneumothorax is quickly fatal.

- Assess for and document:
  1. Asymmetry of the thorax
  2. Tracheal movement away from midline to the unaffected side
  3. Respiratory distress
  4. Absence of breath sounds on one side
  5. Distended neck veins
  6. Cyanosis
  7. Hypertympanic sound on percussion over the affected side
- Initial management includes insertion of a large-bore needle into the second intercostal space in the midclavicular line of the affected side.
- Chest tube placement into the fourth intercostal space then follows, with water seal drainage until the lung reinflates.

POLYNEUROPATHY

OVERVIEW

- The terms *polyneuritis*, *polyneuropathy*, and *peripheral neuropathy* may be used interchangeably.
- The disorders are characterized by muscle weakness with or without atrophy; pain that is described as stabbing, cutting, or searing; paresthesia or loss of sensation; impaired reflexes; autonomic manifestations; or a combination of these symptoms.
- The most common type is a symmetric polyneuropathy in which the patient experiences decreased sensation along with a feeling that the extremity is asleep. Tingling, burning, tightness, or aching sensations usually start in the feet and progress to the level of the knee before affecting the hands ("glove and stocking" neuropathy).
- The disorders can result from inflammatory or noninflammatory processes; both can damage cranial and peripheral nerves.
- Factors associated with polyneuropathy include diabetes; kidney or hepatic failure; alcoholism; vascular disease; vitamin B_1, B_6, and B_{12} deficiencies; and exposure to heavy metals or industrial solvents.

PATIENT-CENTERED COLLABORATIVE CARE

- Assess for and document:
  1. Light touch sensation and pain in the distal extremities
  2. Position sense and kinesthetic sensation
  3. Any signs of injury

    4. Indications of autonomic dysfunction, such as orthostatic hypotension, abnormal sweating, and miosis
- Treatment consists of elimination or treatment of the underlying cause and symptomatic therapy.
  1. Treat the underlying cause.
  2. Supplement the patient's diet with vitamins.
  3. Provide pain management as needed.
  4. Provide health teaching, including the importance of foot care and of inspecting the extremities for injuries.
  5. Stress the importance of wearing shoes at all times and of purchasing well-fitting shoes.
  6. Teach the patient how to recognize potential hazards, such as exposure to extremes of environmental temperature.
  7. Discourage smoking.
  8. Promote glycemic control.

POLYPS, GASTROINTESTINAL

- Polyps in the intestinal tract are small growths covered with mucosa that are attached to the surface; polyps have the potential to become malignant.
- Two forms of inherited GI polyps are particularly concerning to the health care provider: (1) familial adenomatous polyposis (FAP); and (2) hereditary nonpolyposis colorectal cancer (HNPCC). See *Cancer (Colorectal)* for more information. If these conditions are left untreated, colorectal cancer will occur.
- Polyps are usually asymptomatic but can cause rectal bleeding, intestinal obstruction, and intussusception.
- Polyps can usually be removed with a snare or by electrocautery during colonoscopy. After the procedure, monitor for abdominal distention, pain, and bleeding.
- Teach the patient about the need for regular, routine monitoring if polyps were found (removed) during colonoscopy because there is a risk for new/recurrent polyp formation, particularly with a positive family history of polyps. The specific follow-up time frame varies but generally occurs within 3 years.

PRESSURE ULCERS

OVERVIEW

- A pressure ulcer is a loss of tissue integrity caused when the skin and underlying tissue are compressed between a bony prominence and external surface for an extended period.
- They form most commonly over the sacrum, hips, and ankles but can occur on any body surface.
- Tissue injury and compression result in reduced tissue perfusion and oxygenation leading to cell death of skin and underlying anatomy.

- The forces that lead to pressure ulcer formation include:
  1. *Pressure:* A mechanical force occurring as a result of gravity, compressing blood vessels at the point of contact and leading to ischemia, inflammation, and tissue necrosis
  2. *Friction:* A mechanical force occurring when surfaces rub the skin and irritate or directly pull off epithelial tissue (as when the patient is dragged or pulled across bed linen)
  3. *Shear* or *shearing forces:* Mechanical forces occurring when the skin itself is stationary and the tissues below the skin (e.g., fat, muscle) shift or move, reducing the blood supply to the skin

Considerations for Older Adults

- Older adults are at particular risk for pressure ulcers because of the presence of age-related skin changes such as epidermal thinning, reduced strength and elasticity, and increased fragility of capillaries in the dermal layer.
- Flattening of the cells in the dermal-epidermal junction increases risk for injury from mechanical shearing forces, such as removal of tape or friction from restraints.
- Skin moisture and irritation resulting from incontinence can contribute to early pressure ulcer formation.

- Once formed, these chronic wounds are slow to heal, resulting in increased morbidity and health care costs.
- Complications include sepsis, kidney failure, infectious arthritis, and osteomyelitis.
- Pressure ulcers are categorized using the following descriptors:
  1. *Stage I:* The skin is intact and red and does not blanch with external pressure.
  2. *Stage II:* The skin is not intact, and there is a partial-thickness skin loss of the epidermis or dermis. It may appear as an abrasion, a blister (open or fluid-filled), or a shallow crater, and bruising is not present.
  3. *Stage III:* Skin loss is full thickness and subcutaneous tissues may be damaged or necrotic. Bone, tendon, and muscle are not exposed, but the fat may show a deep, crater-like appearance. Undermining and tunneling may or may not be present.
  4. *Stage IV:* Skin loss is full thickness with exposed or palpable muscle, tendon, or bone. Undermining, tunneling, and sinus tracts may be present. Slough and eschar are often present on at least part of the wound.
  5. *Unstageable:* Skin loss is full thickness, and the base is completely covered with slough or eschar, obscuring the true depth of the wound.

6. *Suspected deep tissue injury:* The intact skin area appears purple or maroon and blood-filled blisters may be present. Other changes that may have preceded the discoloration include that the area may have felt more firm, boggy, mushy, warmer, or cooler than the surrounding tissue.

- Health promotion and maintenance
  1. Intervene early when risk is present to prevent pressure ulcers.
  2. Identify patients at risk for pressure ulcer formation, commonly with a valid and reliable tool such as the Braden Scale. Risk factors include:
     a. Mental status changes
     b. Decreased sensory perception
     c. Impaired mobility
     d. Poor nutritional status
     e. Incontinence
- Implement prevention interventions.
  1. Perform proper positioning by:
     a. Padding contact surfaces with pressure-relieving devices
     b. Re-positioning an immobile patient at least every 2 hours
     c. Using a designated slide board or a mechanical lift when moving an immobile patient from a bed to another surface
     d. Keeping the patient's heels off the bed surface with the use of a bed pillow under the ankles
  2. Ensure adequate nutrition by:
     a. Providing sufficient fluid intake to maintain urine output of 0.5 to 1 mL/kg/hr
     b. Helping the patient maintain an adequate intake of protein and calories
  3. Provide skin care, including:
     a. Performing a daily inspection of the patient's entire skin
     b. Documenting and reporting any manifestations of skin infection
     c. Using moisturizers daily on dry skin and applying them when skin is damp
     d. Keeping moisture from prolonged contact with skin
     e. Using a wicking cloth where two moist skin surfaces touch or where perspiration collects
     f. Using moisture barriers on skin areas where wound drainage or incontinence occurs
  4. Ensure appropriate skin cleaning by:
     a. Cleaning the skin as soon as possible after soiling occurs and at routine intervals
     b. Using a mild, heavily fatted soap or gentle commercial cleanser for incontinence
     c. Using tepid rather than hot water

P

    d. Using a disposable cleaning cloth that contains a skin barrier agent when cleaning the perineal area

    e. Using the minimal scrubbing force necessary to remove soil

    f. Patting gently rather than rubbing the skin dry

    g. Avoiding the use of powders or talcs directly on the perineum

    h. Applying a commercial skin barrier after cleansing to those areas in frequent contact with urine or feces

5. Use appropriate pressure-relieving and pressure-reducing devices.

    a. Pressure-relieving devices consistently reduce pressure to less than the capillary closing pressure.

    b. Pressure-reducing devices lower pressure to less than that of a standard hospital mattress or chair surface but do not consistently reduce pressure to less than the capillary closing pressure.

PATIENT-CENTERED COLLABORATIVE CARE
Assessment

- Obtain patient information about:
  1. The cause and specific circumstances of skin loss or injury
  2. Whether any contributing factors are present, such as prolonged bedrest, immobility, incontinence, diabetes mellitus, inadequate nutrition or hydration, altered mental status (decreased sensory perception), or peripheral vascular disease
- Assess for and document:
  1. The entire body for areas of skin injury or pressure
  2. General appearance for body weight and the proportion of weight to height
  3. Overall cleanliness of the skin, hair, and nails
  4. Any loss of mobility or range of joint motion
- Assess existing wounds daily for:
  1. Location, size, color, and extent of tissue involvement, using a clock face approach to the wound, with 12 o'clock in the direction of the patient's head and 6 o'clock in the direction of the patient's feet:
     a. Length
     b. Width
     c. Depth
  2. Exudate
  3. Condition of surrounding tissue
  4. Presence of foreign bodies
  5. Whether reddened areas blanch with pressure
  6. Texture of the wound
  7. Presence of undermining and tunneling

8. Comparison of existing wound features with those documented previously to determine the current state of healing or deterioration
9. Presence of wound infection
   a. Inflammation
   b. Induration
   c. Redness
   d. Foul odor
   e. Moderate to heavy exudate
   f. Cellulitis
   g. Progressive increase in ulcer size or depth
   h. Fever (systemic infection)
   i. Elevated WBC count (systemic infection)
- Assess for psychosocial issues, including:
  1. Altered body image
  2. Coping patterns
  3. Changes in lifestyle and ADLs
  4. Financial resources
  5. Patient's and family's willingness and skill in cleaning the wound and applying a dressing
- Assess laboratory data for:
  1. Wound contamination, which is the presence of organisms without any manifestation of infection
  2. Wound infection, which is contamination with pathogenic organisms to the degree that growth and spread cannot be controlled by the body's immune defenses
  3. Systemic infection with bacteremia and sepsis

PLANNING AND IMPLEMENTATION
Impaired Skin Integrity
Nonsurgical Management
- Dressing and wound care are the basis for pressure ulcer management. A properly designed dressing can speed healing by removing unwanted debris from the ulcer surface, protecting exposed healthy tissues, and creating a barrier between the body and the environment until the ulcer is closed.
  1. *Hydrophobic* (nonabsorbent, waterproof) dressing materials are used when the wound is relatively free of drainage. They protect the ulcer from external contamination.
  2. *Hydrophilic* (absorbent) materials draw excessive drainage away from the ulcer surface, preventing maceration.
- The frequency of dressing changes depends on the amount of necrotic material or exudate.
  1. Dry gauze dressings are changed when "strike-through" occurs or when the outer layer of the dressing first becomes saturated with exudate.

2. Gauze dressings used for débridement, such as those that are wetted and placed on a wound, allowed to become damp, and then removed, are changed often enough to take off any loose debris or exudate, usually every 4 to 6 hours.

3. Synthetic dressings are changed when exudate causes the adhesive seal to break and leakage to occur.

- Before reapplying any dressing, gently clean the ulcer surface with saline or a nontoxic wound cleanser as prescribed.
- Drug therapy with topical antibacterial agents is often needed to control bacterial growth.
- Nutrition therapy requires adequate nutritional intake of calories, protein, vitamins, minerals, and water.
  1. Perform a nutritional assessment at least weekly.
  2. Coordinate with the dietitian to encourage the patient to eat a well-balanced diet, emphasizing protein, vegetables, fruit, whole-grain breads and cereals, and vitamins.
- New technologies may be useful for chronic ulcers that remain open for months.
  1. *Electrical stimulation* is the application of a low-voltage current to a wound area to increase blood vessel growth and promote granulation.
  2. *Vacuum-assisted wound closure* (VAC) is the use of a suction tube that is covered by a special sponge and sealed in place for 48 hours. During that time, continuous low-level negative pressure is applied through the suction tube.
  3. *Hyperbaric oxygen* (HBO) therapy is the administration of oxygen under high pressure, which raises the tissue oxygen concentration.
  4. *Topical growth factors* are biologically active substances that stimulate cell movement and growth and are applied to the wound.
  5. *Skin substitutes* are engineered products that aid in the temporary or permanent closure of various types of wounds.

Surgical Management
- Surgical management includes removal of necrotic tissue (surgical débridement) and skin grafting or use of muscle flaps to close wounds that cannot heal by epithelialization and contraction.
- Provide preoperative care.
  1. Implement routine preoperative care as described in Part One.
  2. Monitor potential donor sites.
  3. Maintain the integrity of the donor skin.
  4. Avoid minor injuries that may result in infection and graft loss.
- Provide postoperative care, including:
  1. Implementing routine postoperative care as described in Part One

2. Elevating and resting the grafted area to allow revascularization
3. Maintaining graft site immobilization with bulky cotton pressure dressings for 3 to 5 days
4. After dressings are removed, monitoring the graft for indications of failure to vascularize, nonadherence to the wound, or graft necrosis
   a. A pale flap with delayed capillary filling when blanched
   b. A dusky color or sharp line of color change
5. Caring for donor sites
   a. Protect the area from injury and infection
   b. Position the patient to avoid pressure on the site
   c. Use an overbed cradle to tent the sheets
   d. Trimming the separating gauze (when gauze dressings are used) close to the skin surface reduces the chance of accidentally moving the still adherent gauze before healing is complete
   e. Administer analgesics as prescribed
   f. Use special low-pressure or air-fluidized mattresses when grafts or donor sites are on posterior body surface

POTENTIAL FOR WOUND DETERIORATION
- Priority nursing interventions focus on preventing wound infections and promoting progression to complete wound healing.
  1. Monitor the ulcer's appearance using objective criteria.
  2. Re-evaluate the treatment plan if an ulcer worsens or shows no progress toward healing within 7 to 10 days.
  3. Check for manifestations of wound infection.
     a. Increased redness at the wound margins
     b. Edema
     c. Purulent and malodorous drainage
     d. Tenderness of the wound margins
     e. Increase in the size or depth of the lesion
     f. Changes in the color or texture of the granulation tissue
  4. Maintain a safe environment by:
     a. Performing meticulous wound care
     b. Teaching all personnel to use standard precautions
     c. Disposing properly of soiled dressings and linens

Community-Based Care
- Teach the patient and family how to modify the home and obtain supplies to manage wound care.
- Ensure that the patient or the person who will be performing the wound care demonstrates facility in removing the dressing, cleaning the wound, and applying the dressing.
- Explain the manifestations of wound infection, and remind the patient and family to report these to the health care provider or wound care clinic.

- Work with the social worker or case manager to obtain special beds or mattress overlays for the home and assistance for complex care.
- Encourage the patient to eat a balanced diet with frequent high-protein snacks.
- Emphasize the need to keep the skin of an incontinent patient clean and dry.
- Make referrals for home care nursing visits, if needed, to monitor wound progress or provide assistance with activity or rehabilitation.

PROLAPSE, MITRAL VALVE

- Mitral valve prolapse occurs when the heart valve leaflets prolapse into the left atrium during systole.
- Mitral valve prolapse is usually benign (asymptomatic) but may progress to pronounced mitral regurgitation.
- Assess for and document:
  1. Chest pain; typically sharp pain localized in the left side of the chest
  2. Palpitations, dizziness, or syncope
  3. Family history of mitral valve disease
  4. Midsystolic click or a late systolic murmur audible at the apex
- Valve repair or replacement surgery is indicated for symptomatic mitral prolapse.

PROLAPSE, PELVIC ORGAN

- The pelvic organs are supported by a sling of muscles and tendons, which sometimes become weak and are no longer able to hold an organ in place.
- *Uterine prolapse* is the downward displacement of the uterus. It can be caused by neuromuscular damage of childbirth; increased intra-abdominal pressure related to pregnancy, obesity, or physical exertion; or weakening of pelvic support due to decreased estrogen.
- A *cystocele* is a protrusion of the bladder through the vaginal wall (urinary bladder prolapse), which can lead to stress urinary incontinence (SUI) and urinary tract infections (UTIs).
- A *rectocele* is a protrusion of the rectum through a weakened vaginal wall (rectal prolapse).
- Assessment findings include:
  1. Patient's report of feeling as if "something is falling out"
  2. Dyspareunia (painful intercourse)
  3. Backache
  4. Feeling of heaviness or pressure in the pelvis

5. Protrusion of the cervix when the woman is asked to bear down
6. Bowel or bladder problems, such as urinary incontinence, constipation, hemorrhoids, or fecal impaction
- Interventions are based on the degree of prolapse.
  1. Nonsurgical management may include:
     a. Teaching women to improve pelvic support and tone by pelvic floor muscle exercises (PFME, also called *Kegel exercises*)
     b. Using space-filling devices such as pessaries or spheres worn intravaginally to elevate the uterine prolapse
     c. Administering intravaginal estrogen therapy
     d. Promoting bladder training and attention to complete emptying
     e. Promoting bowel elimination with high-fiber diet and a stool softener or laxative
  2. Surgical management, usually with a vaginal approach, may be recommended for severe symptoms.
     a. Transvaginal repair can be completed using vaginal mesh or tape.
     b. Anterior colporrhaphy (anterior repair) tightens the pelvic muscles for better bladder support.
     c. Posterior colporrhaphy (posterior repair) reduces rectal bulging.
     d. If both a cystocele and a rectocele are present, an anterior and posterior colporrhaphy (A&P repair) is performed.
  3. Nursing care is similar to that for a woman undergoing a vaginal hysterectomy (see *Surgical Management* under *Leiomyomas [Uterine Fibroids]*):
     a. Warn the patient to avoid lifting anything heavier than 5 pounds, strenuous exercises, and sexual intercourse for 6 weeks.
     b. Instruct her to notify her surgeon if she has signs of infection, such as fever, persistent pain, or purulent, foul-smelling discharge.

PROSTATIC HYPERPLASIA, BENIGN

OVERVIEW

- The exact cause of benign prostatic hyperplasia (BPH) is unclear. It is likely the result of a combination of aging and the influence of androgens that are present in prostate tissue, such as dihydrotestosterone (DHT). With aging, the glandular units in the prostate undergo nodular hyperplasia (an increase in the number of cells), resulting in prostatic hypertrophy (enlargement).
- The enlarged prostate extends upward into the bladder and inward, causing bladder outlet obstruction.

- The patient has an increased residual urine (stasis) or acute or chronic urinary retention.
- Increased residual urine causes overflow urinary incontinence in which the urine "leaks" around the enlarged prostate, causing dribbling.
- Urinary stasis can result in urinary tract infections and bladder calculi (stones).

PATIENT-CENTERED COLLABORATIVE CARE
Assessment
- Use a standardized tool such as the International Prostate Symptom Score (I-PSS) to determine the severity of lower urinary tract symptoms.
- Assess for and document:
  1. Current urinary patterns such as frequency, straining to begin urination, number of nocturnal voids (nocturia), hesitancy, force and size of urinary stream, sensation of bladder fullness after voiding, and post-void dribbling or leaking
  2. Bladder distention (by palpation or bedside ultrasound)
  3. History or finding by the provider of an enlarged prostate
  4. Laboratory findings
     a. Evidence of urinary tract infection and hematuria (WBCs and RBCs in the urine)
     b. Prostate-specific antigen (PSA) and a serum acid phosphatase level to rule out prostate cancer

Interventions
Nonsurgical Management
- "Watchful waiting" observation period with yearly examination
- Drug therapy
  1. Drugs to lower dihydrotestosterone (DHT) levels
     a. Finasteride (Proscar)
     b. Dutasteride (Avodart)
  2. Alpha-blocking agents to reduce urethral pressure and improve flow
     a. Tamsulosin (Flomax) (OTC)
     b. Alfuzosin (Uroxatral)
     c. Doxazosin (Cardura)
     d. Terazosin (Hytrin)
     e. Silodosin (Rapaflo)
- Prostatic fluid can be released and obstructive symptoms reduced with frequent sexual intercourse.
- Teach the patient about ways to prevent bladder distention, such as:
  1. Avoiding drinking large amounts of fluid in a short period
  2. Avoiding alcohol, diuretics, and caffeine
  3. Voiding as soon as the urge is felt

! NURSING SAFETY PRIORITY: Drug Alert

If you are giving alpha blockers in an inpatient setting, assess for orthostatic (postural) hypotension, tachycardia, and syncope ("blackout"), especially after the first dose. If the patient is taking the drug at home, teach him or her to be careful when changing positions and report any weakness, light-headedness, or dizziness to the health care provider immediately. Bedtime dosing may decrease the risk for problems related to hypotension. Drugs used to treat erection problems (e.g., Viagra) can worsen these side effects. Teach patients taking a 5-alpha-reductase inhibitor (5-ARI) or alpha-blocking drug to keep all appointments for follow-up laboratory testing, because both drug classes can cause liver dysfunction.

4. Avoiding drugs that can cause urinary retention, especially anticholinergics, antihistamines, and decongestants
- Minimally invasive techniques to reduce prostate tissue include:
    1. *Transurethral needle ablation* (TUNA), in which low radiofrequency energy shrinks the prostate
    2. *Transurethral microwave therapy* (TUMT), in which high temperatures heat and destroy excess tissue
    3. *Interstitial laser coagulation* (ILC), also called *contact laser prostatectomy* (CLP), in which laser energy coagulates excess tissue
    4. *Electrovaporization of the prostate,* in which high-frequency electrical current cuts and vaporizes excess tissue
    5. *Prostatic stents,* which may be placed into the urethra to maintain permanent patency after a procedure for destroying or removing prostatic tissue

Surgical Management
- The most common surgery for BPH is a *transurethral resection of the prostate* (TURP), in which the enlarged portion of the prostate is cut into pieces and removed through the urethra by an endoscopic instrument. A similar procedure is the *transurethral incision of the prostate* (TIUP), in which small cuts are made into the prostate to relieve pressure on the urethra.
- Newer surgical technologies include *holmium laser enucleation of the prostate* (HoLEP) and *transurethral ultrasound-guided laser incision of the prostate* (TULIP).
- Provide preoperative care as described in Part One and:
    1. Correct any misconceptions about the surgery.
    2. Inform the patient that he will have an indwelling bladder catheter for at least 24 hours and may have traction on the catheter.

3. Explain that the patient will feel the urge to void while the catheter is in place.
4. Reassure the patient that it is normal for the urine to be blood-tinged after surgery.
- Provide postoperative care described in Part One and:
  1. Monitor the patient's urine output every 2 to 4 hours with vital signs.

❗ NURSING SAFETY PRIORITY: Critical Rescue

If arterial bleeding occurs, notify the surgeon immediately, and increase the continuous bladder irrigation (CBI) rate or intermittently irrigate the catheter with normal saline solution according to physician or hospital protocol.

---

2. Monitor for severe bleeding, including serum hemoglobin and hematocrit levels, presence of hematuria, and signs of hypovolemia from blood loss in the first 24 postoperative hours.
3. Administer antispasmodic drugs as prescribed.
4. Keep the catheter free of obstruction and kinks, monitoring for clots and sudden cessation of urine output.
5. Instruct the patient to increase fluid intake to keep the urine clear.
6. Teach the patient that sexual function should not be affected after TURP, but that retrograde ejaculation is possible.
7. Reassure the patient that loss of urine control or dribbling is usually temporary and will resolve.
8. Assist the patient and his family in finding ways to keep his clothing dry until sphincter control returns.

PROSTATITIS

OVERVIEW
- Prostatitis is an inflammation of the prostate gland.
- Bacterial prostatitis often occurs with urethritis or an infection of the urinary tract.
- Chronic prostatitis may also be associated with a urinary infection but has a less dramatic presentation and few or no systemic manifestations.

PATIENT-CENTERED COLLABORATIVE CARE
- Assess for:
  1. Urinary urgency, frequency, difficulty starting or stopping urine flow, and dysuria
  2. Urine with threads, pus, or blood and urine malodor

3. Fever, chills, and elevated WBCs
4. Backache or perineal pain
5. History of enlarged prostate
- Treatment includes:
    1. Drug therapy with antimicrobials, which may last from weeks to many months because of poor penetration of antibiotics into prostatic tissue
    2. Comfort measures such as sitz baths, muscle relaxants, and NSAIDs
    3. Stool softeners to prevent straining and rectal irritation of the prostate during a bowel movement
    4. Drug therapy with alpha blockers such as tamsulosin (Flomax) to promote voiding
- Teach patients about:
    1. Avoiding alcohol, coffee, tea, and spicy foods that aggravate symptoms
    2. Avoiding cold preparations containing decongestants or antihistamines that may cause urinary retention
    3. The importance of adequate fluid intake to dilute urine
    4. The fact that prostatitis is not contagious
    5. The importance of adhering to long-term antibiotic therapy for CBP

PSEUDOCYSTS, PANCREATIC

- Pancreatic pseudocysts develop as a complication of acute or chronic pancreatitis or abdominal trauma.
- These "false cysts" do not have an epithelial lining and are encapsulated, saclike structures that form on or surround the pancreas.
- The pancreatic wall is inflamed, vascular, and fibrotic and contains large amounts of straw-colored or dark brown viscous fluid (enzyme exudate from the pancreas).
- The pseudocyst may be palpated as an epigastric mass.
- The primary symptoms are epigastric pain radiating to the back, abdominal fullness, nausea, vomiting, and jaundice. Serum amylase and lipase levels may be elevated.
- Complications include rupture; hemorrhage; infection; obstruction of the bowel, biliary tract, or splenic vein; abscess or fistula formation; and pancreatic ascites.
- A pseudocyst may spontaneously resolve.
- Surgical intervention with internal drainage is accomplished by creating an ostomy between the pseudocyst and the stomach, jejunum, or duodenum; external drainage is provided by the insertion of a sump drainage tube to remove pancreatic exudate and secretions.

PSORIASIS

OVERVIEW

- Psoriasis is a chronic, autoimmune scaling skin disorder with underlying dermal inflammation that has exacerbations and remissions.
- Langerhans cells in the skin activate T-lymphocytes that, in turn, target increased cell division of keratinocytes. Normally, cells at the basement membrane of the epidermis take about 28 days to reach the outermost layer where they are shed. In a person with psoriasis, the rate of cell division is speeded up so that cells are shed every 4 to 5 days.

🧬 Genetic/Genomic Considerations

A genetic predisposition is associated with psoriasis as indicated by the observation that when one identical (monozygotic) twin develops the disease, the second twin also develops the disease about 70% of the time. Variation in many gene sequences, labeled PSORS1 through PSORS13, influence the development of this autoimmune disorder. It is likely that different variations of these gene loci also influence individual patient responses to therapy. Always ask about a family history of the disorder when assessing the patient with psoriasis.

- Factors like trauma, sunburn, and injury influence whether the disease occurs, its severity, and its response to various treatments.
- Some patients with psoriasis also develop a debilitating arthritis.

PATIENT-CENTERED COLLABORATIVE CARE

Assessment

- Obtain patient information about:
  1. Any family history of psoriasis
  2. Current status
     a. Age at onset
     b. Description of the disease progression
     c. Pattern of recurrences
     d. Whether fever and itching are present
     e. Exposure to precipitating factors, including skin trauma or surgery
- Assess for and document the appearance of psoriasis and its course.
  1. *Psoriasis vulgaris* is the most common type of psoriasis.
     a. Thick, reddened papules or plaques covered by silvery white scales
     b. Sharply defined borders between the lesions and normal skin

  c. Lesions are usually present in the same areas on both sides of the body
  d. Common lesion sites are the scalp, elbows, trunk, knees, sacrum, and outside surfaces of the limbs
2. *Exfoliative psoriasis* (erythrodermic psoriasis) has generalized erythema and scaling that do not form obvious lesions.

Interventions

- Teach the patient about the disease and its treatment, and provide emotional support for the changes in body image often experienced with psoriasis.
- Topical therapy includes:
  1. Corticosteroids applied to skin lesions, followed by warm, moist dressings to increase absorption
  2. Tar preparations applied to the skin lesions as solutions, ointments, lotions, gels, and shampoos
  3. Anthralin (Anthraforte, Drithocreme, Lasan) application alone or in combination with coal tar baths and ultraviolet (UV) light
  4. Calcipotriene (Dovonex), a synthetic form of vitamin D that regulates skin cell division
  5. Tazarotene (Tazorac), which can cause birth defects even when used topically
- UV radiation therapy decreases dermal growth rates.
  1. Ultraviolet B (UV-B) light
  2. Ultraviolet A (UV-A) light
  3. Psoralen and UV-A (PUVA) treatments involve the ingestion of a photosensitizing agent (psoralen) 2 hours before exposure to UV-A light.
- Systemic therapy
  1. Oral vitamin A derivatives
  2. Immunosuppressants like methotrexate and cyclosporine
  3. Immunomodulating biologic agents including adalimumab (Humira), alefacept (Amevive), infliximab (Remicade), ustekinumab (Stelara), and etanercept (Enbrel)
- Provide emotional support when the patient suffers because of the presence of skin lesions and the unpleasantness of some of the treatments.
  1. Encourage the patient and family members to express their feelings about having an incurable skin problem that can alter appearance.
  2. Urge patients to contact other people with the disorder.
  3. Use touch without gloves during social interactions to communicate acceptance of the person and the skin problem.
- Teach women of childbearing age who are taking vitamin A derivatives or immunosuppressive or immunomodulating drugs to

use a reliable method of contraception, because these agents can cause birth defects when taken during pregnancy.

PULMONARY ARTERIAL HYPERTENSION

OVERVIEW

- Primary pulmonary arterial hypertension (PAH) is a problem of the pulmonary blood vessel constriction in the absence of lung disease.
- Primary PAH is considered idiopathic, because the causes of this life-threatening disorder are unclear.
- Primary PAH is rare and occurs mostly in women between the ages of 20 and 40 years.
- Without treatment for primary PAH death usually occurs within 2 years after diagnosis.
- Secondary PAH can occur as a complication of other lung disorders.
- As PAH increases, blood flow decreases, leading to poor lung perfusion and hypoxemia. Eventually, the right side of the heart fails *(cor pulmonale)* because of the continuous workload of pumping against the high pulmonary pressures.

☒ Genetic/Genomic Considerations

- About 50% of patients with primary PAH have a genetic mutation in the *BMPR2* gene, which codes for a growth factor receptor. Excessive activation of this receptor allows increased growth of arterial smooth muscle in the lungs, making these arteries thicker.
- Because many more people have mutations in this gene than have PAH, it is thought that the mutations increase susceptibility to PAH when other, often unknown, environmental factors also are present.
- Teach women who have a first-degree relative (parent or sibling) with PAH to have regular health checkups and to consult a health care provider whenever pulmonary problems are present.

PATIENT-CENTERED COLLABORATIVE CARE

Assessment

- Assess for and document:
  1. Dyspnea and fatigue in an otherwise healthy adult
  2. Angina-like chest pain
- Diagnosis is made from the results of right-sided heart catheterization showing elevated pulmonary pressures.

Interventions

- Drug therapy can reduce pulmonary pressures and slow the development of *cor pulmonale* by dilating pulmonary vessels and preventing clot formation.
  1. Natural and synthetic prostacyclin agents provide the best specific dilation of pulmonary blood vessels (e.g., epoprostenol [Flolan] or treprostinil [Remodulin])

> ### ! NURSING SAFETY PRIORITY: Critical Rescue
>
> Although IV prostacyclin therapy is very effective, deaths have been reported if intravenous drug delivery is interrupted for even a few minutes. Teach the patient to always have backup drug cassettes and battery packs. If these are not available or the line is disrupted the patient should go to the emergency department immediately.

  2. Endothelin-receptor antagonists, bosentan (Tracleer)
  3. Warfarin (Coumadin), low–molecular-weight heparin and antiplatelet drugs
  4. Calcium channel blockers such as nifedipine (Procardia) and diltiazem (Cardizem)
  5. Sildenafil (Revatio, Viagra) administered orally or intravenously with prostacyclins therapy
- Secondary pulmonary hypertension is usually managed by treating the underlying lung pathology. When lung pathology is terminal or untreatable, then management of symptoms or palliative care becomes the focus of care.
- Teach patients about the need to:
  1. Use strict aseptic technique in all aspects of manipulating the drug delivery system
  2. Notify the pulmonologist at the first sign of any respiratory or systemic infection
- Surgical management of PAH involves single-lung or whole-lung transplantation.
- If *cor pulmonale* also is present, the patient may need combined heart-lung transplantation.

PULMONARY CONTUSION

- Pulmonary contusion most often follows injuries caused by rapid deceleration during vehicular accidents. Hemorrhage and edema occur in and between the alveoli, decreasing lung movement and reducing the area for gas exchange.
- Respiratory failure often develops over time rather than immediately after the trauma.

- Manifestations include:
  1. Dyspnea
  2. Hypoxemia
  3. Bloody sputum
  4. Decreased breath sounds
  5. Crackles and wheezes
  6. Hazy opacity on chest x-ray in the lobes or parenchyma
- Management is aimed at maintenance of ventilation and oxygenation.
  1. Use central venous pressure (CVP) to monitor response to fluid therapy and limit overhydration.
  2. Provide oxygen therapy and mechanical ventilation with positive end-expiratory pressure (PEEP) to maintain open alveoli.
  3. Monitor the work of breathing and maintain vigilance for early detection of the onset of acute respiratory distress syndrome (ARDS), a relatively common complication of extensive lung contusion.

PULMONARY EMBOLISM

OVERVIEW

- Pulmonary embolism (PE) is a collection of particulate matter (solids, liquids, or air), most commonly a blood clot, that lodges in the pulmonary vessels.
- Large emboli obstruct pulmonary blood flow, leading to reduced oxygenation of the whole body, pulmonary tissue hypoxia, and, potentially, death.
- The local response includes blood vessel constriction and pulmonary hypertension that impair gas exchange and tissue perfusion.
- Major risk factors for venous thromboembolism (VTE), leading to PE are:
  1. Prolonged immobility
  2. Central venous catheters
  3. Surgery (especially pelvic or leg surgery)
  4. Obesity
  5. Older age
  6. Conditions that increase blood clotting
  7. History of thromboembolism
- Smoking, pregnancy, estrogen therapy, heart failure, stroke, cancer (particularly lung or prostate), and trauma increase the risk for VTE and PE.

PATIENT-CENTERED COLLABORATIVE CARE
Assessment

- Obtain patient information about:
  1. Risk factors for VTE and PE

- Assess for manifestations.
  1. Pulmonary manifestations
     a. Dyspnea
     b. Pleuritic chest pain (sharp, stabbing pain on inspiration)
     c. Crackles, wheezes, pleuritic rub
     d. Dry or productive cough
     e. Hemoptysis (bloody sputum)
  2. Cardiac manifestations
     a. Rapid heart rate
     b. Distended neck veins
     c. Syncope (fainting or loss of consciousness)
     d. Cyanosis
     e. Hypotension

! NURSING SAFETY PRIORITY: Critical Rescue

Any patient who has shortness of breath, chest pain, and or/ hypotension without an obvious cause should be assessed for PE and the Rapid Response Team notified. If PE is strongly suspected, prompt oxygenation and management are started before diagnostic studies have been completed.

     f. Abnormal heart sounds, such as an S_3 or S_4
     g. Electrocardiographic (ECG) abnormalities (nonspecific and transient)
  3. Miscellaneous manifestations
     a. Low-grade fever
     b. Petechiae on the skin over the chest and in the axillae
     c. Nausea, vomiting, and general malaise
     d. Low $Paco_2$ with tachypnea may be an early symptom
     e. Low Pao_2 with high $Paco_2$ and acidosis (low pH) are late symptoms
     f. Anxiety and restlessness or confusion from hypoxemia
- Diagnosis is most commonly made with chest computed tomography (CT) scan using a PE protocol.

PLANNING AND IMPLEMENTATION
Hypoxemia
- Increase gas exchange, improve lung perfusion, reduce the risk for further clot formation, and prevent complications.
  Nonsurgical Management
- Oxygen therapy
  1. Apply oxygen by nasal cannula or by mask in less severe cases.
  2. Institute intubation and mechanical ventilation for the severely hypoxemic patient.

   3. Monitor:
      a. Oxygen saturation continually
      b. Vital signs, lung sounds, and cardiac status hourly
   4. Assess for and document increasing or decreasing:
      a. Dyspnea
      b. Dysrhythmias
      c. Distended neck veins
      d. Abnormal lung sounds
      e. Peripheral perfusion
- Drug therapy
   1. Anticoagulants keep the embolus from enlarging and prevent
      the formation of new clots.
      a. Heparin initially for 5 to 10 days, with oral anticoagulants
         started and overlapping with heparin around days 3 to 5.
      b. Fibrinolytic drugs
   2. Review the patient's partial coagulation profile.

! NURSING SAFETY PRIORITY: Drug Alert

Heparin comes in a variety of concentrations in vials that have
differing amounts. Similar packaging or labeling contribute to
possible medication errors. Check the prescribed dose carefully and ensure the correct concentration is being used to
prevent overdosing or underdosing.

Surgical Management
- *Embolectomy* is the surgical removal of the embolus from pulmonary blood vessels using special thrombectomy catheters that can
  mechanically break up clots (e.g., AngioJet).
- *Inferior vena cava interruption* with placement of a vena cava filter
  is a lifesaving measure that prevents further embolus formation
  for some patients.

Hypotension
- Hypotension is related to inadequate circulation to the left ventricle and/or reduced circulation from bleeding due to anticoagulant or antifibrinolytic therapy.
- IV fluid therapy involves giving crystalloid solutions to restore
  plasma volume and prevent shock.
   1. Continuously monitor:
      a. ECG
      b. Central venous or right atrial pressure
   2. Assess for signs of right-sided heart failure
      a. Hypoxemia
      b. Dependent edema
- Drug therapy with intravenous vasopressors or agents that
  increase myocardial contractility may be used.

- Monitor the patient's response to anticoagulant and antifibrinolytic therapy to reduce the risk for unintended hemorrhage from
  excess anticoagulation or recurrent clot formation from inadequate anticoagulation therapy.

Anxiety
- Anxiety is related to hypoxemia and life-threatening illness.
- Reduce anxiety with communication.
    1. Acknowledge the anxiety and the patient's perception of a
       life-threatening situation.
    2. Stay with the patient and speak calmly and clearly, providing
       reassurance that appropriate measures are being taken.
    3. Explain the rationale and share information with the patient
       regarding any procedure, assessment, or intervention.
- Drug therapy with an antianxiety drug may be prescribed if the
  patient's anxiety increases or prevents adequate rest.

Risk for Bleeding
- Assess at least every 2 to 4 hours for evidence of bleeding in the
  form of oozing, bruises that cluster, petechiae, or purpura, includ-
  ing IV sites.
- Examine all stools, urine, drainage, and vomitus visually for gross
  blood and test for occult blood.
- Measure any blood loss as accurately as possible.
- Implement best practices for bleeding prevention.
    1. Handle the patient gently.
    2. Use and teach unlicensed assistive personnel (UAP) to use a
       lift sheet when moving and positioning the patient in bed.
    3. Avoid intramuscular injections and venipunctures.
    4. If injections or venipunctures are necessary, use the smallest
       gauge needle for the task.
    5. Apply firm pressure to the needle stick site for 10 minutes or
       until the site no longer oozes blood.
    6. Apply ice to areas of trauma.
    7. Instruct patients to notify nursing personnel immediately if
       any trauma occurs or if bleeding or bruising is noticed.
    8. Avoid trauma to rectal tissues by not taking rectal tempera-
       ture, and not administering enemas or rectal drugs.
    9. Instruct the patient and UAP to use an electric shaver rather
       than a razor.
    10. When providing mouth care or supervising others in provid-
        ing mouth care:
        a. Use a soft-bristled toothbrush or tooth sponges.
        b. Do not use floss.
        c. Check to make certain that dentures fit and do not rub.
    11. Instruct the patient not to blow the nose forcefully or insert
        objects into the nose.

12. Instruct UAP and the patient to wear shoes with firm soles whenever he or she is ambulating.
13. Ensure that antidotes to anticoagulation therapy are on the unit.
- Monitor laboratory values daily.
  1. Complete blood count (CBC): hematocrit, hemoglobin, and platelet count
  2. Prothrombin time (PT), activated PTT (aPTT), international normalized ratio (INR)

Community-Based Care
- The patient with PE is discharged after hypoxemia and hemodynamic instability have been resolved and adequate anticoagulation has been achieved.
- Anticoagulation therapy usually continues after discharge.
- Teach the patient and family about:
  1. Bleeding precautions
  2. Activities to reduce the risk for VTE
  3. Need for follow-up care

PULMONARY EMPYEMA

OVERVIEW
- Pulmonary empyema is a collection of pus in the pleural space; the fluid is thick, opaque, exudative, and foul smelling.
- The most common cause is pulmonary infection (pneumonia), lung abscess, or infected pleural effusion that can spread across the pleura, obstructing lymph nodes and leading to a retrograde (backward) flood of infected lymph into the pleural space.
- Other causes include liver or abdominal abscesses that spread infection through the lymphatic system into the lung area, thoracic surgery, and chest trauma.

PATIENT-CENTERED COLLABORATIVE CARE
Assessment
- Obtain patient information about:
  1. Recent febrile illness (including pneumonia)
  2. Chest pain
  3. Dyspnea
  4. Cough and sputum
  5. Chest trauma
  6. Fever, chills, night sweats
- Assess for and document:
  1. Reduced chest wall motion
  2. Decreased or abnormal breath sounds
  3. Dyspnea, labored breathing, or tachypnea
  4. Weight loss
  5. Hypotension
  6. Hypoxia, decreased Spo_2

- Diagnosis is made by chest x-ray and analysis of pleural fluid is obtained by thoracentesis.

Interventions

- Therapy for empyema is focused on emptying the empyema cavity, re-expanding the lung, and controlling the infection.
- Antibiotics that are appropriate for the identified organism are prescribed.
- Closed–chest drainage is used to promote lung expansion.
- Open thoracotomy and removal of a portion of the pleura may be needed for thick pus or marked pleural thickening.
- Nursing care is the same as for patients with a pleural effusion, pneumothorax, or infection.

PYELONEPHRITIS

OVERVIEW

- Pyelonephritis is an infection or inflammation of the kidney and renal pelvis.
- Microorganisms enter the renal pelvis and activate the inflammatory response, which results in mobilization of white blood cells (WBCs) and local edema.
- Pyelonephritis is generally classified as acute or chronic. Acute pyelonephritis is the active bacterial infection, whereas chronic pyelonephritis results from repeated or continued upper urinary tract infections (UTIs) or the effects of such infections.
- Complications include abscess formation and septicemia.
- Pregnancy, diabetes mellitus, and chronic renal calculi increase the risk for pyelonephritis.
- Structural deformities or obstruction with reflux caused by stones, obstruction, and neurogenic impairment involving the voiding mechanism often lead to chronic pyelonephritis.

PATIENT-CENTERED COLLABORATIVE CARE

Assessment

- Obtain patient information about:
  1. History of urinary tract and kidney infections
  2. History of diabetes mellitus or other conditions and treatment associated with immunocompromise
  3. History of stone disease or other structural or functional abnormalities of the genitourinary tract
- Assess for:
  1. Pregnancy because pyelonephritis is associated with early onset of labor, compromising fetal health
  2. Flank or abdominal discomfort
  3. Hematuria, cloudy urine
  4. Signs of infection: general malaise, fever, chills

    5. Asymmetry, edema, or erythema at the costovertebral angle
    6. Presence of leukoesterase, nitrogen, WBCs, or bacteria in the urine
- Diagnostic testing may include:
    1. Urinalysis and urine for culture and sensitivity
    2. WBC count with differential, basic metabolic panel for kidney function
    3. X-ray, CT, or cystourethrogram to diagnose stones or obstruction. *Ensure that the patient is not pregnant before any imaging study is performed.*

Interventions
- Administer antibiotics. Drug therapy initially includes broad-spectrum antibiotics. With urine and blood culture sensitivity results, a single antibiotic may be ordered.
- Surgical procedures include:
    1. Pyelolithotomy (removal of a stone from the renal pelvis)
    2. Nephrectomy (removal of a kidney)
    3. Ureteral diversion or reimplantation of the ureter to restore the bladder drainage mechanism
- Maintain sufficient perfusion to the kidneys to prevent hypotensive or hypertensive kidney injury.
- Maintain sufficient fluid intake to promote urine output greater than 1 mL/kg/hr.
- Assess for signs of acute kidney injury, such as increasing blood urea nitrogen (BUN) or creatinine level or decreased urinary output.

Community-Based Care
- Health teaching includes:
    1. Antibiotic self-administration including effects, side effects, and importance of following the prescribed duration of therapy
    2. Planning and implementing healthy choices for fluid intake
    3. Monitoring urine output and manifestations of disease recurrence such as fever, urgency, frequency, or incontinence

R

RAYNAUD'S PHENOMENON AND RAYNAUD'S DISEASE

- *Raynaud's phenomenon* is caused by vasospasm of the arterioles and arteries of the upper and lower extremities, usually unilaterally.
- *Raynaud's disease* occurs bilaterally. It is more common in women and occurs between the ages of 17 and 50 years.
- The pathophysiology is the same for both entities: vasospasm of the arterioles and arteries of the upper and lower extremities.
- Cutaneous vessels are constricted, causing blanching of the extremities followed by cyanosis.

- When the vasospasm is relieved, the tissue becomes reddened or hyperemic.
- Patients often have an associated systemic connective tissue disease such as systemic lupus erythematosus (SLE) or progressive systemic sclerosis.
- Assess for:
  1. Color changes in the extremity or digits, ranging from blanched to reddened to cyanotic
  2. Numbness of the extremity or digits
  3. Coldness of the extremity or digits
  4. Pain
  5. Swelling
  6. Ulcerations
  7. Aggravation of symptoms by cold or stress
  8. Gangrene of digits in severe cases
- Interventions include:
  1. Drug therapy to prevent vasoconstriction, including calcium channel blockers
  2. Lumbar sympathectomy to relieve severe symptoms in the feet
  3. Sympathetic ganglionectomy to relieve severe symptoms in the upper extremities
- Health teaching emphasizes methods to minimize vasoconstriction.
  1. Smoking cessation and caffeine reduction
  2. Minimizing exposure to cold by wearing warm clothes, socks, and gloves and maintaining a warm indoor ambient temperature
  3. Stress management

REGURGITATION, AORTIC

- In aortic regurgitation (insufficiency), the aortic valve leaflets do not close properly during diastole, and the annulus may become dilated, loose, or deformed.
- Regurgitation of blood from the aorta into the left ventricle occurs during diastole; the left ventricle dilates to accommodate the greater blood volume and hypertrophies.
- Causes include infective endocarditis, congenital anatomic aortic valvular abnormalities, hypertension, and Marfan syndrome (a rare, inherited systemic connective tissue disease).
- Patients with aortic insufficiency remain asymptomatic for many years because of the compensatory mechanisms of the left ventricle.
- Signs and symptoms include:
  1. Palpitations (severe disease)
  2. Dyspnea on exertion
  3. Orthopnea and paroxysmal nocturnal dyspnea

4. Nocturnal angina with diaphoresis
5. Widened pulse pressure
6. High-pitched, blowing, decrescendo diastolic murmur

- Nonsurgical therapy focuses on drug therapy to reduce heart failure progression.
- Surgical treatment is performed after symptoms of left ventricular failure have developed but before irreversible dysfunction occurs.
- Aortic valve repair or replacement surgery is performed to improve cardiac function in symptomatic patients.
- Repair procedures include valvuloplasty, commissurotomy, and annuloplasty (reconstruction).
- Replacement with a synthetic or biologic valve occurs during cardiopulmonary bypass surgery and requires lifetime anticoagulation therapy to prevent thrombus formation on the valve postoperatively.
- Perioperative care reflects the best practices outlined in Part One and is similar to care for patients having other open heart/heart-lung bypass procedures such as coronary artery bypass surgery.

REGURGITATION, MITRAL

- Mitral regurgitation (insufficiency) results from fibrotic and calcific changes that prevent the mitral valve from closing completely during systole, allowing backflow of blood into the left atrium during both contraction (systole) and rest (diastole).
- To compensate for the increased volume and pressure, the left atrium and ventricle dilate and hypertrophy.
- Degeneration (age-related damage) followed by infective endocarditis are the most common causes of mitral regurgitation. When the cause is rheumatic carditis, regurgitation often coexists with mitral stenosis.
- Signs and symptoms include:
  1. Right heart failure with neck vein distention, liver enlargement (hepatomegaly), and peripheral edema
  2. Fatigue and weakness
  3. Dyspnea, orthopnea
  4. Anxiety
  5. Atypical chest pains and palpitations
  6. Atrial fibrillation
  7. High-pitched, systolic murmur
- Drug therapy is instituted to maintain normal cardiac output.
- The reparative surgical procedure is mitral annuloplasty. Mitral valve leaflets and annuli are reconstructed to narrow the valve orifice.
- Perioperative care reflects the best practices outlined in Part One and is similar to care for patients having other open heart/

heart-lung bypass procedures such as coronary artery bypass surgery.
- The patient with mitral valve replacement requires lifetime anti-coagulation therapy to prevent thrombus formation on the biosynthetic valve.

! NURSING SAFETY PRIORITY: Drug Alert

Teach patients with valve replacement the importance of prophylactic antibiotic therapy before any invasive dental or respiratory procedure. Prophylactic antibiotics are not recommended prior to gastrointestinal procedures such as upper GI endoscopy, colonoscopy, or procedures requiring genitourinary instrumentation.

R

RESPIRATORY FAILURE, ACUTE
OVERVIEW
- Acute respiratory failure can be defined in three ways, based on the underlying problem.
  1. *Ventilatory failure* occurs when air movement into/out of the lungs is inadequate. As a result, too little oxygen reaches the alveoli and carbon dioxide is retained. Problems included respiratory center depression (e.g., sedation, anesthesia, opioid overdose, brain damage), a lung problem (e.g., adult respiratory distress syndrome, severe pneumonia), or poor function of respiratory muscles (e.g., chronic degenerative neurologic disorders like amyotrophic lateral syndrome [ALS] or diaphragmatic injury). In addition to reduced arterial oxygen, this type of acute respiratory failure is characterized by significant hypercarbia ($Paco_2$ greater than 50 mm Hg) and acidemia (pH less than 7.35).
  2. *Oxygenation failure* is a problem in which air moves in and out of lungs without difficulty but does not oxygenate the pulmonary blood sufficiently. Generally, lung blood flow (perfusion or Q) is decreased. Problems leading to this type of failure include impaired diffusion of oxygen at the alveolar level (e.g., lung fibrosis), right-to-left shunting of blood in the pulmonary vessels (e.g., atelectasis), and failure of hemoglobin to bind oxygen (e.g., inherited hemoglobin disorders, carbon monoxide poisoning).
  3. *Combined ventilatory and oxygenation failure* involves hypoventilation and impairment of oxygenation at the alveolar-capillary membrane. This type of respiratory failure leads to a

more profound hypoxemia than either ventilatory failure or oxygenation failure alone. It is seen in patients who have abnormal lungs (chronic bronchitis, emphysema, or during asthma attacks) and in patients who have both cardiac failure and respiratory disease.

- Regardless of the underlying cause, the patient in acute respiratory failure is always hypoxemic.

PATIENT-CENTERED COLLABORATIVE CARE
Assessment
- Assess for and document:
  1. Dyspnea (the hallmark of respiratory failure)
  2. Changes in the respiratory rate or pattern
  3. Abnormal lung sounds
  4. Manifestations of hypoxemia
     a. Pallor or cyanosis
     b. Tachypnea
     c. Restlessness, anxiety, or confusion
  5. Hypoxia (decreased arterial oxygen levels [Pao_2] and decreased peripheral oxygenation [Spo_2])
  6. Hypercarbia (high arterial carbon dioxide levels or Pao_2)

Interventions
- Management of acute respiratory failure of any origin includes:
  1. Applying oxygen therapy to keep the Spo_2 92% or greater and Pao_2 greater than 60 mm Hg. These values may be modified if the patient has a lung condition like chronic obstructive pulmonary disease (COPD).
  2. Implementing invasive or noninvasive mechanical ventilation if other measures do not increase oxygenation
  3. Reducing hypercarbia to patient baseline. Patients with chronic respiratory conditions that include carbon dioxide retention may have a baseline $Paco_2$ greater than 45 mm Hg.
  4. Assisting the patient to find a position of comfort that allows easier breathing, usually a more upright position
  5. Assisting the patient to use relaxation, diversion, and guided imagery to reduce anxiety
  6. Instituting energy-conserving measures of minimal self-care and no unnecessary procedures
  7. Administering drug therapy given systemically or by metered dose inhaler (MDI) to resolve bronchoconstriction contributing to poor air exchange
  8. Encouraging deep-breathing techniques or incentive spirometer use to increase oxygen intake or reduce carbon dioxide retention

RETINAL HOLES, TEARS, AND DETACHMENTS
OVERVIEW
- A *retinal hole* is a break in the retina, usually caused by trauma or aging.
- A *retinal tear* is a more jagged and irregularly shaped break, often caused by traction on the retina.
- A *retinal detachment* is the separation of the retina from the epithelium. Detachments are classified by the nature of their development.

PATIENT-CENTERED COLLABORATIVE CARE
Assessment
- Subjective manifestations
  1. Bright flashes of light (*photopsia*) or floating dark spots in the affected eye
  2. The sensation of a curtain being pulled over part of the visual field
  3. No pain
- Ophthalmoscopic manifestations
  1. Gray bulges or folds in the retina that quiver
  2. Possibly a hole or tear at the edge of the detachment

Interventions
- For an actual detachment, surgical repair is needed to place the retina in contact with the underlying structures. A common repair procedure is scleral buckling.
  1. Preoperative care includes applying prescribed topical drugs to inhibit pupil constriction and accommodation and allaying fears about visual loss.
  2. Postoperative care as outlined in Part One and:
     a. Monitor the patient's vital signs and check the eye patch and shield for any drainage.
     b. If gas or oil has been placed in the eye, teach the patient to keep his or her head in the position prescribed by the surgeon to promote reattachment.
     c. Remind the patient to avoid activities that increase intraocular pressure (IOP).
     d. Teach the patient to avoid reading, writing, and close work such as sewing during the first week after surgery, because these activities cause rapid eye movements and promote detachment.
     e. Teach the patient the manifestations of infection and detachment (sudden reduced visual acuity, eye pain, pupil that does not respond to light by constricting) and the need to notify the provider immediately if symptoms occur.

ROTATOR CUFF INJURIES

- The function of the rotator cuff is to stabilize the head of the humerus during shoulder abduction.
- It may be injured by substantial trauma or the accumulation of many small tears related to aging, repetitive motions, or falls.
- Manifestations include shoulder pain and the inability to achieve or maintain abduction of the arm at the shoulder.
- Conservative management involves the use of NSAIDs, physical therapy, sling or immobilizer support, and ice or heat applications while the injury heals.
- Surgical cuff repair may be needed for patients who do not respond to conservative treatment over a 3 to 6 month period and for those who have a complete tear.

S

SARCOIDOSIS

- Sarcoidosis is a granulomatous disorder of unknown cause that can affect any organ, especially the lung.
- It develops over time as an autoimmune disorder in which the normally protective T-lymphocytes increase and cause damaging actions in lung tissue.
- Alveolar inflammation (alveolitis) results from the presence of immune cells in the alveoli and the chronic inflammation causes fibrosis that reduces lung compliance (elasticity) and the ability to exchange gases.
- *Cor pulmonale* (right-sided cardiac failure) is often present, because the heart can no longer pump effectively against the stiff, fibrotic lung.
- The disease usually affects young adults.
- Manifestations include enlarged lymph nodes in the hilar area of the lungs, lung infiltrate on chest x-ray, skin lesions, eye lesions, cough, dyspnea, hemoptysis, and chest discomfort.
- The disease may resolve permanently or may lead to progressive pulmonary fibrosis and severe systemic disease.
- The goal of therapy is to lessen symptoms and prevent fibrosis and includes immunomodulating drugs such as corticosteroids and cytokine mediators.

SCABIES

- Scabies is a contagious skin infection caused by mite infestations.
- It is transmitted by close contact with an infested person or infested bedding. Infestation is common among patients with poor hygiene or crowded living conditions. Treatment involves

the use of scabicides, such as permethrin (Acticin), lindane (Kwell, Kildane, Scabene, Thionex), malathion (Ovide), or benzyl benzoate (Ascabiol).

- Laundering clothes and personal items with hot water and detergent is sufficient to eliminate the mites.

SEIZURE DISORDERS

OVERVIEW

- A seizure is an abnormal, sudden, excessive, uncontrolled electrical discharge of neurons within the brain that may result in alterations in consciousness, motor or sensory ability, or behavior.
- Epilepsy is a chronic disorder characterized by two or more seizures.
- Three major categories and associated subclasses of seizures are:
  1. Generalized seizures that involve both cerebral hemispheres
     a. *Tonic-clonic seizure* (formerly called a *grand mal seizure*) is characterized by stiffening or rigidity of the muscles (tonic phase), followed by rhythmic jerking of the extremities (clonic phase). Immediate unconsciousness occurs, and the patient may be incontinent of urine or feces and may bite his or her tongue.
     b. *Clonic* seizures are repetitive, rhythmic jerks that involve both sides of the body at the same time.
     c. *Tonic* seizures are characterized by stiffening of the muscles.
     d. *Absence seizure* (formerly called *petit mal seizure*) consists of a brief (often seconds) period of loss of consciousness and blank staring, as if the patient were daydreaming.
     e. *Myoclonic seizure* is a brief, generalized jerking or stiffening of the extremities and may occur singly or in groups.
     f. *Atonic seizures* (formerly called *drop attacks*) are characterized by sudden loss of muscle tone, which in most cases causes the patient to fall.
  2. Focal (partial) seizures that begin in one cerebral hemisphere
     a. During a *simple seizure* awareness is retained. There may be symptoms of jerking, muscle rigidity, spasms, and head-turning; unusual sensations affecting vision, hearing, smell, taste, or touch; or memory or emotional disturbances.
     b. *Complex seizure* (often called a *psychomotor seizure* or a *temporal lobe seizure*) causes the patient to lose consciousness. Characteristic behavior, known as automatism, may occur (e.g., lip smacking, patting, picking at clothes).
     c. *Partial seizure with secondary generalization* involves symptoms that are initially associated with a preservation of consciousness followed by a loss of consciousness and tonic/clonic muscle contractions.

S

3. Unclassified seizures have too few observations to classify as either generalized or focal.

- *Status epilepticus* is a seizure that lasts longer than 10 minutes or repeated seizures over the course of 30 minutes. It is a neurologic emergency and must be treated promptly, or brain damage and possibly death from anoxia, cardiac dysrhythmias, or lactic acidosis may occur.
- Status epilepticus is usually caused by:
  1. Sudden withdrawal from anticonvulsant drugs
  2. Acute alcohol withdrawal
  3. Head trauma
  4. Cerebral edema
  5. Metabolic disturbances
- An epileptic seizure occurs because of abnormal excessive or synchronous neuronal activity in the brain. Epilepsy is a disorder of the brain characterized by an enduring predisposition to recurrent seizures and by the neurobiologic, cognitive, psychological, and social consequences of this condition.
- Genetic, structural, and metabolic abnormalities contribute to seizure occurrence.

Considerations for Older Adults

Seizures in older adults can appear to have symptoms similar to dementia, psychosis, or Alzheimer's disease (AD), especially in the postictal stage (after the seizure). New-onset seizures in older adults are typically associated with conditions such as hypertension, cardiac disease, diabetes mellitus, stroke, or AD.

PATIENT-CENTERED COLLABORATIVE CARE
Assessment

- Obtain patient information about:
  1. Frequency, duration, and pattern of occurrence for seizure activity
  2. Description of preictal symptoms and postictal activity (aura, motor activity, sequence of progression, eye signs, consciousness, respiratory patterns) and events surrounding the seizure
  3. Current drugs, including dosage, frequency of administration, and the time at which the drug was last taken
  4. Compliance with the antiepileptic drug schedule and reasons for noncompliance, if a diagnosis of epilepsy has been made
- Note whether an observed seizure is new (first occurrence) or recurrent. Seizures occurring in greater intensity, number, or length than the patient's usual seizures are considered *acute.* New

or acute seizures may also appear in clusters that are different from the patient's typical seizure pattern.

Interventions

Nonsurgical Management

- Administer antiepileptic drugs and monitor the patient's response with serum levels for effectiveness. Anticipate multiple drug-drug interactions with antiepileptic drugs and other medications.
- When providing care for the patient during a tonic-clonic or complete focal seizure:
  1. Protect the patient from injury.
  2. Do not force anything into the patient's mouth.
  3. Turn the patient to the side.
  4. Loosen any restrictive clothing.
  5. Maintain the airway, and suction as needed.
  6. Do not restrain the patient; rather, guide the patient's movements.
  7. At the completion of the seizure:
     a. Take vital signs.
     b. Perform neurologic assessment.
     c. Allow the patient to rest.
- Nursing observations and documentation of a seizure include:
  1. Onset and cessation of seizure activity: date, time, and duration
  2. Sequence and type of movement and whether more than one activity occurs
  3. Observations during the seizure:
     a. Changes in pupil size and any eye deviation
     b. Level of consciousness (LOC)
     c. Presence of apnea, cyanosis, salivation
     d. Incontinence of bowel or bladder
     e. Eye fluttering
     f. Movement and progression of motor activity
     g. Lip smacking or other automatism
     h. Tongue or lip biting
  4. How long the seizure lasted
  5. Presence and description of aura or precipitating events
  6. Postictal status
  7. Length of time before the patient returns to pre-seizure status
- Drug therapy is the major component of management; the health care provider introduces one anticonvulsant at a time to achieve seizure control.
- Serum drug levels are monitored for the first 3 days after the start of anticonvulsants and thereafter as needed.
- Follow agency policy for the implementation of Seizure Precautions.

1. Keep oxygen, suctioning equipment, and an airway available at the bedside.
2. Maintain IV access (a saline lock) for patients at risk for tonic-clonic seizures.
3. Padded tongue blades do not belong at the bedside; nothing should be inserted into the patient's mouth after a seizure begins.
4. Keep the bed in the low position. Use of padded siderails is controversial; siderails are rarely the source of significant injury and the use of padded siderails may embarrass the patient and family.

- Status epilepticus is a neurologic emergency and must be treated promptly and aggressively. Notify the health care provider immediately. Immediate treatment of status epilepticus includes:
  1. Establishing an airway (intubation may be necessary)
  2. Monitoring the patient's respiratory status carefully
  3. Administering oxygen
  4. Establishing an IV line and starting 0.9% saline infusion
  5. Drawing blood for arterial blood gas analysis and identifying metabolic, toxic, and other causes of uncontrolled seizures
  6. Administering drugs such as IV lorazepam (Ativan, Apo-Lorazepam) or possibly diazepam (Valium) to stop motor movement, followed by phenytoin (Dilantin) or fosphenytoin (Cerebyx) to prevent recurrence. General anesthesia may be used as a last resort to stop the seizure activity.
  7. Monitoring vital signs every 15 minutes or more frequently until the patient's condition stabilizes

❗ NURSING SAFETY PRIORITY: Critical Rescue

Ensure that oxygen and suction are available at the bedside of any patient who is at risk for seizure activity. Maintaining oxygen/gas exchange can prevent brain injury during a seizure.

Surgical Management

- Several procedures may be performed when traditional methods fail to maintain seizure control.
  1. Vagal nerve stimulation involves surgically implanting a vagal nerve–stimulating device below the left clavicle to control partial seizures.
  2. Corpus callosotomy involves severing the corpus callosum to prevent neuronal discharges from passing through the two hemispheres of the brain. It is used to treat tonic-clonic or atonic seizures.
  3. Other procedures may be performed, including anterior temporal lobe resection for complex partial seizures of temporal

origin, cortical resection, and removal of part or all of a cerebral hemisphere.

- Perioperative care is as outlined in Part One, with the addition of assessing neurologic status with vital signs postoperatively.

Community-Based Care

- Health teaching includes:
  1. The importance of taking all drugs consistently as prescribed and monitoring for effects and side effects; dosage or effectiveness may change over time or with the occurrence of comorbid conditions
  2. The importance of not taking any herbal remedies or over-the-counter (OTC) drugs without notifying the health care provider; antiseizure medications have multiple and serious drug-drug and drug-herb interactions
  3. Components of a balanced diet and the effects of alcohol (alcohol should be avoided)
  4. The role of rest, time management, and stress management in health promotion
  5. The utility of keeping a seizure diary to determine whether there are factors that tend to be associated with seizure activity
  6. Restrictions (if any), such as driving or operating dangerous equipment and participating in certain physical activities or sports
  7. The importance of follow-up visits with the health care provider
  8. The value of wearing a medical alert bracelet or necklace
- Inform the patient that state laws prohibit discrimination against people who have epilepsy.
- Refer the patient to the state Vocational Rehabilitative Services, Epilepsy Foundation of America, National Epilepsy League, National Association to Control Epilepsy, and local support groups.

SEVERE ACUTE RESPIRATORY SYNDROME

OVERVIEW

- Severe acute respiratory syndrome (SARS) is a respiratory infection with a high mortality rate, caused by a new coronavirus known as *SARS-CoV,* which is highly contagious.
- The manifestations of SARS are the same as those of any respiratory infection and include fever, cough, and dyspnea with potential for rapid progression to respiratory failure.
- Diagnosis is made by the manifestations and the use of a rapid SARS test that detects SARS-CoV RNA in the blood.
- Interventions include quarantine or isolation and support with oxygen and bronchodilators.

SHOCK

OVERVIEW

- Shock is a widespread abnormal cellular metabolism that occurs when oxygenation and tissue perfusion are not sufficient to maintain cell function. All body organs are affected by shock.
- Any problem that impairs oxygen delivery to tissues and organs can start the condition of shock and lead to a life-threatening emergency.
- Shock is classified as one of four types, and more than one type may be present.
  1. *Hypovolemic shock* occurs when too little circulating blood volume causes a decrease in perfusion so that the body's total need for oxygen is not met. Common problems leading to hypovolemic shock are hemorrhage (external or internal) and dehydration.
  2. *Cardiogenic shock* occurs when the heart muscle is unhealthy and pumping is impaired. Heart failure from myocardial infarction (MI) is the most common cause of cardiogenic shock.
  3. *Distributive shock* occurs when blood volume is not lost from the body but is distributed to the interstitial tissues, where it cannot circulate and deliver oxygen. It has several origins, including:
     a. In neural-induced distributive shock, sympathetic nerve impulses controlling smooth muscle in blood vessels are disrupted, causing widespread vasodilation.
     b. Chemical-induced distributive shock occurs when certain chemicals or foreign substances within the blood and blood vessels initiate widespread changes in blood vessel walls. Common conditions leading to this type of shock include:
        (1) Anaphylaxis after exposure to a specific allergen in a susceptible person, which results in widespread loss of blood vessel tone and decreased cardiac output
        (2) Sepsis resulting from widespread infection, which triggers a whole-body inflammatory response when pathologic microorganisms are present in the blood (also called *septic shock*)
        (3) Capillary leak syndrome, which is the response of capillaries to the presence of biologic chemicals (mediators) that change blood vessel integrity and allow fluid to leak from the blood in the vascular space into the interstitial tissues. Once in the interstitial tissue, these fluids are stagnant and not able to deliver oxygen or

remove tissue waste products. Problems causing fluid shifts include severe burns, liver disorders, ascites, peritonitis, paralytic ileus, severe malnutrition, large wounds, hyperglycemia, kidney disease, hypoproteinemia, and trauma.

4. *Obstructive shock* occurs when the normal heart muscle is prevented from pumping effectively. The heart itself remains normal, but conditions outside the heart prevent adequate filling of the heart or adequate contraction of the healthy heart muscle. Common causes of obstructive shock are pericarditis and cardiac tamponade.

- Although the causes and initial manifestations associated with the different types of shock vary, eventually the effects of hypotension and anaerobic cellular metabolism result in the common key features:
  1. Cardiovascular manifestations
     a. Decreased cardiac output
     b. Decreased systolic blood pressure and mean arterial pressure (MAP)
     c. Narrowed pulse pressure
     d. Postural hypotension
     e. Slow capillary refill in nail beds and reduced peripheral pulses
  2. Respiratory manifestations
     a. Increased respiratory rate
     b. Shallow depth of respirations
     c. Decreased Pao_2 or Spo_2
  3. Neuromuscular manifestations
     a. Early
        (1) Anxiety and restlessness
        (2) Increased thirst
     b. Late
        (1) Lethargy to coma
        (2) Generalized muscle weakness
        (3) Sluggish pupillary response to light
     c. Kidney manifestations
        (1) Decreased and concentrated urine output
  4. Skin and mucous membrane manifestations
     a. Cool, pale, mottled, or cyanotic changes
- Hypovolemic shock
  1. The basic problem of hypovolemic shock is a loss of blood volume from the vascular space, causing a decreased MAP and reduced oxygen-carrying capacity from the loss of circulating red blood cells (RBCs).
  2. These problems decrease tissue perfusion and oxygenation, leading to anaerobic cellular metabolism.

S

3. The most common problems leading to hypovolemic shock are hemorrhage (external or internal) and dehydration.
4. Uncorrected hypovolemic shock progresses in four stages as poor cellular oxygenation continues.
   a. *Initial stage of shock (early shock)* occurs when the patient's baseline MAP is decreased by less than 10 mm Hg. Adaptive (compensatory) mechanisms are effective at returning MAP to normal levels, and oxygenated blood flow to all vital organs is maintained. Heart and respiratory rates are increased from the patient's baseline level, or a slight increase in diastolic blood pressure may be the only objective manifestation.
   b. *Nonprogressive stage (compensatory stage)* occurs when MAP decreases by 10 to 15 mm Hg from baseline. Kidney and hormonal adaptive (compensatory) mechanisms are activated because cardiovascular adjustments alone are not enough to maintain MAP and supply needed oxygen to the vital organs. Tissue hypoxia occurs in the skin, GI tract, and kidney but is not great enough to cause permanent damage. The cellular effects of this stage are reversible if the problem is recognized and appropriate interventions are started.
   c. *Progressive stage of shock (intermediate stage)* occurs when there is a sustained decrease in MAP of more than 20 mm Hg from baseline. Adaptive (compensatory) mechanisms are functioning but can no longer deliver sufficient oxygen, even to vital organs. Some tissues have severe cell damage and die because of poor oxygenation and a buildup of toxic metabolites.
   d. *Refractory stage of shock (irreversible stage)* occurs when too much cell death and tissue damage results from too little oxygen reaching the tissues. Vital organs have overwhelming damage, the body can no longer respond effectively to interventions, and shock continues. Widespread release of toxic metabolites and destructive enzymes causes cell damage in vital organs to continue despite aggressive interventions, and multiple organ dysfunction syndrome (MODS) leads to death.

PATIENT-CENTERED COLLABORATIVE CARE
Assessment
- Obtain patient information about:
  1. Recent illness, trauma, procedures, or chronic health problems that may contribute to decreased intake, excessive output, or bleeding

2. Document:
   a. Volume of blood loss
   b. Swelling or skin discoloration that may indicate an internal hemorrhage
   c. Provide trend information about cardiovascular changes, particularly blood pressure, heart rate, and peripheral pulse quality
3. Include trends in systolic and mean arterial blood pressure and pulse pressure

! NURSING SAFETY PRIORITY: Action Alert

Changes in systolic blood pressure are not always present in the initial stage of shock and should not be used as the main indicator of shock presence or progression.

4. Record respiratory changes
   a. Increased rate
   b. Decreased depth
   c. Peripheral oxygenation (Spo_2)
5. Record and communicate kidney and urine changes
   a. Decreased urine output
   b. Increased urine specific gravity
6. Document skin perfusion changes
   a. Cool or clammy sensation
   b. Pallor or cyanosis, especially oral mucous membranes
   c. Slow or sluggish capillary refill
7. Recognize and communicate central nervous system (CNS) changes
   a. Decreasing alertness and LOC
   b. Restlessness or apprehension
   c. Decreasing orientation or cognition
8. Identify and communicate significant laboratory changes
   a. Decreased hematocrit and hemoglobin levels if shock is caused by hemorrhage
   b. Increased hematocrit, sodium, and BUN levels if shock is caused by dehydration or a fluid shift

Interventions for Hemorrhagic or Hypovolemic Shock
Nonsurgical Management
- Oxygen therapy is useful whenever shock is present. It can be delivered by mask, hood, nasal cannula, nasopharyngeal tube, endotracheal tube, or tracheostomy tube.
- Intravenous fluid resuscitation is initiated as prescribed.
  1. Crystalloid solutions are first-line treatment and include normal saline in lactated Ringer's.

2. If the patient is bleeding, anticipate infusing packed RBCs, plasma, plasma fractions, and clotting factors.
   a. Drug therapy is used when the patient does not respond to the replacement of fluid volume and blood products and can include intravenous vasoconstricting agents like norepinephrine (Levophed) and vasopressin.

- Additional nursing interventions include assessing the patient's response to therapy.
  1. Until shock is controlled, monitor the following every 30 to 60 minutes:
     a. Blood pressure, pulse pressure, and MAP
     b. Heart rate and pulse quality
     c. Skin and mucosal color
     d. Urine output
     e. LOC
     f. Respiratory rate and Spo_2

Surgical Management

- After a cause has been established, surgical intervention may be needed to correct the cause of shock. Such procedures include vascular repair or revision, surgical hemostasis of major wounds, closure of bleeding ulcers, and chemical scarring (chemical sclerosis) of varicosities.
- Sepsis and septic shock are a complex type of distributive shock that usually begins as a bacterial or fungal infection and progresses to a dangerous condition over a period of days.
- Sepsis is a widespread infection coupled with a general inflammatory response, known as *systemic inflammatory response syndrome* (SIRS), which is triggered when an infection escapes local control.
  1. When infection is confined to a local area it should not lead to sepsis and shock. In the person whose immune system and inflammatory responses are effective, the presence of organism invasion first starts a helpful, local response of inflammation to confine and eliminate the organism and to prevent the infection from becoming worse or widespread.
- When organisms and their toxins or endotoxins enter multiple organs or the bloodstream, the generalized inflammatory response contributes to extensive tissue and vascular changes that further impair oxygenation and tissue perfusion.
  1. WBCs produce many pro-inflammatory molecular messengers, leading to widespread immune system activation, vasodilation, and impaired perfusion to tissues.
  2. Microthrombi begin to form within the capillaries of some organs. The microthrombi increase the number of cells that are operating under anaerobic conditions, which results in the generation of more toxic metabolites.

3. Increased cell, tissue, and organ damage promotes additional inflammatory and immune response, leading to a cycle of poor oxygenation and tissue perfusion.

- The patient with SIRS and sepsis has a low-grade fever, mild hypotension, a urine output that is lower than expected for fluid intake, and an increased respiratory rate.
- These subtle manifestations indicate early sepsis and usually progress unless intervention occurs at this time:
  1. If early sepsis is identified and treated aggressively, the cycle of progression to septic shock is stopped and the outcome is good.
  2. If early sepsis is not identified and treated at this stage it usually progresses to severe sepsis, which is much harder to control.

SEPTIC SHOCK
- The amplified inflammatory response causes capillary leak, injures cells (especially endothelial cells of blood vessels), and increases cell metabolism.
- Damage to endothelial cells alters coagulation with the formation of even more small clots.
- Anaerobic metabolism continues and is manifested by lactic acidosis. Lactic acidosis is manifested with serum lactate levels above 2 mg/dL, and levels above 4 mg/dL are associated with death from septic shock.
- The hypoxic stress response triggers hyperglycemia. The more severe the response, the higher the blood glucose level.
- Septic shock is the stage of sepsis and SIRS in which multiple organ failure is evident and uncontrolled bleeding can occur. *Even with appropriate intervention, the death rate is very high.*

INTERVENTIONS TO PREVENT SEPSIS AND SEPTIC SHOCK
- Evaluate all patients for their risk for sepsis.
- Use aseptic technique during invasive procedures and when working with nonintact skin and mucous membranes in immunocompromised patients.
- Remove indwelling urinary catheters and IV access lines as soon as they are no longer needed.
- Assess vital signs often (at least twice per shift) for changes from baseline levels.
- Review laboratory data for changes associated with sepsis and septic shock.
  1. The hallmark of sepsis is leukocytosis (elevated WBCs), an increase in band neutrophils, and a detectable serum lactate level.
  2. Derangements in coagulation parameters (e.g., D-dimer, INR, aPTT) may also occur.

3. Elevated markers of kidney injury such as rising serum BUN or creatinine and decreased urine output may indicate shock from infection and inflammation.

MANAGEMENT OF SEPSIS AND SEPTIC SHOCK

- The health care team implements the sepsis resuscitation bundle by:
  1. Administering broad-spectrum antibiotics within 1 to 3 hours of suspected sepsis/septic shock
  2. Obtaining blood cultures before administering antibiotics unless this intervention delays antibiotic administration
  3. Administering IV fluids to maintain MAP greater than 65 mm Hg
     a. Institute IV delivery of 20 mL/kg of crystalloid fluids (or the colloid equivalent).
     b. If MAP is not 65 mm Hg after initial fluid resuscitation, start IV vasopressor therapy.
  4. Supporting respiratory effort and avoiding sustained hypoxemia with oxygen therapy
  5. Using central venous oxygen saturation ($Scvo_2$) of at least 70% or a mixed venous oxygen saturation (Svo_2) of at least 65% to monitor the effectiveness of therapy
  6. Using serum lactate to guide diagnosis and treatment of sepsis
  7. Obtaining procalcitonin (PCT) serum level; PCT shows a rapid elevation at early stages of bloodstream infection and decreases nearly as rapidly as bloodstream infections clear
  8. When septic shock is present, administering low-dose steroids (200 to 300 mg hydrocortisone IV daily in divided doses) in accordance with intensive care unit (ICU) protocol
  9. Administering insulin to maintain blood glucose levels 120 to 180 mg/dL

SICKLE CELL DISEASE AND TRAIT

OVERVIEW

- *Sickle cell disease* (SCD) is a genetic disorder that results in chronic anemia, pain, disability, organ damage, increased risk for infection, and early death.
- The disorder results in the formation of abnormal hemoglobin chains. SCD is an autosomal recessive trait. Inheritance of two sickle-type alleles results in 80% to 100% of hemoglobin formed as abnormal beta chains, known as *hemoglobin S (HbS)*.
- In *sickle cell trait,* one normal gene and one abnormal gene for hemoglobin are inherited, so that less than half of the hemoglobin chains produced are abnormal, resulting in mild manifestations of the disease.

- When RBCs having large amounts of HbS are exposed to decreased oxygen conditions, the abnormal beta chains contract and pile together within the cell, distorting the shape of the RBC, resulting in a sickle-shaped RBC. The distorted RBC is rigid, becomes "sticky" and fragile, and forms a clump that blocks blood flow.
- Episodes of vascular occlusion from sickled, clumped RBCs cause ischemia, leading to potential organ damage from anoxia and infarction. Episodes of severe sickling are called *crisis.*
- Conditions that cause sickling include hypoxia, dehydration, infections, venous stasis, pregnancy, alcohol consumption, high altitudes, low environmental or body temperatures, acidosis, strenuous exercise, and anesthesia.

PATIENT-CENTERED COLLABORATIVE CARE

Assessment
- Family history
- Previous crises, what led to the crises, severity, and usual treatments
- Onset of pain and events leading to current symptoms
- Symptoms or anemia from RBC destruction
- Potential organ damage (e.g., chronic kidney disease or acute kidney injury, heart failure, lung damage, cirrhosis/liver damage, joint swelling, bone necrosis, muscle damage, and open sores from poor skin perfusion and stroke or seizure) from occlusive events

Interventions
- Evaluate the presence of HbS in a newly diagnosed patient.
- Manage pain from ischemia; severe pain can cause/prolong crisis.
- Administer hydroxyurea (Droxia) to reduce sickling episodes and pain.
- Provide hydration by the oral or IV route to reduce the duration of pain episodes.
- Use oxygen therapy and optimize perfusion to prevent or minimize multiorgan dysfunction because of occlusion and ischemia during sickling episodes.
- Reduce the risk for infection because splanchnic injury can result in immunocompromise; consider reverse isolation precautions during crisis.
- Monitor vital signs, temperature, and other indicators of perfusion impairment regularly to detect early signs of organ damage.

SJÖGREN'S SYNDROME

- Sjögren's syndrome (SS) is a group of problems that often appear with other autoimmune disorders, typically rheumatoid arthritis or fibromyalgia. Inflammation and autoimmune responses obstruct certain secretory ducts and glands.

- Problems include dry eyes (sicca syndrome), dry mucous membranes of the nose and mouth (xerostomia), and vaginal dryness.
    1. Insufficient tears cause ulceration of the cornea. Other manifestations include blurred vision, burning and itching of the eyes, and thick mattering in the conjunctiva.
    2. Insufficient saliva decreases digestion of carbohydrates, promotes tooth decay, and increases the incidence of oral and nasal infections. Difficulty swallowing food, changes in taste sensation, nosebleeds, and upper respiratory infections may also occur.
    3. Vaginal dryness may cause pain during sexual intercourse and increase risk for infection.
- There is no cure, and management focuses on slowing the intensity and the progression of the disorder by suppressing immune and inflammatory responses.
- Dry eye and mouth symptoms may be managed with artificial tears and saliva.
- Use of water-soluble vaginal lubricants or moisturizers can increase patient comfort.

SKIN INFECTIONS

OVERVIEW

- Skin infections can be bacterial, viral, or fungal, but most are bacterial, caused by *Staphylococcus* or *Streptococcus* microorganisms.
- *Folliculitis* is a superficial infection involving only the upper portion of the follicle. It usually manifests as a raised, red rash with small pustules.
- *Furuncles* (boils) are deeper follicle infections with a large, sore-looking, raised bump that may or may not have a pustular "head" at its point.
- *Cellulitis* is a generalized infection and involves the deeper connective tissue.
- The major cause of bacterial skin infection is minor skin trauma.
- Viral skin infections are commonly caused by the herpes simplex virus (HSV) and include type I infections (common cold sore), type II infections (genital herpes), and herpes zoster (shingles) (see *Herpes, Genital*). Viral infections differ from bacterial infections in two ways.
    1. After the first infection, the virus remains in the body in a dormant state in the nerve ganglia, and the patient has no symptoms.
    2. Re-activation stimulates the virus to travel the pathways of sensory nerves to the skin, where lesions reappear.

- Many fungal infections also affect the skin
  1. Superficial dermatophyte infections include:
     a. Tinea pedis ("athlete's foot")
     b. Tinea manus (hands)
     c. Tinea cruris (groin, "jock itch")
     d. Tinea capitis (head)
     e. Tinea corporis (ringworm)
  2. *Candida albicans,* also known as *yeast infection,* is another common superficial fungal infection of skin and mucous membranes.
     a. Risk factors include immunosuppression, long-term antibiotic therapy, diabetes mellitus, and obesity.
     b. The incidence is higher in hot, humid climates.
     c. Infected skin (most often in skin folds such as under the breasts) has a moist, red, irritated appearance, usually with itching and burning.
- Prevention of skin infections, especially bacterial and fungal infections, involves avoiding the offending organism and good personal hygiene to remove the organism before infection can occur.

S

> **! NURSING SAFETY PRIORITY: Action Alert**
>
> Handwashing and not sharing personal items with others are the best ways to avoid contact with some of the most easily transmitted organisms.

PATIENT-CENTERED COLLABORATIVE CARE
Assessment
- Obtain patient information about:
  1. Recent history of skin trauma
  2. Living conditions, home sanitation, personal hygiene habits, and leisure or sport activities
  3. Whether fever and malaise are also present
  4. Lesion locations, especially skin folds, lips, mouth, or genital region
  5. History of similar lesions in the same location
  6. Presence of burning, tingling, or pain
  7. Recent contact with an infected person
  8. Whether the patient has ever had chickenpox or shingles
  9. Whether the patient has received Zostavax, the shingles prevention vaccine
  10. Social and environmental factors
      a. Direct contact with an infected person
      b. Personal hygiene practices

    c. Frequent contact with animals

    d. Type and frequency of athletic activities

- Assess for and document the condition of the skin, including local or general:
    1. Redness
    2. Warmth
    3. Edema
    4. Tenderness
    5. Pain
    6. Itching
    7. Stinging
    8. Location of areas of inflammation, rash, or infection
    9. Presence of:
        a. Blisters or vesicles
        b. Pustules
        c. Papules
        d. Scaling
        e. Single or multiple lesions

Interventions

- Most skin infections heal well with nonsurgical management, but surgery may be required if an infectious agent is present in deep tissue layers.
- Nursing interventions include:
    1. Skin care instructions
        a. Showering daily with soap; chlorhexidine gluconate showers or dilute bleach baths can reduce bacterial load
        b. Not squeezing any pustules or crusts but removing them gently
        c. Applying warm compresses twice a day to furuncles or areas of cellulitis
        d. Avoiding constricting garments that might rub the lesions
        e. Keeping the skin dry between treatments
        f. Positioning for optimal air circulation to the area
    2. Prevention of transmission
        a. Using handwashing and antimicrobial hand solutions to prevent cross-contamination
        b. Isolating the patient if infections are colonized with bacteria that is resistant to antibiotic therapy (e.g., *methicillin-resistant staphylococcus;* see *Multidrug-Resistant Organisms [MDRO]*).
        c. Teaching patients to avoid sharing personal items such as hairbrushes, articles of clothing, or footwear
        d. Teaching patients to avoid skin-to-skin and sexual contact when infectious skin lesions are present

- Drug therapy includes:
    1. Topical agents for superficial infections and mild bacterial infections
    2. Systemic antibiotic therapy for extensive infections, especially if fever or lymphadenopathy is present
    3. Antiviral agents such as acyclovir (Zovirax), valacyclovir (Valtrex), or famciclovir (Famvir)
    4. Antifungal agents such as ketoconazole (Nizoral) or fluconazole

SPINAL CORD INJURY

OVERVIEW

- As a result of spinal cord injury (SCI), losses of or decreases in motor function, sensation, reflex activity, and bowel and bladder function may occur.
- The extent of the injury can be classified as:
    1. *Complete* if the spinal cord is severed or damaged in a way that eliminates all innervation below the level of injury, and total motor and sensory loss occurs
    2. *Incomplete* (more common) if there is preservation of a mixed pattern of motor, sensory, and reflex function
- Cervical SCIs may result in specific syndromes
    1. Anterior cord injury is characterized by loss of motor function, pain, and temperature sensation below the level of the injury; sensations of touch, position, and vibration remain intact.
    2. Posterior cord injury is characterized by intact motor function and loss of vibratory sense, crude touch, and position sense.
    3. Central cord injury is characterized by loss of motor function that is more pronounced in the upper extremities than in the lower extremities.
- Complications of SCI include pressure ulcers, contractures, and deep vein thrombosis (DVT) or pulmonary emboli. Muscle spasticity and bone loss can occur over time.

PATIENT-CENTERED COLLABORATIVE CARE

Assessment

- Obtain information about:
    1. How the injury occurred and the probable mechanism of injury
    2. The patient's position immediately after the injury
    3. Symptoms that occurred after the injury and what changes have occurred since
    4. Prehospital rescue personnel should be questioned about:
        a. Problems encountered during the extrication and transport

    b. Type of immobilization devices used

    c. Medical treatment given at the scene

  5. Medical history, with particular attention to a history of arthritis of the spine, congenital deformities, osteoarthritis or osteomyelitis, cancer, previous back or spinal cord injury, and respiratory problems

- Assess for and document:

  1. Adequacy of airway, breathing, and circulation

  2. Vital signs and indication of hemorrhage or other non-CNS injury

---

! NURSING SAFETY PRIORITY: Critical Rescue

Monitor the patient at least hourly for:

- Severe bradycardia
- Severe hypotension

Notify the physician immediately if these symptoms occur, because this problem is an emergency. Neurogenic shock is treated symptomatically by restoring fluids to the circulating blood volume and providing supportive care to stabilize the patient.

---

  3. Indications of a head injury, such as a change in LOC, abnormal pupil size and reaction to light, and change in behavior or ability to respond to directions

  4. The presence of spinal shock. Spinal shock is characterized by complete but temporary loss of motor, sensory, reflex, and autonomic function that often lasts less than 48 hours but may continue for several weeks. Assessment of spinal shock includes:

    a. Evaluate motor strength, comparing bilateral movement, the ability to shrug the shoulders, flex and extend the arms, elevate the arms and legs off the bed, extend the wrist, wiggle the toes, and flex and extend the feet and legs; and deep tendon reflexes.

    b. Evaluate sensation, comparing bilaterally and documenting decreased or absent tactile sensation.

    c. Evaluate cardiovascular dysfunction such as bradycardia, hypotension, and cardiac dysrhythmias.

  5. Change in thermoregulatory capacity, with the patient's body tending to assume the temperature of the environment (hypothermia)

  6. Breathing problems resulting from an interruption of spinal innervation to the respiratory muscles, assessing for atelectasis and/or pneumonia symptoms; *patients with injuries at or*

above T6 are especially at risk for respiratory complications and pulmonary embolus during the first 5 days after injury

7. Evaluation of the patient's abdomen for manifestations of internal bleeding, distention, or paralytic ileus; paralytic ileus is manifested by decreased or absent bowel sounds and distended abdomen, usually 72 hours or longer after injury

8. Bladder fullness and/or urinary tract infection. Autonomic dysfunction initially causes an areflexic (neurogenic) bladder (no reflex ability for bladder contraction), which later leads to urinary retention. The patient is at risk for UTI from an indwelling urinary catheter, intermittent catheterizations, or bladder distention, stasis, and/or overflow.

9. Coping strategies used in the past to deal with illness, difficult situations, or disappointments; initial hospitalization after SCI lasts for 3 or more months to include rehabilitation

Planning and Implementation

- The patient with an acute SCI has the following prioritized problems:

1. Risk for respiratory distress/failure related to aspiration or diaphragmatic denervation (e.g., impaired phrenic nerve impulses in patients with cervical injury)

2. Potential for cardiovascular instability related to loss or interruption of sympathetic innervation or hemorrhage

3. Potential for secondary spinal cord injury related to hypoperfusion, edema, or delayed spinal column stabilization

4. Impaired physical mobility related to spinal compression and edema

5. Spastic or flaccid bladder and bowel related to direct neurologic damage or disruption in nerve impulses

6. Risk for compromised resilience from injury requiring the need for life change

❗ NURSING SAFETY PRIORITY: Critical Rescue

Assess breath sounds every 2 to 4 hours during the first few days after injury and document and report any adventitious or diminished sounds. Monitor vital signs carefully, and watch for changes in respiratory pattern, effort, and secretions. Note also tachycardia, bradycardia, and changes in LOC with respiratory evaluation.

- There is a potential for further spinal cord injury related to swelling and/or fractures.

1. Immobilize the fracture to prevent further damage to the spinal cord from bone fragments. Skeletal traction (e.g., halo fixator) may be used.

2. Log roll the patient to avoid an in-bed position that bends the spine. Use reverse Trendelenburg position to elevate the head rather than pillows or back rest elevation.
3. Anticipate surgery to reduce or repair vertebral fractures.

- The patient with an established SCI is at risk for pressure ulcers, contractures, venous thromboembolism (DVT and/or pulmonary embolus), and fractures related to osteoporosis. Patients with high SCIs are also at risk for orthostatic hypotension.
  1. Provide safe, effective positioning and re-positioning.
  2. Use pressure-relieving devices, implementing pressure ulcer prevention strategies at all times.
  3. Assist with slow transitions to upright posture, especially after a period of supine positioning.
- The patient may have spastic or flaccid bladder and bowel related to direct neurologic damage or disruption in nerve impulses.
  1. The type of bladder emptying program depends on the usual elimination pattern and whether the injury involved upper motor neurons (UMNs) or lower motor neurons (LMNs).
  2. Use a bedside bladder ultrasound device to measure bladder residual and determine effectiveness of bladder emptying strategies.
  3. Teach the patient that the essential elements of a bowel program include stool softeners, increased fluid intake (unless medically contraindicated), high-fiber diet, and a consistent time for elimination.
  4. Evaluate for UTI, particularly foul-smelling urine; the SCI patient may not develop flank pain, urgency, frequency, or other signs of UTI.

❗ NURSING SAFETY PRIORITY: Critical Rescue

Observe the patient with an upper SCI (above the level of T6) for signs of autonomic dysreflexia (hyperreflexia). Although it does not occur often, autonomic dysreflexia is an excessive, uncontrolled sympathetic output. It is characterized by severe hypertension, bradycardia, severe headache, nasal stuffiness, and flushing. The cause of this syndrome is a noxious stimulus, usually a distended bladder or constipation. *This is a neurologic emergency and must be treated promptly to prevent a hypertensive stroke.*

- Treatment of autonomic dysreflexia includes:
  1. Consideration of contacting the Rapid Response Team
  2. Raising the head of the bed to a high Fowler's position
  3. Loosening tight clothing

4. Checking the urinary drainage system (if present) for kinks or obstruction
5. Checking for bladder distention and catheterizing immediately if a urinary catheter is not in place,
6. Checking the patient for fecal impaction and, if present, disimpacting immediately using anesthetic ointment
7. Checking the room temperature to ensure that it is not too cool or drafty
8. Monitoring blood pressure every 15 minutes; hypertension may be treated with nitrates or hydralazine

- The patient may experience impaired adjustment related to disability, requiring the need for life change.
  1. Help to set and reinforce realistic goals for managing self-care while promoting independence and decision making daily.
  2. Provide opportunities for emotional and spiritual support.
  3. Collaborate with the case manager or discharge planner for a review of the patient's insurance and financial status.
- Drug therapy during the acute phase may include:
  1. Methylprednisolone (Solu-Medrol)
  2. IV fluids and vasopressors to maintain a MAP greater than 70 mm Hg.
- Drug therapy for chronic SCI may include treatments to manage the effects of prolonged immobility and denervation of the motor system.
  1. Dantrolene (Dantrium) or baclofen (Lioresal) to treat spasticity
  2. Drugs to prevent osteoporosis and abnormal bony overgrowth associated with disuse
  3. Drugs to prevent VTE
  4. Drugs to promote regular bowel evacuation

Community-Based Care

- Discharge planning: Most patients are discharged to a rehabilitation setting, where they learn processes to enable self-care, mobility, and bladder and bowel management.
  1. Psychosocial adaptation is a crucial factor in determining the success of rehabilitation.
     a. Assist the patient to verbalize feelings and fears about body image, self-concept, role performance, and self-esteem.
     b. Talk to the patient about the expected reactions of those outside the hospital environment.
- To prepare for discharge to home or for a weekend home visit:
  1. Collaborate with the patient, family, case manager, and rehabilitation professionals to assess the home environment to ensure that it is free from hazards and can accommodate the patient's special needs.

  2. Ensure that the patient can correctly use all adaptive devices ordered for home use.
  3. Ensure that adaptive equipment is installed in the home before discharge.
- Teach the patient and family, in collaboration with health care team members:
  1. Mobility and self-management skills
  2. Bowel and bladder program
  3. Drug regimen
  4. Pressure ulcer prevention strategies
  5. Sexual functioning

STENOSIS, AORTIC
OVERVIEW
- The most common cause of aortic stenosis (AS) is age ("wear and tear"). Other causes include congenital bicuspid valves and mitral valve disease.
- In AS the aortic valve opening narrows, obstructing left ventricular outflow (afterload) during systole, resulting in left ventricle hypertrophy and heart failure.
- As stenosis progresses cardiac output becomes fixed and unable to meet the demands of the body during exertion and symptoms of angina, dyspnea, and syncope develop.

Considerations for Older Adults

Atherosclerosis and degenerative calcification of the aortic valve are the predominant causative factors in people older than 70 years. Aortic stenosis has become the most common valvular disorder in countries with an aging population.

PATIENT-CENTERED COLLABORATIVE CARE
- Assess for and document:
  1. Dyspnea, angina, and syncope on exertion
  2. Systolic crescendo-decrescendo murmur
  3. Dysrhythmias and signs of left heart failure: fatigue and pulmonary edema
- Aortic valve surgery is the treatment of choice when the patient is symptomatic with AS.
  1. Balloon valvuloplasty may be performed to enlarge the valve opening. A catheter inserted through the femoral artery is advanced to the aortic valve where the balloon is inflated then removed.
  2. Transcatheter aortic valve replacement procedures place a bioprosthetic valve using a catheter inserted from the femoral or other arterial route.

! **NURSING SAFETY PRIORITY: Action Alert**

After valvuloplasty observe the patient closely for bleeding from the catheter insertion site and institute post-angiogram precautions. Bleeding is likely because of the large size of the catheter. Assess for signs of a regurgitant valve by closely monitoring heart sounds, cardiac output, and heart rhythm. Because vegetation (thrombi) may have been dislodged from the valve, observe for any indication of systemic emboli.

3. In aortic valve replacement surgery, the valve is excised during cardiopulmonary bypass surgery and replaced with a prosthetic (synthetic) or biologic (tissue) valve.
- The postoperative patient requires lifetime anticoagulation therapy to prevent thrombus formation on the replacement valve.
- Perioperative care reflects the best practices outlined in Part One and is similar to patients having other open heart/heart-lung bypass procedures such as coronary artery bypass surgery, including pain management, incisional care, prevention of respiratory complications, and monitoring for excessive bleeding or clotting.

STENOSIS, MITRAL
OVERVIEW
- Mitral stenosis usually results from rheumatic carditis or congenital cardiac anomalies.
- Valve leaflets fuse together, becoming stiff; the chordae tendineae contract and shorten; the valve opening narrows, preventing normal blood flow from the left atrium to the left ventricle; and as a result, the left atrial pressure rises, the left ventricle dilates, pulmonary artery pressures increase, and the right ventricle hypertrophies.
- Pulmonary congestion and right-sided heart failure occur; later, preload is decreased and cardiac output declines.

PATIENT-CENTERED COLLABORATIVE CARE
Assessment
- Assess for and document:
  1. Changes in respiratory patterns: orthopnea, dyspnea with exertion, paroxysmal nocturnal dyspnea, cough
  2. Symptoms of right ventricular failure: hepatomegaly, neck vein distention, peripheral pitting edema
  3. Symptoms of left ventricular failure that occur later in disease progression: pulmonary edema, S_3 heart sound, crackles in lungs, frothy sputum

4. Atrial fibrillation resulting from right atrial hypertrophy
5. Rumbling, apical diastolic murmur
6. A history of rheumatic fever

Interventions

- Mitral valve repair or replacement surgery is the treatment of choice for symptomatic mitral valve stenosis.
    1. Balloon valvuloplasty, an invasive nonsurgical procedure, involves passing a balloon catheter from the femoral vein through the atrial septum to the mitral valve. The balloon is inflated to enlarge the mitral orifice.
    2. Mitral commissurotomy is performed during cardiopulmonary bypass surgery. The surgeon removes thrombi from the atria, incises the fused commissures (leaflets), and débrides calcium from the leaflets, thus widening the orifice.
    3. Mitral annuloplasty is a reconstruction and repair of the valve leaflets and the valve ring that attaches to the leaflets
    4. Mitral valve replacement is indicated if the leaflets are calcified and immobile. The valve is excised during cardiopulmonary bypass surgery, and a new valve is sutured into place.
- The postoperative patient requires lifetime anticoagulant therapy to prevent the formation of a thrombus on the valve.
- Perioperative care reflects the best practices outlined in Part One and is similar to patients having other open heart/heart-lung bypass procedures such as coronary artery bypass surgery.
    1. Observe for signs of reduced cardiac output or a regurgitant valve by closely monitoring for change in the quality of a murmuring heart sound, heart rhythm, reduced urine output, decreased cognition, or other signs of decreased perfusion.
    2. Anticipate the need for increased vigilance and more frequent interventions (such as deep-breathing exercises and use of incentive spirometer) since mitral stenosis leads to respiratory system changes similar to those caused by pulmonary hypertension and emphysema.
    3. Observe for signs of vascular occlusion (reduced peripheral pulses, stroke, and acute coronary syndrome) from emboli while establishing anticoagulation therapy.

Community-Based Care

- Provide health teaching information regarding:
    1. Drugs, especially anticoagulant therapy
    2. Plan of work, activity, and rest to conserve energy
    3. The potential need for an antibiotic before invasive procedures (e.g., dental work, surgery)

❗ NURSING SAFETY PRIORITY: Drug Alert

Heparin and warfarin (Coumadin) are two drugs commonly associated with significant errors in administration. Be especially vigilant in verifying the correct patient, dose, route, time of administration, and drug concentration when giving these powerful drugs.

❗ NURSING SAFETY PRIORITY: Critical Rescue

Patients with mitral stenosis often have pulmonary hypertension and stiff lungs. Therefore monitor respiratory status closely during weaning from the ventilator. Be especially alert for bleeding in patients following aortic valve replacements because of a higher risk for postoperative hemorrhage. *If heart rate or blood pressure decreases, call the Rapid Response Team or other health care provider immediately.*

STENOSIS, RENAL ARTERY

- Renal artery stenosis involves narrowing of the lumen and reduced blood flow to the kidney tissues. Uncorrected stenosis leads to ischemia and atrophy of kidneys.
- Renal artery stenosis is suspected when a sudden onset of hypertension occurs. Low renal blood flow from stenosis results in neurohormonal changes (such as activation of the renin-angiotensin-aldosterone system) that elevate blood pressure in a compensatory response to improve renal blood flow.
- Pathology may be fibrotic, atherosclerotic, or both.
- Treatment includes:
  1. Antihypertensive drugs
  2. Percutaneous transluminal balloon angioplasty or stent placement in the renal artery
  3. Renal artery bypass surgery

STOMATITIS

- Stomatitis is a broad term that refers to inflammation within the oral cavity that impairs the protective lining of the mouth.
- It can result from infection, allergy, vitamin deficiency, systemic disease, and irritants like tobacco and alcohol.
- Primary stomatitis includes noninfectious aphthous ("canker sores"), infection from herpes simplex, and traumatic insults.
- Secondary stomatitis results from infection by opportunistic viruses, fungi, or bacteria in patients who are immunocompromised.
- The patient is instructed to:
  1. Use a soft-bristled brush to gently clean teeth, gums, and the oral cavity.

2. Rinse the mouth often with sodium bicarbonate solution, warm saline, or hydrogen peroxide solution. Avoid alcohol-based commercial mouthwashes.
3. Take drugs (antimicrobials, immune modulators, and symptomatic topical agents) as prescribed.
4. Use topical agents (with benzocaine or lidocaine) and diet modification (avoid salty, spicy, acidic, and other irritating foods) to control pain and promote healing.

STROKE (BRAIN ATTACK)

OVERVIEW

- Stroke is caused by an interruption of perfusion to any part of the brain. The National Stroke Association uses the term *brain attack* to describe a stroke to convey the urgency for activation of the emergency medical system for care.
- A stroke is a medical emergency that strikes suddenly, and it should be treated immediately to prevent neurologic deficit and permanent disability.
- Strokes may be classified as:
  1. *Acute ischemic stroke,* which is caused by the occlusion of a cerebral artery; types of ischemic strokes include:
     a. A *thrombotic stroke* is commonly associated with the development of atherosclerosis of the blood vessel wall. Rupture of one or more atherosclerotic plaque exposes foam cells to clot-promoting elements in the blood. The result is clot formation. The artery becomes occluded, and blood flow to the area is markedly diminished, causing transient ischemia and then complete ischemia and infarction of brain tissue. Signs and symptoms occur over minutes to hours.
     b. A *lacunar stroke* is a type of thrombotic stroke that causes a soft area or cavity to develop in the white matter or deep gray matter of the brain.
     c. An *embolic stroke* is caused by a thrombus or group of thrombi that travel to the cerebral arteries through the carotid artery and block the artery, resulting in ischemia. Sudden and rapid development of focal neurologic deficits occurs. Cerebral hemorrhage may result if the vessel wall is damaged. Embolic strokes are associated with atrial fibrillation, coronary disease, and heart valve disease or repair.
     d. Ischemic stroke may be preceded by warning signs, including *transient ischemic attack* (TIA), a reversible neurologic deficit such as vertigo or blurred vision that lasts a few minutes to fewer than 24 hours
  2. *Hemorrhagic stroke,* in which the integrity of the vessel wall is interrupted and bleeding occurs into the brain tissue

(intracerebral) or spaces surrounding the brain (ventricular, subdural, subarachnoid); causes include hypertension, ruptured aneurysm, and arteriovenous malformation (AVM)

a. An *aneurysm* is an abnormal ballooning or blister on the involved artery that may become stretched or thinned and rupture.

b. *AVM* is a tangled or spaghetti-like mass of malformed, thin-walled, dilated vessels that form an abnormal communication between the arterial and venous systems.

c. *Vasospasm,* a sudden and periodic constriction of a cerebral artery, often results from a cerebral hemorrhage caused by aneurysm rupture. Blood flow to distal areas of the brain supplied by the artery is markedly diminished, leading to cerebral ischemia and infarction and further neurologic dysfunction.

PATIENT-CENTERED COLLABORATIVE CARE
Assessment

- Obtain patient information about:
  1. Time of symptom onset
  2. Progression and severity of symptoms, including the presence of a previous TIA
  3. LOC, orientation, and other measures of cognitive function
  4. Motor status: gait, balance, reading and writing abilities
  5. Sensory status: speech, hearing, vision
  6. Medical history with attention to identifying risk factors such as hypertension, hyperlipidemia, cardiovascular disease, diabetes, smoking, sedentary lifestyle, alcohol use, obesity, high fat diet, conditions that alter coagulation, and the presence of atrial fibrillation (dysrhythmia)
  7. Social history, with attention to identifying sources of support
  8. Current drugs and nonprescribed drugs, especially anticoagulants, aspirin, vasodilators, and illegal drugs
- Assess for and document:
  1. Neurologic function using a standard stroke screening tool such as the National Institutes of Health (NIH) Stroke Scale, including:
     a. LOC
     b. Orientation
     c. Motor ability
     d. Pupil size and reaction to light, extraocular movement, visual field deficits, ptosis (drooping eyelid)
     e. Speech and language
  2. Vital signs
  3. Blood glucose

4. Additional assessment includes:
    a. Cognition, memory, judgment, and problem-solving and decision-making abilities
    b. Ability to concentrate and attend to tasks
    c. Range of motion (ROM), proprioception, head and trunk control, balance, gait, coordination, bowel and bladder control
    d. Sensory status (response to touch and painful stimuli; ability to distinguish between two tactile stimuli presented simultaneously; ability to read, write, and follow verbal directions; and ability to name objects and use them correctly)
    e. Speech pattern (rhythm, clarity, aphasia)
    f. Visual system (homonymous hemianopsia, bitemporal hemianopsia, amaurosis fugax)
    g. Cranial nerve function
    h. Cardiac system (dysrhythmias and murmurs)
    i. Coping mechanisms or personality changes
5. Emotional lability and screen for depression
6. Nutritional status
7. Social support, financial status, and occupation
- Diagnostic tests
    1. CT scan of the head without contrast is performed within 30 minutes after arrival at the emergency department. This study is essential to determine patient eligibility for fibrinolytic therapy.
    2. Magnetic resonance imaging (MRI) and related multimodal imaging demonstrate ischemia earlier than CT scan and are used to identify the presence of hemorrhage or a cerebral aneurysm. Results also help differentiate stroke from other pathologic changes that mimic a stroke.
    3. CBC, serum electrolytes, and coagulation factors
    4. Carotid ultrasound
    5. ECG and echocardiography to determine whether cardiac disease or dysrhythmia is a contributing factor to stroke

PLANNING AND IMPLEMENTATION
Ineffective Cerebral Tissue Perfusion
Nonsurgical Management
- Management includes either fibrinolytic therapy or endovascular procedures.
- Monitor for neurologic changes or complications before, during, and after medical interventions.
    1. Perform a neurologic assessment at least every 2 to 4 hours, checking:
        a. Verbal ability, orientation
        b. Eye opening, pupil size, and reaction to light
        c. Motor response

2. Monitor vital signs with neurologic checks.
   a. Ask the physician for acceptable limits for blood pressure.

! NURSING SAFETY PRIORITY: Critical Rescue

Be alert for symptoms of increased intracranial pressure (ICP) and report any deterioration in the patient's neurologic status to the health care provider immediately. The first sign of increased ICP is a declining LOC.

3. Perform a cardiac assessment.
   a. Monitor the patient for dysrhythmias; auscultate the heart and palpate peripheral pulses to identify new irregular heart rhythms in the absence of a cardiac monitor.
4. Position the back rest to promote cerebral perfusion. In the presence of ischemic stroke, a flat back rest may be preferred initially.
5. Avoid activities that may increase ICP.
   a. Maintain the patient's head in a midline neutral position.
   b. Position the patient to avoid extreme hip or neck flexion.
   c. Avoid clustering of nursing procedures.
   d. Provide a quiet environment; room lights should be low.
   e. Assess the need for suctioning; hyperoxygenate the patient before suctioning.

- Drug therapy
  1. Fibrinolytic therapy may be used for an acute ischemic stroke.
     a. Recombinant tissue plasminogen activator (rtPA) may be given IV within 3 to 4.5 hours after the onset of symptoms.
        (1) Patients who have had a stroke or serious head trauma in the past 3 months, a hemorrhagic stroke, recent MI, increased partial thromboplastin time (PTT), anticoagulant therapy, or who are pregnant are not candidates for this therapy.
     b. Catheter-directed fibrinolytic therapy may be performed as an alternative treatment for up to 6 hours after initial symptoms.
  2. Anticoagulant therapy and antiplatelet therapy may be prescribed depending on the health care provider's preference.
     a. Obtain a baseline CBC, INR, and activated partial thromboplastin (aPTT) before initiating therapy.
     b. Oral drugs to manage ischemic stroke include aspirin and other antiplatelet drugs like clopidogrel and dabigatran or warfarin to prevent progression or future thrombotic and embolic strokes.

S

3. Other drugs used to treat symptoms associated with stroke include:
   a. Calcium channel blockers (nimodipine [Nimotop]), which may be administered to treat vasospasm or chronic spasm of the vessel that inhibits blood flow to the area
   b. Stool softeners, analgesics for pain, and antianxiety drugs
   c. Antihypertensives to maintain blood perfusion within prescribed limits

- Monitor the patient for complications such as:
  1. Vasospasm, or narrowing of the cerebral arteries, which leads to cerebral ischemia and infarction and is manifested by a decreased LOC, motor and reflex changes, and increased neurologic deficits (cranial nerve deficits, aphasia)
  2. Bleeding following fibrinolytic therapy or rebleeding with hemorrhagic stroke
  3. Bleeding caused by thrombolytic, anticoagulant, or antiplatelet therapy; observe for blood in the urine and stool, epistaxis (nosebleed), bleeding gums, and easy bruising
  4. Hydrocephalus-enlarged ventricles manifested by a change in the LOC, gait disturbances, and behavior changes
- Carotid artery angioplasty is a nonsurgical intervention used to treat certain types of ischemic stroke. A distal protection device may be placed beyond the stenosis to catch any debris that breaks off during the angioplasty or stenting procedure.

Surgical Management

- Two surgical procedures that may be used for ischemic stroke are:
  1. Carotid endarterectomy to remove atherosclerotic plaque from the inner lining of the carotid artery
  2. Extracranial-intracranial bypass to bypass the occluded area and re-establish blood flow to the affected area
- Surgical and interventional radiologic procedures to treat intracranial aneurysm or AVM are:
  1. Surgical ligation or resection, removing involved vessels through sterotactic, gamma knife, or conventional approaches
  2. Placing a clip to clamp the base or neck of an aneurysm
  3. Placing a coil under fluoroscopy with either stent or balloon assist
  4. Creating flow diversion with stentlike devices delivered under fluoroscopy
  5. Using liquid polymer embolization, generally prior to surgical ligation
- The nursing care for these procedures is similar to that discussed in *Perioperative Care* (Part One) including neurologic assessment with vital signs.

IMPAIRED SWALLOWING
- Nursing interventions include:
  1. Initiating aspiration precautions
  2. Before feeding, assessing the patient's ability to swallow using an evidence-based tool
     a. Observe for facial drooping, drooling, impaired voluntary cough, hoarseness, incomplete mouth closure, or cranial nerve palsies.
     b. A runny nose may also indicate impaired swallowing with saliva discharged through the nasal passages.
     c. Next check the gag and cough reflex.
  3. Positioning the patient to facilitate swallowing
     a. Place the patient in a chair or sitting straight up in bed.
     b. Position the patient's head and neck slightly forward and flexed.
  4. Providing soft or semisoft foods and thickened fluids (e.g., mechanical soft, dental diet; custards, scrambled eggs)
  5. Maintaining a quiet room with few distractions while the patient is eating
  6. Providing nutritional supplementation if needed
  7. Encouraging family members to participate in mealtimes and feeding
  8. Weighing the patient twice a week
  9. Consultation with speech pathology specialist for additional evaluation

IMPAIRED PHYSICAL MOBILITY AND SELF-CARE DEFICITS
- Nursing care includes:
  1. Performing ROM exercises and progressing to chair and ambulation
  2. Consulting with the physical therapist and occupational therapist to evaluate strength and ability, promote mobility, and evaluate for discharge placement
  3. Carefully positioning the patient in proper body alignment using a splint or brace if needed
  4. Using sequential compression devices or pneumatic compression boots to prevent VTE when limited mobility is present
  5. Monitoring the patient for signs of VTE and iatrogenic pneumonia
  6. Supporting nutritional intake

APHASIA OR DYSARTHRIA
- Interventions to help the patient with impaired speech to develop communication strategies include:
  1. Presenting one idea or thought in a sentence (e.g., "I am going to help you get into the chair.")
  2. Using simple one-step commands rather than asking patients to do multiple tasks

3. Speaking slowly but not loudly; using cues or gestures as needed
4. Avoiding "yes" and "no" questions for patients with expressive aphasia, because they often give automatic responses that may be incorrect
5. Using alternative forms of communication if needed, such as a computer, communication board, or flash cards (often with pictures)
6. Collaborating with the speech-language pathologist or therapist

BOWEL AND BLADDER INCONTINENCE

• Interventions to help the patient become continent include:
1. Establishing the type (bowel or bladder) and cause of the problem
   a. Altered LOC
   b. Impaired innervation
   c. Inability to communicate the need to urinate or defecate
2. Determining the patient's usual voiding or bowel movement pattern
3. Implementing an individualized bladder training program (see *Urinary Incontinence*)
   a. Place the patient on a bedpan or commode every 2 hours; encourage fluid intake to 2000 mL daily unless contraindicated.
   b. Use an intermittent catheterization program if retraining is not feasible.
4. Implementing an individualized bowel training program
   a. Determine the normal time or routine for bowel elimination.
   b. Place the patient on a bedpan or commode at the same time each day; use a suppository or stool softener, if needed.
   c. Provide a diet high in bulk or fiber (may require consultation with a nutritionist).

SENSORY CHANGES

• Nursing interventions include:
1. Providing frequent verbal and tactile cues to help the patient perform activities of daily living (ADLs)
2. Breaking down tasks into small steps when cueing
3. Approaching the patient from the nonaffected side
4. Placing objects within the patient's field of vision
5. Placing a patch over the affected eye if diplopia is present
6. Removing clutter from the room
7. Orienting the patient to time, place, and event with each encounter
8. Providing a structured, repetitious, and consistent routine or schedule
9. Presenting information in a clear, simple, concise manner

10. Using a step-by-step approach
11. Placing pictures and other familiar objects in the room

UNILATERAL NEGLECT

- Interventions include:
  1. Teaching the patient to use both sides of the body
  2. Teaching the patient to scan with the eyes and turn the head from side to side

Community-Based Care

- Provide a detailed plan of care at the time of discharge for patients to be transferred to a rehabilitation center or long-term care facility.
- If possible, a case manager should be assigned to help coordinate plans for the patient discharged to the home setting. The case manager should collaborate with the home health agency and with physical and occupational therapists to:
  1. Identify and suggest corrections of hazards in the home before discharge.
  2. Ensure that the patient and family can correctly use all adaptive devices ordered for home use.
  3. Arrange follow-up appointments as needed.
- Discharge teaching includes:
  1. Providing drug information as needed
  2. Reinforcing mobility skills (in collaboration with other therapists) such as:
     a. How to safely climb stairs, transfer from bed to chair, and get into and out of a car
     b. How to use adaptive equipment
  3. Teaching the family that depression and emotional lability may occur
     a. Depression is usually self-limited; antidepressants may be needed.
     b. Advise the family to avoid being overprotective.
     c. Assist the family and patient to develop realistic and achievable goals.
- Depending on the location of the stroke, the patient may be anxious, slow, cautious, hesitant, or impulsive; may lack initiative; or may be seemingly unaware of the deficit.
- Refer the family to a social worker for further support and counseling. Family members may need a referral for respite care.
- Provide the patient and family with information (including written materials) about ongoing therapy that alters coagulation.

SUBCLAVIAN STEAL

- Subclavian steal occurs in the upper extremities from a subclavian artery occlusion or stenosis and results in altered blood flow and ischemia in the arm.

QSEN TEAMWORK AND COLLABORATION

Hand-off errors lead to patient harm. Be sure that clear, consistent communication and complete documentation are available when the patient transfers between in-hospital care units or procedural suites or to rehabilitative or home care.

- The disorder can occur at any age but is more common when the patient also has risk factors for atherosclerosis.
- Assess for:
  1. Paresthesias
  2. Light-headedness
  3. Dizziness
  4. Pain and discomfort when the arms are elevated
  5. Difference in blood pressure between arms
  6. Subclavian bruit or decreased pulse on the occluded side
  7. Edema, redness or cyanosis, and delayed capillary refill of the affected arm
- Surgical intervention involves one of three procedures.
  1. Endarterectomy of the subclavian artery
  2. Carotid-subclavian bypass
  3. Dilation of the subclavian artery

SYNDROME OF INAPPROPRIATE ANTIDIURETIC HORMONE

OVERVIEW

- Syndrome of inappropriate antidiuretic hormone (SIADH) occurs when antidiuretic hormone (ADH; also known as vasopressin) is secreted even when plasma osmolarity is low or normal.
- Water is retained, which results in dilutional hyponatremia (a decreased serum sodium level) and expansion of the extracellular fluid volume.
- SIADH occurs with many pathologic conditions and some drugs, including:
  1. Malignancies: associated with small cell lung cancer; pancreatic, duodenal, and genitourinary carcinomas; thymoma; and Hodgkin's lymphoma and non-Hodgkin's lymphoma
  2. Pulmonary disorders: pneumonia, lung abscesses, active tuberculosis, pneumothorax, and chronic lung diseases
  3. CNS disorders: brain trauma, infection, tumors, and strokes
  4. Drugs: selective serotonin reuptake inhibitors, quinolone antibiotics, some antiepileptics, and opioids

PATIENT-CENTERED COLLABORATIVE CARE
Assessment
- Obtain patient information about:
  1. Recent head injury or brain trauma
  2. Cerebrovascular disease or stroke
  3. Tuberculosis, pneumonia, or other pulmonary disease
  4. Cancer
  5. All past and current drug use
  6. Loss of appetite, nausea, and vomiting
  7. Recent weight gain
- Assess for fluid overload, electrolyte derangements, pulmonary edema, and heart failure.
  1. Increased pulse quality
  2. Increasing neck vein distention
  3. Presence of crackles in lungs
  4. Increasing peripheral edema
  5. Altered serum sodium, potassium, calcium, phosphate, and magnesium levels
  6. Reduced and concentrated urine output
  7. Lethargy or decreased mental status
  8. Hyponatremia and hypo-osmolarity, leading to neurological or neuromuscular changes

! NURSING SAFETY PRIORITY: Critical Rescue

Pulmonary edema can occur very quickly and can lead to death. Notify the health care provider about any change that indicates the fluid overload from SIADH is not responding to therapy or is becoming worse.

Interventions
- Fluid restriction
  1. Intake may be restricted to 500 to 1000 mL/24 hr.
  2. Use saline to irrigate and dilute medications when using an enteral or gastric tube.
- Assess therapy for fluid excretion and sodium replacement.
  1. Measure intake and output; anticipate output goal greater than intake.
  2. Weigh the patient daily.
  3. Monitor serum sodium and osmolarity.
- Drug therapy may include:
  1. Administering ADH antagonists to promote water loss without urinary sodium excretion: tolvaptan (oral) (Samsca) or conivaptan (IV) (Vaprisol)
  2. Using loop diuretics if heart failure results from fluid overload

> **! NURSING SAFETY PRIORITY: Drug Alert**
>
> Administer tolvaptan or conivaptan only in the hospital setting, so serum sodium levels can be monitored closely for the development of hypernatremia.

    3. Hypertonic saline (i.e., 3% sodium chloride [3% NaCl]) infusions

    4. Demeclocycline (Declomycin), an antibiotic with ADH antagonist properties

- Provide a safe environment when serum sodium is below 120 mEq/L.
  1. Initiate seizure precautions.
  2. Increase patient surveillance to prevent falls or harm during a period of disorientation.
- Include comfort measures during oral fluid restriction, including saliva substitute or stimulant.

SYPHILIS

OVERVIEW

- Syphilis is a complex sexually transmitted disease (STD) that can become systemic and can cause serious complications, including death.
- The causative organism is a spirochete called *Treponema pallidum.*
- Syphilis progresses through four stages: primary, secondary, latent, and tertiary.
  1. In *primary syphilis* a chancre develops (typically within 3 weeks) at the site of entry (inoculation) of the organism. Without treatment the chancre disappears within 6 weeks; however, the organism spreads throughout the body, and the patient is highly infectious.
  2. *Secondary syphilis* develops 6 weeks to 6 months after the onset of primary syphilis. Manifestations are typical of systemic infections: fever, malaise, and generalized aches; and a rash, often manifested on palms and soles, that progresses to contagious pustules.
  3. *Latent syphilis* is a later stage of the disease and has two phases.
     a. *Early latent syphilis* occurs during the first year after infection, and infectious lesions can recur.
     b. *Late latent syphilis* is a disease occurring more than 1 year after infection. It is not infectious except to the fetus of a pregnant woman.
  4. *Tertiary syphilis,* or *late syphilis,* occurs after 4 to 20 years in untreated cases. Any organ system can be affected, and manifestations vary widely. Manifestations include benign lesions

(gummas) of the skin, mucous membranes, and bones; aortic valvular disease and aortic aneurysms; and neurosyphilis with CNS problems (e.g., meningitis, hearing loss, or generalized paresis).

PATIENT-CENTERED COLLABORATIVE CARE

* Diagnosis of primary or secondary syphilis is confirmed by a finding of *T. pallidum* on microscopic examination, by a positive Venereal Disease Research Laboratory (VDRL) serum test, or by a positive rapid plasma reagin (RPR) test result. Latent and tertiary syphilis may be confirmed by the fluorescent treponemal antibody absorption (FTA-ABS) test or the microhemagglutination assay for *T. pallidum* (MHA-TP).

Interventions

* Antibiotic therapy is the treatment for all stages of syphilis. A prolonged course of intravenous antibiotics for the late latent stage may be required.

! NURSING SAFETY PRIORITY: Drug Alert

Discuss with the patient the importance of partner notification and treatment, including the risk for re-infection if the partner goes untreated. All sexual partners must be prophylactically treated as soon as possible, preferably within 90 days of the syphilis diagnosis.

---

* Provide education about safe sex practices.
* It is essential to teach patient to follow up at 6, 12, and 24 months after initial treatment.
* Inform the patient that the disease will be reported to the local health authority and that all information will be held in strict confidence.
* Encourage the patient to provide accurate information for this follow-up to ensure that all at-risk partners are treated appropriately.
* Provide a setting that offers privacy and encourages open discussion.

SYSTEMIC LUPUS ERYTHEMATOSUS

OVERVIEW

* *Systemic lupus erythematosus* (SLE) is a chronic, progressive, inflammatory connective tissue disease that can cause major body organs and systems to fail.
* The main mechanism of organ damage is the formation of immune complexes in organ tissues and in blood vessels, which deprive the organ of essential oxygen.

- It is classified as an autoimmune disease and has periods of spontaneous remissions and exacerbations (flares) with a wide variation in symptoms. However, most patients with SLE have kidney involvement, because the immune complexes tend to aggregate in that system.
- *Discoid lupus erythematosus* (DLE) affects only the skin and is not as common as SLE.
- The cause is unknown, although like many autoimmune disorders, a genetic predisposition with environmental interactions is likely.

🌐 Cultural Considerations

Lupus affects women 10 times more often than men; women of color are affected far more often than Euro-Americans. The reason for this difference is unknown.

PATIENT-CENTERED COLLABORATIVE CARE
Assessment
- Assess for and document:
  1. Dry, scaly, raised rash on the face (butterfly rash) or upper body
  2. Individual round lesions (scarring lesions of discoid lupus)
  3. Joint involvement
     a. Initial changes are similar to rheumatoid arthritis.
     b. Later changes may include joint deformity.
  4. Muscle aches and atrophy
  5. Fever
  6. Various degrees of weakness, fatigue, anorexia, and weight loss
  7. Kidney insufficiency characterized by reduced urine output, proteinuria, hematuria, and fluid retention
  8. Pulmonary effusions or pneumonia
  9. Pericarditis (the most common cardiovascular change)
     a. Tachycardia
     b. Chest pain
     c. Myocardial ischemia
  10. Neurologic changes
     a. Psychoses
     b. Seizures
     c. Paresis
     d. Migraine headaches
     e. Cranial nerve palsies
  11. Raynaud's phenomenon or other manifestations of vasculitis
  12. Abdominal pain from peritoneal and blood vessel inflammation

13. Body image changes
14. Social isolation
15. Fear, anxiety
- Diagnostic tests include:
  1. Skin biopsy
  2. Positive blood tests for immune dysfunction and autoimmunity dysregulation
     a. Rheumatoid factor
     b. Antinuclear antibodies
     c. Erythrocyte sedimentation rate
     d. Serum complement
     e. Anti-SS-A (Ro), anti-SS-B (La), anti-Smith (anti-SM), anti-DNA, extractable nuclear antigens (ENA)
     f. Serum protein electrophoresis
  3. CBC showing pancytopenia
  4. Complete metabolic panel to evaluate kidney function
  5. Cardiac and liver enzymes

Interventions

- Drug therapy may include:
  1. Topical or oral steroid therapy
  2. Hydroxychloroquine (Plaquenil) to reduce inflammatory skin responses
  3. Immunosuppressive agents, such as methotrexate (Rheumatrex) or azathioprine (Imuran)
  4. Antineoplastic drugs, such as cyclophosphamide (Cytoxan, Procytox)
  5. Belimumab (Benlysta), an intravenous agent to reduce B-lymphocyte activity and the production of autoantibodies

❗ NURSING SAFETY PRIORITY: Action Alert

When patients are taking immunosuppressants or steroids, stress the importance of avoiding large crowds and people who are ill. Teach patients to report any early sign of infection to their health care provider. Observe for side effects and toxic effects of these drugs and report their occurrence immediately. Remind patients to take their medication early in the morning before breakfast because that is the time when the body's natural corticosteroid level is the lowest.

- Teach the patient how to protect the skin by:
  1. Minimizing exposure to sunlight and other forms of ultraviolet light by:
     a. Wearing long sleeves and wide-brimmed hats
     b. Using sun-blocking agents with a sun protective factor of at least 30

    2. Cleaning the skin with a mild soap and avoiding harsh, perfumed products

    3. Using moisturizers and sun protectants

    4. Using mild protein shampoo and avoiding hair bleaching agents, permanents, and dyes

- Reinforce measures for joint protection and energy conservation (see *Arthritis, Rheumatoid*).
- Help the patient identify coping strategies and support systems that can help him or her deal with the unpredictable nature of the exacerbations.
- Teach the patient about:
  1. Informing his or her provider at the onset of symptoms signaling exacerbation
  2. Monitoring for infection, particularly the onset of fever
  3. Protecting joints and conserving energy
  4. Risks related to pregnancy and for contraception options
  5. Resources such as the Lupus Foundation and the Arthritis Foundation
  6. Drug therapy information for scheduling, side effects, and any precautions

Planning and Implementation
- The priority for patient care is to provide supportive care by relieving symptoms, decreasing inflammation, and anticipating or treating complications. As for any patient, continually assess for and support the ABCs (airway, breathing, and circulation).

Acute Pain

Nonsurgical Management
- Diet therapy includes:
  1. Withholding food and fluids in the acute period; maintaining hydration with IV fluids
  2. Maintaining nasogastric (NG) intubation to decrease gastric distention and suppress pancreatic secretion
  3. Initiating nasojejunal enteral nutrition
  4. Assessing frequently for the presence of bowel sounds
- Drug therapy may include:
  1. Opioids such as morphine or hydromorphone, often with a patient-controlled analgesia (PCA) device
  2. Proton pump inhibitors or H_2-histamine receptor blockers to decrease gastric hydrochloric acid production during fasting
  3. Antibiotics for patients with acute necrotizing pancreatitis
- Comfort measures include:
  1. Helping the patient assume a sidelying position to decrease abdominal pain
  2. Avoiding oral stimulation while providing measures to keep mucous membranes from drying

SYSTEMIC SCLEROSIS
OVERVIEW
- Systemic sclerosis (SSc), also called *scleroderma,* is a chronic, inflammatory, autoimmune connective tissue disease that usually first manifests with hardening of the skin.
- The disease is often confused with systemic lupus erythematosus (SLE) but is less common and has a higher mortality rate.
- The manifestations vary widely from person to person.
- It is classified as:
  1. *Diffuse cutaneous SSc,* with skin thickening on the trunk, face, and proximal and distal extremities (over most of the body); the first symptom is hand and forearm edema, which may exist with bilateral carpal tunnel syndrome.
  2. *Limited cutaneous SSc,* with thick skin limited to sites distal to the elbow and knee but also involving the face and neck; patients have the *CREST syndrome.*
     a. *C*alcinosis (calcium deposits)
     b. *R*aynaud's phenomenon
     c. *E*sophageal dysmotility
     d. *S*clerodactyly (scleroderma of the digits)
     e. *T*elangiectasia (spider-like hemangiomas)
- Women are affected more often than men and usually are between 25 and 65 years old.

PATIENT-CENTERED COLLABORATIVE CARE
Assessment
- SSc manifests with joint pain and stiffness; painless, symmetric, pitting edema of the hands and fingers that may progress to include the entire upper and lower extremities and face; and taut, shiny skin that is free of wrinkles.
- When scleroderma progresses, swelling is replaced by tightening, hardening, and thickening of skin tissue with loss of elasticity and greatly decreased ROM.
- Ulcerations and joint contractures may develop, and the patient may be unable to perform ADLs.
- Major organ involvement is manifested by:
  1. GI tract changes with dysphagia and esophageal reflux (GERD); a small, sliding hiatal hernia may be present. Intestinal peristalsis is diminished, leading to partial bowel obstruction and malabsorption.
  2. Cardiovascular system changes, especially Raynaud's phenomenon with digit necrosis, excruciating pain, and autoamputation of the distal digits; myocardial fibrosis may be present with cardiac dysrhythmias and chest pain.

   3. Lung changes include fibrosis of the alveoli and interstitial tissues, and pulmonary hypertension may develop.
   4. Vascular involvement may lead to pulmonary arterial hypertension and renal artery–induced malignant hypertension.

Interventions

- The focus of medical management is to induce disease remission and slow disease progression.
- Systemic steroids and immunosuppressants are used in large doses and often in combination.
- Nursing management includes:
   1. Local skin protective measures
      a. Teaching the patient to use mild soap and lotions and gentle cleaning techniques
      b. Inspecting the skin for further changes or open lesions
      c. Caring for skin ulcers according to their type and location
      d. Using bed cradles and foot boards
      e. Adjusting room temperature to prevent chilling
   2. Implementing and teaching about drug therapy
   3. Teaching patients to avoid or minimize cigarette smoking with associated vasoconstriction
   4. Promoting nutrition
      a. Providing small, frequent meals
      b. Instructing the patient to avoid foods that may exacerbate GERD (e.g., spicy foods, caffeine, alcohol)
      c. Teaching the patient to keep the head elevated for 1 to 2 hours after a meal
   5. Reducing pain and maintaining joint mobility using interventions similar to those for rheumatoid arthritis
   6. Referring patients and families to community resources

T

TETANUS

- Tetanus, also known as *lockjaw,* is caused by *Clostridium tetani.*
- Tetanus vaccination is initiated in childhood and re-administered every 10 years ("booster") to provide protection against this infection. A booster dose may be given at 5 to 7 years if an injury with a high risk for tetanus infection is present. In addition, tetanus vaccination is given with trauma injuries, burns, and animal/spider bites to prevent secondary infection. Tetanus is preventable with vaccination.
- Tetanus is characterized by muscle rigidity, opisthotonos (abnormal posturing that includes arching the back), cramps, muscle spasms, stiffness, and headache.

- When infection occurs, treatment includes prompt (within 72 hours) IM administration of antitoxin: human tetanus immune globulin or hyperimmune equine or bovine serum.
- Sedation, antianxiety agents, and muscle relaxants are provided to decrease muscle spasms and increase comfort.
- Beta blockers or another antidysrhythmic agent may be given to treat cardiac irregularities, and the patient may need aggressive respiratory support.

THORACIC OUTLET SYNDROME

- Thoracic outlet syndrome is a compression of the subclavian artery at the thoracic outlet by anatomic structures, such as a rib or muscle.
- Damage to the arterial wall can produce thrombosis or embolization in distal arteries of the arm.
- Assess for:
  1. Neck, shoulder, and arm pain or numbness that increases when the arm is extended or held above the shoulder
  2. Recent trauma or moderate edema of the arm
- Conservative treatment includes:
  1. Physical therapy
  2. Avoidance of aggravating positions, typically arm above head
- Surgical treatment involves resection of the anatomic structures that are compressing the artery.

THROMBOCYTOPENIA PURPURA, AUTOIMMUNE

OVERVIEW

- In autoimmune thrombocytopenic purpura, also called *idiopathic thrombocytopenic purpura* (ITP), there is a greatly reduced number of circulating platelets, increasing the patient's risk for hemorrhage and death.
- In this type of thrombocytopenia, platelet production in the bone marrow is normal, but an antiplatelet antibody causes increased platelet destruction and impaired clotting.
- The problem is most common among women between the ages of 20 and 40 years and among people who have other autoimmune disorders.

PATIENT-CENTERED COLLABORATIVE CARE

- Assess for and document:
  1. Large bruises or petechial rash on the arms, legs, upper chest, and neck
  2. Mucosal bleeding
  3. Anemia

    4. Neurologic impairment as a result of an intracranial bleed-induced stroke

    5. Laboratory findings: decreased platelet count, large numbers of megakaryocytes in the bone marrow, presence of antiplatelet antibodies in the blood, low hematocrit, and low hemoglobin levels

- Interventions include:
  1. Drug therapy to suppress immune function
     a. Corticosteroids
     b. Immunomodulators like azathioprine (Imuran), eltrombopag, rituximab (Rituxan), and romiplostim
  2. Administration of IV immunoglobulin and IV anti-Rho to prevent the destruction of antibody-coated platelets
  3. Platelet transfusions when platelet counts are less than 10,000/mm^3 or patient is actively bleeding
  4. Preventing or minimizing injury to avoid bleeding
  5. A possible splenectomy if there is no response to drug therapy

TONSILLITIS

- Tonsillitis is an inflammation and infection of the tonsils and lymphatic tissues located on each side of the throat.
- It is a contagious airborne infection.
- The acute form usually lasts 7 to 10 days and often is caused by bacteria, most commonly *Streptococcus,* or by viruses.
- Manifestations of acute tonsillitis include the sudden onset of:
  1. A mild to severe sore throat
  2. Fever, muscle aches, chills
  3. Dysphagia, odynophagia (painful swallowing of food)
  4. Pain in the ears
  5. Headache, anorexia, malaise
  6. "Hot potato" voice (thickened voice of poor quality)
  7. Tonsils visually swollen and red with white or yellow exudate
  8. Edematous or inflamed uvula
  9. Enlarged cervical lymph nodes
- Treatment includes:
  1. Oral antibiotics for 7 to 10 days
  2. Teaching the patient about:
     a. Supportive care (rest, increasing fluid intake, humidifying the air, analgesics for pain, gargling several times daily with warm saline, throat lozenges containing mild anesthetics)
     b. The importance of completing antibiotic therapy
- Surgical intervention (e.g., tonsillectomy and adenoidectomy) may be needed for recurrent acute or chronic infections, a peritonsillar abscess, or enlarged tonsils or adenoids that obstruct the airway.

TOXIC EPIDERMAL NECROLYSIS

- Toxic epidermal necrolysis (TEN) is a rare acute drug reaction of the skin resulting in diffuse erythema and large blister formation. Mucous membranes are often involved, and systemic toxicity is evident.
- The most common causative drugs are chemotherapy agents, sulfonamides, pyrazolones, barbiturates, and antibiotics. Removal of the drug is usually followed by gradual healing in 2 to 3 weeks, with widespread peeling of the epidermis.

TOXIC SHOCK SYNDROME

- Toxic shock syndrome (TSS) is a form of septic shock caused by *Staphylococcus aureus* or *Streptococcus* infection and is related to menstruation and tampon use.
- Other conditions associated with TSS include internal contraceptive devices, surgical wound infection, nonsurgical infections, and gynecologic surgeries.
- In menstrual-related infection, menstrual blood provides a growth medium for the bacteria, which produces endotoxins that cross the vaginal mucosa to the bloodstream. Tampon insertion or prolonged use can cause vaginal dryness and microabrasions that provide an entry for the microorganisms.
- Assess for:
  1. Abrupt onset of a high fever
  2. Headache and flu-like symptoms
  3. Severe hypotension
  4. Sunburn-like rash with broken capillaries in the eyes and on the skin
- Management includes:
  1. Removal of the infection source
  2. Management of fluids and electrolyte imbalances, avoiding hypotension
  3. IV antibiotics and other measures included in the management of sepsis and septic shock
- Patient education focuses on prevention by teaching all women about the proper use of tampons, internal contraceptive devices such as vaginal sponges and diaphragms, and prompt treatment of gynecologic infections.

TRACHOMA

- Trachoma is a chronic, bilateral scarring form of conjunctivitis caused by *Chlamydia trachomatis*. It is the chief cause of preventable blindness in the world.
- Manifestations include tears, photophobia, edema of the eyelids and conjunctiva, and follicles on the upper eyelid conjunctiva.

With disease progression, the eyelid scars and turns inward, causing the eyelashes to damage the cornea.
- Drug therapy management involves oral or topical (eye drop) antibiotics; teach patients to complete the entire course of antibiotics.
- Infection control prevents transmission. Teach patients to:
  1. Wash the hands before and after touching the eyes.
  2. Keep washcloths separate from those of unaffected people and launder them separately.

TRAUMA, ABDOMINAL
OVERVIEW
- Abdominal trauma is an injury to the structures located between the diaphragm and the pelvis that occurs when the abdomen is subjected to blunt or penetrating force.
  1. Blunt trauma is also caused by motor vehicle crashes, falls, assaults, and contact sports.
  2. Penetrating trauma is most often caused by bullets, knives, or other objects that open the abdomen.
- Organs that may be injured include the large and small bowel, liver, spleen, duodenum, pancreas, kidneys, and urinary bladder.

PATIENT-CENTERED COLLABORATIVE CARE
Assessment
- Assess for airway, breathing, and circulation (ABCs).
- Identify the mechanism (force and type) of injury.
  1. The spleen is vulnerable to blunt trauma and contributes to significant blood loss.
  2. The liver is the most commonly injured organ with penetrating trauma.
- Evaluate for symptoms of hypovolemia and shock. The key assessment factors related to early shock detection are decreased mental status, hypotension, tachycardia, tachypnea, decreased Spo_2, and decreased skin perfusion (see *Shock* for discussions of hemorrhagic and hypovolemic forms of shock).
- Assess for and document:
  1. Mental status, vital signs (HR, BP, RR, and Spo_2), bowel sounds, urinary output, and changes in clinical findings every 15 to 30 minutes until stable, then hourly; report any deterioration immediately to the physician.
  2. The patient's report about the presence, location, and quality of pain, including referred pain (e.g., right shoulder) and nausea
  3. Inspection of the abdomen, back, flanks, genitalia, and rectum for contusions, abrasions, lacerations, ecchymoses, penetrating injuries, and symmetry. Ecchymosis around the umbilicus

(Cullen's sign) and ecchymosis in either flank (Turner's sign) may indicate retroperitoneal bleeding into the abdominal wall. Be aware that a large volume of blood can accumulate in the abdominal cavity before there is a change in the size or color during inspection.

4. Auscultation of the abdomen for absent or diminished bowel sounds and bruits
5. Percussion for abnormal sounds such as resonance over the liver or dullness over the stomach or intestines (Ballance's sign)
6. Results from light palpation of the abdomen to identify areas of tenderness, guarding, rigidity, and spasm
7. Kehr's sign, indicating splenic injury, which is left shoulder pain resulting from diaphragmatic irritation
8. Blood in peritoneal lavage, NG tube output, or emesis

Interventions

Nonsurgical Management

- Interventions include:
  1. Placing two peripheral IV catheters to provide rapid fluid resuscitation
  2. Infusing IV fluids at a rapid rate, as ordered, and monitoring patient responses
  3. Inserting an indwelling Foley catheter and monitoring urine output hourly for at least 24 hours
  4. Inserting an NG tube to prevent vomiting and reduce intra-abdominal pressure
  5. Monitoring intra-abdominal pressure (in some facilities) to detect compartment syndrome, which is compression of structures in the abdominal cavity (see *Compartment Syndrome*)
- Diagnostic studies may include:
  1. Abdominal ultrasound in the presence of blunt trauma
  2. Peritoneal lavage
  3. Abdominal CT scan
  4. Chest x-ray
  5. ECG and ongoing ECG monitoring
  6. Serum analyses: CBC, basic metabolic panel, coagulation factors, tests for liver function and blood typing with antibody screening for possible transfusion
  7. Continuous intra-abdominal pressure monitoring
- Analgesics are used for pain, with careful attention to maintaining airway and breathing.

Surgical Management

- For patients with severe abdominal trauma, an exploratory laparotomy with repair of abdominal injuries is performed.

- Most patients with gunshot or stab wounds require an exploratory laparotomy to assess for internal damage.
- Perioperative care is performed as outlined in Part One.
- A colostomy, either temporary or permanent, may be required (see *Surgical Management* under *Cancer, Colorectal*).

QSEN SAFETY

Before administering medications or implementing procedures, ensure that the right patient is receiving interventions by using at least two identifiers. This process is challenging to implement in the emergency department, where the fast pace of admissions and rapidly changing condition of the patient may not prioritize "routine" admission activities such as placing an identification wrist band. Nonetheless, accurate identification is essential for risk reduction and avoidance of adverse drug errors.

TRAUMA, BLADDER

- Bladder trauma occurs as a result of blunt or penetrating injury to the lower abdomen.
- The most common cause is a fractured pelvis (bone fragments puncture the bladder).
- Assess:
  1. Urinary output, particularly the presence of hematuria and anuria
  2. Bloody urinary meatus
  3. Results of cystogram and voiding cystourethrogram
- Patients with bladder trauma other than a simple contusion require surgical intervention, including closure repair of the bladder wall and peritoneal membrane.
- Recovery may include prolonged use of a urinary ureteral or suprapubic catheter while the repaired bladder heals.

TRAUMA, BRAIN (ACUTE BRAIN INJURY WITH OR WITHOUT SKULL FRACTURE)

OVERVIEW

- A brain injury that occurs from an external mechanical force is considered traumatic. Examples of mechanical force include a blow to the head or penetration of the brain by a bullet.
  1. In a closed brain injury, the integrity of the skull remains intact.
  2. In an open brain injury, the skull is fractured or penetrated by an object (e.g., bullet, projectile, or knife), violating the integrity of brain and dura and exposing brain tissue to extracranial contaminants.

- Traumatic brain injury (TBI) may produce a diminished state of consciousness and changes in cognitive abilities, physical functioning, or behavioral and emotional functioning. These changes may be immediate or delayed and may resolve or persist long after the original injury.
- Primary injury occurs at the time force occurs with potential for additional primary injury from contrecoup forces when the intracranial tissue "bounces" against the skull opposite the site of direct injury. Primary traumatic brain injury involves the frontal or temporal lobes.
- Secondary brain injury can occur from physiologic, vascular, and biochemical events that extend the area of the primary injury and involve cellular changes that contribute to tissue injury. The most common responses are hypotension, hypoxia, ischemia, and cerebral edema. Prevention of secondary injury is a major focus of acute care.
- Damage to brain tissue depends on the location, degree, and mechanism of injury.
  1. Brain injury can be classified as mild, moderate, or severe, depending on the initial Glasgow Coma Scale (GCS) score, which has implications for both treatment and prognosis.
  2. It may be also described by the degree of apparent damage to the brain.
     a. A *concussion* is a brain injury that temporarily changes how the brain functions as a result of mechanical force or trauma. It may or may not be associated with a brief loss of consciousness. Typically, no brain tissue damage is visible by CT.
     b. A *contusion* causes bruising of the brain tissue.
     c. A *laceration* causes tearing of the cortical surface vessels and may lead to secondary hemorrhage
     d. A *diffuse axonal injury* occurs when axons of the CNS neurons are stretched and damaged, resulting in widespread inflammation and CNS cell damage or death.
- Types of skull fractures associated with open brain injuries include:
  1. *Linear,* a simple, clean break
  2. *Depressed,* in which bone is pressed inward into brain tissue
  3. *Open,* in which the scalp is lacerated along with the skull fracture
  4. *Comminuted,* in which the skull is fragmented and bone is depressed into the brain tissue
  5. *Basilar,* which occurs at the base of the skull, usually along the paranasal sinus, and which may result in a cerebrospinal fluid (CSF) leak from the nose or ear and potential damage to cranial nerves I, II, VII, and VIII

PATIENT-CENTERED COLLABORATIVE CARE
Assessment
- Obtain patient information about:
  1. When, where, and how the injury occurred
  2. The patient's LOC immediately after the injury and on admission to the hospital or unit and whether there have been any changes or fluctuations
  3. Presence of seizure activity at the scene of injury
  4. Medical and social history, especially presence of alcohol or drug use
  5. Hand dominance
- Assess for:
  1. Impaired airway or breathing pattern: respiratory rate, depth, and quality with peripheral oxygenation (SpO_2)
  2. Signs and symptoms of hypovolemic shock or hemorrhage, which may indicate additional traumatic injuries such as abdominal bleeding or bleeding into soft tissue around major fractures
  3. Heart rate and rhythm, blood pressure, peripheral pulses, and core temperature
  4. Baseline and ongoing neurologic status with a standard assessment tool such as the GCS
     a. Decreased or garbled verbal response to auditory or tactile stimulus; new aphasia
     b. Inability to follow commands; confusion
     c. Pupils that are large, pinpoint, or ovoid, and nonreactive to light (indicates cranial nerve dysfunction, especially III, IV, and VII; may indicate brainstem dysfunction)
     d. Decreased or absent motor strength in the extremities; hemiparesis or hemiplegia
     e. Complaints of severe headache, nausea, or vomiting
     f. Seizure activity
     g. Drainage of CSF from the ear or nose ("halo sign")
  5. Indications of post-traumatic sequelae in the patient who experienced a brain injury (symptoms may persist for weeks or months)
     a. Persistent headache
     b. Weakness
     c. Dizziness
     d. Loss of memory
     e. Personality and behavioral changes
     f. Problems with perception, reasoning abilities, and concept formation
  6. Changes in personality, behavior, and abilities, such as:
     a. Increased incidence of temper outbursts, risk-taking behavior, depression, and denial of disability

   b. Becoming more talkative and developing a very outgoing personality
   c. Decreased ability to learn new information, to concentrate, and to plan
   d. Impaired memory, especially recent or short-term memory; this should not be confused with problems of aphasia
- Assess family dynamics. Family members may be angry with the patient for being injured, especially if the patient's behavior resulted in an injury that could have been prevented, or they may feel guilty that they could not prevent the injury.
- Diagnostic studies may include:
   1. CBC, basic metabolic panel, coagulation studies, arterial blood gases (ABGs), and toxicology screen
   2. CT scan
   3. Chest x-ray and abdominal x-ray to evaluate for the presence of additional injuries

❗ NURSING SAFETY PRIORITY: Critical Rescue

LOC is the most sensitive and specific indicator of neurologic deterioration. Immediately inform the physician about changes in mentation, orientation, or behavior. A decrease in GCS score of 2 points or more should be reported immediately.

Interventions
Nonsurgical Management
- Assess vital signs with a standard neurologic assessment every 1 to 2 hours to detect early signs of decreased levels of consciousness, poor perfusion, hypovolemia, and dangerous elevations of blood pressure that may cause further brain damage. Cardiac monitoring to detect cardiac dysrhythmias may be implemented. Report derangements immediately.
- Maintain normothermia; fever may extend the area of brain damage during the acute phase.
   1. The patient may be placed in systemic or local (cranial) hypothermia devices (blanket, helmet) to slow brain metabolism during the acute phase.
- Position the patient to avoid extreme flexion or extension of the neck, which interferes with CSF outflow. Maintain the head in a midline, central position; log roll the patient and elevate the back rest 30 degrees unless contraindicated; use reverse Trendelenburg position if spinal cord injury is still being evaluated.
- Maintain the Pao$_2$ at 85 to 100 mm Hg and Spo$_2$ at greater than 92% to maintain sufficient oxygen to brain cells, preventing secondary brain injury.

- The patient receiving mechanical ventilation may have settings to maintain the $Paco_2$ at 35 to 38 mm Hg after the 24 hours to promote cerebral vasoconstriction and reduce intracranial hypertension.
- Monitor ICP with a specialized device in the ICU if the patient presents with coma; manage ICP and cerebral perfusion pressure to maintain adequate blood flow to brain tissue. Maintain infection control/prevention processes specific to the use of ICP monitoring devices to prevent secondary brain injury from infection.
- Monitor brain tissue oxygenation with jugular venous oxygen apparatus (Sjo_2).
- Drug therapy
  1. Administer hypertonic saline or osmotic diuretics (mannitol) and use a filter to eliminate microscopic crystals when removing mannitol from its vial. Mannitol is used to pull fluid out of the intracranial space and into the vasculature for excretion. Osmotics are most effective when given as a bolus rather than a continuous infusion.
  2. Use opioids or sedatives if the patient is mechanically ventilated to control restlessness and agitation that causes increased ICP.
  3. Use antiepileptic drugs and seizure precautions for actual or potential seizure activity.
  4. Barbiturate coma (with severe injury and use of mechanical ventilation) may be induced to reduce the oxygen demands of the brain during acute injury and subsequent increases in ICP.
- Pulmonary management includes:
  1. Encouraging the conscious patient to breathe deeply every hour while awake and to avoid coughing, which can increase ICP
  2. Turning and re-positioning the patient at least once every 2 hours; consider the use of continuous lateral rotational therapy if the patient is comatose, hypoxic, and mechanically ventilated
- Fluid and electrolyte management includes:
  1. Monitoring electrolytes and serum and urine osmolarity to maintain/replace a normal range of values, particularly during diuretic/osmotic treatment
  2. Measuring intake and output every hour to avoid overhydration and subsequent increased ICP or dehydration and subsequent poor perfusion
  3. Measuring urine osmolality, sodium, and specific gravity when there is a significant increase in urine output (greater than 300 mL/hr for 2 hours) to evaluate for syndrome of inappropriate antidiuretic hormone (SIADH)

4. Using a urinary catheter to monitor hourly output if acute moderate or severe brain injury is diagnosed
5. Monitoring daily weight

- Sensory, cognitive, and behavioral management includes:
  1. Providing a balance between sensory stimulation and quiet rest to promote brain recovery
  2. Monitoring the patient for nutritional deficits that may occur secondary to the loss of smell and loss of ability to taste, swallow, or feel food in the oral cavity
     a. Ensure that mealtime is a pleasant experience.
     b. Check the temperature of food and beverages on the tray before serving.
     c. Position the patient to maximize swallowing ability.
     d. Collaborate with the speech-language pathologist to develop and implement a swallowing program for the patient as needed.
  3. Providing a safe environment with frequent monitoring, use of a sitter, or if needed, use of restraints following institutional policy
  4. Initiating a sensory stimulation program, such as audio recordings used for no longer than 10 to 15 minutes for patients in coma; awake or alert patients may enjoy longer tapes
  5. Orienting the patient to environment, time, place, and the reason for hospitalization with each encounter if short-term memory loss or coma is present
  6. Reassuring the patient realistically about concerns, visitation, and plan for care at least once per shift
  7. Providing simple, short explanations of procedures and activities immediately before any interventions
  8. Collaborating with physical and occupational therapists to plan exercise and ADL programs
  9. Maintaining the patient on a normal sleep-wake cycle for mild brain injury, and providing periods of rest for patients with moderate or severe injury
  10. Asking the family to bring in familiar objects, such as pictures or music
  11. Monitoring the patient's reaction to television or radio to promote rest or comfort
  12. Keeping the bed in the low position if the patient is awake
  13. Observing and documenting behavior; providing constant supervision if the patient is unable to consistently follow directions or is unsafe because of short-term memory failure

- Nutrition management includes:
  1. Beginning nutritional support as soon as possible with oral, enteral, or intravenous feeding

2. Monitoring the patient's weight and serum albumin, prealbumin, and transferrin levels to ensure adequate protein intake

Surgical Management

- A craniotomy may be indicated to:
  1. Evacuate a subdural or epidural hematoma
  2. Treat uncontrolled increased ICP by excising the tips of the temporal lobe or removing ischemic tissue
  3. Treat hydrocephalus
- An alternative to a craniotomy is surgical burr holes in which a hole is drilled into the skull to expose the dura mater, usually to relieve intracranial hypertension.
- Bedside surgical insertion of an ICP-monitoring device is often performed. Types of devices include:
  1. Intraventricular catheter
  2. Epidural catheter or sensor
  3. Subarachnoid bolt or screw
  4. Fiberoptic transducer-tipped sensor

Community-Based Care

- Respite care may be needed to help the family cope with feelings of isolation, increased responsibility, financial or emotional stress, or role reversal; refer them to support groups.
- The patient may experience a sense of isolation and loneliness, because personality and behavior changes make it difficult to resume or maintain preinjury social contacts.
- Discharge planning for moderate to severe brain injury often involves transition to rehabilitation and includes:
  1. Providing a detailed plan of care at the time of transfer to a rehabilitation or long-term care facility:
     a. Drugs, including dosage and possible side effects
     b. Current patient activity
     c. Techniques used to motivate or calm the patient
     d. Successful coping strategies identified by the patient or family
  2. For patients returning home, consider home care referral and follow-up appointments to promote recovery and adjustment.
     a. Inform the patient and family about resources such as the National Head Injury Foundation or a local brain injury support group
     b. Provide the patient and family with information about:
        (1) Strategies to adapt to sensory dysfunction and to cope with the personality or behavior problems that may arise
        (2) The purpose, dosage, schedule, and route of administration of drugs
        (3) Participation in activities as tolerated

3. For minor head injury, discuss symptoms of post-traumatic stress disorder and mild cognitive deficit disorder. Inform the patient that these symptoms are common and refer the patient and family to a specialist in brain injury or cognitive therapy and a support group if symptoms persist. Symptoms include:
   a. Personality changes
   b. Irritability
   c. Headaches
   d. Dizziness
   e. Restlessness
   f. Nervousness
   g. Insomnia
   h. Memory loss
   i. Depression

TRAUMA, ESOPHAGEAL

- Trauma to the esophagus can result from blunt injuries, chemical burns, surgery or endoscopy, or the stress of protracted severe vomiting.
- Trauma may affect the esophagus directly, impairing swallowing and nutrition, or it may create problems and complications in related structures such as the lungs or mediastinum.
- Assess for and document:
  1. Airway patency, breathing
  2. Chest pain
  3. Dysphagia
  4. Vomiting, hematemesis
  5. Results of x-ray examination, CT, and endoscopy
- Treatment includes:
  1. Maintaining NPO status to prevent further leakage of esophageal secretions
  2. Maintaining NG or gastrostomy tube drainage to heal ("rest") the esophagus
  3. Administering total parenteral nutrition (TPN) during esophageal rest (usually for at least 10 days)
  4. Administering broad-spectrum antibiotics, corticosteroids, and analgesics
- Surgery may be needed to remove the damaged tissue. A resection or replacement of the damaged esophageal segment with small bowel tissue may be required.

TRAUMA, FACIAL

OVERVIEW

- Facial trauma is described by the specific bones (e.g., mandibular, maxillary, orbital, or nasal fractures) and the side of the face involved.

T

- Mandibular (lower jaw) fractures can occur at any point on the mandible and are the most common facial fractures.
- The rich blood supply of the face leads to extensive bleeding and bruising with facial trauma.

PATIENT-CENTERED COLLABORATIVE CARE
Assessment
- The first action to take for a patient with facial trauma is airway assessment.
- Assess for:
  1. Manifestations of airway obstruction
     a. Stridor
     b. Shortness of breath
     c. Anxiety and restlessness or decreased consciousness
     d. Hypoxia and decreased oxygen saturation
     e. Hypercarbia
  2. Soft tissue edema
  3. Facial asymmetry
  4. Pain
  5. Leakage of spinal fluid through the ears or nose
  6. Vision and eye movement
  7. Bruising behind the ears in the mastoid area ("battle sign")

Interventions
- The priority action is to establish and maintain a patent airway.
  1. Provide suction at the bedside.
  2. Anticipate the need for emergency intubation, tracheotomy, or cricothyroidotomy.
- Other interventions include:
  1. Controlling hemorrhage
  2. Assessing for the extent of injury
  3. Establishing IV access and initiating fluid resuscitation
  4. Assisting in the stabilization of fractures
  5. Administering prescribed antibiotics
  6. For mandibular fixation with plates, teaching the patient about:
     a. Oral care with an irrigating device
     b. Soft diet or dental liquid diet restrictions
     c. How to cut the wires if emesis occurs

! NURSING SAFETY PRIORITY: Critical Rescue

Instruct the patient to keep wire cutters with him or her at all times in case emergent aspiration occurs.

TRAUMA, KIDNEY

- Kidney (renal) trauma is injury to one or both kidneys. Injury can be blunt or penetrating.
- Injuries
  1. Minor injuries (contusion, small lacerations, tearing of the parenchyma and the calyx) are likely to follow falls, contact sports, and blows to the back or torso.
  2. Major injuries (lacerations to the cortex, medulla, or one of the branches of the renal artery or vein) are likely to follow penetrating abdominal, flank, or back wounds.
  3. Pedicle injuries (laceration or disruption of the renal artery or vein) result in rapid and extensive hemorrhage and death unless diagnosis and intervention are prompt.
- Obtain patient information about:
  1. The mechanism of injury, including the events surrounding the trauma
  2. History of kidney or urologic disease, including previous surgical intervention
  3. History of diabetes, hypertension, or atherosclerosis
- Assess for and document:
  1. Vital signs, particularly derangements in HR, BP, RR, and SpO_2 indicating poor perfusion or reduced gas exchange that contribute to hypovolemic or hypoxic kidney damage
  2. Abdominal or flank pain
  3. Penetrating injuries of the lower thorax, back, or abdomen
  4. Abdominal or flank distension, bruising, or asymmetry
  5. Urine output hourly and abnormal urine, especially blood in the urine
  6. Decreased serum hemoglobin and hematocrit values
- Treatment may include fluids and drugs for perfusion and surgery.
  1. Administer fluids, such as crystalloids or packed RBCs, to restore circulatory blood volume; plasma volume expanders may also be given.
  2. Assess the need for clotting factors such as vitamin K and platelets.
- Interventional radiology techniques may be used to drain fluid around the urinary tract or to stent or embolize a renal artery.
- Nephrectomy (surgical removal of the kidney) may be required with extensive trauma.

TRAUMA, KNEE

- There are two semilunar cartilaginous structures (menisci) in the knee joint, the medial meniscus and the lateral meniscus, which act as shock absorbers.

- Meniscus injuries are usually tears and occur more often in the medial meniscus, usually causing the knee to lock.
  1. Manifestations include pain, swelling, tenderness in the knee, and a clicking or snapping sound when the knee is moved.
  2. Management of a locked knee is manipulation followed by splinting or casting for 3 to 6 weeks.
  3. A partial or total meniscectomy may be required and is usually performed by arthroscopy.
- The cruciate and collateral ligaments of the knee are prone to injury.
  1. Manifestations of an anterior cruciate ligament (ACL) tear include feeling a snap and the knee giving way, swelling and stiffness, and pain.
  2. Management may be nonsurgical (exercises, bracing, activity limitation) or surgical, depending on the severity of the injury and the anticipated activity of the patient.

TRAUMA, LARYNGEAL

- Laryngeal trauma occurs with a crushing or direct blow, fracture, or by prolonged endotracheal intubation.
- Manifestations include dyspnea, aphonia, hoarseness, subcutaneous emphysema, and hemoptysis.
- Management consists of assessing the effectiveness of gas exchange.
  1. Monitor vital signs and pulse oximetry every 15 to 30 minutes.
  2. Communicate increased respiratory difficulty immediately to the provider.
     a. Tachypnea, especially rates greater than 28 breaths/minute
     b. Nasal flaring or use of accessory respiratory muscles
     c. Anxiety, restlessness, or a decreased LOC
     d. Dyspnea or new-onset voice weakness or hoarseness
     e. Decreased oxygen saturation (SpO_2)
     f. Stridor

! NURSING SAFETY PRIORITY: Critical Rescue

If the patient has respiratory difficulty, stay with him or her and instruct trauma team members or the Rapid Response Team to prepare for an emergency intubation or tracheostomy.

- Surgical intervention is necessary for lacerations of the mucous membranes, cartilage exposure, or paralysis of the cords.
- An artificial airway may be needed.

TRAUMA, LIVER

- The liver is one of the organs most commonly injured in patients with abdominal trauma. Damage or injury should be suspected whenever any upper abdominal or lower chest trauma is sustained.

- Common injuries to the liver include simple lacerations, multiple lacerations, avulsions (tears), and crush injuries.
- Because the liver is a vascular organ, blood loss is massive when trauma occurs (see *Shock*, especially the discussion of hemorrhagic and hypovolemic shock).
- Clinical manifestations of liver trauma include right upper quadrant pain with abdominal tenderness, distention, guarding, rigidity, and abdominal pain that is aggravated by deep breathing and is referred to the right shoulder.
- Ultrasonography or CT is done to determine injury and clot formation.
- Anticipate bleeding and prolonged coagulopathy with severe liver injury. The patient with liver trauma may require infusion of multiple blood products, packed RBCs, fresh-frozen plasma, and massive volume replacement to maintain hydration.

TRAUMA, PERIPHERAL NERVE

- The peripheral nerves are subject to injuries associated with mechanical or vehicular accidents, sports, the injection of particular drugs, military conflicts, and acts of violence (e.g., knife or gunshot wounds).
- Specific mechanisms of injury include:
  1. Partial or complete severance of a nerve or nerves
  2. Contusion, stretching, constriction, or compression of a nerve or nerves
  3. Ischemia
  4. Electrical, thermal, or radiation injury
- Most commonly affected are the median, ulnar, and radial nerves of the arms and the peroneal, femoral, and sciatic nerves of the legs.
- Nerve damage is characterized by pain, burning, or other abnormal sensations distal to the trauma; weakness or flaccid paralysis; and change in skin color and temperature (a warm phase and a cold phase).
- Nonsurgical treatment consists of immobilization of the area with a splint, cast, or traction followed by physical and occupational therapy.
- Surgery may include resection and suturing to reapproximate the severed nerve ends, nerve grafting, and nerve and tendon transplantation.
- Regeneration of the damaged nerve and return of sensation may occur several years after the injury; motor movement is less likely to recover long after the event.

- Postoperative nursing care is directed toward frequent skin care and assessment, management of pain, and instructing the patient to protect the involved area from new trauma.

TRAUMA, TRACHEOBRONCHIAL

- Most tears of the tracheobronchial tree result from severe blunt trauma or rapid deceleration and primarily involve the trachea at the cricoid or mainstem bronchi.
- Patients with tracheobronchial trauma develop massive air leaks, causing air to enter the mediastinum and leading to extensive subcutaneous emphysema.
- Upper airway obstruction may occur, causing severe respiratory distress and inspiratory stridor.
- Large tracheal tears are managed by cricothyroidotomy or tracheotomy below the level of injury.
- Management includes:
  1. Assessing oxygenation, ventilation, and work of breathing along with lung sounds
  2. Administering oxygen or initiating mechanical ventilation as needed
  3. Assessing for subcutaneous emphysema
  4. Providing tracheostomy care if surgical repair was needed

TUBERCULOSIS

OVERVIEW

- Pulmonary tuberculosis (TB) is a highly communicable disease caused by *Mycobacterium tuberculosis* infection.
- The organism is transmitted by aerosolization (airborne route) from an infected person during coughing, laughing, sneezing, whistling, or singing.
- When the bacillus is inhaled into a susceptible site, it multiplies freely, causing an exudative pneumonitis.
- While exposure may lead to infection, few people manifest active TB after exposure to the organism.
- Initial infection is seen more often in the middle or lower lobes of the lung, and re-activation occurs more in the upper lobes.
- Progression of infection leads to an inflammatory lump that surrounds the bacilli and is filled with collagen, fibroblasts, and lymphocytes. The lump necroses, causing calcification or liquefaction and leading to destruction of lung tissue with cavity formation.
- *Miliary,* or *hematogenous,* TB is the spread of TB throughout the body when a large number of organisms enter the blood and can then infect the brain, liver, kidney, or bone marrow.
- An infected individual is not infectious to others until manifestations of disease occur.

- People at greatest risk for developing TB are:
  1. Those in constant, frequent contact with an untreated individual with active TB
  2. Those who have decreased immune function
  3. Those who live in crowded areas such as long-term care facilities, prisons, and mental health facilities
  4. Older homeless people
  5. Abusers of injection drugs or alcohol
  6. Members of lower socioeconomic groups
  7. Foreign immigrants (especially from Mexico, the Philippines, and Vietnam)

PATIENT-CENTERED COLLABORATIVE CARE
Assessment
- Obtain patient information about:
  1. Persistent cough
  2. Weight loss
  3. Anorexia
  4. Night sweats
  5. Fever or chills
  6. Dyspnea or hemoptysis
  7. Past exposure to TB
  8. Country of origin and travel to foreign countries
  9. History of bacillus Calmette-Guérin (BCG) vaccination
- Assess for and document:
  1. Dullness with percussion over involved lung fields
  2. Bronchial breath sounds
  3. Crackles, wheezes
  4. Enlarged lymph nodes
- TB is diagnosed on the basis of manifestations and/or a positive nucleic acid amplification test (NAAT). Blood analysis by an enzyme-linked immunosorbent assay using the QuantiFERON-TB Gold (QFT-G) may be used for testing in the acute care setting. A purified protein derivative (PPD) two-step test may be used for screening purposes.

T

! NURSING SAFETY PRIORITY: Action Alert
- Do not assume that a positive PPD reaction of 10 mm induration 48 to 72 hours after injection means that active disease is present. It only indicates exposure to TB, TB vaccination, or the presence of inactive (dormant) disease.
- A reduced PPD skin reaction or a negative PPD skin test result does not rule out TB disease or infection in the very old or in anyone who is severely immunocompromised.

Interventions

- Combination drug therapy is the most effective method of treating TB and preventing transmission. Current first-line therapy uses four medications.
  1. Isoniazid (INH) for 6 months
  2. Rifampin for 6 months
  3. Pyrazinamide for the first 2 months
  4. Ethambutol for 6 months

! NURSING SAFETY PRIORITY: Drug Alert

The first-line drugs used as therapy for tuberculosis all can damage the liver. Warn the patient to not drink any alcoholic beverages for the entire duration of TB therapy. Duration of therapy is usually 6 months but can be as long as 2 years for multidrug-resistant TB.

- Variations of the first-line drugs along with other drug types are used if the patient does not tolerate the standard first-line therapy.
- Nursing interventions include:
  1. Caring for the hospitalized patient using strict Airborne Precautions
  2. Ensuring that the patient understands drug therapy
     a. Explain the actions, side effects, dosing, and scheduling of the drugs and request that the patient summarize information accurately.
     b. Stress the importance of taking each drug regularly, exactly as prescribed.
     c. Present drug information in multiple formats, such as pamphlets, videos, and drug-schedule worksheets.
     d. Explain that nausea can be prevented by taking the drugs at bedtime.
  3. Informing the patient about multidrug-resistant strains of TB; higher doses of some drugs for longer periods and absolute adherence to therapy are required for survival and cure of the disease
  4. Providing information about infection control
     a. Remind patients that Airborne Precautions are not necessary in the home, because family members have already been exposed.
     b. Teach family members in the household about the need to undergo TB testing.
     c. Teach the patient to cover the mouth and nose with a tissue when coughing or sneezing and to place used tissues in plastic bags.

    d. Teach the patient to wear a mask when in contact with crowds until the drugs suppress infection.

5. Teaching about health and general care issues
    a. Fatigue will diminish as the treatment progresses.
    b. Avoid exposure to any inhalation irritants, because they can cause further lung damage.
    c. Incorporate a well-balanced diet and adequate rest to promote recovery.

6. Reporting the TB infection to the local public health department

Community-Based Care

- Consult with the social service worker in the hospital or the community health nursing agency to ensure that the patient is discharged to the appropriate environment.
- Teach the patient to follow the drug regimen exactly as prescribed and always to have a supply on hand.
- Remind the patient that the disease is usually no longer contagious after drugs have been taken for 2 to 3 consecutive weeks and clinical improvement is seen; however, he or she *must continue with the drugs for 6 months or longer as prescribed.*
- Determine the need for *directly observed therapy* (DOT), in which the nurse or other health care provider watches the patient swallow the drugs.
- Remind the patient to receive follow-up care by a health care provider for at least 1 year during active treatment.
- Urge smokers to quit, and assist them in finding an appropriate smoking-cessation program.
- Ensure that active cases are reported to the local public health department or agency.

TUMORS, BRAIN

OVERVIEW

- Brain tumors can arise anywhere within the brain structures and are named according to the cell or tissue where they are located.
- *Primary tumors* originate within the CNS.
- *Secondary tumors (metastatic tumors)* spread to the brain from cancers in other body areas, such as the lungs, breast, kidney, and GI tract.
- Regardless of brain tumor type or location, the tumor expands and invades, infiltrates, compresses, and displaces normal brain tissue, leading to one or more problems, including:
  1. Cerebral edema/brain tissue inflammation
  2. Increased intracranial pressure, intracranial hypertension
  3. Neurologic deficits: sensory, motor, or cranial nerve dysfunction

4. Hydrocephalus
5. Pituitary dysfunction
6. Seizure activity
- *Supratentorial tumors* are located within the cerebral hemispheres, and *infratentorial tumors* are located in the brainstem structures and cerebellum.
- Some brain tumors are benign (noninvasive), and others are cancerous. Regardless of type, most brain tumors must be treated or death will occur.
- Classification by cell type or tissue type includes tumors arising from:
  1. Neurons, which are responsible for nerve impulse conduction
  2. Neuroglial cells (glial cells), which provide support, nourishment, and protection
     a. Astrocytes (astrocytomas)
     b. Oligodendroglia
     c. Ependymal cells
     d. Microglia (gliomas, which are malignant)
  3. Meninges, which are the coverings of the brain (meningiomas)
  4. Pituitary (pituitary adenomas)
  5. The sheath of Schwann cells in cranial nerve VII (acoustic neuromas)
- Metastatic, or secondary, tumors from other body areas make up about 30% of brain tumors.
- The exact cause of brain tumors is unknown but may be related to genetic changes, heredity, errors in fetal development, ionizing radiation, electromagnetic fields, environmental hazards, diet, viruses, or injury.

PATIENT-CENTERED COLLABORATIVE CARE
Assessment
- Obtain patient information about general symptoms of a brain tumor, including:
  1. Headaches that are usually more severe on awakening in the morning
  2. Nausea and vomiting
  3. Vision changes (blurred or double vision)
  4. Seizures
  5. Changes in mentation or personality
  6. Papilledema (swelling of the optic disc)
  7. Specific neurologic deficits
     a. Supratentorial (cerebral) tumors usually result in paralysis, seizures, memory loss, cognitive impairment, language impairment, or vision problems.

b. Infratentorial tumors produce ataxia, autonomic nervous system dysfunction, vomiting, drooling, hearing loss, and vision impairment.
- Diagnosis is based on the history, neurologic assessment, clinical examination, results of neurodiagnostic testing, CT, magnetic resonance imaging (MRI), and skull x-rays. Cerebral angiography, electroencephalography (EEG), lumbar puncture (LP), brain scan, and positron emission tomography (PET) may be also be used to further define the tumor.

Interventions

Nonsurgical Management

- Management depends on tumor size and location, patient symptoms and general condition, and whether the tumor is primary or has recurred.
- Drug therapy for symptom management may include:
  1. Analgesics for headache
     a. Codeine
     b. Acetaminophen
  2. Agents to control cerebral edema
     a. Dexamethasone (Decadron)
     b. Corticosteroids
  3. Phenytoin (Dilantin) or other antiepileptic drug for seizure activity
  4. Agents to prevent stress ulcers, typically proton pump inhibitors (e.g., pantoprazole [Protonix])
  5. Institution-specific seizure precautions
- Chemotherapy may be given alone, in combination with radiation therapy and surgery, and with tumor progression. More than one agent may be given orally, IV, intra-arterially, or intrathecally through an Ommaya reservoir placed in a cranial ventricle. Both cytotoxic and targeted therapy agents may be used.
  1. An emerging practice is direct drug delivery to the tumor using a disk-shaped drug wafer (polifeprosan 20 with carmustine implant [Gliadel]) placed directly into the cavity created during surgical tumor removal (interstitial chemotherapy).
  2. General management issues for care of patients undergoing chemotherapy are presented in Part One, under *Cancer Treatment*.
- Radiation therapy may be used alone, after surgery, or in combination with chemotherapy and surgery.
  1. Traditional external beam radiation may be used.
  2. A radioactive monoclonal antibody may be directly injected into the cavity from which the tumor was removed.
  3. General management issues for care of patients undergoing radiation therapy are presented in Part One under *Cancer Treatment*.

T

- Stereotactic radiosurgery (SRS) is an alternative to traditional surgery. Techniques used may include:
  1. Modified linear accelerator using accelerated x-rays (LINAC)
  2. Particle accelerator using beams of protons (cyclotron)
  3. Isotope seeds implanted in the tumor (brachytherapy)
  4. Gamma knife using a single high dose of ionized radiation to focus 201 beams of gamma radiation produced by the radio-isotope cobalt 60
  5. CyberKnife

  Surgical Management
- Brain biopsy is done to determine the specific pathology. Then a craniotomy (incision into the cranium) may be performed to improve symptoms related to the lesion or to decrease pressure effect from the tumor. Complete removal is possible with some tumors, which results in a "surgical cure."
  1. Minimally invasive surgery (MIS) may involve:
     a. The trans-nasal approach with endoscopy for pituitary tumors
     b. Stereotactic surgery using burr holes and local anesthesia
     c. Laser surgery
  2. In traditional open craniotomy, the patient's head is placed in a skull fixation device, and a piece of bone (bone flap) is removed to expose the tumor area. The tumor is removed, the bone flap is replaced, and a drain or monitoring device may be inserted.
- Provide preoperative care, including:
  1. Implementing routine preoperative care as described in Part One
  2. Allowing the patient to express anxiety and concerns about:
     a. Surgery into the brain
     b. Possibility of neurologic deficits
     c. Changes in appearance and self-image
  3. Teaching the patient and family about what to expect immediately after surgery and throughout the recovery period
  4. Ensuring that the patient has refrained from alcohol, tobacco, anticoagulants, or NSAIDs for at least 5 days before surgery
- Provide postoperative care, including:

❗ NURSING SAFETY PRIORITY: Action Alert

The focus of postoperative care is to monitor the patient to detect changes in status and to prevent or minimize complications, especially increased ICP.

  1. Implementing routine postoperative care as described in Part One
  2. Assessing neurologic (LOC) and vital signs every 15 to 30 minutes for the first 4 to 6 hours after surgery and then every hour

3. Assessing for:
   a. Decreased LOC
   b. Motor weakness or paralysis
   c. Aphasia
   d. Visual changes
   e. Personality changes
4. Ensuring appropriate positioning
   a. After supratentorial surgery:
      (1) Elevate the head of the bed 30 degrees
      (2) Avoid extreme hip or neck flexion
      (3) Maintain the head in a midline, neutral position
      (4) Place the patient on the nonoperative side
   b. After infratentorial (brainstem) craniotomy:
      (1) Keep the patient flat
      (2) Position the patient on either side for 24 to 48 hours
5. Maintaining NPO status for at least the first 24 hours after surgery
6. Administering prescribed drug therapy
   a. Antiepileptic drugs
   b. Proton pump inhibitors
   c. Corticosteroids
   d. Analgesics
7. Monitoring the dressing every 1 to 2 hours for:
   a. Amount, type, and color of drainage
   b. Suction of drains maintained as prescribed

! NURSING SAFETY PRIORITY: Critical Rescue

Immediately report to the surgeon a saturated head dressing or drainage greater than 50 mL in 8 hours.

8. Applying cold compresses for periorbital edema and ecchymosis of one or both eyes
9. Irrigating the affected eye with warm saline solution or artificial tears
10. Assessing the airway and managing mechanical ventilation
    a. Keeping $Paco_2$ at about 35 mm Hg
    b. Keeping the arterial oxygen levels higher than 95 mm Hg
    c. Hyperoxygenating the patient carefully before suctioning
11. Assessing the cardiac monitor for dysrhythmias
12. Precisely measuring intake and output to maintain a balance, avoiding overhydration and underhydration
13. Implementing any prescribed fluid restriction
14. Ensuring that ROM exercises are performed with all extremities at least every 2 to 3 hours
15. Ensuring that the patient turns, coughs, and breathes deeply every 2 hours (if permitted)

16. Maintaining VTE prophylaxis until the patient ambulates
17. Monitoring laboratory values for changes and abnormalities
    a. CBC
    b. Serum electrolyte levels and osmolarity
    c. Coagulation studies
    d. ABGs
18. Assessing for fluid volume overload or syndrome of inappropriate antidiuretic hormone (SIADH)
    a. Irritability
    b. Rapid weight gain
    c. Low serum sodium and potassium values
    d. Low urine output in relation to fluid intake
19. Assessing for diabetes insipidus (DI)
    a. High serum sodium and osmolarity
    b. Muscle weakness and restlessness
    c. Extreme thirst and dry mouth
    d. High output of dilute urine
20. Assessing for cerebral salt wasting (CSW)
    a. Low serum sodium and decreased osmolarity
    b. No dilution of other electrolytes or of hematocrit and hemoglobin
21. Preventing and assessing for other postoperative complications, including:
    a. Increased ICP
       (1) Severe headache
       (2) Deteriorating LOC
       (3) Restlessness and irritability
       (4) Dilated or pinpoint pupils that are slow to react or nonreactive to light
    b. Subdural and epidural hematomas and intracranial hemorrhage
       (1) Severe headache
       (2) Rapid change in LOC
       (3) Progressive neurologic deficits
       (4) Sudden cardiovascular and respiratory arrest
    c. Hydrocephalus (increased CSF in the brain)
    d. Respiratory complications:
       (1) Atelectasis
       (2) Pneumonia
       (3) Neurogenic pulmonary edema
    e. Wound infections:
       (1) Reddened and puffy wound appearance
       (2) Area sensitive to touch
       (3) Area warm
    f. Meningitis

Community-Based Care

- Assist the family to make the environment safe for prevention of falls (e.g., remove scatter rugs, install grab bars in the bathroom).
- When needed, work with the case manager or discharge planner to help the family select a facility with experience in providing care for neurologically impaired patients.
- Teach patients and families about:
  1. Seizure precautions and what to do if a seizure occurs
  2. Drug therapy and person to call if adverse drug events occur
  3. Avoiding any OTC drugs unless approved by the health care provider
  4. The importance of recommended follow-up health care appointments
  5. The need for adequate caloric intake during radiation therapy or chemotherapy
- Refer the patient and family to support groups and community resources such as the American Brain Tumor Association, the National Brain Tumor Foundation, the American Cancer Society, home care agencies, and hospice services or palliative care services (for those who are terminally ill).

U

ULCERS, PEPTIC

OVERVIEW

- A peptic ulcer is a mucosal lesion of the stomach or duodenum. The term is used to describe both gastric and duodenal ulcers.
- Peptic ulcer disease (PUD) results when mucosal defenses become impaired and no longer protect the epithelium from the effects of acid and pepsin.
- Peptic ulcer development is primarily associated with bacterial infection with *Helicobacter pylori* and NSAID use. Caffeine, gluco-corticoid drugs, smoking, and radiation therapy also contribute to PUD.
- Types of peptic ulcers include:
  1. *Gastric ulcer,* which occurs when there is a break in the mucosal barrier and hydrochloric acid injures the stomach, usually near the antrum; gastric emptying is often delayed with gastric ulceration, worsening the injury.
  2. *Duodenal ulcer,* a chronic break in the duodenal mucosa that extends through the muscularis mucosa and most commonly

occurs in the upper portion of the duodenum; it is characterized by high gastric acid secretion and is the most common type of peptic ulcer.
3. *Stress ulcer,* which occurs with acute and chronic diseases or major trauma; bleeding resulting from gastric erosion is the principal manifestation, and multiple lesions occur in the proximal portion of the stomach, beginning with the area of ischemia and evolving into erosions.

- Complications of PUD include:
  1. Gastrointestinal (GI) bleeding
  2. Perforation, with the gastroduodenal contents emptying through the anterior wall of the stomach or duodenum into the peritoneal cavity
  3. Pyloric obstruction
  4. Intractable disease, which is characterized by a lack of response to conservative management and with symptoms that interfere with ADLs

PATIENT-CENTERED COLLABORATIVE CARE
Assessment
- Obtain patient information about:
  1. Symptoms, including epigastric discomfort, abdominal tenderness, cramps, indigestion, nausea, or vomiting and their onset, duration, location, and frequency, as well as aggravating and alleviating factors, including meal and sleep patterns
     a. Gastric ulcer pain may be relieved by food
     b. Duodenal ulcer pain occurs 1.5 to 3 hours after eating and often awakens the patient at night
  2. Tobacco, alcohol, caffeine, and intake of foods known to cause gastric irritation
  3. Medical history focusing on GI problems, particularly *H. pylori* infection
  4. Prescribed and OTC drugs, such as corticosteroids and NSAIDs
  5. Recent severe, serious, complex, or traumatic illness
  6. Presence of chronic disease and recent changes in flares or medications
- Assess for and document:
  1. Epigastric pain and tenderness; rigid, board-like abdomen accompanied by rebound tenderness (if perforation occurred)
  2. Secretions (emesis, sputum, stool, urine, and nasogastric drainage) for frank or occult blood
  3. Color, amount, and character of stools; note the presence of melena or occult blood
  4. Vital signs, including orthostatic blood pressure indicating hypovolemia or bleeding

5. Impact of chronic disease on the patient
- Diagnostic studies may include:
  1. Hemoglobin and hematocrit levels
  2. Testing for *H. pylori*
  3. Esophagogastroduodenoscopy (EGD), which is the major diagnostic test for PUD; direct visualization of the ulcer crater by EGD allows the health care provider to take specimens for *H. pylori* testing and for biopsy and cytologic studies for ruling out gastric cancer

Planning and Implementation
ACUTE OR CHRONIC PAIN
- Perform a comprehensive pain assessment. Carefully assess changes in the characteristic or location of peptic ulcer pain, because this may indicate the development of complications.
- Drug therapy includes:
  1. Proton pump inhibitors (PPI) are the drug class of choice for treating patients with acid-related GI disorders
  2. Alternatives are H_2 blockers or prostaglandin analogues to inhibit acid secretion and contribute to the mucosal barrier
  3. Antacids as buffering agents to decrease pain (given 2 hours after meals)
  4. Mucosal barrier fortifiers to provide a protective coat, preventing digestive action
  5. *H. pylori* infection treatment with antibiotics and a drug to reduce gastric acidity; antibiotics may include metronidazole, tetracycline, and amoxicillin for 10 to 14 days
- Monitor for gastric outflow or pyloric obstruction caused by edema, spasm, or scar tissue. Obstruction may be manifested by abdominal pain, bloating, distention, tenderness, and reduced bowel sounds.
- Surgery, either in a minimally invasive approach or an open approach, may be used to remove a chronic ulcer or provide a subtotal gastrectomy (partial stomach removal) and/or vagotomy (cutting of the vagus nerve) to reduce acid production.

RISK FOR GI BLEEDING
- For patients with persistent upper GI bleeding, embolization during endoscopy is done. An interventional radiologist may complete a catheter-directed embolization for small or persistent bleeding. For patients with a perforation, a surgical intervention may be needed to remove the ulcer site.
- The patient is at risk for fluid volume deficit (hypovolemia) and symptomatic blood loss.
  1. Management of hypovolemia and hemorrhage includes:
     a. Monitoring vital signs to detect hypovolemia manifested by tachycardia, hypotension, increased rate and depth of respirations, decreased Spo_2, and reduced LOC

U

b. Recording intake and output, including output from bleeding or vomiting
c. Monitoring serum electrolytes, coagulation factors, hematocrit, and hemoglobin and reporting abnormal values to the provider in a timely manner
d. Replacing fluids with IV fluids such as normal saline or lactated Ringer's solution
e. Transfusing blood products safely in the presence of symptomatic anemia or hypoxemia from low hemoglobin
f. Inserting an NG tube to ascertain the presence of blood in the stomach, assess the rate of bleeding, prevent gastric dilation, and provide lavage or removal of blood in the stomach
g. Keeping the patient NPO during periods of active bleeding

Community-Based Care

- Collaborate with the patient and family to identify gastric irritants.
- Instruct the patient about symptoms that should be brought to the attention of the health care provider.
  1. Abdominal pain
  2. Nausea and vomiting
  3. Black, tarry stools
  4. Weakness and dizziness
- Instruct the patient to avoid NSAIDs unless under the care of a health care provider who may prescribe concurrent acid-reducing medication.
- Teach dietary management to the postoperative patient, especially the patient who has had a partial stomach removal. Management should include:
  1. Eating small-volume meals
  2. Avoiding drinking liquids with meals
  3. Abstaining from foods that contribute to discomfort
  4. Receiving vitamin B_{12} injections as appropriate
- Teach the patient and family to recognize symptoms of pyloric obstruction that can occur from edema, spasm, or scar tissue. Symptoms of obstruction related to difficulty in emptying the stomach include feelings of fullness, distention, nausea after eating, and vomiting copious amounts of undigested food.

URETHRITIS

- Urethritis is inflammation or infection of the urethra.
- Symptoms of urethritis are:
  1. Burning, painful urination similar to cystitis/UTI symptoms
  2. Urgency and frequency
  3. Weak urine stream (men)

4. Incontinence
5. Discharge from the urethral meatus, especially in men
6. Pyuria (cloudy) or foul-smelling urine
- The most common cause of urethritis in males is sexually transmitted disease (STD).
- In postmenopausal women, urethritis may be caused by tissue changes related to low estrogen levels and it is treated with estrogen vaginal cream.
- Noninfectious urethritis may be caused by increased serum urea levels.
- STDs and infectious processes are treated with appropriate antibiotic therapy.

URINARY INCONTINENCE

OVERVIEW

- Urinary incontinence (UI) is the involuntary loss of urine that is severe enough to cause social or hygienic problems. It may be transient or permanent. It is not a normal change associated with aging.
- Common forms of urinary incontinence (UI)
  1. *Stress incontinence* is the loss of small amounts of urine during coughing, sneezing, jogging, or lifting. Patients are unable to tighten the urethra sufficiently to overcome the increased detrusor pressure, and leakage of urine results.
  2. *Urge incontinence* is the involuntary loss of urine associated with a sudden, strong desire to urinate. Patients are unable to suppress the signal for bladder contractions. It is also known as *overactive bladder.*
  3. *Mixed incontinence* is a combination of stress and urge incontinence.
  4. *Overflow incontinence* occurs when the bladder has reached a specific bladder volume. There is a decreased or absent ability to sense a full bladder.
  5. *Functional incontinence* is leakage of urine caused by factors other than pathology of the lower urinary tract, such as impaired cognition, impaired vision, or inability to reach a toilet.

PATIENT-CENTERED COLLABORATIVE CARE

Assessment

- Obtain patient information
  1. Determine the presence and severity of incontinence with effective screening questions. Ask the patient to respond with *always, sometimes,* or *never* to the following questions:
     a. Do you ever leak urine when you do not want to?
     b. Do you ever leak urine or water when you cough, laugh, or exercise?
     c. Do you ever leak urine on the way to the bathroom?

    d. Do you ever use pads, tissue, or cloth in your underwear to catch urine?

  2. Risk factors for UI

    a. Age, menopausal status

    b. Conditions that may affect the autonomic nervous system, cognition, or communication

    c. Childbirth

    d. Urologic procedures

    e. Drugs, especially drugs that affect the autonomic nervous system

    f. Bowel pattern

    g. Stress or anxiety level

  3. Limited mobility, reduced ability to ambulate and to transfer to a chair or toilet

  4. Inability to communicate the need for toileting

  5. Presence of UTI (cystitis)

- Assess for and document the findings of the following:

  1. Palpate the abdominal area for evidence of bladder fullness.

  2. Percuss the abdomen, and listen for the dull sound of a distended bladder.

  3. Observe for urine leakage while the patient strains by coughing or bearing down in the standing position.

  4. Determine the amount of residual urine by portable ultrasound or by catheterizing the patient immediately after voiding.

  5. Inspect the external genitalia of women to determine uterine prolapse, cystocele, or rectocele.

  6. Describe any secretions from the genitourinary openings.

  7. Inspect the urinary meatus of men for the presence of discharge or other characteristics.

  8. Query the patient regarding the effects of incontinence on socialization, family relationships, and emotional status.

  9. Monitor the urine for color, odor, and presence of sediment or cloudiness, and report abnormal results of a urinalysis in a timely manner to the prescribing health care provider.

  10. Review the results of the voiding cystourethrogram, which detects the anatomic structure and function of the bladder, and the postvoiding residual.

Planning and Implementation
REDUCING STRESS URINARY INCONTINENCE
Nonsurgical Management

- Nonsurgical management of incontinence may include:

  1. Drug therapy to reduce urgency and frequency

  2. Dietary counseling, in collaboration with the dietitian, to assist the obese patient with weight loss and to encourage all patients to avoid alcohol and caffeine (bladder irritants)

3. Exercise therapy
   a. Teach women how to do Kegel exercises to strengthen the muscles of the pelvic floor; biofeedback devices may be used to help the patient detect the effectiveness of the exercises.
   b. Instruct the patient in the correct use of vaginal cones.
      (1) The lightest cone is inserted into the vagina with the string to the outside for a 1-minute test period and repeated with heavier cones until one is not retained. Treatment begins with the heaviest cone the patient is able to retain while walking for one minute.
      (2) The treatment is for 15 minutes twice daily; when the patient can hold the cone comfortably in her vagina for 15 minutes, proceed to the next heaviest weight.
4. Other treatments include behavior modification, psychotherapy, and electrical devices for the inhibition of bladder contraction.

Surgical Management

- Operative procedures for women are used to elevate the bladder and urethra into a normal intra-abdominal position, increase the length of the urethra, and decrease hypermobility of the bladder neck. These procedures are:
  1. A surgical procedure that suspends the bladder with a sling made from mesh.
  2. Injection of a bulking agent into the urethral wall to provide resistance or urine outflow.
  3. Placement of an artificial sphincter, a mechanical device that opens and closes the urethra, around the anatomic urethra. This procedure is used for men more often than for women.
- Provide preoperative and postoperative care as described in Part One and:
  1. Secure the urethral catheter to prevent unnecessary movement or traction on the bladder neck.
  2. Monitor the suprapubic catheter, if present, for leakage of urine and serosanguineous drainage.

REDUCING URGE URINARY INCONTINENCE

- Interventions for urge UI include drug and behavioral interventions such as bladder and habit training. Surgery is not recommended.
  1. Drug therapy includes:
     a. Anticholinergic agents and anticholinergics with smooth muscle relaxant properties
     b. Tricyclic antidepressants
  2. Diet therapy includes:
     a. Instructing the patient to avoid foods that have a bladder-stimulating effect, such as caffeine and alcohol

U

     b. Instructing the patient to space fluids throughout the day and to limit fluids after dinner

3. Bladder training is an educational program to help patients gain control of their bladder.
   a. A regular schedule of voiding is established.
   b. The patient is instructed to void during the established time frame and to ignore any urge to urinate that occurs between the mandated intervals.
   c. After the patient is comfortable with the initial interval, the interval time is increased by 15 to 30 minutes.
4. Habit training is a variation of bladder training that is useful for cognitively impaired patients. The caregiver assists the patient to void every 2 hours.
5. Exercise therapies, such as Kegel exercises and vaginal cone therapy, are also useful.
6. Electrical stimulation with a variety of intravaginal and intrarectal devices has been used to treat both stress and urge UI.

REDUCING OVERFLOW URINARY INCONTINENCE

- Interventions for reflex incontinence include surgery, drugs, and teaching the patient interventions to empty the bladder. Avoid urine volumes greater than 300 mL to maintain continence in this condition.
  1. Surgery, which includes removal of the prostate and repair of genital prolapse to relieve the obstruction of the bladder outlet
  2. Drug therapy, which includes bethanechol chloride for the short-term management of urinary retention
  3. Interventions can assist with bladder emptying
     a. Use or teach the Credé maneuver, Valsalva maneuver, or double-voiding technique to assist in promoting bladder contraction.
     b. Teaching intermittent self-catheterization to patients with neurogenic bladder disorders and other long-term problems of incomplete bladder emptying.

REDUCING FUNCTIONAL URINARY INCONTINENCE

- The primary focus of the intervention is to treat reversible causes of incontinence. When that is not possible, the goal is to contain the urine and protect the patient's skin. Interventions include:
  1. Altering the environment so the patient can reach the toilet easily
  2. Implementing habit training for the cognitively impaired patient
  3. Using absorbent pads and briefs to collect urine and keep the patient's skin and clothing dry
  4. Using an external catheter for men or any patient, inserting a Foley catheter, or implementing intermittent catheterization, especially when perineal skin impairment is present

Community-Based Care

- Discharge planning includes:
  1. Assessing the home environment for barriers that impede access to the toileting facilities
  2. Considering the patient's personal, physical, emotional, and social resources that can promote bladder training or toileting
  3. Assisting the patient to control or manage fears and anxieties related to incontinence while in public
- Teach the patient and family about:
  1. The causes of incontinence and treatment options available
  2. Prescribed drugs (purpose, dosage, method, route of administration, and expected and potential side effects)
  3. The importance of weight reduction and dietary modification
  4. Options available for external devices or incontinence pads, considering the patient's lifestyle and resources
  5. The technique of self-catheterization, ensuring that a return demonstration is correct

UROLITHIASIS
OVERVIEW

- Urolithiasis is the presence of calculi (stones) in the urinary tract. Stones often do not cause symptoms until they pass into the lower urinary tract, where they can cause excruciating pain. *Nephrolithiasis* is the formation of stones in the kidney. *Ureterolithiasis* is the formation of stones in the ureter.
- The exact mechanism of formation is not known, but three conditions contribute to stone formation.
  1. Slow urine flow, resulting in supersaturation of the urine with the particular element (e.g., calcium) that first becomes crystallized and later becomes the stone
  2. Damage to the lining of the urinary tract (from crystals)
  3. Decreased inhibitor substances in the urine that would otherwise prevent supersaturation and crystal aggregation; high urine acidity (as with uric acid and cystine stones), high alkalinity (as with calcium phosphate and struvite stones), and drugs (triamterene, indinavir, and acetazolamide)
- Calculi may be formed from calcium, phosphate, oxalate, uric acid, struvite, and cystine crystals, but most stones contain calcium as one component.

PATIENT-CENTERED COLLABORATIVE CARE
Assessment

- Obtain patient information about:
  1. Personal and family history of kidney stones
  2. Metabolic disorders and diet history

☣ Genetic/Genomic Considerations

Family history has a strong association with stone formation and recurrence. More than 30 genetic variations are associated with the formation of kidney stones. Single gene disorders are rare. More commonly, nephrolithiasis is a complex disease, with genetic variation in intestinal calcium absorption, kidney calcium transport, or kidney phosphate transport. Always ask a patient with a renal stone whether other family members have also had this problem.

- Assess for and document:
  1. The location and duration of pain, which is often described as severe, unbearable, spasmodic (colic), and in the region of the trunk, back, and thighs ("flank" pain)
  2. Nausea and vomiting
  3. Hematuria, oliguria, or anuria
  4. Increased turbidity and odor of urine
  5. Bladder distention

Planning and Implementation
MANAGE ACUTE PAIN
  Nonsurgical Management
- Drug therapy includes:
  1. Opioid agents, such as hydromorphone or morphine
  2. NSAIDs, such as ketorolac (Toradol)
  3. Spasmolytic agents, such as oxybutynin chloride (Ditropan) and propantheline bromide (Pro-Banthine, Propanthel)
- Assess the patient's response to drug interventions.
- Encourage ambulation and an upright position to drain the renal calyx and pass renal calculi.
- Assist the patient in finding a comfortable position; distraction or relaxation techniques such as hypnosis, imagery, or acupuncture can be used to relieve pain.
- Lithotripsy, or *extracorporeal shock wave lithotripsy* (ESWL), is the application of ultrasound or dry shock wave energies to fragment the calculus. The patient receives conscious sedation as the lithotriptor and fluoroscope locate and break up the calculus. After lithotripsy, implement routine postoperative care with additional monitoring for urine output (quantity, quality, and presence of sediment or stones).
  Surgical Management
- Stone removal procedures include:
  1. *Ureteroscopy,* which is the use of an endoscope through the urethra to visualize stones and to extract stones with a basket,

or the use of a laser to fragment stones; stents may be used to dilate the ureter and create a passageway for the stone

2. *Percutaneous ureterolithotomy* and *nephrolithotomy,* or the use of an endoscope to visualize the stone with a special attachment to extract the calculus through a small flank incision

3. *Laparoscopic* or *open ureterolithotomy, pyelolithotomy,* or *nephrolithotomy,* which is the use of a laparoscope or a retroperitoneal incision to remove the stone(s)

- Preoperative care includes routine care described in Part One and:
  1. Providing individualized instructions, depending on the procedure to be performed
  2. Preparing bowel according to the physician's preference
- Postoperative care includes routine care described in Part One and:
  1. Monitoring the urine amount and character (color, presence of sediment or clots, volume) every 1 to 2 hours for 24 hours and preventing urinary obstruction from stone fragments or clots
  2. Straining the patient's urine to capture stones for analysis
  3. Reducing the risk for infection including administering antibiotics and monitoring vital signs for fever or urosepsis
  4. Ensuring adequate nutrition and fluid intake, which may include additional fluid intake to "flush" the kidneys for the first 24 hours after diagnosis
  5. Administering drug therapy to promote the elimination of chemicals contributing to stone formation and assessing for adverse effects, including:
     a. Acetohydroxamic acid (Lithostat) and hydroxyurea (Hydrea) for patients with struvite stones; monitoring serum creatinine levels (contraindicated for levels above 2 mg/dL)
     b. Thiazide diuretics to treat hypercalciuria (high levels of calcium in the urine)
     c. Allopurinol (Zyloprim) and vitamin B_6 (pyridoxine) to treat hyperoxaluria (high levels of oxalic acid in the urine) or gout
     d. Alpha-mercaptopropionylglycine (AMPG) and captopril (Capoten) to treat cystinuria (high levels of cystine in the urine)

Community-Based Care
- Inform the patient that:
  1. Extensive bruising may occur after lithotripsy and may take several weeks to resolve.
  2. Urine may be bloody for several days after surgical intervention.

- Instruct the patient about:
    1. The importance of following the prescribed drug regimen
    2. Diet, depending on metabolic evaluation or stone type
    3. The rationale for preventing dehydration, stressing the importance of dilute urine from adequate fluid intake
    4. The importance of reporting symptoms of infection or formation of another stone, such as pain, fever, chills, and difficulty with urination
    5. The importance of keeping follow-up appointments to check on the resolution of symptoms or postoperative recovery

UTERINE BLEEDING (DYSFUNCTIONAL)

OVERVIEW

- Dysfunctional uterine bleeding (DUB) is abnormal bleeding from the vagina. Most women have menstrual cycles every 24-34 days and a cycle that lasts 4-7 days. When bleeding or spotting between cycles occurs, when bleeding is very heavy or lasts more than 7 days, or when the time between cycles is less than 21 days, DUB may be diagnosed.
- Most cases of DUB are classified into two types: anovulatory DUB (most common) and ovulatory DUB.
- Risk factors for DUB are obesity, extreme weight loss or gain, age older than 40 years, high stress levels, polycystic ovary disease, long-term use of oral contraceptives, excessive exercise, and anatomic abnormalities including leiomyomas (fibroids) or cancer.

PATIENT-CENTERED COLLABORATIVE CARE

Assessment

- Ask about:
    1. Changes in weight, exercise, and health
    2. Abdominal or pelvic pain
    3. History of contraceptive use
- Determine whether there are systemic symptoms from blood loss (anemia).

Interventions

Nonsurgical Management

- Treatment is hormone therapy with progestin or combined estrogen-progestin therapy.
- Evaluate the patient's knowledge about the effects, dosage, and administration schedule of her prescribed hormone therapy.
- Teach the patient the information she needs to know about her prescribed hormone therapy.

Surgical Management

- Surgical management includes laser endometrial ablation, uterine artery embolization, dilation and curettage, and hysterectomy.

- Nursing care is similar to that for a woman undergoing a vaginal hysterectomy (see *Surgical Management* under *Leiomyomas [Uterine Fibroids]*).

UTERINE FIBROIDS (LEIOMYOMAS)

See *Leiomyomas (Uterine Fibroids)*.

V

VASCULAR DISEASE, PERIPHERAL

- Peripheral vascular disease (PVD) includes disorders that alter the natural flow of blood through the arteries and veins of the peripheral circulation.
- It affects the lower extremities much more commonly than the upper extremities.
- A diagnosis of PVD usually implies arterial disease rather than venous involvement. Some patients have both arterial and venous disease (see *Peripheral Arterial Disease* and *Peripheral Venous Disease*).

VEINS, VARICOSE

- Varicose veins are distended, protruding veins that appear darkened or tortuous.
- The vein walls weaken and dilate. Venous pressure increases, and the valves become incompetent. Incompetent valves contribute to venous insufficiency (see *Peripheral Venous Disease*). Both superficial and deep veins can become dilated.
- Varicose veins occur primarily in patients subjected to prolonged standing. They also occur in pregnant women and in patients with systemic problems, such as heart disease or obesity, and a family history of varicose veins.
- Conservative treatment measures include:
  1. Wearing elastic stockings
  2. Elevating the legs as often as possible
- Surgical management includes endovascular ablation to occlude the bulging vein.
  1. This is generally completed as a same-day surgery with routine perioperative care and restrictions to weight bearing for several days.
  2. Other surgical procedures include:
     a. Sclerotherapy, in which the physician injects a chemical to sclerose the vein, performed on small or a limited number of varicosities
     b. Laser treatment, using a laser to heat and close the main vessel that is contributing to the varicosity

      c. Surgical ligation (tying) and stripping (removal) the affected veins with the patient under general anesthesia
- Collateral veins take over supplying blood to tissues after laser, radiofrequency, or surgical interventions.

VENOUS THROMBOEMBOLISM

Venous thromboembolism (VTE) includes both deep vein thrombosis (DVT) and pulmonary embolism (PE) or occlusion to the pulmonary artery. A thrombus (also called a *thrombosis*) is a blood clot typically associated with endothelial injury, venous stasis, or hypercoagulability. An embolus is a clot that travels and lodges in a new area.

VISUAL IMPAIRMENT (REDUCED VISION)

OVERVIEW

- Visual impairment can range from total blindness in both eyes to various degrees and types of partial impairment.
- Patients are legally blind if their best visual acuity with corrective lenses is 20/200 or less in the better eye or if the widest diameter of the visual field in that eye is 20 degrees or less.
- Blindness can occur in one or both eyes. When one eye is affected, the field of vision is narrowed, and depth perception is impaired.
- Central vision can be impaired by diseases involving the macula, such as macular edema or macular degeneration.
- Peripheral vision loss affects the patient's ability to drive and awareness of hazards in the periphery.

PATIENT-CENTERED COLLABORATIVE CARE

- Test the visual acuity of both eyes immediately of any person who experiences an eye injury or any sudden change in vision.
- Ask the patient about vision problems in any other members of the family, because some vision problems have a genetic component.
- Urge all patients to wear eye protection when they are performing yard work, working in a woodshop or metal shop, using chemicals, or are in any environment in which drops or particulate matter are airborne.
- Nursing interventions for the patient with reduced sight focus on communication, safety, ambulation, self-management, and support.
  1. Communicate and listen to the patient's preferences for safety.
     a. Stress to hospital staff, family, and friends that changes in item location should not be made without input from the person with reduced vision.
     b. Orient the patient to the immediate environment, including the size of the room. Use one object in the room, such as a chair or hospital bed, as the focal point during your description. Guide the person to the focal point and describe all other objects in relation to the focal point.

! NURSING SAFETY PRIORITY: Action Alert

Never leave the patient with reduced vision in the center of an unfamiliar room.

    c. Allow the patient to establish the location of important objects, such as the call light, water pitcher, and clock.

    d. Set up food trays using imaginary clock placement to orient the patient to the location of specific items.

2. Teach safe ambulation.

    a. Allow the patient to grasp your arm at the elbow while keeping the arm close to your body so that he or she can detect your direction of movement.

    b. Alert the patient when obstacles are in the path ahead.

    c. Assist with the correct use of a cane to detect obstacles (the cane is held in the dominant hand several inches off the floor and sweeps the ground where the patient's foot will be placed next).

    d. Go with the patient to other important areas, such as the bathroom. Count steps and highlight landmarks such as the location of the toilet, sink, and toilet paper holder.

3. Promote self-management.

    a. To make better use of existing vision, teach the patient:

        (1) To move the head slightly up and down to enhance a three-dimensional effect

        (2) To line up the object and move toward it when shaking hands or pouring water

        (3) To choose a position that favors the good eye; for example, people with vision in the right eye should position people and items on their right

    b. Knock on the door before entering the room and state your name and the reason for visiting when entering the room. Use a normal tone of voice unless there is a hearing problem.

    c. Encourage mastery of one task at a time and provide positive reinforcement for each success when adapting to visual loss or impairment.

    d. Use local resources that provide adaptive items such as large print books for reduced vision or talking clocks for any impaired vision.

4. Provide support.

    a. Provide opportunities for the patient and family to express their concerns about a possible change in vision status.

    b. Allow the newly blind person a period of grieving for loss of vision.

V

W

WEST NILE VIRUS

* West Nile virus infection is typically spread by infected mosquitoes; blood products, breast milk, or organ transplantation can also transmit the disease.
* The infection is generally mild, and the patient usually is asymptomatic or has only flu-like symptoms (e.g., fever, body aches, nausea, vomiting).
* A small percentage of patients develop encephalitis with symptoms that include:
  1. High fever
  2. Severe headache
  3. Decreased LOC
  4. Vision loss
  5. Seizures
  6. Tremors and muscle weakness or paralysis
* Diagnostic tests include enzyme-linked immunosorbent assay (ELISA) and West Nile virus-specific IgM antibody in serum or cerebrospinal fluid (CSF).
* Management is symptomatic, as for any other type of viral encephalitis.
* For the severe form of the disease, manifestations may last for several weeks, and neurologic deficits may be permanent.
* To prevent West Nile virus infection, avoid mosquito bites.
  1. Use an insect repellent containing an Environmental Protection Agency (EPA)-registered active ingredient such as DEET or Picaridin.
  2. Wear long sleeves and pants at dusk when mosquitoes abound.
  3. Keep mosquitoes out of homes and sleeping areas with screens.
  4. Destroy mosquito breeding sites by emptying standing water from flower pots, buckets, wading pools, and barrels.

Guide to Head-to-Toe Physical Assessment of Adults

Guide to Head-to-Toe Physical Assessment of Adults*

Nursing Activity	Typical Finding	Changes Associated with Aging
NEUROLOGIC SYSTEM		
1. Determine level of consciousness.	1. Awake, alert	1. None
2. Test for orientation.	2. States name, place, and time	2. None
SKIN		
1. Inspect skin.	1. Intact, warm, dry, elastic skin without lesions	1a. Excessive dryness; wrinkles; discolorations from ultraviolet exposure ("age spots") and hemangiomas; inelastic, sagging skin
		1b. Ecchymotic areas as a result of increased capillary fragility
HEAD AND FACE		
1. Inspect and palpate the scalp, hair, and skull.	1. No lesions, shiny hair	1. Alopecia, thinning and dullness of hair
2. Inspect the face for symmetry of expression.	2. Symmetric expression	2. None

Continued

Guide to Head-to-Toe Physical Assessment of Adults—cont'd

Nursing Activity	Typical Finding	Changes Associated with Aging
EYE		
1. Inspect the external eye structures.	1. No structural abnormalities	1. Entropion (inverted eyelid) or ectropion (everted eyelid)
2. Inspect the conjunctivae, sclerae, corneas, and irides.	2. No abnormalities; round irides	2. None
3. Use a penlight to test pupillary response (direct and consensual).	3. Pupils are equal and round and react to light and accommodation	3. None
4. Test vision by asking the client to read (if able) or interpret an eye chart. **NOTE:** Be sure that glasses or contact lenses are in place, if used.	4. No vision impairment	4. Presbyopia (farsightedness)
EAR		
1. Inspect the external structure.	1. No structural abnormalities	1. No major change
2. Inspect the auditory meatus for drainage.	2. No drainage; small amount of cerumen may be present	2. None
3. Test hearing by whispering to the client while turning head away. **NOTE:** Be sure that hearing aid, if used, is in place.	3. No difficulty in hearing	3. Hearing loss, especially high-frequency sounds

Guide to Head-to-Toe Physical Assessment of Adults—cont'd

Nursing Activity	Typical Finding	Changes Associated with Aging
MOUTH		
1. Use a penlight to inspect mouth, teeth, and gums.	1. No lesions, extensive dental caries, or gum disease	1. None
NECK		
1. Inspect for symmetry, lesions, pulsations, and JVD.	1. Symmetric, without lesions or JVD	1. None
2. Palpate the carotid pulse, one side at a time; check for bruits.	2. No bruits; pulses equal	2. None
3. Palpate the cervical lymph nodes.	3. Unable to palpate	3. None
4. Test ROM.	4. No limitations	4. Possible reduced neck flexion and extension; possible crepitus
CHEST (POSTERIOR, ANTERIOR, AND LATERAL)		
1. Inspect the chest for deformity, symmetry, expansion, and lesions; note pulsations or heaves (lifts).	1. Symmetric; without lesions; anteroposterior-lateral ratio of 1:2; no heaves	1. Slight change in anteroposterior-lateral ratio (1:1.5)
2. Palpate any chest lesions.	2. No lesions	2. None
3. Locate the PMI.	3. PMI at the left MCL, fifth ICS	3. None
4. Palpate each vertebra of the spine.	4. No tenderness or bony spurs	4. Thoracic kyphosis

Continued

Guide to Head-to-Toe Physical Assessment of Adults—cont'd

Nursing Activity	Typical Finding	Changes Associated with Aging
5. Auscultate breath sounds throughout all lung fields.	5. Unlabored excursion of air; no adventitious sounds	5. Shallow respirations
6. Auscultate apical rate and rhythm; auscultate heart sounds.	6. S_1 and S_2 heart sounds	6. Possible S_4 heart sound
UPPER EXTREMITIES		
1. Inspect and palpate joints for swelling, tenderness, and deformity.	1. No swelling, tenderness, or deformity	1. Tenderness of one or more joints
2. Palpate brachial and radial arteries; assess for pulse deficit.	2. Pulses equal and within normal limits	2. None
3. Test ROM in all joints and sensation.	3. No restriction	3. Slight decrease in ROM; possible crepitus
4. Test muscle strength of arms, hands, and shoulders.	4. Movement against both gravity and resistance (5/5)	4. None or slight decrease (4+/5)
5. Palpate axillary nodes.	5. Nodes not palpable	5. None
ABDOMEN		
1. Inspect for contour, symmetry, lesions, and pulsations.	1. Symmetric; without lesions or pulsations	1. None
2. Auscultate bowel sounds in all four quadrants.	2. 5-15 sounds/min in each quadrant	2. May be slightly decreased (hypoactive)
3. Auscultate over abdominal aorta for bruit.	3. No bruit	3. None

Guide to Head-to-Toe Physical Assessment of Adults—cont'd

Nursing Activity	Typical Finding	Changes Associated with Aging
4. Palpate for liver enlargement.	4. Liver not below costal margin	4. None
LOWER EXTREMITIES		
1. Inspect and palpate for swelling, tenderness, and deformity.	1. No swelling, tenderness, or deformity	1. Tenderness of one or more joints
2. Test ROM and sensation.	2. No limitation	2. Slight decrease in ROM; possible crepitus
3. Test muscle strength.	3. Movement against gravity and resistance (5/5)	3. None or slight decrease (4+/5)
4. Palpate femoral, popliteal, and pedal pulses.	4. Pulses equal and within normal range	4. Pedal pulses may be weak or not palpable.
5. Palpate inguinal nodes.	5. Nodes not palpable	5. None
GENITALIA		
1. Inspect external genitalia for lesions or drainage.	1. No lesions or drainage	1. None

For more information on physical assessment, see Ignatavicius, D. D., & Workman, M. L. (2016). *Medical-Surgical Nursing: Patient-Centered Collaborative Care* (8th ed.). Philadelphia: Saunders.

ICS, intercostal space; *JVD,* jugular venous distension; *MCL,* mid-clavicular line; *PMI,* point of maximal impulse; *ROM,* range of motion.

*Additional assessments may be needed, depending on the patient's concerns and the medical diagnoses.

Interventions for Common Environmental Emergencies

Interventions for Common Environmental Emergencies

	Clinical Manifestations	Collaborative Management
HEAT-RELATED ILLNESS		
Heat exhaustion, a syndrome resulting mainly from dehydration	Patient complains of flu-like symptoms: Headache Weakness Nausea, vomiting Hypotension, tachycardia May have normal temperature	Stop physical activity. Move to cool environment or fan while spraying water on skin. Remove constrictive clothing. Rehydrate with an oral solution such as a sports drink. Place cool packs on neck, chest, abdomen, and groin. If symptoms persist, transport to the hospital. Monitor vital signs and consider intravenous fluid replacement based on serum electrolyte analysis.
Heat stroke: Medical emergency with thermoregulatory failure	Profoundly elevated body temperature >104° F (40°C) Hot, dry skin although sweating can be present	Ensure patent airway, effective breathing, and adequate circulation (ABCs). Anticipate emergency transport to hospital. Administer oxygen as needed. Provide rapid cooling to achieve rectal temperature of 102° F (37.8°C) by: Removing clothing Placing ice packs on neck, axillae, chest, and groin Immersing in cold water or spraying body with cold water and fanning rapidly

Continued

Interventions for Common Environmental Emergencies—cont'd

	Clinical Manifestations	Collaborative Management
Two types: Exertional occurs as a sudden onset and during strenuous activity Classic occurs over a longer time period with chronic exposure to a hot, humid environment	Mental status changes: Confusion Bizarre behavior Seizures Coma Vital sign abnormalities: Hypotension Tachycardia Tachypnea	Provide intravenous (IV) access and cool IV fluids. Monitor for multiple organ dysfunction syndrome and electrolyte imbalances during treatment and recovery phases.
COLD-RELATED INJURIES Hypothermia: core body temperature below 95°F (35°C) Mild: 32°-35°C, 89.6°-95 F	*Mild:* Shivering Tachycardia, tachypnea Muscular incoordination Impaired cognition Diuresis	*Mild:* Shelter from cold environment. Remove wet clothes and apply warm clothes or blankets; warm room. Provide liquids that do not contain alcohol or caffeine. Monitor skin to avoid rewarming damage.

Interventions for Common Environmental Emergencies—cont'd

	Clinical Manifestations	Collaborative Management
Moderate: 28°-32° C, 82.4°-89.6° F	*Moderate:* Obvious motor impairment such as stumbling, falling Irrational, incoherent progressing to stupor or coma Shivering stops Patient may perceive warmth and undress Bradycardia and hypotension Decreased respiratory rate and cardiac output Dysrhythmias Coagulopathy Thrombocytopenia	*Moderate and severe:* Hospital care is required. Monitor and support ABCs. Rewarm trunk first to avoid "after drop," which is a continued decrease in core body temperature from cold peripheral blood returning to the trunk after the victim is removed from the cold environment. Core rewarming methods include administration of warm IV fluids, heated oxygen, and inspired gas.
Severe: <28° C, <82.4° F	*Severe:* Absent neurologic reflexes; no response to pain Hypotension	*Severe:* Rewarm core as with moderate hypothermia using internal and external warming devices.

Continued

Interventions for Common Environmental Emergencies—cont'd

	Clinical Manifestations	Collaborative Management
	Acid-base abnormalities Ventricular fibrillation, asystole Coagulopathy Thrombocytopenia	Extracorporeal rewarming methods used for severe hypothermia such as cardiopulmonary bypass, hemodialysis, or continuous arteriovenous rewarming Administer medications cautiously because metabolism is unpredictable. A drug can accumulate without obvious therapeutic effect while the patient is cold, becoming active or toxic with effective rewarming.
Frostbite	*Frostnip:* superficial frostbite without tissue injury, with pain, numbness, and pallor of the affected area (white or waxy appearance)	*Frostnip:* Apply warmth. Use body heat to warm the affected area. For example, place warm hands over cold ears or cold hands under axillary region.

Interventions for Common Environmental Emergencies—cont'd

Clinical Manifestations	Collaborative Management
Superficial frostbite: Hyperemia and edema *Partial frostbite:* Large, fluid-filled blisters with partial-thickness skin necrosis *Full-thickness frostbite:* Small blisters that contain dark fluid Full-thickness and subcutaneous necrosis Affected area cool, numb, blue, or red that does not blanch *Fourth-degree frostbite:* No blisters or edema Affected area is numb, cold, and bloodless. Full-thickness necrosis extends into muscle and bone	*Frostbite:* Hospital care is required. Rapidly rewarm in a water bath at temperature 104°-108°F (40°-42°C) for partial and full-thickness injuries. Premedicate for pain before rewarming. Do not apply dry heat or rub affected area. After rewarming, elevate an involved extremity above the heart to decrease tissue edema. Administer tetanus prophylaxis if needed. Surgical management may be necessary for deep wounds. Amputation may be necessary.

Continued

Interventions for Common Environmental Emergencies—cont'd

	Clinical Manifestations	Collaborative Management
SNAKEBITES North American pit viper: Rattlesnake Copperhead Water moccasin (cottonmouth)	One or more puncture wounds Severe pain, massive local tissue swelling with redness or bruising at the bite Later: vesicles or hemorrhagic bullae Tingling or paresthesias of scalp, face, and lips Muscle fasciculations and weakness Nausea, vomiting Hypotension Seizures Coagulopathy	Move patient to safe location and encourage rest to decrease venom circulation. Remove jewelry and constrictive clothes before swelling occurs. Call for help; take a picture of the snake if possible. If extremity is affected, immobilize and keep below level of heart without touching the wound; ice the site or use a tourniquet. Provide intravenous fluid and oxygen. Start cardiac and blood pressure monitoring. Manage pain. Give tetanus prophylaxis.

Interventions for Common Environmental Emergencies—cont'd

Clinical Manifestations	Collaborative Management
	Administer antibiotic to reduce risk of infection.
	Obtain laboratory studies:
	CBC, electrolytes
	Coagulation studies
	Creatinine kinase
	Type and crossmatch
	Urinalysis
	Measure and record circumference of bite site and monitor distal circulation every 15-30 minutes.
	Monitor for bleeding because of potential of coagulopathy.
	Contact the poison control center.
	Administer antivenom if ordered and monitor for adverse reactions.

Continued

Interventions for Common Environmental Emergencies—cont'd

	Clinical Manifestations	Collaborative Management
Coral snake	Coral snake venom is neurotoxic, producing: Pain Weakness Cranial nerve deficits particularly swallowing difficulties Altered consciousness Respiratory paralysis Toxic effect may be delayed 12-13 hours Patient may develop total flaccid paralysis and/or cardiovascular collapse	Limit venom spread with pressure and immobilization. Take a picture of the snake. Provide continuous cardiac, blood pressure, and pulse oximetry monitoring. Monitor and initiate interventions to prevent aspiration. Contact the poison control center. Intubate and provide breathing support as needed; the patient may require prolonged mechanical ventilatory support while the venom is cleared.

Interventions for Common Environmental Emergencies—cont'd

	Clinical Manifestations	Collaborative Management
ARTHROPOD (SPIDER) BITES		
Brown recluse spider	Bite is painless or stinging to sharply painful	Apply cold compresses—never use heat.
	Intense local aching and pruritus develops over minutes to hours	Contact health care provider.
	Central bite site appears as a bleb or vesicle surrounded by edema and erythema, which may expand	Wound care includes oral or topical antibiotics, antiseptic cream, and a sterile dressing to cover the bite area.
	Over 1-3 days, central lesion becomes dark and necrotic; eschar forms.	Surgical evaluation to determine the need for débridement and skin grafting
	When the eschar sloughs, an open wound or ulcer can remain for weeks to months.	
	Systemic toxicity manifested by:	
	Renal failure	
	Thrombocytopenia	
	Hemolytic anemia	

Continued

Interventions for Common Environmental Emergencies—cont'd

	Clinical Manifestations	Collaborative Management

Black widow spider	Pain from bite can be nearly painless to severe
	Tiny papule or small, red punctate mark
	Systemic effects:
	  Severe abdominal pain
	  Muscle rigidity/spasm
	  Facial edema, ptosis
	  Diaphoresis, increased salivation
	  Fasciculations and paresthesias
		Apply ice pack.
		Monitor ABCs and support as needed.
		Transport to tertiary care center if systemic manifestations of toxicity occur.
		Manage pain.
		Manage spasticity.
		Maintain ABCs as needed.

Scorpions	Pain and inflammation Mild systemic symptoms	Call primary care provider. Analgesics, supportive management Clean wound and apply moist dressing for 24 hours.

Interventions for Common Environmental Emergencies—cont'd

	Clinical Manifestations	Collaborative Management
Bees and wasps	Sting produces discomfort to severe pain Allergy is manifested by hives, itching, and tongue or lip swelling Anaphylaxis can occur in allergic people and is manifested by: Respiratory distress Bronchospasm Laryngeal edema Hypotension Loss of consciousness Cardiac dysrhythmias Systemic effects depend on the venom load or the number of stings and person's sensitivity to the venom	Remove stingers. Provide ice packs. Monitor ABCs and support as needed. Establish cardiac and frequent vital sign monitoring if systemic allergy or anaphylaxis occurs. Anaphylaxis treatment includes immediate administration of epinephrine, generally intramuscularly via an autoinjector (EpiPen) or intravenously (IV) followed by oral or IV diphenhydramine.

Continued

Interventions for Common Environmental Emergencies—cont'd

Clinical Manifestations	Collaborative Management
LIGHTNING INJURIES	
Cardiac arrest	Initiate basic life support; monitor ABCs.
Central nervous system	Follow advanced life support guidelines.
Temporary paralysis lasting from	Monitor vital signs and cardiac rhythm.
minutes to hours	Immobilize for spinal cord injury.
Loss of consciousness	Note entrance and exit site injuries to
Amnesia	evaluate internal pathway damage.
Confusion, disorientation	Initiate burn care if needed.
Seizures	Monitor laboratory studies for muscle
Cerebellar dysfunction	damage such as creatinine kinase (CK) and
Spinal cord injury	anion gap.
Integumentary	Provide tetanus prophylaxis if needed.
Burns (superficial to full thickness)	Monitor kidney injury with serial serum and
	urine laboratory analyses of blood urea
	nitrogen (BUN), creatinine, and hourly
	urine output.

Interventions for Common Environmental Emergencies—cont'd

Clinical Manifestations	Collaborative Management
ALTITUDE-RELATED ILLNESSES	
Altitude sickness can occur at elevations of 2500 feet and above. Elevations 5000 feet above sea level are high altitudes.	
Elevations of greater than 18,000 feet are extreme altitudes.	
Acute mountain sickness (AMS)	Rest and allow time to acclimate to altitude.
Throbbing headache	Remove to lower altitude.
Anorexia	Administer oxygen if available.
Nausea and vomiting	Medications
Irritability, apathy	Acetazolamide (Diamox) to prevent and treat AMS
Variable vital signs	Dexamethasone (Decadron) may be given
Dyspnea on exertion, at rest	while patient moves to lower altitude

Continued

Interventions for Common Environmental Emergencies—cont'd

	Clinical Manifestations	Collaborative Management

High altitude cerebral edema (HACE)	Extreme apathy
	Confusion, lack of judgment
	Cranial nerve dysfunction
	Seizures
	Stupor, coma, death
		Rapid descent to lower altitude
		Supplemental oxygen
		Keep patient warm
		Medications, if available, during descent
		    Dexamethasone (Decadron)
		    Loop diuretics
		Hospital care required
		Monitor ABCs

High altitude pulmonary edema (HAPE)	Dyspnea on exertion Cyanosis of nails and lips Tachycardia, tachypnea Crackles on lung auscultation Pink frothy sputum	Symptom management As above

ABCs, Airway, breathing, circulation.

Chemical and Biological Agents of Terrorism

A bioterrorism attack is the deliberate release of viruses, bacteria, or other agents to cause illness or death. Bioterrorism agents are typically found in nature; some have been changed to increase their virulence. Biological agents can be spread through the air, through water, or in food.

Information on bioterrorism agents and general clinical management in this appendix is from the Centers for Disease Control and Prevention (CDC) website: www.bt.cdc.gov/bioterrorism.

Pathogen or Agent and Disease Information	Clinical Management

ANTHRAX (BACILLUS ANTHRACIS)
 	
Cutaneous: 1-7 days after contact, exposed skin itching, progressing to papular and vesicular lesions, eschar, edema, ulceration, and sloughing. If untreated, may spread to lymph nodes and bloodstream. Fatality 5%-20%.
 	
Inhalation: 48 hr after organism or spore inhalation, flu-like illness with possible brief improvement. 2-4 days from initial symptoms, abrupt onset of severe cardiopulmonary illness (dyspnea, tachycardia, fever, diaphoresis, thoracic edema, shock, and respiratory failure). If antibiotics are delayed until onset of cardiopulmonary symptoms, mortality is high. May be confused with common upper respiratory infection (URI).
 	
Other forms: Gastrointestinal (GI), meningeal, and sepsis.
	For cutaneous and inhaled anthrax: No person-to-person spread.
	Contact Precautions are not needed unless patient presents directly from exposure.
	Standard Precautions for:
	  Prescribed wound cleansing and management of lesions
	  Ventilator support for respiratory failure
	  Postmortem care

Pathogen or Agent and Disease Information	Clinical Management
BOTULISM (*CLOSTRIDIUM BOTULINUM* AND NEUROTOXIN) Toxin ingestion results in dysphasia, dry mouth, drooping eyelids, and blurred or double vision. Vomiting and constipation or diarrhea may be present initially, extending to symmetric flaccid paralysis in an alert person. Acute bilateral cranial nerve impairment and descending weakness or paralysis follow. Neurologic symptoms after 12-36 hr for foodborne botulism and in 24-72 hr after aerosol exposure. Case fatality up to 10%. Recovery may take months.	Standard Precautions: Decontamination of patient is not required. No person-to-person spread. Consider outbreak with suspicion of a single case. Consult with Centers for Disease Control and Prevention (CDC) and health departments. Advise careful cleanup and disposal of suspected contaminated food source *after* consultation with health department about any needed laboratory sampling. Interdisciplinary planning for nutrition and rehabilitation support during lengthy neuromuscular and respiratory recovery.

Continued

Pathogen or Agent and Disease Information	Clinical Management
PLAGUE (YERSINIA PESTIS) **Lymphatic infection:** 2-8 days after bites from fleas of an infected rodent (rarely after infected tissue or body fluid contact), onset of fever and chills, painful lymphadenopathy (or bubo—usually inguinal, axillary, or cervical lymph nodes), headache, GI symptoms, and rapidly progressive weakness. 50%-60% fatality if untreated. **Pneumonic:** 1-3 days after aerosolized organism inhalation, fever and chills, productive cough, hemoptysis, rapidly progressive weakness, GI symptoms, and bronchopneumonia. Survival unlikely if not treated within 18 hr of symptom onset. **Other forms:** Sepsis with coagulopathy, rarely meningitis.	Droplet Precautions: required for pneumonic plague (until 72 hr of antibiotic therapy). Contact Precautions until decontamination is complete: For any suspected gross contamination. See documentation information listed above under Anthrax. For prescribed management of bubo(s) if incised to drain. Community and other environmental modifications: Apply insecticide to infested environment and pets (to kill fleas). Reduce food and water supply for rodents. Avoid sick or dead animals.

Pathogen or Agent and Disease Information	Clinical Management
SMALLPOX (VARIOLA VIRUS) (VARIOLA MAJOR AND MINOR) 10-17 days after droplet or airborne virus inhalation or contact with bleeding lesions is onset of severe myalgias, headache, and high fever. 2-3 days later, a papular rash appears on face and spreads to extremities (and palms and soles). The rash quickly (simultaneously) becomes vesicular, then painful and pustular (contrasted to varicella rash that crops and concentrates more on trunk with various stages of macules to vesicles seen at one time). Patients are infectious at onset of rash until scabs separate (3 wk). Historically, variola major kills 20%. May be confused with varicella.	Standard, Contact, and Airborne Precautions for patients with vesicular rash pending diagnosis are the same for varicella and variola. Also, avoid contact with organism while handling contaminated clothes and bedding. Wear protective attire (gloves, gown, and N95 respirator). One case is a public health emergency—highly communicable. Consult CDC and health departments at earliest suspicion. Vaccine does not give reliable lifelong immunity. Previously vaccinated persons are considered susceptible. *Following exposure:* Initiate Airborne Precautions, and observe for unprotected contacts (from days 10-17). Vaccinate within 2-3 days of exposure.

Continued

Pathogen or Agent and Disease Information	Clinical Management

OTHER KEY POINTS

Assessment: Include account of symptoms, patient's incident (what, where, when, how, others exposed or ill, and officials aware).

Treatment: Antibiotic-resistance possible. Vaccine and postexposure prophylaxis are subject to change. If any of the above diseases are suspected, consult infection control practitioner for coordination with community health officials and CDC about current recommendations and specimen collection. *If bioterrorism suspected,* Federal Bureau of Investigation (FBI) will coordinate evidence collection and delivery.

Multiple exposures planning: Emergency and critical care managers must address availability and acquisition of stocks of medications, vaccines, equipment (e.g., ventilators), and communications with officials and public information needs.

Terminology Associated with Fluid and Electrolyte Balance

Active transport: assisted movement of a substance through a permeable membrane between two fluid compartments; occurs against a concentration, or electrical or pressure gradient; requires the expenditure of chemical energy.

Adenosine triphosphate (ATP): a substance generated by the metabolism of glucose or fat within cells; chemical energy for physiologic function of cells.

Aldosterone: a hormone secreted by the adrenal cortex that stimulates the renal reabsorption of sodium and water and the renal excretion of potassium.

Anion: a molecule (electrolyte) that carries a negative charge when dissolved.

Antidiuretic hormone (ADH): a hormone secreted from the posterior pituitary gland that increases the renal reabsorption of pure water and decreases urine output; also known as *vasopressin.*

Atrial natriuretic peptide (ANP): a hormone secreted by cardiac atrial cells that increases the renal excretion of sodium and water.

B-type natriuretic peptide (BNP) (sometimes called brain-natriuretic peptide): a hormone produced mainly in the cardiac ventricle cells that increases the excretion of sodium and water. BNP correlates to left ventricular pressures; the higher the BNP the higher the pressure and, by implication, the volume. Thus, high levels of BNP indicate worsening heart failure.

Capillary (plasma) hydrostatic pressure: the force generated by fluid within a capillary that tends to move fluid out from the capillary and into the interstitial space.

Capillary (plasma) osmotic pressure: the force generated by the concentration of plasma solutes (osmotic and oncotic pressures) that maintains fluid balance in vasculature.

Cation: a molecule (electrolyte) that carries a positive charge when dissolved.

Cofactor: a substance required to enhance the activity of an enzyme or a physiologic reaction.

Colloidal oncotic pressure: the osmotic pressure exerted by the concentration of colloids (proteins) within a solution; also known as *oncotic pressure.*

Diffusion: unimpeded movement of a substance through a permeable membrane between two fluid compartments; occurs down a concentration gradient; does not require the expenditure of chemical energy.

Disequilibrium: a state in which two fluid compartments are unequal in at least one characteristic.

Electrolytes: substances that carry an electrical charge when dissolved.

Electroneutrality: an equal number of cations and anions so that the cell, tissue, or fluid does not express an electrical charge.

Equilibrium: a state in which two fluid compartments are equal in one or more characteristics.

Extracellular fluid (ECF): body fluid present outside of cells, including plasma and interstitial fluid.

Facilitated diffusion: assisted movement of a substance through a permeable membrane between two fluid compartments; occurs down a concentration gradient; does not require the expenditure of chemical energy.

Filtration: the movement of fluid through a biologic membrane as a result of hydrostatic pressure differences on the two sides of the membrane.

Gradient: a difference in some characteristic between two fluid compartments.

Hydrostatic pressure: the force of pressure exerted by static water in a confined space; "water-pushing" pressure.

Hypertonic (hyperosmotic): any solution with a solute concentration (osmolarity) greater than that of normal body fluids (greater than 310 mOsm/L).

Hypotonic (hypo-osmotic): any solution with a solute concentration (osmolarity) less than that of normal body fluids (less than 270 mOsm/L).

Impermeable membrane: a membrane separating two fluid compartments that does not permit the movement of one or more substances through the membrane by diffusion.

Insensible fluid loss: fluid losses from the skin, gastrointestinal tract, wounds, and pulmonary epithelium.

Interstitial fluid: fluid in the spaces between cells.

Intracellular fluid (ICF): fluid found inside cells.

Isotonic (isosmotic): any solution with a solute concentration equal to the osmolarity of normal body fluids or normal saline (0.9% NaCl), or about 300 mOsm/L.

Obligatory urine output: the minimal amount of urine output necessary to ensure the excretion of metabolic wastes (approximately 400 mL/day); a clinical goal for urine output may be higher.

Osmolality: the concentration of particles (solutes) within a solution as measured per kilogram of solution.

Osmolarity: the concentration of particles (solutes) within a solution as measured per liter of solution.

Osmoreceptor: specialized sensory nerve cells in the thalamus or hypothalamus that are sensitive to changes in the osmolarity of extracellular fluid.

Osmosis: diffusion of water (no other substance) through a selectively permeable membrane from an area of lower osmotic pressure to an area of greater osmotic pressure.

Osmotic pressure: the pressure exerted by a solution with particles (solutes); this pressure draws water from areas or compartments with lower concentrations of solute into the areas or compartments with higher concentrations of solute; "water-pulling" pressure.

Permeable membrane: a membrane separating two fluid compartments that permits the movement of one or more substances through the membrane (by diffusion) from one compartment to the other.

Solubility: the degree to which any given solute completely dissolves (dissociates) in water.

Solute: particle or compound dissolved in a solution.

Solvent: the fluid (water) portion of a solution.

Tissue hydrostatic pressure (THP): the force generated by fluid within the interstitial spaces that tends to move fluid into the capillary from the interstitial space.

Tissue osmotic pressure (TOP): the force generated by the concentration of interstitial fluid solutes that tend to retain fluid in the interstitial space or move fluid from the capillary into the interstitial space.

Transcellular fluid: extracellular fluid confined to a specific area or region of the body (cerebrospinal fluid, pericardial fluid, visceral fluid, aqueous humor, peritoneal fluid, and pleural fluid).

Viscosity: fluidity or ability of a fluid to flow.

Electrocardiographic Complexes, Segments, Intervals

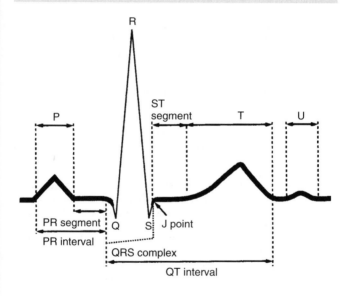

The electrocardiogram (ECG) is the graphic record of electrical activity of the heart. The spread of electrical current in the heart is detected by surface electrodes, and the amplified electrical signals are recorded on calibrated paper.

Cardiac dysrhythmias are abnormal rhythms of the heart's electrical system that can affect its ability to effectively pump oxygenated blood throughout the body. Some dysrhythmias are life threatening, and others are not. They are the result of disturbances of cardiac electrical impulse formation, conduction, or both. When the heart does not work effectively as a pump, perfusion to vital organs and peripheral tissues can be impaired, resulting in organ dysfunction or failure.

The first step in reading an ECG is to analyze the rhythm and rate. Determine whether the rhythm is regular or irregular, then calculate the heart rate by counting the number of PP or RR intervals that occur in 6 seconds, and multiply that number by 10. A normal rate is 60 to 100 beats per minute. The rhythm is either regular or irregular.

The second step is to systematically examine the waveforms, intervals, and segments:

P wave represents atrial depolarization.

PR segment represents the time required for the impulse to travel through the atrioventricular (AV) node (where the impulse is delayed).

PR interval represents the time required for atrial depolarization and impulse travel through the AV node, inclusive of the P wave and PR segment. It is measured from the beginning of the P wave to the end of the PR segment, and a normal time in adults is 0.12 to 0.2 second.

QRS complex represents depolarization of both ventricles and is measured from the point at which the complex first leaves the baseline to the end of the last appearing wave (from the end of the PR interval to the J point). This is normally 0.04 to 0.1 second. A wide (i.e., greater than 0.12 second) QRS complex indicates a delay in the conduction time in the ventricles. Delay in ventricular depolarization (i.e., a wide QRS) can be the result of myocardial ischemia, injury, or infarct; it may also result from ventricular hypertrophy or electrolytes imbalances.

J point represents the junction where the QRS complex ends and the ST segment begins.

ST segment represents early ventricular repolarization. It is measured from the J point to the beginning of the T wave.

T wave represents ventricular repolarization.

U wave represents late ventricular repolarization. It is not normally seen in all leads.

QT interval represents the total time required for ventricular depolarization and repolarization. It is measured from the beginning of the QRS complex to the end of the T wave. It varies with age, gender, and heart rate. It must be corrected to a heart rate of 60 after measurement (QTc). The upper limit of normal QTc is less than 0.43 second in men and less than 0.45 second in women with a normal rate of 60 to 100 beats/min.

The third and final step is to interpret the recording. Rhythm strips in this appendix illustrate common and clinically important ECG patterns.

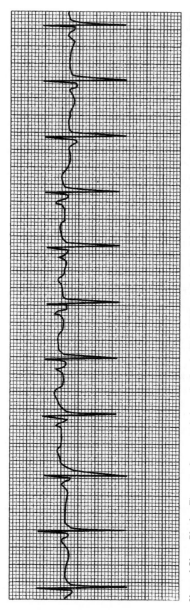

Normal Sinus Rhythm The rate for normal sinus rhythm is 60 to 100 beats/min (bpm) for both atria (i.e., P waves) and ventricles (i.e., QRS waveforms); in this illustration the rate is 92 beats/min. Notice that the atrial and ventricular rhythms are essentially regular (a slight variation in rhythm is normal). One P wave occurs before each QRS complex, and all P waves are of a consistent morphology (shape). The PR interval measures 0.14 second and is constant; the QRS complex measures 0.08 second and is constant. The T waves vary in amplitude because of respirations; they are flat with inspiration and positive with expiration.

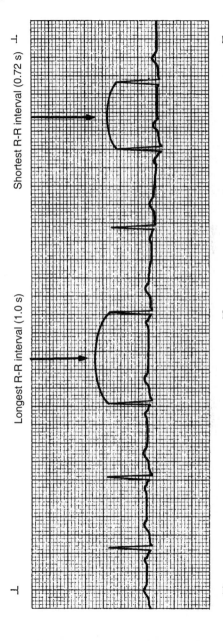

Sinus Arrhythmia or Sinus Dysrhythmia Caused by Respiratory Variation All P waves have the same shape and PR interval, indicating that they are from the sinus node. The rhythm is slightly irregular with the shortest RR interval at 0.74 second and the longest at 1 second. Sinus dysrhythmia most commonly originates from respiratory causes (inhalation/exhalation) and is considered normal. Abnormal causes of RR variation include drugs and acid-base imbalances.

Shortest R-R interval (0.72 s)

Longest R-R interval (1.0 s)

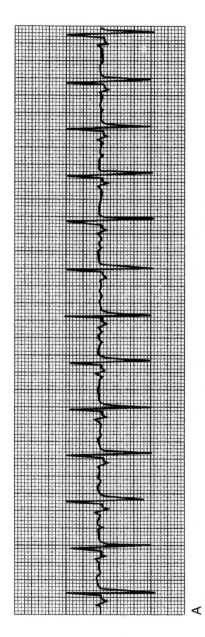

Sinus Rhythms A, Sinus tachycardia is defined as a heart rate (HR) faster than 100 beats/min with normal waves and intervals (HR = 100 beats/min, PR = 0.12 second, QRS = 0.08 second).

A

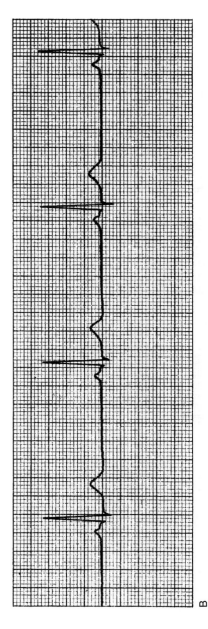

Sinus Rhythms—cont'd B, Sinus bradycardia is defined as a heart rate less than 60 beats/min with all other waves and segments within normal values (HR = 35 beats/min, PR = 0.16 second, QRS = 0.10 second).

B

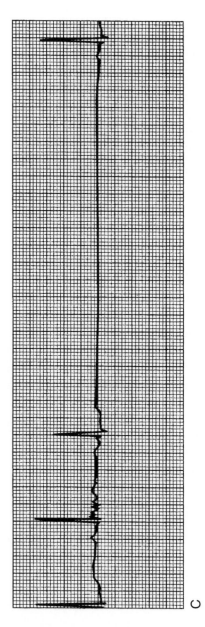

C

Sinus Rhythms—cont'd C, Sinus pause (underlying HR = 60 beats/min, PR = 0.20 second, QRS = 0.08 second, with just under a 5-second pause).

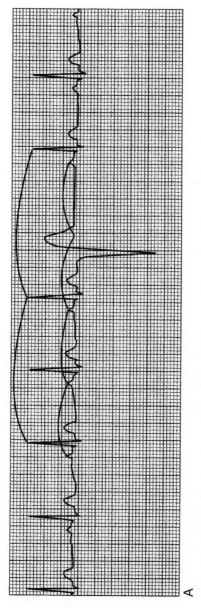

Normal Sinus Rhythm with a Premature Contraction A, Normal sinus rhythm with a premature ventricular contraction (PVC). A complete compensatory pause follows the PVC, indicated by the fact that the sinus P wave after the pause comes exactly when it was due to occur.

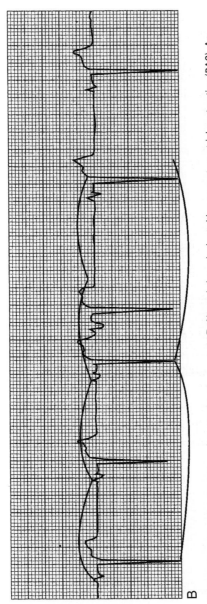

Normal Sinus Rhythm with a Premature Contraction—cont'd B, Normal sinus rhythm with a premature atrial contraction (PAC). An incomplete or noncompensatory pause follows the PAC, indicated by the sinus P wave after the pause coming before it was originally due to occur. The QRS complex also comes before it was due.

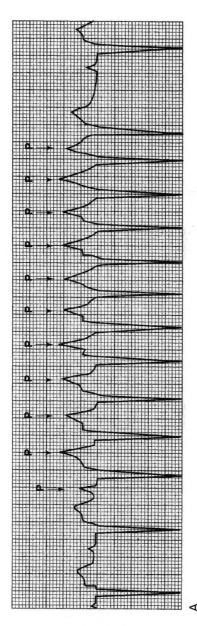

Atrial Dysrhythmias An atrial dysrhythmia implies that the source of the irregular rate or rhythm originates in the atria. **A,** Normal sinus rhythm with an 11-beat run of paroxysmal atrial tachycardia (PAT) with 1:1 conduction.

A

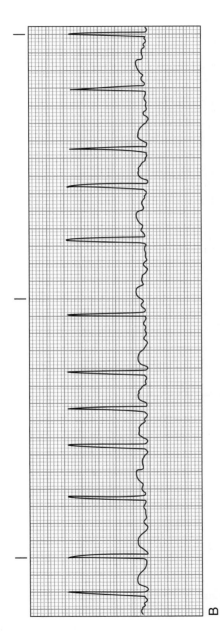

Atrial Dysrhythmias—cont'd B, Atrial fibrillation (AF). Multiple pacemaker sites in the atria cause atrial depolarization at 350 to 600 times per minute. The result is an irregular, wavy baseline between each QRS rather than organized P waves. Atrial fibrillation is often but not universally characterized by an irregular ventricular response, seen in this figure.

B

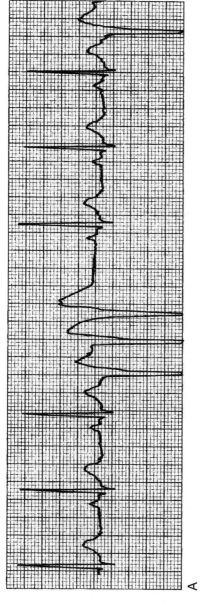

Ventricular Dysrhythmias A, Normal sinus rhythm with a three-beat run of ventricular tachycardia and one unifocal premature ventricular complex.

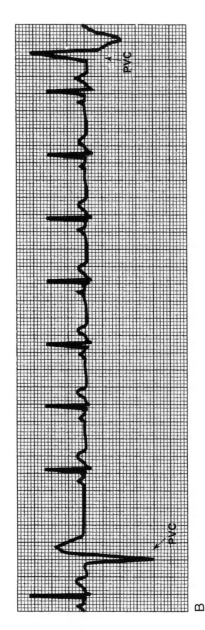

Ventricular Dysrhythmias—cont'd B, Normal sinus rhythm with multifocal PVCs (one negative and the other positive).

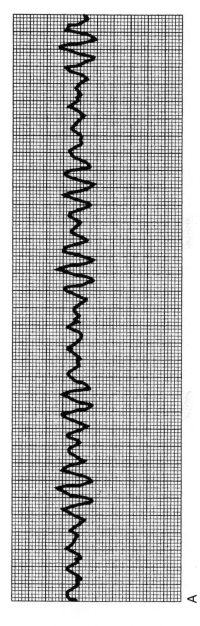

Ventricular Dysrhythmias The dysrhythmia originates in the ventricle. Sustained ventricular tachycardia, ventricular fibrillation, and a systole are all associated with sudden cardiac death as they do not support a blood pressure or perfusion. **A,** Coarse ventricular fibrillation.

A

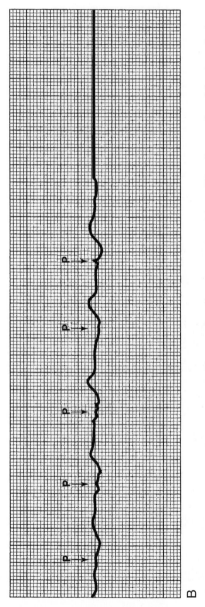

Ventricular Dysrhythmias—cont'd B, Ventricular asystole, initially with five P waves and then with no P waves (arterial and ventricular standstill).

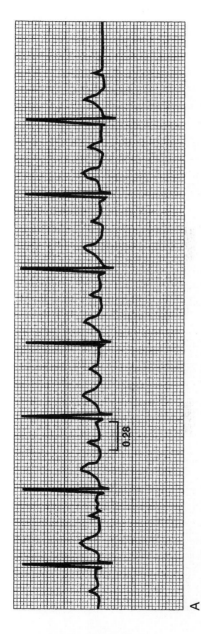

Atrioventricular Block A heart block implies a disruption in the normal conduction of a pacemaker signal that originates in the sinoatrial (SA) node. **A,** Normal sinus rhythm with a first-degree AV block (PR interval = 0.28 second). First- and second-degree heart block imply a delay at the AV node.

0.28

A

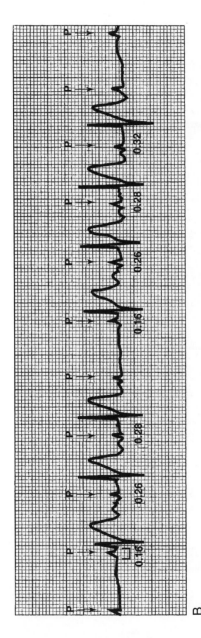

Atrioventricular Block—cont'd B, Second-degree AV block type 1 (Wenckebach) with an irregular rhythm, grouped beating, and progressive prolongation of the PR interval until a P wave is completely blocked and not followed by a QRS complex.

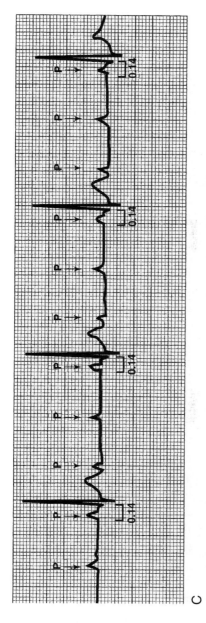

Atrioventricular Block—cont'd C, Second-degree AV block type 2 (Mobitz II) with 3:1 conduction and a constant PR interval. A type 2 second-degree block is more serious and indicates the need for more urgent intervention, such as placing a transcutaneous pacemaker and anticipating the placement of a permanent pacemaker.

C

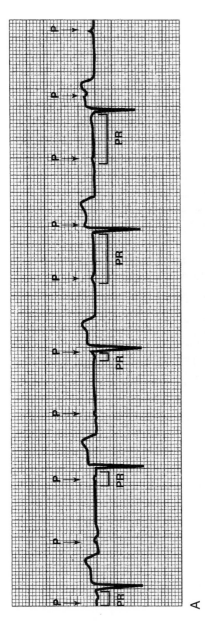

Atrioventricular Block A, Third-degree AV block (complete heart block) with regular atrial and ventricular rhythms. This dysrhythmia indicates no communication between the atria and ventricles at the AV node and is typically treated with a pacemaker. Note the inconsistent PR intervals (AV dissociation) and a junctional escape focus (normal QRS complexes) pacing the ventricles at a rate of 38 beats/min.

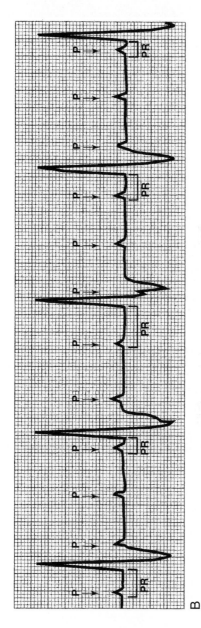

Atrioventricular Block—cont'd B, Third-degree AV block with regular atrial and ventricular rhythms, inconsistent PR intervals (AV dissociation), and ventricular escape focus pacing the ventricles at a rate of 35 beats/min, with wide QRS complexes. Third-degree heart block implies a more serious condition and a delay low in the AV node or along the bundle of His. New onset of this rhythm should be communicated to the physician immediately and a transcutaneous pacemaker should be placed until the patient can be fully evaluated for possible permanent pacemaker placement.

The Patient Requiring Intubation and Ventilation

OVERVIEW

- Mechanical ventilation is usually a temporary life-support technique, although it may be lifelong for those with severe, restrictive lung disease such as fibrotic pneumonitis and for those with chronic, progressive neuromuscular diseases such as amyotrophic lateral sclerosis that reduce effective ventilation.
- It is most often used for patients with hypoxemia and progressive alveolar hypoventilation with respiratory acidosis.
- Invasive mechanical ventilation requires intubation to establish an artificial airway, typically an endotracheal (ET) tube. A tracheotomy tube may be used for prolonged invasive mechanical ventilation.
- The purposes of intubation are to maintain a patent airway, to provide a means to remove secretions, and to provide ventilation and oxygen.
- Some patients receive noninvasive mechanical ventilation through a face, mouth, or nose mask. A common application of noninvasive mechanical ventilation is the device used to maintain an airway in patients with obstructive sleep apnea (e.g., continuous positive airway pressure [CPAP] or bi-level positive airway pressure [BiPAP] delivery).

PATIENT-CENTERED COLLABORATIVE CARE

- Endotracheal intubation
  1. The polyvinyl chloride ET tube is passed through the mouth into the trachea, usually by an anesthesiologist, nurse anesthetist, pulmonologist, or advanced practice nurse. The nasal route is used for facial anomalies, facial or oral trauma, and surgeries when oral intubation is not possible.
  2. When properly positioned, the tip of the ET tube rests about 2 cm above the carina.
  3. The main parts of the ET tube are:
     a. The shaft, with a radiopaque line running its length and short horizontal markings to identify the depth of tube insertion

      b. The cuff at the distal end, which is inflated after placement to create a seal between the trachea and the cuff; the pilot balloon is connected to the cuff and has a one-way valve to prevent air from leaving the balloon

4. Prepare for emergency intubation by:
   a. Summoning intubation personnel in the facility to the bedside in an emergency situation
   b. Explaining the procedure to the patient as clearly as possible
   c. Ensuring that airway equipment box or code ("crash") cart with the airway equipment drawer is at the bedside
   d. Setting up suction and providing both oral and endotracheal suction devices; the code cart usually has this equipment stored in one drawer
   e. Maintaining a patent airway through positioning and inserting an oral or nasopharyngeal airway when indicated
   f. During the intubation, continuously monitoring for changes in vital signs, signs of hypoxia or hypoxemia, dysrhythmias, and aspiration
   g. Ensuring that each intubation attempt lasts no longer than 30 seconds, preferably fewer than 15 seconds, and after 30 seconds, providing oxygen by means of a mask and manual resuscitation bag to prevent hypoxia and cardiac arrest
   h. Suctioning as necessary
   i. Verifying tube placement by assessing for:
      (1) End-tidal carbon dioxide levels
      (2) Bilateral breath sounds
      (3) Symmetrical chest movement
      (4) Air emerging from the ET tube
      (5) Chest x-ray confirmation
   j. Stabilizing ET tube at the mouth or nose and marking the tube where it touches the lip, incisor tooth, or naris

5. Provide nursing care, including:
   a. Regularly assessing tube placement via chest x-ray and landmark (e.g., "23 cm at the lips"), minimal cuff leak, breath sounds, and chest wall movement
   b. Preventing pulling or tugging on the tube to prevent dislodgment
   c. Maintaining a patent airway
   d. Avoiding or identifying complications from endotracheal intubation early including airway obstruction, trauma, pressure-related injury, and infections

- Mechanical ventilation
   1. The purposes of mechanical ventilation are to support and maintain gas exchange and to decrease the work needed for an effective breathing pattern.

2. Mechanical ventilation does not cure diseased lungs; it provides ventilation until the patient is able to resume the process of breathing.

3. In acute care, positive-pressure ventilators generate pressure that pushes air into the lungs and expands the chest. There are four types.

   a. *Pressure-cycled ventilators* push air into the lungs until a preset airway pressure is reached.

   b. *Time-cycled ventilators* push air into the lungs until a preset time has elapsed.

   c. *Volume-cycled ventilators* push air into the lungs until a preset volume is delivered.

   d. *Microprocessor ventilators* are computer-managed, positive-pressure ventilators that often have the components of volume-, time-, and pressure-cycled ventilators.

4. High-frequency ventilation and oscillation are delivered through special mechanical ventilators.

5. Small portable compressors with an oxygen or air source are used to deliver noninvasive mechanical ventilatory support such as BiPAP or CPAP when an endotracheal tube is not used or needed for breathing.

! NURSING SAFETY PRIORITY: Critical Rescue

If the patient develops respiratory distress during mechanical ventilation, immediately remove the ventilator and provide ventilation with a bag-valve-mask device. This action allows quick determination of whether the problem is with the ventilator or with the patient.

6. Modes of ventilation are the way in which the patient receives breaths from the ventilator. Some common modes are:

   a. *Assist-control ventilation* (ACV), in which the ventilator takes over the work of breathing for the patient; the tidal volume and ventilatory rate are preset to establish a minimal ventilatory pattern if the patient does not trigger spontaneous breaths.

   b. *Synchronized intermittent mandatory ventilation* (SIMV), in which the tidal volume and ventilatory rate are preset to establish a minimal ventilatory pattern when the patient does not trigger breaths, but it also allows spontaneous breathing at the patient's own rate and tidal volume between the ventilator breaths.

   c. Additional modes include maximum mandatory ventilation airway pressure release ventilation, proportional assist ventilation, and inverse inspiration-expiration ratio ventilation.

7. Ventilator settings are prescribed by the provider and adjusted or maintained by the respiratory therapist in most settings. Common ventilator settings include:

   a. *Tidal volume* (V_T) is the volume of air the patient receives with each breath. In the presence of acute respiratory distress syndrome (ARDS), a tidal volume of 5 to 6 mL/kg is used to prevent lung injury from "overstretching" or hyperinflating alveoli.

   b. *Rate* is the number of ventilator breaths delivered per minute, typically 12 to 20.

   c. *Fraction of inspired oxygen* (Fio_2) is the oxygen level delivered to the patient, which can range between 21% and 100% oxygen.

   d. *PEEP:* Positive pressure is exerted during the expiratory phase of invasive ventilation to improve oxygenation by preventing atelectasis. The amount of PEEP is usually 5 to 15 cm H_2O.

      (1) Continuous positive airway pressure (CPAP) is airway pressure applied throughout the entire respiratory cycle for patients *who are breathing spontaneously.* It keeps the alveoli open during inspiration and prevents alveolar collapse during expiration. Normal levels of CPAP are 5 to 15 cm H_2O.

   e. *Flow rate:* This rate is how fast each breath is delivered; it is usually set at 40 L/min.

   f. *Pressure support:* The set inspiratory pressure support level is kept constant and there is a decelerating flow.

❗ NURSING SAFETY PRIORITY: Safety Alert

The nursing priorities in caring for the patient during mechanical ventilation are monitoring and evaluating patient responses, managing the ventilator system safely, and preventing complications.

---

8. Provide nursing care, including:

   a. Assessing respiratory status, including auscultating lung sounds, assessing respiratory rate and quality, evaluating Spo_2, secretions, and patient comfort with mechanical ventilation settings. Coordinate respiratory assessment with:

      (1) Taking vital signs

      (2) Placement and security of the ET tube

      (3) Noting the peak and plateau inspiratory pressures from the ventilator; increasing pressures may indicate worsening lung disease or a need for suctioning

    (4) Reviewing the ventilator and alarm settings every 4 hours to ensure they reflect what is prescribed or are adjusted using a protocol to promote liberation from mechanical ventilation

    (5) Observing the exhaled tidal volume to be sure the patient is receiving the prescribed volume; a low tidal volume may indicate a leak from the ET cuff. A high tidal volume may indicate barotrauma or other serious condition needing an intervention.

    (6) Draining water in tubing away from the humidifier and the ventilator

  b. Explaining all procedures and treatments and checking the patient often

  c. Promoting communication with a light touch or blow-by call light; a magic slate, letter/picture board, or pencil and paper for communication is also essential

! NURSING SAFETY PRIORITY: Critical Rescue

Never empty fluid in the tubing back into the ventilator or humidification reservoir.

  d. Responding rapidly to ventilator alarms

  e. Implementing a ventilator care bundle

    (1) Maintaining head of bed elevation of 30 to 45 degrees or more to prevent aspiration during intubation

    (2) Performing oral care per institutional policy (usually with chlorhexidine rinse at least every 12 hours)

    (3) Performing suctioning as needed, considering tracheal, oral, and nasal secretions

    (4) Considering subglottic fluid collection as the major risk for aspiration and perform subglottic suctioning about every 2 hours; some endotracheal tubes have a subglottic lumen and suction port

    (5) Using chest physiotherapy, turning and positioning to promote lung expansion

    (6) Some ventilator bundles include gastrointestinal ulcer prophylaxis and venous thromboembolism prophylaxis

  f. Inspecting the patient's mouth for internal and external pressure ulcers, especially at the point of contact with the ET tube

  g. Changing the airway anchor (e.g., tape or commercial device) per institutional policy, whenever airway device is not secure and as needed for hygiene

   h. Carefully moving the oral ET tube to the opposite side of the mouth once daily to prevent ulcers
   i. Repositioning the patient at least every 2 hours; consider continuous lateral rotation therapy if the patient is comatose or at high risk for or experiences acute respiratory distress syndrome
   j. Positioning the patient to facilitate ventilation-perfusion matching ("good lung down"), as appropriate
   k. Monitoring for adverse effects of mechanical ventilation: infection, barotrauma, and reduced cardiac output
   l. Administering prescribed muscle-paralyzing agents, sedatives, and narcotic analgesics for comfort or to improve oxygenation and decrease ventilator asynchrony

9. Provide a daily weaning evaluation. Incorporate best practices related to a spontaneous breathing trial combined with a sedation vacation daily.

10. Prevent complications (most are caused by the positive pressure from the ventilator).
   a. Cardiac problems include hypotension and fluid retention.
      (1) Establish intake and output goals.
      (2) Monitor the patient's fluid intake and output, weight, hydration, and signs of hypovolemia.
   b. Lung problems include barotrauma (damage to the lungs by positive pressure), volutrauma (damage to the lung by excess volume delivered to one lung over the other), and acid-base imbalance.
      (1) Review ventilator settings with the respiratory therapist at the start of the shift and with every change in setting or when the patient's condition changes, necessitating a change in setting.
   c. GI and nutritional problems include stress ulcer formation, constipation, and electrolyte derangements from NPO status.
      (1) Administer prescribed GI prophylactic drug therapy (antacids, sucralfate [Carafate, Sulcrate ✦], histamine blockers such as ranitidine [Zantac], or proton-pump inhibitors such as esomeprazole [Nexium]).
      (2) Consult with a nutritionist to provide balanced nutrition through the diet, enteral feedings, or parenteral feedings.
      (3) Verify that an initial x-ray has been obtained to confirm the placement of any nasogastric tube before instilling drugs, fluids, or feedings into the tube.
      (4) Closely monitor potassium, calcium, magnesium, and phosphate levels, and replenish deficits as prescribed.

    d. Renal problems include fluid and electrolyte imbalances. Positive pressure ventilation causes diuresis initially.

       (1) Monitor sodium and renal function (i.e., BUN, creatinine, urine output, peripheral edema) because fluid overload and dehydration can impair optimal respiratory function.

    e. Other

       (1) Monitor for anemia in patients with chronic ventilation. Reduced oxygen-carrying capacity in anemia can contribute to delayed weaning from mechanical ventilation.

       (2) Monitor for infection, especially ventilator-associated pneumonia (VAP) and sepsis.

❗ NURSING SAFETY PRIORITY: Safety Alert

The "ABCDE bundle" incorporates the best available evidence for weaning the mechanically ventilated adult (www .ICULiberation.org). Successful implementation of the ABCDE bundle requires effective, frequent communication among a number of different ICU team members.

Awakening trials of stopping sedation for 20 minutes or longer; if sedation is resumed, it is restarted at half the previous dose and titrated to a shared goal based on a valid tool for assessing patient sedation like the Richmond Agitation and Sedation Scale (RASS).

Breathing by providing a daily trial of spontaneous patient breathing while intubated, once the underlying condition requiring mechanical ventilation is resolved or resolving.

Coordination of the awakening and breathing trials so they occur simultaneously.

Delirium monitoring and management using a valid assessment tool like the ICU-Confusion Assessment Method (ICU-CAM).

Early mobility by enabling patients to become active and even walk while intubated; muscle deconditioning, loss of joint range of motion, and weakness are caused by immobility. Premedicate with analgesics before initiating activity if pain interferes with mobility. Consult with physical and occupational therapists to provide assistive devices, positioning devices, and splints to maintain function in weak or comatose patients.

- When weaning is delayed beyond 21 days or is unlikely to be successful because of the patient's condition, anticipate a surgical tracheostomy with subsequent placement of a tracheostomy tube.

Considerations for Older Adults

The older patient, especially one who has smoked or who has a chronic lung problem such as COPD, is at risk for ventilator dependence and failure to wean. Age-related changes, such as chest wall stiffness, reduced ventilatory muscle strength, and decreased lung elasticity, reduce the likelihood of weaning. The usual manifestations of ventilatory failure—hypoxemia and hypercarbia—may be less obvious in the older adult, and other clinical measures of gas exchange and oxygenation, such as a change in mental status, should be used to determine breathing effectiveness.

1. Maintain a clean surgical site, following institutional policy for new tracheostomy site care.
2. Inform the surgeon of bright red or copious or recurrent bleeding immediately and about the presence of persistent blood at the site or in endotracheal secretions beyond 3 to 4 days after surgery.
3. Provide tracheostomy tube management per institutional policy.
   a. If using inline suction equipment, use tracheostomy-compatible equipment. It is shorter, reflecting the decreased length of the airway.
4. In some cases, a patient may progress to a permanent tracheotomy without tubing to mechanical ventilation. A tracheotomy may close over time if it is not needed to maintain an airway.
- Weaning from mechanical ventilation ultimately results in extubation or removal of the ET tube. Nursing responsibilities include:
  1. Explaining the procedure to the patient
  2. Ensuring that the post-extubation prescribed oxygen delivery system is set up
  3. Being able to readily access the equipment for emergency reintubation if needed
  4. Hyperoxygenating the patient
  5. Thoroughly suctioning the ET tube and the oral cavity
  6. Rapidly deflating the cuff of the ET tube, and removing the tube with exhalation immediately after a peak inspiration
  7. Instructing the patient to cough after ET tube removal
  8. Giving oxygen by facemask or nasal cannula
  9. Assessing the patient's responses, particularly the ability to clear his or her airway, respiratory rate, effort, and Sp_{O_2} (ability to maintain adequate gas exchange)

! NURSING SAFETY PRIORITY: Critical Rescue

Monitor vital signs every 5 minutes at first, and assess ventilatory pattern for manifestations of respiratory distress (dyspnea, coughing, and the inability to expectorate secretions). Notify the physician or Rapid Response Team at the onset of these problems.

! NURSING SAFETY PRIORITY: Critical Rescue

If stridor (high-pitched, crowing noise during inspiration) develops at any time, immediately call the Rapid Response Team.

The Patient Requiring Chest Tubes

OVERVIEW

- A chest tube is a drain placed in the pleural space to drain air or fluid from the pleural space.
    1. The overall goal is to promote lung re-expansion, restore oxygenation and ventilation, and prevent complications after chest surgery or trauma.
- The drainage system consists of one or more chest tubes or drains, a collection container placed below the chest level, and a water seal to keep air from entering the chest.
- Chest tubes are used to treat conditions that disrupt the pleural space.
    1. The tip of the tube used to drain air is placed near the front lung's apex and usually sutured in place.
    2. The tube that drains liquid is placed on the side near the base of the lung.
- The chest tube is connected to about 6 feet (2 meters) of tubing that leads to a collection device placed several feet below the chest.
- Integrated chest drainage units have three chambers connected to each other.
    1. A water seal chamber prevents air from entering the patient's pleural space.
        a. Bubbling of the fluid in this chamber indicates air drainage from the patient and is usually seen when the patient exhales, coughs, or sneezes.
        b. Bubbling stops when the air in the pleural space has been removed and the pleural space reseals. A blocked or kinked chest tube also can cause bubbling to stop.
    2. A suction-control chamber that contains sterile water and is connected to vacuum to provide suction or negative pressure.
        a. The amount of fluid, not the amount of vacuum pressure, creates the negative pressure to draw air out of the pleural space.
        b. The health care provider prescribes the amount of suction (typically about −20 mm Hg).
    3. Chamber 3 is the collection chamber.

PATIENT-CENTERED COLLABORATIVE CARE

- Initial care includes:
  1. Checking hourly to ensure the sterility and patency of any chest drainage system
     a. Assess drainage color.
     b. Don't milk, strip, or clamp the tube.
  2. Taping tubing junctions to prevent accidental disconnections
  3. Keeping an occlusive dressing at the chest tube insertion site
  4. Keeping sterile gauze at the bedside to cover the insertion site immediately if the chest tube becomes dislodged
- Ongoing nursing care includes:
  1. Assessing breathing effectiveness by respiratory rate, rhythm, lung sounds, and pulse oximetry
  2. Ensuring that the dressing on the chest around the tube is dry and intact; reinforce or replace according to institutional policy or practice
  3. Checking the surrounding skin for intactness and palpating the area for puffiness or crackling that may indicate subcutaneous emphysema
  4. Inspecting the site for signs of infection (redness, purulent drainage) or excessive bleeding
  5. Assessing and documenting the depth of tube placement
  6. Assessing for pain and its location and intensity, re-positioning for comfort, and administering drugs for pain as prescribed
  7. Assisting the patient to deep breathe, cough, perform maximal sustained inhalations, and use incentive spirometry
- Manage the drainage system by:
  1. Keeping the drainage system lower than the level of the patient's chest
  2. Keeping the chest tube as straight as possible, avoiding kinks and dependent loops
  3. Assessing the water seal chamber for gentle bubbles during the patient's exhalation, forceful cough, or position changes; assessing fluctuation of the sealed chamber
  4. Assessing for normal "tidaling" (water in the long tube of the second chamber rises and falls 2 to 4 inches during inhalation and exhalation)
  5. Checking that the prescribed suction pressure is maintained with appropriate fluid amount in the suction chamber and connection to wall vacuum
  6. Checking and documenting the amount, color, and characteristics of fluid in the collection chamber as often as needed according to the patient's condition and agency policy

7. Changing the system if the collection chamber becomes more than 75% full
8. Obtaining drainage samples (when prescribed) using institutional or manufacturer practice guidelines
9. Immediately notifying the physician or Rapid Response Team about:
   a. Tracheal deviation
   b. Sudden onset or increased intensity of dyspnea
   c. Oxygen saturation less than 90%
   d. Drainage greater than 70 mL/hr for 2 or more hours or sudden cessation of chest drainage in the first 24 hours
   e. Visible eyelets on the chest tube or the chest tube falling out of the patient's chest; cover the area with dry, sterile gauze.
   f. Chest tube disconnecting from the drainage system; first put the end of tube in a container of sterile water and keep it below the level of the patient's chest before reporting this situation.

Communication Quick Reference for Spanish-Speaking Patients

THE BODY · EL CUERPO (EHL KOO-EHR-POH)

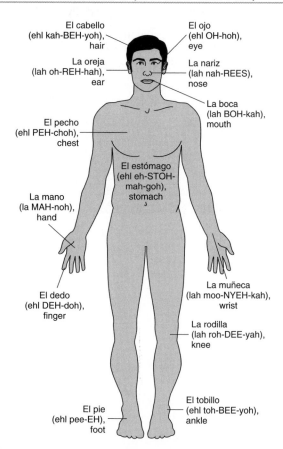

El cabello
(ehl kah-BEH-yoh),
hair

El ojo
(ehl OH-hoh),
eye

La oreja
(lah oh-REH-hah),
ear

La nariz
(lah nah-REES),
nose

La boca
(lah BOH-kah),
mouth

El pecho
(ehl PEH-choh),
chest

El estómago
(ehl eh-STOH-mah-goh),
stomach

La mano
(la MAH-noh),
hand

El dedo
(ehl DEH-doh),
finger

La muñeca
(lah moo-NYEH-kah),
wrist

La rodilla
(lah roh-DEE-yah),
knee

El pie
(ehl pee-EH),
foot

El tobillo
(ehl toh-BEE-yoh),
ankle

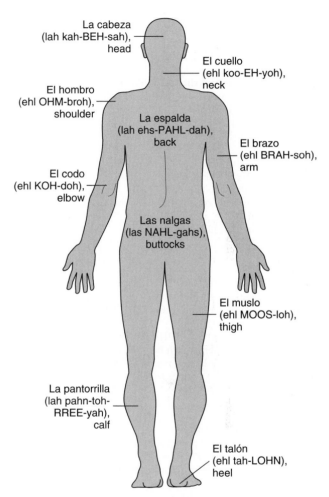

La cabeza
(lah kah-BEH-sah),
head

El cuello
(ehl koo-EH-yoh),
neck

El hombro
(ehl OHM-broh),
shoulder

La espalda
(lah ehs-PAHL-dah),
back

El brazo
(ehl BRAH-soh),
arm

El codo
(ehl KOH-doh),
elbow

Las nalgas
(las NAHL-gahs),
buttocks

El muslo
(ehl MOOS-loh),
thigh

La pantorrilla
(lah pahn-toh-
RREE-yah),
calf

El talón
(ehl tah-LOHN),
heel

COMMON TERMS

Move, mueva (mooh-EH-bah)
Touch, toque (TOH-keh)
Point to, señale (seh-NYAH-leh)

MORE PARTS OF THE BODY

Armpit, la axila (lah ahk-SEE-lah)
Breasts, los senos (lohs SEH-nohs)
Collarbone, la clavícula (lah klah-BEE-koo-lah)
Diaphragm, el diafragma (ehl dee-ah-FRAHG-mah)
Forearm, el antebrazo (ehl ahn-teh-BRAH-soh)
Groin, la ingle (lah EEN-gleh)
Hip, la cadera (lah kah-DEH-rah)
Kneecap, la rótula (lah ROH-too-lah)
Nail, la uña (lah OO-nyah)
Pelvis, la pelvis (lah PEHL-bees)
Rectum, el recto (ehl REHK-toh)
Rib, la costilla (lah kohs-TEE-yah)
Spine, la espina dorsal (lah ehs-PEE-nah dor-SAHL)
Throat, la garganta (lah gahr-GAHN-tah)
Tongue, le lengua (lah LEHN-goo-ah)

ORGANS

Appendix, el apéndice (ehl ah-PEHN-dee-seh)
Bladder, la vejiga (lah beh-HEE-gah)
Brain, el cerebro (ehl seh-REH-broh)
Colon, el colon (ehl KOH-lohn)
Esophagus, el esófago (ehl eh-SOH-fah-goh)
Gallbladder, la vesícula biliar (lah beh-SEE-koo-lah bee-lee-AHR)
Genitals, los genitales (lohs heh-nee-TAH-lehs)
Heart, el corazón (ehl koh-rah-SOHN)
Kidney, el riñón (ehl ree-NYOHN)
Large intestine, el intestino grueso (ehl een-tehs-TEE-noh groo-EH-soh)
Liver, el hígado (ehl EE-gah-doh)
Lungs, los pulmones (lohs pool-MOH-nehs)
Pancreas, el páncreas (ehl PAHN-kreh-ahs)
Small intestine, el intestino delgado (ehl een-tehs-TEE-noh dehl-GAH-doh)
Spleen, el bazo (ehl BAH-soh)
Thyroid gland, la tiroides (lah tee-ROH-ee-dehs)
Tonsils, las amígdalas (lahs ah-MEEG-dah-lahs)
Uterus, el útero (ehl OO-teh-roh)

ESSENTIAL PHRASES

Good morning.	*Buenos días.*	Boo-EH-nohs DEE-ahs.
Good afternoon.	*Buenas tardes.*	Boo-EH-nahs TAHR-dehs.
Good night.	*Buenas noches.*	Boo-EH-nahs NOH-chehs.
Hello.	*Hola.*	OH-lah.
How are you?	*¿Cómo está?*	¿Koh-moh ehs-TAH?
Good (fine).	*Bien.*	Bee-EHN.
Bad, Better, Worse	*Mal, Mejor, Peor*	Mahl, Meh-OHR, peh-OHR
The same	*Igual*	Ee-GOO-ahl
Do you speak English?	*¿Habla inglés?*	¿Ah-blah een-GLEHS?
I don't understand.	*No comprendo.*	Noh kom-PREHN-doh.
Excuse me.	*Discúlpeme.*	Dees-KOOL-peh-meh.
Please speak slowly.	*Por favor, hable más lento.*	Pohr fah-VOHR, AH-bleh mahs LEHN-toh.
Are you in pain?	*¿Está adolorido(a)?*	¿Ehs-TAH ah-doh-loh-REE-doh(dah)?
Yes, No	*Sí, No*	SEE, Noh
Tell me where it hurts.	*Dígame donde le duele.*	DEE-gah-meh DOHN-deh leh doo-EH-leh.
Here, there	*Aquí, ahí*	Ah-KEE, ah-EE

DESCRIPTION OF PAIN

Is your pain ... burning?	*Tiene un dolor ...*	Tee-EH-neh oon doh-LOHR ...
	¿que arde?	¿keh AHR-deh?
constant?	*¿constante?*	¿kohns-TAHN-teh?
dull?	*¿amortiguado?*	¿ah-MOHR-tee-goo-AH-doh?
intermittent?	*¿intermitente?*	¿een-tehr-mee-TEHN-teh?
mild?	*¿moderado?*	¿moh-deh-RAH-doh?
severe?	*¿muy fuerte?*	¿MOO-ee foo-EHR-teh?
sharp?	*¿agudo?*	¿ah-GOO-doh?
throbbing?	*¿pulsante?*	¿pool-SAHN-teh?
worse?	*¿peor?*	¿peh-OHR?

Continued

Are you allergic to any medication?	*¿Es usted alérgico(a) a algún medicamento?*	¿Ehs oos-TEHD ah-LEHR-hee-koh(kah) ah ahl-GOON meh-dee-kah-MEHN-toh?
I'm here to help you.	*Estoy aquí para ayudarle.*	Ehs-TOH-ee ah-KEE pah-rah ah-yoo-DAHR-leh.
Calm down.	*Cálmese.*	KAHL-meh-seh.
Please.	*Por favor.*	Pohr fah-VOHR.
Thank you.	*Gracias.*	GRAH-see-ahs.
You're welcome.	*De nada.*	Deh NAH-dah.
May I?	*¿Puedo?*	¿Poo-EH-doh?
Who, What, When, Where?	*¿Quién, Qué, Cuándo, Dónde?*	¿Kee-ehn, Keh, Koo-AHN-doh, DOHN-deh?
Zero, one, two, three, four	*Cero, uno, dos, tres, cuatro*	SEH-roh, OO-noh, dohs, trehs, koo-AH-troh
Five, six, seven, eight, nine, ten	*Cinco, seis, siete, ocho, nueve, diez*	SEEN-koh, SEH-ees, see-EH-teh, OH-choh, noo-EH-beh, dee-EHS

PRELIMINARY EXAMINATION

My name is _____, and I am your nurse.	*Me llamo _____, y soy su enfermera(o).*	Meh YAH-moh ___, ee SOH-ee soo ehn-fehr-MEH-rah(roh).
I'm going to ...	*Le voy a ...*	Leh VOH-ee ah ...
take your vital signs.	*tomar los signos vitales.*	toh-MAHR lohs SEEG-nohs vee-TAH-lehs.
weigh you.	*pesar.*	peh-SAHR.
take your blood pressure.	*tomar la presión.*	toh-MAHR lah preh-see-OHN.
Extend your arm and relax.	*Extienda su brazo y descánselo.*	Ehks-tee-EHN-dah soo BRAH-soh ee dehs-KAHN-seh-loh.
I'm going to take your ... pulse.	*Le voy a tomar ... el pulso.*	Leh voy ah toh-MAHR ... ehl POOL-soh.
temperature.	*su temperatura.*	soo tehm-peh-rah-TOO-rah.
I'm going to count your respirations.	*Voy a contar sus respiraciones.*	VOH-ee ah kohn-TAHR soos rehs-pee-rah-see-OH-nehs.

OBTAINING A BLOOD SAMPLE

I need to draw a blood sample.	*Necesito tomar una muestra de la sangre.*	Neh-seh-SEE-toh toh-MAHR OO-nah MOO-ehs-trah deh lah SAHN-greh.
Please give me your arm.	*Por favor, déme el brazo.*	Pohr fah-VOHR, DEH-meh ehl BRAH-soh.
It may cause a little discomfort.	*Le puede causar alguna molestia.*	Leh poo-EH-deh kah-OO-sahr ahl-GOO-nah moh-LEHS-tee-ah.
I am going to put a tourniquet around your arm.	*Le voy a poner una liga alrededor del brazo.*	Leh VOH-ee ah poh-NEHR OO-nah LEE-gah ahl-reh-deh-DOHR dehl BRAH-soh.
I am going to draw blood from this vein.	*Voy a sacar la sangre de esta vena.*	Voy ah sah-KAHR lah SAHN-greh deh EHS-tah VEH-nah.

OBTAINING BLOOD FROM A FINGER STICK

| I need to take a few drops of blood from your finger. | *Necesito sacar unas gotas de sangre de uno de sus dedos.* | Neh-seh-SEE-toh sah-KAHR OO-nahs GOH-tahs deh SAHN-greh deh OO-noh deh soos DEH-dohs. |

OBTAINING A URINE SAMPLE

We also need a urine sample.	*También necesitamos una muestra de la orina.*	Tahm-bee-EHN neh-seh-see-TAH-mohs OO-nah moo-EHS-trah deh lah oh-REE-nah.
It has to be from the middle of the stream.	*Tiene que ser de la mitad del chorro.*	Tee-EH-neh keh sehr deh lah mee-TAHD dehl CHOH-rroh.
Put the urine in this cup.	*Ponga la orina en esta tasa.*	POHN-gah lah oh-REE-nah ehn EHS-tah TAH-sah.

OBTAINING A STOOL SPECIMEN

I need a sample of your stool.	*Necesito una muestra de su excremento.*	Neh-seh-SEE-toh OO-nah moo-EHS-trah deh soo ehks-kreh-MEN-toh.
Please put a small amount in this cup.	*Por favor ponga un poco en esta tasa.*	Pohr fah-VOHR POHN-gah oon POH-koh ehn EHS-tah TAH-sah.

OBTAINING A SPUTUM SPECIMEN

I need a sample of your sputum.	*Necesito una muestra de su esputo.*	Neh-seh-SEE-toh OO-nah MOO-ehs-trah deh soo ehs-POO-toh.
Please spit in this cup.	*Por favor, escupa en este vaso.*	Pohr fah-VOHR, ehs-KOO-pah ehn EHS-tah VAH-soh.

ORDERS

You need ... a bandage.	*Necesita ... un vendaje.*	Neh-seh-SEE-tah ... oon behn-DAH-heh.
a blood transfusion.	*una transfusión de sangre.*	OO-nah trahns-foo-see-OHN deh SAHN-greh.
a cast.	*un molde de yeso.*	oon MOHL-deh deh YEH-soh.
gauze.	*la gasa.*	lah GAH-sah.
intensive care.	*cuidado intensivo.*	koo-ee-DAH-doh een-tehn-SEE-boh.
intravenous fluids.	*líquidos intravenosos.*	LEE-kee-dohs een-trah-beh-NOH-sohs.
an operation.	*una operación.*	OO-nah oh-peh-rah-see-OHN.
physical therapy.	*terapia física.*	teh-RAH-pee-ah FEE-see-kah.
a shot.	*una inyección.*	OO-nah een-yehk-see-OHN.
x-rays.	*rayos equis.*	RAH-yohs EH-kees.
We're going to ...	*Vamos a ...*	VAH-mohs ah ...
change the bandage.	*cambiarle el vendaje.*	kahm-bee-AHR-leh ehl behn-DAH-heh.
give you a bath.	*darle un baño.*	DAHR-leh oon BAH-nyoh.
take out the IV.	*sacarle el tubo intravenoso.*	sah-KAHR-leh ehl TOO-boh een-trah-beh-NOH-soh.

DESCRIPTION OF TUBES

The tube in your ...	*El tubo en su ...*	Ehl TOO-boh ehn soo ...
arm is for IV fluids.	*brazo es para líquidos intravenosos.*	BRAH-soh ehs PAH-rah LEE-kee-dohs een-trah-beh-NOH-sohs.
bladder is for urinating.	*vejiga es para orinar.*	beh-HEE-gah ehs PAH-rah oh-ree-NAHR.
stomach is for food.	*estómago es para los alimentos.*	ehs-TOH-mah-goh ehs PAH-rah lohs ah-lee-MEN-tohs.
throat is for breathing.	*garganta es para respirar.*	gahr-GAHN-tah ehs PAH-rah rehs-pee-RAHR.

INDEX

Page numbers followed by "f" indicate figures, "t" indicate tables, and "b" indicate boxes.